Miguel A. Cuesta
Editor

Minimally Invasive Surgery for Upper Abdominal Cancer

Springer

Editor
Miguel A. Cuesta
Department of Surgery
VU University Medical Center
Amsterdam
The Netherlands

ISBN 978-3-319-54300-0   ISBN 978-3-319-54301-7 (eBook)
DOI 10.1007/978-3-319-54301-7

Library of Congress Control Number: 2017946480

Printed on acid-free paper

This Springer imprint is published by Springer Nature
The registered company is Springer International Publishing AG
The registered company address is: Gewerbestrasse 11, 6330 Cham, Switzerland

Preface

Since the publication in 1993 of our book *Minimally Invasive Surgery in Gastrointestinal Cancer*, our interest has been the implementation of minimally invasive procedures in gastrointestinal cancer.

Surgeons continually strive to provide the best care possible for their patients. This focus on enhancing the quality of surgery brings them to employ the minimally invasive surgical (MIS) approach. Doing so, it reduces postoperative pain, lowers the risk of postoperative complications and increases the quality of life.

Surgeons have in the past decades demonstrated major progress in improving surgery. We have seen diagnostic invasive procedures replaced by a variety of imaging techniques providing high-resolution insight in the anatomical aspects of the disease, thereby allowing surgical teams to refine their surgical indications and approaches. We have seen large abdominal incisions replaced by minimal incisions, thus allowing patients to ambulate very early after surgery and reassume their activities within days instead of long postoperative stays in the hospital. We have seen endoluminal and image-guided percutaneous placement of stents or drains for relieving obstructions or fluid collections that impede the recovery of patients.

Hence it is no surprise that MIS is currently the standard surgical treatment in many areas of abdominal surgery, such as gallbladder surgery, the whole benign gastrointestinal surgery and colon and rectum cancer surgery.

Studies do continue to determine the quality of MIS. To be sure, the notion that minimally invasive procedures in upper gastrointestinal surgery, especially the oncological processes, are as efficient or even better than their counterpart of open surgery still follows different phases of becoming evident. For some procedures, like esophageal resection and partial gastrectomy for cancer, the evidence of the supremacy of MIS is now reasonably certain. High evidence even suggests that MIS may be superior to the counterpart open resections by providing clearer short-term advantages and equal oncologic safety. Other procedures, such as total gastrectomies, hepatic resections and duodenopancreatectomies for pancreatic head cancer, are still subject to high-level studies for determining how evidence-based these standard procedures are. Significant is that the introductions of high-definition imaging, 3D technology and robot-assisted surgery demonstrate the advantages of having a better visualization and ergonomy. These techniques involve the capacity to dissect and reconstruct tissues in difficult to locate places and suffice with a relative short learning curve.

Despite successes, upper abdominal MIS procedures remain difficult to standardize because of the complicated and tortuous surgical anatomy and due to the limited numbers of patients undergoing these procedures in comparison with, for example, the high numbers in colorectal surgery.

The philosophy of surgery we follow is that once a good indication exists for surgery, the combination of an optimal use of neoadjuvant therapy with minimally invasive surgery will achieve the best outcome for the patient, offering a high quality of life. Our objective in this book is to depict the current situation of minimal upper GI surgery in oncology. By doing so, we demonstrate how to perform these procedures with the minimum risk for the patients and simultaneously obtaining as many advantages as is feasible.

The setup for this book has five sections: the esophageal, the gastric, the duodeno-pancreas, the hepatic and splenic surgery. Each section starts with a chapter dedicated to surgical anatomy of the different areas that configure the upper abdomen, followed by different possibilities of neoadjuvant treatment of a specific cancer. After dealing with neoadjuvant treatment, a chapter compares the outcome of minimally invasive procedures in comparison with their counterpart open approach. More chapters treat the specific operative techniques of MIS, its outcome and the current situation whereby the robot-assisted minimally invasive surgery is used.

Knowledge of the surgical anatomy is very important for each surgeon and helps to standardize the use of convenient dissection planes and to perform a standard oncological resection.

The call for achieving higher proficiencies in MIS is clear. Mastering the MIS procedures is arduous and may take time. We realize that surgeons dedicated to upper abdominal surgery may have to gain proficiencies involving a lengthy learning curve while under the control and assistance of a master.

Moreover, readers of this book will be aided by a well-chosen collection of videos that describe the accomplishment of the surgical procedures in MIS.

Our gratitude for the splendid contributions of all authors is great. Their dedication to the design and implementation of the procedures treated in this volume is encouraging.

We hope that this book will enrich the knowledge and understanding of surgeons and surgical residents around the world who are dedicated to upper gastrointestinal cancer surgery and will inspire these professionals to persist in improving on surgery.

Amsterdam, The Netherlands Miguel A. Cuesta

Contents

Contributors

M. Abu Hilal University of Southampton, Southampton University Hospital, Southampton, UK

M.D. Ayllon Unit of Hepatobiliary Surgery and Liver Transplantation, IMIBIC, CIBERehd, University Hospital Reina Sofia, Córdoba, Spain

S. Barbaro Southampton University Hospital, University of Southampton, Southampton, UK

R.E. Beard Division of Hepatobiliary and Pancreatic Surgery, University of Pittsburgh Medical Center, Pittsburgh, PA, USA

J.W. van den Berg Department of Surgery, Erasmus Medical Center, Rotterdam, The Netherlands

M.I. van Berge Henegouwen Department of Surgery, Academic Medical Center, Amsterdam, The Netherlands

P.A. Bertulucci Department of Upper GI Surgery, Americas Medical City Hospital, Rio de Janeiro, Brazil

M.G.H. Besselink Department of Surgery, Academic Medical Center, Amsterdam, The Netherlands

R.L.A.W. Bleys Department of Anatomy, University Medical Center, Utrecht, The Netherlands

U. Boggi Division of General and Transplant Surgery, University of Pisa, Pisa, Italy

H.J.F. Brenkman Department of Surgical Oncology, University Medical Center, Utrecht, The Netherlands

J. Briceño Unit of Hepatobiliary Surgery and Liver Transplantation, IMIBIC, CIBERehd, University Hospital Reina Sofia, Córdoba, Spain

O.R.C. Busch Department of Surgery, Academic Medical Center, Amsterdam, The Netherlands

T.T. Cheung Department of Surgery, Hepatobiliary and Pancreatic Surgery, Queen Mary Hospital, The University of Hong Kong, Hong Kong SAR, China

R. Ciria Unit of Hepatobiliary Surgery and Liver Transplantation, IMIBIC, CIBERehd, University Hospital Reina Sofia, Córdoba, Spain

Y.H.M. Claassen Department of Surgery, Leiden University Medical Center, Leiden, The Netherlands

M.A. Cuesta Emeritus professor, Department of Surgery, VU University Medical Center, Amsterdam, The Netherlands

A. Sa Cunha Hepato-biliary Center, Paul Brousse Hospital, University of Paris-Sud, Villejuif, France

F. Daams Department of Surgery, VU University Medical Center, Amsterdam, The Netherlands

B.H. Edil Department of Surgical Oncology, Pancreas and Biliary, University of Colorado School of Medicine, Aurora, CO, USA

C.H.J. van Eijck Department of Surgery, Erasmus Medical Center, Rotterdam, The Netherlands

S. Festen Department of Surgery, OLVG Hospital, Amsterdam, The Netherlands

A. van der Gaast Department of Medical Oncology, Erasmus Medical Center, Rotterdam, The Netherlands

M.F. Gerhards Department of Surgery, OLVG Hospital, Amsterdam, The Netherlands

S.S. Gisbertz Department of Surgery, Academic Medical Center, Amsterdam, The Netherlands

I. Gómez-Luque Unit of Hepatobiliary Surgery and Liver Transplantation, IMIBIC, CIBERehd, University Hospital Reina Sofia, Córdoba, Spain

A. Guner Department of Surgery, Yonsei University College of Medicine, Seoul, South Korea

Department of General Surgery, Karadeniz Technical University College of Medicine, Farabi Hospital, Trabzon, Turkey

M. Halls Southampton University Hospital, University of Southampton, Southampton, UK

H.H. Hartgrink Department of Surgery, Leiden University Medical Center, Leiden, The Netherlands

R. van Hillegersberg Department of Surgical Oncology, University Medical Center Utrecht, Utrecht, The Netherlands

K. Honselmann Department of Surgery, University Medical Center Schleswig-Holstein, Luebeck, Germany

S. van der Horst Department of Surgical Oncology, University Medical Center Utrecht, Utrecht, The Netherlands

W.J. Hyung Department of Surgery, Yonsei University College of Medicine, Seoul, South Korea

Gastric Cancer Center, Yonsei Cancer Center, Yonsei University Health System, Seoul, South Korea

M.N.J. Vanegas University of Pittsburgh Medical Center, Health System, Pittsburgh, PA, USA

University of Pittsburgh Medical Center, Pittsburgh, PA, USA

T. Keck Department of Surgery, University Medical Center Schleswig-Holstein, Luebeck, Germany

S-H Kong Department of Surgery, Seoul National University Hospital, Seoul National University College of Medicine, Seoul, South Korea

K. Kudou Department of Surgery, Institute of Gastroenterology, Tokyo Women's Medical University, Tokyo, Japan

C. Franco Lacerda Department of Upper GI Surgery, Americas Medical City Hospital, Rio de Janeiro, Brazil

S.M. Lagarde Department of Surgery, Erasmus Medical Center, Rotterdam, The Netherlands

J.J.B. van Lanschot Department of Surgery, Erasmus Medical Center, Rotterdam, The Netherlands

A. Laurenzi Hepato-biliary Center, Paul Brousse Hospital, University of Paris-Sud, Villejuif, France

H-J Lee Department of Surgery, Seoul National University Hospital, Seoul National University College of Medicine, Seoul, South Korea

M.S. van Leeuwen Department Radiology, University medical Center, Utrecht, The Netherlands

C. Lombardo Division of General and Transplant Surgery, University of Pisa, Pisa, Italy

J.D. Luketich University of Pittsburgh Medical Center, Health System, Pittsburgh, PA, USA

University of Pittsburgh Medical Center, Pittsburgh, PA, USA

C. Rodriguez Luppi Universidad Autónoma de Barcelona, Servicio de Cirugía General y del Aparato Digestivo, Hospital de la Santa Creu i Santpau, Barcelona, Spain

C. Mariette Department of Digestive and Oncological Surgery, Claude Huriez University Hospital, University Lille, Lille, France

Centre de Recherche Jean-Pierre AUBERT Neurosciences et Cancer, Lille, France

Inserm, Lille, France

ONCOLille, Lille, France

D. Martinez-Cecilia Servicio Cirugía General, Hospital Virgen de la Salud, Toledo, Spain

J. Lopez Monclova Universidad Autónoma de Barcelona, Servicio de Cirugía General y del Aparato Digestivo, Hospital de la Santa Creu i Santpau, Barcelona, Spain

Mexican Institute for Social Security, Delicias, Mexico

C. Moreno-Sanz Department of General and Digestive Surgery, Hospital General La Mancha Centro, Ciudad Real, Spain

K. Narumiya Department of Surgery, Institute of Gastroenterology, Tokyo Women's Medical University, Tokyo, Japan

L.M. Ocuin Division of Hepatobiliary and Pancreatic Surgery, University of Pittsburgh Medical Center, Pittsburgh, PA, USA

A. Talvane Torres de Oliveira Department of Upper GI Surgery, Americas Medical City Hospital, Rio de Janeiro, Brazil

H. Osugi Department of Surgery, Institute of Gastroenterology, Tokyo Women's Medical University, Tokyo, Japan

D.L. van der Peet Department of Surgery, VU University Medical Center, Amsterdam, The Netherlands

D. Pietrasz Hepato-biliary Center, Paul Brousse Hospital, University of Paris-Sud, Villejuif, France

G. Pittau Hepato-biliary Center, Paul Brousse Hospital, University of Paris-Sud, Villejuif, France

M.J. van der Poel Department of Surgery, Academic Medical Center, Amsterdam, The Netherlands

R.E. Pouw Department of Gastroenterology and Hepatology, Academic Medical Center, Amsterdam, The Netherlands

T. de Rooij Department of Surgery, Academic Medical Center, Amsterdam, The Netherlands

J.P.H. Ruurda Department of Surgical Oncology, University Medical Center Utrecht, Utrecht, The Netherlands

J.J. Scheepers Department of Surgery, Reinier de Graaf Hospital, Delft, The Netherlands

A.E. Slaman Department of Surgery, Academic Medical Center, Amsterdam, The Netherlands

M. Slingerland Department of Medical Oncology, Leiden University Medical Center, Leiden, The Netherlands

J.W. Dekker Department of Surgery, Reinier de Graaf Hospital, Delft, The Netherlands

P.C. van der Sluis Department of Surgical Oncology, University Medical Center Utrecht, Utrecht, The Netherlands

W.O. De Steur Department of Surgery, Leiden University Medical Center, Leiden, The Netherlands

J. Straatman Department of Surgery, VU University Medical Center, Amsterdam, The Netherlands

M. Suker Department of Surgery, Erasmus Medical Center, Rotterdam, The Netherlands

P.J. Tanis Department of Surgery, Academic Medical Center, Amsterdam, The Netherlands

E.M[a]. Targarona Soler Universidad Autónoma de Barcelona, Servicio de Cirugía General y del Aparato Digestivo, Hospital de la Santa Creu i Santpau, Barcelona, Spain

R.J. Torphy Department of Surgical Oncology, Pancreas and Biliary, University of Colorado School of Medicine, Aurora, CO, USA

A. Tsung Department of Surgery, Division of Hepatobiliary and Pancreatic Surgery, University of Pittsburgh School of Medicine, St. Pittsburgh, PA, USA

C.J.H. Van de Velde Department of Surgery, Leiden University Medical Center, Leiden, The Netherlands

T.J. Weijs University Medical Center Utrecht, Utrecht, The Netherlands

U. Wellner Department of Surgery, University Medical Center Schleswig-Holstein, Luebeck, Germany

L.R. van der Werf Department of Surgery, Erasmus University Medical Center, Rotterdam, The Netherlands

B.L.A.M. Weusten Department of Gastroenterology and Hepatology, St. Antonius Hospital, Nieuwegein, The Netherlands

D.A. Wicherts Department of Surgery, Academic Medical Center, Amsterdam, The Netherlands

N.I. van der Wielen Department of Surgery, VU University Medical Center, Amsterdam, The Netherlands

B.P.L. Wijnhoven Department of Surgery, Erasmus University Medical Center, Rotterdam, The Netherlands

H-K Yang Department of Surgery, Seoul National University Hospital, Seoul National University College of Medicine, Seoul, South Korea

M.W.W. Zwart Department of Surgery, Academic Medical Center, Amsterdam, The Netherlands

Part I

Advantages of Minimally Invasive Surgery

Advantages of Minimally Invasive Surgery in Upper Abdominal Surgery

1

Miguel A. Cuesta

The postoperative advantages of the Minimally Invasive Surgical (MIS) approach in comparison with Open approach in Upper Gastrointestinal Oncology concern: (1) The stress and immune responses, (2) the surgical intervention, (3) the postoperative short-term effects and morbidity, (4) the postoperative Quality of Life and (5) the oncological consequences.

1.1 Advantages Holding for Stress and Immune Responses

All surgical traumas are followed by unanticipated side effects such as pain and infection. A theory regarding the onset of these side effects pertains to the surgical stress response entailing subsequently increased demands on the patient's reserves and immune status. The demand on organ functions is increased following surgery and it is thought to be mediated by trauma-induced endocrine and metabolic changes. To circumvent this problem and reduce surgical trauma, the first minimally invasive colectomy was described by Jacobs et al. in 1991 [1]. Since, many studies have shown the clinical short-term benefits for laparoscopic colectomy over open procedures without compromising oncological outcomes [2–5].

HLA-DR expression on monocytes is correlated to the competence of a patient's specific immune response. C-reactive protein levels are associated with postoperative infectious complications. Interleukin-6 levels are associated with postoperative complications rates and are a predictor of morbidity following surgical intervention. Since the introduction of laparoscopic colectomies, several studies have studied these parameters and compared the postoperative stress response between open and minimally invasive procedures. Wu et al. [6] and Harmon et al. [7] both described lower interleukin-6 levels following laparoscopic colectomy.

Both interleukin-6 levels and C-reactive protein levels were found to be lower for laparoscopic colectomies by Schwenk et al. [8]. Recently, our Department published a series of 40 patients comparing surgical stress response between laparoscopic and open total mesorectal excision (TME) [9]. Only a significant reduction in surgical stress response regarding HLA-DR expression in monocytes and interleukin-6 levels could be found for the laparoscopic TME at 2 h postoperatively. No differences regarding leukocytes, monocytes, C-reactive protein, interleukin-8, cortisol, growth hormone, and prolactin could be found at 24 h and 72 h postoperatively.

M.A. Cuesta
Emeritus Professor, Department of Surgery, VUmc, Amsterdam, The Netherlands
e-mail: ma.cuesta@vumc.nl

M.A. Cuesta (ed.), *Minimally Invasive Surgery for Upper Abdominal Cancer*,
DOI 10.1007/978-3-319-54301-7_1

The conclusion being that only a short-term benefit in surgical stress response for laparoscopic TME procedures could be proven. A similar outcome can be expected after Minimally Upper Abdominal Surgery.

The recent introduction of fast-track postoperative care by Kehlet [10–12] has revived the discussion regarding postoperative immune and stress response. Since the introduction of the fast-track multimodality postoperative care, no studies had yet appeared that investigated the stress response and immune function between fast-track and conventional care. Therefore, two surgical departments in Amsterdam, the AMC and the Vumc, conducted a randomized trial as substudy of the LAFA trial [13] comparing open versus laparoscopic colectomy with fast-track or conventional postoperative care [14]. Patients with nonmetastasized colon cancer were randomized to laparoscopic or open colectomy with fast-track or standard care. A significant difference in HLA-DR expression on monocytes (and therefore immune competence) was observed between the four groups (Fig. 1.1). Patient with laparoscopy and fast-track perioperative care remained the best immune-competent. Patients with open surgery and standard care were found to have higher postoperative C-reactive protein and IL-6 levels when compared to the other groups (Fig. 1.2). Laparoscopy seemed to better preserve immune status and reduce postoperative surgical trauma. On the other hand, in the present study, no clinical benefits such as less postoperative complications could be found.

The ensuing discussion concerns why laparoscopy and fast-track surgery has clinical advantages. Up to date, little evidence exists regarding a reduced-postoperative-surgical stress response explaining enhanced patient-recovery following laparoscopic colorectal surgery with or without fast-track perioperative care.

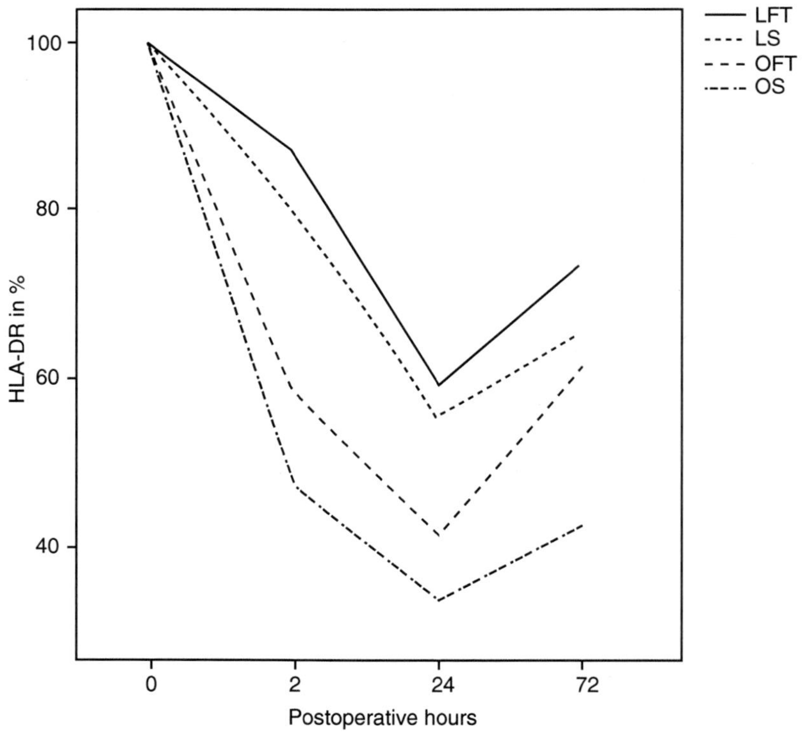

Fig. 1.1 Significant difference in HLA-DR expression on monocytes between the four groups studied in the LAFA trial. The two laparoscopic groups have a higher expression then the two open groups

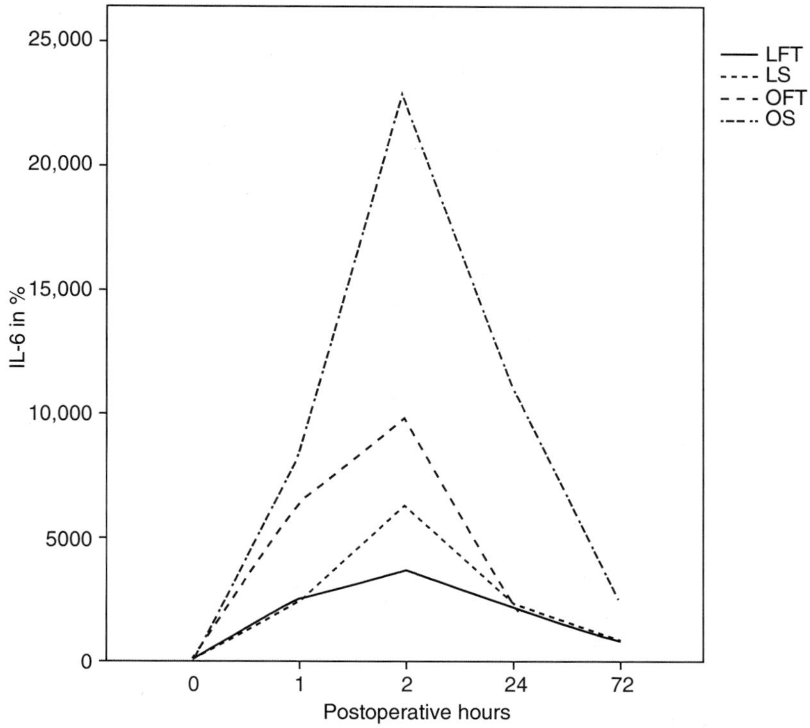

Fig. 1.2 Patients with open surgery and standard care of the LAFA trial have higher postoperative IL-6 levels when compared with the other three groups

1.2 Advantages of the MIS During Surgical Intervention

The advantages derived from the better visualization and the magnification obtained by the laparoscopic camera's are clear. Improvement in 2D-visualization obtained by high definition technologies has been very important in order to increase the quality of MIS and expand these operative techniques worldwide. If you can see better, you can probably dissect better. Moreover, the improvements produced by more advanced techniques—such as 3D-imaging and robot-assisted interventions—are very important but must be evidenced by randomized control studies before their global implementation. In the last 10 years, these imaging improvements have been sustained by new dissection instruments, sealing devices and staplers, which changed the way to operate involving important consequences such as less blood loss, more efficient dissection and new operative protocols. Furthermore, imaging diagnosis has been enormously improved, thereby permitting a better selection of patients and procedures. Hence, surgical anatomy is to be newly described according to the information generated by MIS. These changes will help to define more clearly the surgical planes to be dissected during oncological procedures, and so enhance standardizing the oncological resections [15].

1.3 Advantages on Postoperative Short-Term Effects, Including Morbidity

Short-term advantages of MIS in Upper GI and HPB Surgery are derived from the reduced amount of operative trauma. Advantages of MIS such as less morbidity, short hospital stay and a quicker recovery are frequently found. The reasons for the lower complication rate after MIS as compared to the procedure of its open counterpart are multiple: (a) A careful dissection technique, (b) less blood loss, (c) avoidance of huge-approach wounds such as laparotomy or thoracotomy, and (d) the systematic dissection by planes.

Regarding MI esophagectomy, the published randomized control trial, i.e. the TIME trial, compared open esophagectomy (OE) with Total minimally invasive esophagectomy (MIE). The results demonstrated that MIE results in less blood loss, a lower incidence of pulmonary infections, a shorter hospital stay, and a better short-term quality of life without compromise of the quality of the resected specimen [16]. Concerning gastrectomy, there is evidence that the Minimally Invasive Gastrectomy is a feasible and acceptable surgical technique with short term advantages for partial gastrectomy whereas for total gastrectomy it should still be validated [17].

Laparoscopic total and partial gastrectomy in comparison with the open counterparts for gastric cancer are associated with a longer operative time but lower blood loss, with shorter postoperative hospital stay and faster postoperative recovery. Moreover, there were similar outcomes between both approaches in terms of completeness of the specimen and number of dissected lymph nodes and long-term follow-up (survival).

In Asian countries, the majority of studies (the KLASS studies) refer to a partial gastrectomy. These studies show better short-term outcomes for the minimally invasive approach. For total gastrectomy, hard evidence is lacking and outcomes are based on retrospective databases.

In the Netherlands, two CRTs compare laparoscopic and open gastrectomy: the STOMACH and the LOGICA trial; the STOMACH trial exclusively focused on total gastrectomy. The results of these trials will give more insight into evidence whether minimally invasive gastrectomy is as feasible and safe when performed in the West as it is in the East relating to the treatment of gastric cancer patients [18–22].

Concerning minimally invasive pancreatic surgery, it is demonstrated that for distal pancreatectomy it serves as the standard intervention. The problem involved is to standardize and demonstrate that MI duodenopancreatectomy (LPD) is equal or better than the open procedure. Holding for selected patients, when operated on by expert laparoscopic pancreatic surgeons, LPD seems feasible and safe. Pragmatic and multicenter randomized-control trials will have to demonstrate the superiority of minimally invasive pancreatoduodenectomy (LEOPARD trial). Regarding this operation, it is expected that the robot will give this technique a new and definitive impulse [23–28].

1.4 Consequences for Quality of Life

There is almost no evidence from Quality of Life (QoL) studies pertaining to the Upper GI surgery.

In the TIME trial comparing MIE and OE, QoL questionnaires showed that diverse components concerning physical scores are better-preserved postoperatively in the MIE group in comparison with the open group, and this favourable score remains 1-year postoperatively in favour of MIE. This advantage can be only explained by the avoidance of thoracotomy and the post-thoracotomy syndrome. Such QoL studies should in the future be implemented in every RCT [16, 30].

1.5 Are There Oncological Advantages of the MIS?

All RCT comparing MIS with open colectomies for colorectal cancer have found no differences in overall and disease-free survival and recurrences between the two approaches with the exception of the Barcelona trial for stage 3 colon cancer [2, 29]. Concerning the TIME trial, no differences in overall and disease free survival have been found between the two groups at 1 and 3 years follow-up [30]. Moreover, it seems that CRT and meta-analysis on partial gastrectomies have found no differences in quality of specimen resected and survival, but more evidence concerning survival and the quality of the specimens resected in total gastrectomy is necessary [18, 21, 22].

Pointedly, concerning duodenopancreatectomy and hepatic resections, studies are still ongoing in order to gain evidence that these minimally invasive procedures are oncologically safe [28, 31, 32].

Conclusion

There are potentially rather important advantages to be derived from the implementation of MIS in Upper abdominal surgery. Many advantages stem from reduced operative trauma and the magnificent visualization and magnification obtained. Additionally, acquisition of new instruments has changed the form of dissection and resection. Furthermore, meta-analysis shows that the short-term advantages obtained by MIS in upper abdominal surgery are the same as those produced by the laparoscopic colorectal surgery. These concern less morbidity, shorter hospital stay, faster postoperative recovery and better quality of life. Moreover, completeness of the resection and lymph nodes resected are similar for both procedures. The question remains about long-term oncological safety and survival. Probably, using MIS will by its better visualization and magnification and its dissection through the surgical planes, lead to more radical R0 interventions. Teaching programs designed for this complicated upper abdominal surgery are paramount for obtaining and extending the promising advantages of this approach for all patients.

References

1. Jacobs M, Verdeja JC, Goldstein HS. Minimally invasive colon resection (laparoscopic colectomy). Surg Laparosc Endosc. 1991;1:144–50.
2. Lacy AM, Garcia Valdecasas JC, Delgado S, et al. Laparoscopic-assisted colectomy versus open colectomy for treatment of non metastatic colon cancer: a randomised trial. Lancet. 2002;359:2224–9.
3. Nelson H, Sargent DJ, Wieand S, et al. A comparison of laparoscopically assisted and open colectomy for colon cancer. N Engl J Med. 2004;350:2050–9.
4. The COLOR cancer laparoscopic or Open Resection Study Group. Laparoscopic surgery versus open surgery for colon cancer: short term outcomes of a randomized trial. Lancet Oncol. 2005;6:477–84.
5. Weeks JC, Nelson H, Gelber S, et al. Short term quality-of-life outcomes following laparoscopic assisted vs. open colectomy for colon cancer: a randomised trial. JAMA. 2002;287:321–8.
6. Wu FPK, Sietses C, von Blomberg BME, et al. Systemic and peritoneal inflammatory response after laparoscopic or conventional colon resection in cancer patients: a prospective, randomised trial. Dis Colon Rectum. 2003;46:147–55.
7. Harmon GD, Senagore AJ, Kilbride MJ, Warzynski MJ. Interleukin-6 response to laparoscopic and open colectomy. Dis Colon Rectum. 1994;37:754–9.
8. Schwenk W, Jacobi C, Mansmann U, et al. Inflammatory response after laparoscopic and conventional colorectal resections-results of a prospective randomized trial. Langebecks Arch Surg. 2000;385:2–9.
9. Veenhof AA, Sietses C, von Blomberg BM, et al. The surgical stress response and postoperative immune function after laparoscopic or conventional total mesorectal excision in rectal acncer: a randomized trial. Int J Color Dis. 2011;26:53–9.
10. Wilmore DW, Kehlet H. Management of patients in fast track surgery. BMJ. 2001;322:473–6.
11. Kehlet H. Fast track colorectal surgery. Lancet. 2008;371:791–3.
12. Kehlet H, Wilmore DW. Evidence based surgical care and evolution of fast-track surgery. Ann Surg. 2008;248:189–98.
13. Vlug MS, Wind J, Hollemann MW, et al. Laparoscopy in combination with fast track multimodal management is the best perioperative strategy in patients undergoing colonic surgery: a randomized clinical trial (LAFA study). Ann Surg. 2011;254:868–75.
14. Veenhof AA, Vlug MS, vd Pas MH, et al. Surgical stress response and postoperative immune function after laparoscopy or open surgery with fast track or standard perioperative care: a randomized trial. Ann Surg. 2012;255:216–21.
15. Cuesta MA, Weijs TJ, Bleys RL, van Hillegersberg R, van Berge Henegouwen MI, Gisbertz SS, Ruurda JP, Straatman J, Osugi H, van der Peet DL. A new concept of the anatomy of the thoracic oesophagus: the meso-oesophagus. Observational study during thoracoscopic esophagectomy. Surg Endosc. 2015;29:2576–82.
16. Biere SSAY, van Berge Henegouwen MI, Maas KW, Bonavina L, Rosman C, Roig Garcia J, Gisbertz SS, Klinkenbijl JHG, Hollemann MW, de Lange ESM, Bonjer HJ, van der Peet DL, Cuesta MA. Minimally invasive versus open oesophagectomy for patients with oesophageal cancer: a multicentre, open-label, randomised control trial. Lancet. 2012;379:1887–92.
17. Huscher CGS, Mingoli A, Sgarzini G, Sansonetti A, Di Paola M, Recher A, Ponzano C. Laparosocpic versus open subtotal gastrectomy for distal gastric cancer. Five year results of a randomized prospective trial. Ann Surg. 2005;241(1):232–7.
18. Kim W, Kim HH, Han SU, Kim MC, Hyung WJ, Ryu SW, et al. Decreased morbidity of laparoscopic distal

gastrectomy compared with open distal gastrectomy for stage I gastric cancer: short-term outcomes from a multicenter randomized controlled trial (KLASS-01). Ann Surg. 2016;263(1):28–35.
19. Straatman J, van der Wielen N, Cuesta MA, de Lange-de Klerk ES, Jansma EP, van der Peet DL. Minimally invasive versus open total gastrectomy for gastric cancer: a systematic review and meta-analysis of short-term outcomes and completeness of resection: surgical techniques in gastric cancer. World J Surg. 2016;40:148–57.
20. Martínez-Ramos D, Miralles-Tena JM, Cuesta MA, Escrig-Sos J, van der Peet DL, Hoashi JS, Salvador-Sanchis JL. Laparoscopy versus open surgery for advances and resectable gastric cancer: a meta-analysis. Rev Esp Enferm Dig. 2011;103(3):133–41.
21. Straatman J, van der Wielen N, Cuesta MA, Gisbertz SS, Hartemink KJ, Alonso Poza A, Weitz J, Mateo Vallejo F, Akhtar K, Diez del Val I, Roig Garcia J, van der Peet DL. Surgical techniques, open versus minimally invasive gastrectomy after chemotherapy (STOMACH trial): study protocol for a randomized controlled trial. Trials. 2015;16:123.
22. Haverkamp L, Brenkman HJF, Seesing MFJ, Gisbert SS, van Berge Henegouwen MI, Luyer MDP, Nieuwenhuijzen GAP, Wijnhoven BPL, van Lanschot JJB, de Steur WO, Hartgrink HH, Stoot JHMB, Hulsewé KWE, Spillenaar Bilgen EJ, Rütter JE, Kouwenhoven EA, van Det MJ, van der Peet DL, Daams F, Draaisma WA, Broeders IAMJ, van Stel HF, Lacle MM, Ruurda JP, van Hillegersberg R. Laparoscopic versus open gastrectomy for gastric cancer, a multicenter prospectively randomized controlled trial (LOGICA trial). BMC Cancer. 2015;15:556.
23. Qin H, Qiu J, Zhao Y, Pan G, Zeng Y. Does minimally invasive pancreatoduodenectomy have advantages over its open method. A meta-analysis of retrospective studies. PLoS One. 2014;9(8):e104274.
24. Nakamura M, Nakashima H. Laparoscopic distal pancreatectomy and duodenopancreatectomy: is it worthwhile? J Hepatobiliary Pancreat Sci. 2013;20:421–8.
25. Boggi U, Ugo B, Gabriella A, Fabio V, Fabio C, De Lio N, Vittorio P, Linda B, Mario B, Stefano S, Franco M. Laparoscopic pancreaticoduodenectomy: a systematic literature review. Surg Endosc. 2014;29:9–23.
26. De Rooij T, Besselink M, Shamali A, Butturini G, Busch O, Troisi R, Fernández-Cruz L, Topal B, Dagher I, Bassi C, Abu Hilal M. Pan-European survey on laparoscopic pancreatic surgery. HPB (Oxford). 2016;18:e852–3.
27. Riviere D, Gurusamy KS, Kooby DA, et al. Laparoscopic versus open distal pancreatectomy for pancreatic cancer. Cochrane Database Syst Rev. 2016;4:CD011391. doi:10.1002/14651858.CD011391.pub2.
28. Pancreatic head and peri-ampullary cancer laparoscopic vs. open surgical treatment trial (PLOT). https://clinicaltrials.gov/ct2/show/NCT.
29. Bonjer HJ, Deijnen CL, Abis GA, et al. A randomized trial of laparoscopic versus open surgery for rectal cancer. N Engl J Med. 2015;372:1324–32.
30. Maas KW, Cuesta MA, van Berge Henegouwen MI, et al. Quality of life and late complications after minimally invasive compared to open esophagectomy. results of a randomized trial. World J Surg. 2015; 39:1986–93.
31. The ORANGE II plus trial. Open versus laparoscopic hemihepatectomy. Clinical trials gov. NCT01441856, RM van Dam, updated Sept 2016.
32. Chen J, Bai T, Zhang Y, et al. The safety and efficacy of laparoscopic and open hepatectomy in hepatocellular carcinoma patients with liver cirrhosis: a systematic review. J Clin Exp Med. 2015;8:20679–89.

Part II

Esophagus and Gastro-Esophageal Junction Cancer

2 Surgical Anatomy of Esophagus

Ronald L.A.W. Bleys and Teus J. Weijs

2.1 Introduction

The esophagus is a muscular tube of approximately 25 cm which connects the pharynx to the stomach and serves as a food passage. The greater part lies in the thorax but is has cervical and abdominal parts as well. Except for the vermiform appendix it is the narrowest part of the digestive tract. The esophagus is collapsed at rest and opens during swallowing. Its passage through the thorax with its subatmospheric pressure and the fact that it should be a highly mobile organ, due to its own peristalsis and respiratory movements, sets requirements for its construct and attachments. This chapter discusses its general features, its construction and anchoring, its important topographical relationships, vascular and nerve supply, and lymphatics.

2.2 General Features

The cervical part (3–5 cm) is posterior to the trachea and attached to it by loose connective tissue. Between it and the spine is the prevertebral layer of cervical fascia which is bilayered here, the anterior layer is named alar fascia. Therefore, two narrow pockets with loose connective tissue exist between the esophagus and the spine [1, 2]. These pockets continue into the mediastinum. It is through the loose connective tissue, which acts as a gliding plane, that the esophagus has freedom of movement against the spine. The recurrent laryngeal nerves ascend close to the esophagus and the trachea.

The thoracic part of the esophagus (18–22 cm) traverses the superior mediastinum and the posterior mediastinum. Here it is embedded in loose connective tissue which allows for the movements which are found in the mediastinum: peristalsis of the esophagus, pulsations of the descending aorta and respiratory excursions. Among the main topographical relationships are the spine posteriorly, the trachea and the pericardium anteriorly and the descending aorta to the left.

Where the esophagus traverses the esophageal hiatus of the diaphragm it is connected to it by the phrenico-esophageal ligament. The abdominal part is short (1.5 cm) but of utmost importance. Increase of intra-abdominal pressure results in an increase of the pressure inside the stomach but the same pressure increase simultaneously compresses the abdominal part of the esophagus, thereby minimizing the risk of gastroesophageal reflux.

Inside the thoracic cavity the subatmospheric pressure keeps the elastic lungs expanded. Since it traverses the thorax the intraluminal pressure of the esophagus is lower than the pressures in the pharynx and the stomach. To prevent continuous

R.L.A.W. Bleys (✉) • T.J. Weijs
University Medical Centre Utrecht, Utrecht, The Netherlands
e-mail: R.L.A.W.Bleys@umcutrecht.nl; T.J.Weijs@umcutrecht.nl

M.A. Cuesta (ed.), *Minimally Invasive Surgery for Upper Abdominal Cancer*, DOI 10.1007/978-3-319-54301-7_2

suction of mucus and air from the pharynx and reflux of acid stomach contents, sphincters keep both ends of the esophagus closed except during swallowing. The upper esophageal sphincter (UES) is at the transition of the pharynx to the esophagus and is the caudalmost part of the inferior pharyngeal constrictor. This part has been named cricopharyngeus and can easily be distinguished during anatomical dissections. The lower esophageal sphincter (LES), however, is not a clear morphological entity. It is a so-called functional sphincter which means that it is a part of the esophageal musculature which can generate a high pressure and can therefore have a sphincteric action. It is at the level of passage of the esophagus through the diaphragm and continues to the gastro-esophageal junction [3]. Sphincteric action at this level is reinforced by the right crus of the diaphragm which encircles the esophagus as it traverses the diaphragm. This right crus works as an external sphincter, especially during inspiration when the intra-abdominal pressure increases.

2.3 Structure

The construction of the esophageal wall follows the general pattern of the tissue organization of the digestive tube. There are four layers, from outside inwards: adventitia (external fibrous layer), muscularis, submucosa and mucosa.

The adventitia consists of loose connective tissue which continues as the loose connective tissue elsewhere in the mediastinum. Except for the abdominal part there is no serous lining.

The muscularis consists of an outer longitudinal layer and an inner circular layer. This parallels the plan as found in more distal parts of the digestive tube. However, in the pharynx the opposite is found. An external circular layer consists of the three pharyngeal constrictors while three levators form the inner longitudinal layer. As a consequence a reorganization of muscle layers takes place at the pharynx-esophagus transition. This is the region where areas of sparse muscle exist. Killian's triangle is the area between the thyropharyngeal part of inferior constrictor and cricopharyngeus. Zenker's hypopharyngeal diverticulum arises from here.

At the gastro-esophageal junction the longitudinal and circular muscle layers continue as similar layers in the wall of the stomach. The longitudinal layer continues along the lesser and greater curvatures of the stomach especially. Here the longitudinal muscle layer of the stomach is better developed than over its anterior and posterior surfaces. Inside the circular muscle layer of the stomach a third layer of oblique muscle fibers is present. These fibers form a U-shaped sling left to the oblique implant of the esophagus into the stomach and maintain the cardiac notch, or angle of His, between the esophagus and the greater curvature. It is not certain how much this configuration contributes to the resistance to reflux. Due to the oblique implant of the esophagus a valve-like flap (the flap-valve of Hill) is formed at the cardiac orifice, which also may help to prevent reflux.

Approximately in the upper one-third of the esophagus the muscularis is formed by striated muscle. In the middle one-third smooth muscle cells appear and intermingle with the striated muscle fibers and the lower one-third of the esophagus contains smooth muscle cells only.

The submucosa contains loose connective tissue with elastic and collagen fibers. It contains blood vessels and lymphatics, all in a plexiform arrangement.

The mucosa is thick and consists of a nonkeratinized stratified squamous epithelium, a lamina propria and a muscularis mucosae. There is an abrupt transition into simple columnar epithelium at the gastro-esophageal junction. Because the line of transition is jagged it is often referred to as the Z-line. The esophageal lumen is marked by longitudinal grooves and ridges at rest. These disappear when the lumen is distended during swallowing. Gastric mucosal folds at the cardiac orifice form the so-called mucosal rosette. This may help to form a tight seal, especially for fluid and gas.

In this and the previous sections several structures and mechanisms which help to prevent gastro-esophageal reflux were discussed. To summarize, the following factors may contribute to a greater or lesser extent. (1) The LES in the esophageal wall, (2) the right crus of the diaphragm, (3) the intra-abdominal part of the esophagus, (4) the cardiac notch and the oblique muscle fibers of the stomach, (5) the flap-valve of Hill, (6) the mucosal rosette.

2.4 Anchoring

The cranial half of the esophagus is connected to the trachea, the pleura and the alar fascia by connective tissue strands and small membranes which contain collagen and elastic fibers.

Recently it was described that the esophagus is attached to the descending aorta by the aorto-esophageal ligament (Figs. 2.1 and 2.2) [4, 5]. From this ligament a thin extension courses toward the right pleural reflection, which is the aorto-pleural ligament. The aorto-esophageal ligament contains blood vessels which run from the aorta to the esophagus. The posterior mediastinum is divided in two compartments by the aorto-esophageal and aorto-pleural ligaments. First the peri-esophageal compartment, bounded anteriorly by the pericardium, laterally by the pleura and posteriorly by the aorto-esophageal and aorto-pleural ligaments, containing the esophagus, trachea,

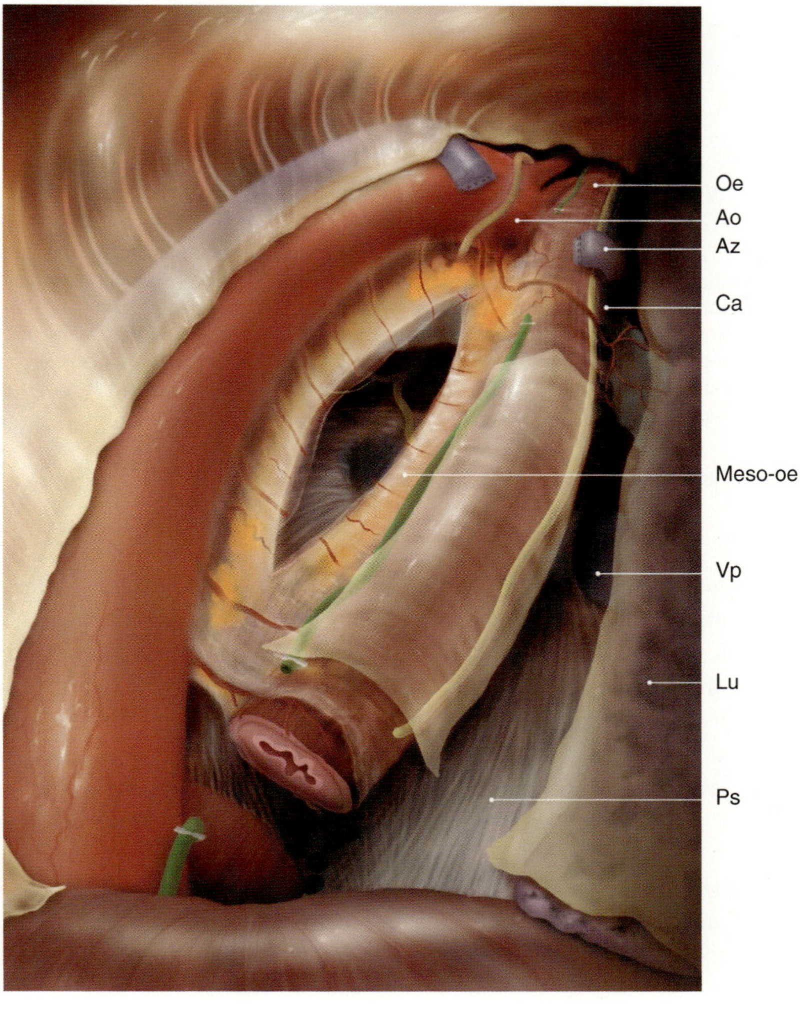

Fig. 2.1 Illustration of the aorto-esophageal ligament, previously named "meso-esophagus". It is a bilayered connective tissue layer with blood vessels coursing from the descending aorta to the esophagus. Abbreviations: *PS* pericardial sac, *Lu* right lung; *Vp* right pulmonary vein, *Ca* carina and right bronchus, *Meso-oe* meso-oesophagus, *Az* azygos vein, *Ao* aorta, *Oe* oesophagus (From [4])

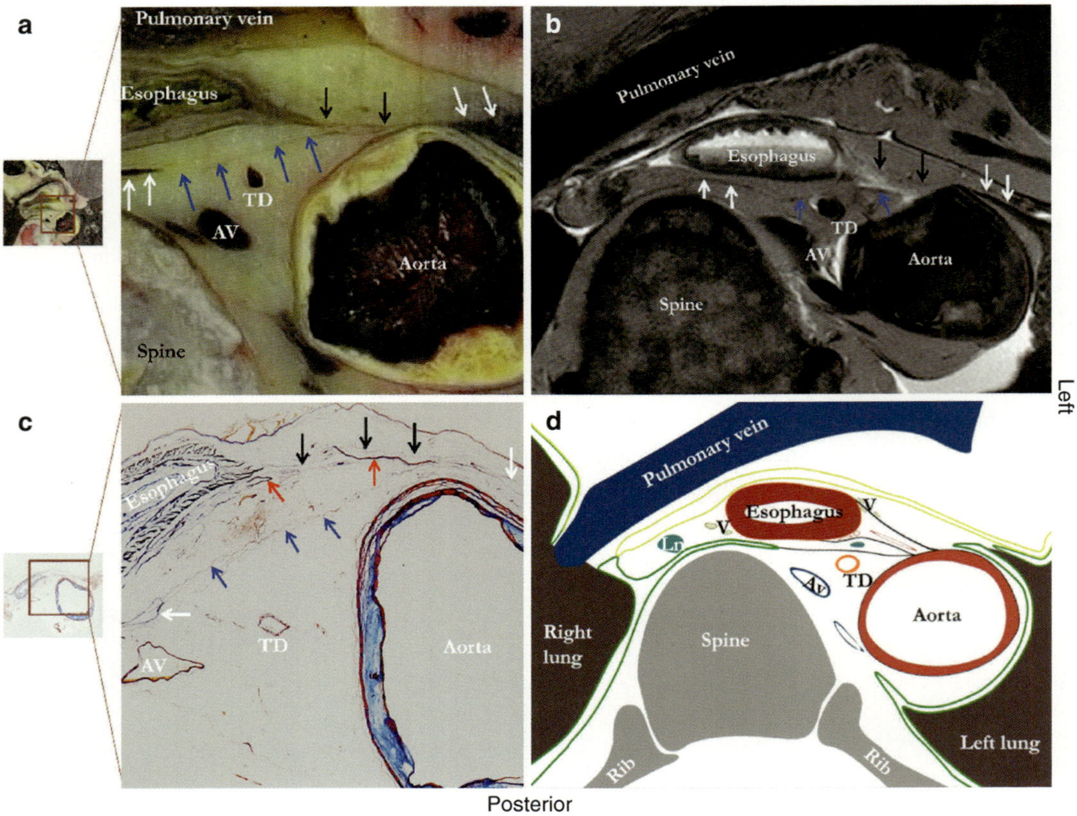

Fig. 2.2 Photograph of a transverse section of the posterior mediastinum between the diaphragm and tracheal bifurcation (**a**) with a magnetic resonance image of the same section (**b**), histology (**c**) and a schematic summary (**d**). For histology the Verhoef-Von Gieson stain was used (elastin stained *black-blue*; collagen stained *light red-pink*). The *black arrows* indicate the aorto-esophageal ligament, the *blue arrows* indicate the aorto-pleural ligament, the *white arrows* indicate the *right* and *left* pleural reflections and the *red arrows* indicate blood vessels. In the schematic drawing the *green line* represents the pleura, the *yellow line* represents pericardium and the *black line* the aorto-esophageal and aorto-pleural ligaments. Abbreviations: *AV* azygos vein, *TD* thoracic duct, *V* vagus nerve (From [5])

vagus nerves and carinal lymph nodes. Second the para-aortic compartment, containing the thoracic duct, azygos vein and lymph nodes.

As the esophagus traverses the diaphragm through the esophageal hiatus it is loosely attached to it by the phrenico-esophageal ligament, also named phrenico-esophageal membrane. This ligament wraps the gastro-esophageal junction like a collar and is derived from the endothoracic and transversalis fascias which run above and below the diaphragm respectively (Fig. 2.3). The space between the ligament and the esophagus is called the para-esophageal space and contains loose connective tissue and some fat. By acting as a gliding plane this tissue enables some movement through the hiatus during respiration and swallowing. Because the ligament, as extensions of the endothoracic and transversalis fascias, also attaches to the esophagus above and below the diaphragm it simultaneously limits upward and downward movements and therefore stabilizes the esophageal passage through the diaphragm. The upper part of the ligament is the longest and firmest and therefore the ligament is

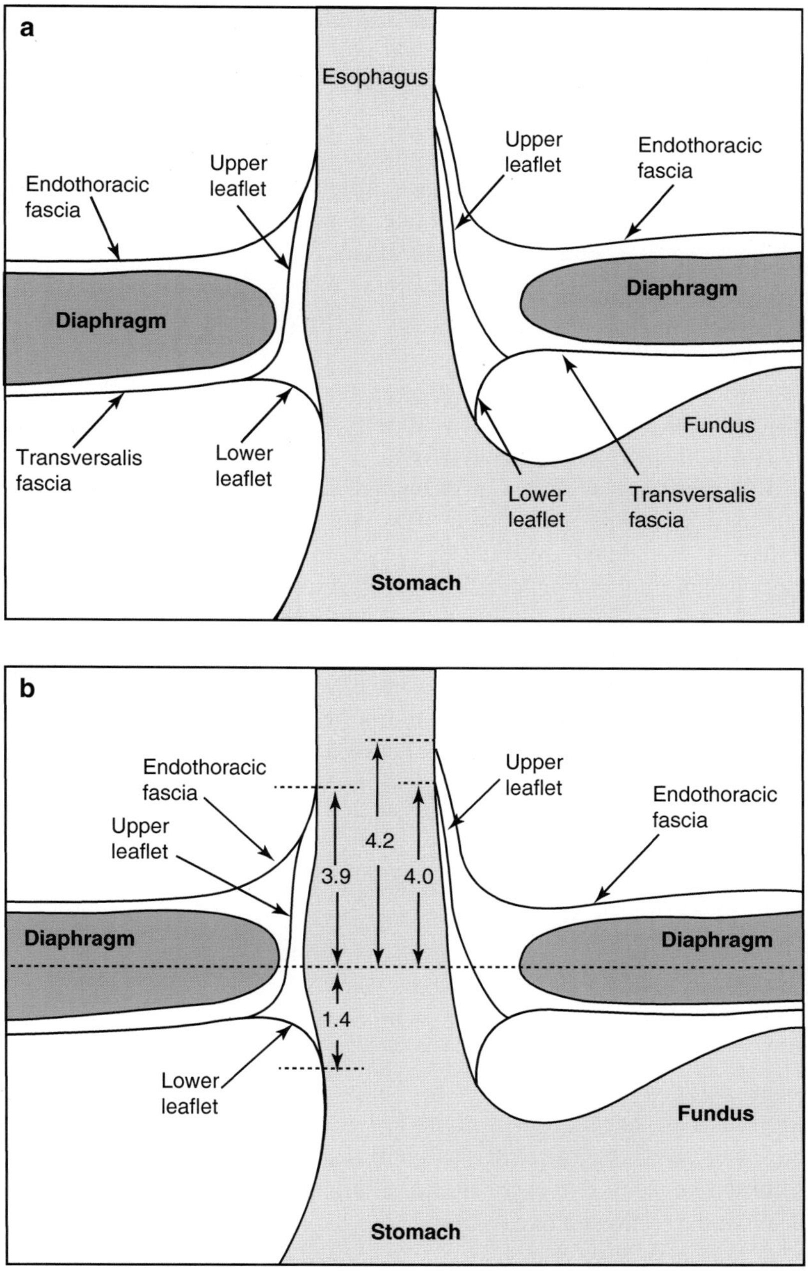

Fig. 2.3 (**a**) Schematic drawing of the gastroesophageal junction demonstrating two ways in which the endothoracic and transversalis fascias may contribute to the phrenico-esophageal ligament. On the right side the endothoracic fascia fuses with the upper leaflet of the transversalis fascia while on the left side they attach separately to the esophagus. (**b**). Mean distances in centimeters between an imaginary horizontal line through the diaphragm and attachment points of the fascial layers of the phrenico-esophageal ligament. It is demonstrated that the upper part of the ligament is the longest part (From [6])

especially important in limiting upward movement of the esophagus during increased intra-abdominal pressure [6]. The phrenico-esophageal ligament contains collagen and elastic fibers. The fiber contents decreases with age and therefore the ligament weakens in the elderly.

2.5 Topographical Relationships

In its course the esophagus has four constrictions. Two of these are caused by the sphincters and are found at its beginning at the pharyngo-esophageal junction and where it traverses the diaphragm. The other constrictions are where the esophagus is crossed by the aortic arch and where it is crossed by left principal bronchus and they are close to each other. In rest the constrictions are not clear but they become obvious during swallowing when the lumen distends. They are of clinical importance in case of swallowing corpora aliena. Radiographs taken during swallowing clearly demonstrate these constrictions. In a lateral radiograph a slight impression in the anterior aspect of the esophagus becomes visible. It is caused by the left atrium which lies directly anterior to the esophagus with the pericardium in between.

In a previous section the main topographical relationships were mentioned. This section describes additional relationships especially those which are important during esophageal surgery. To the right is the mediastinal pleura and the intervening azygos vein which crosses forwards over the right principal bronchus to enter the superior vena cava. Lower in the posterior mediastinum the thoracic duct runs between the esophagus and the azygos vein. At about the level of the fifth thoracic vertebra it crosses to the left behind the esophagus and then ascends on the left. Further posteriorly on the right side the greater splanchnic nerve can be found on its way to the diaphragm. Between the esophagus in front and the azygos vein and spine behind there is a long pleural recess of the right pleural cavity (Fig. 2.2). Below the pulmonary root the right vagus nerve descends along the esophagus and forms an esophageal plexus with its fellow from the other side. The vagus nerves including the recurrent laryngeal nerves are discussed in more detail in the section on innervation.

A left lateral view demonstrates the aortopulmonary window. This is a space between the arch of the aorta and the pulmonary trunk. Its boundaries in front and behind are the ascending and descending aorta respectively, left is the mediastinal pleura and on the right the left principal bronchus. The aortopulmonary window contains the ligamentum arteriosum, lymph nodes and fat. The left recurrent laryngeal nerve passes through it, after branching from the left vagus nerve, and then ascends to the neck.

2.6 Vascular Supply

The esophagus is supplied by many arteries. Since the organ is not involved in absorption of food components all supplying arteries are relatively small. Some of the arteries are shared arteries, they share a blood supply with other structures. The shared arteries are: inferior thyroid arteries, bronchial arteries, left gastric artery and quite often (55%) the left inferior phrenic artery. There are four or five proper arteries as well, these arise from the front of the descending aorta between the tracheal bifurcation and the diaphragm and descend obliquely to the esophagus in the aortopulmonary ligament which was described in a previous section. Inside the wall of the esophagus the proper and shared arteries are connected to each other.

The bronchial arteries deserve special mention. They are relatively large and of great importance for the supply of pulmonary tissues. Normally there are three of them, one on the right side arising from the third posterior intercostal artery and two on the left side which arise directly from the aorta. This 'normal' configuration is found in only 40%. Variations are numerous. In 25% two arteries arise from the aorta through a common trunk but are then distributed normally which means that the left lung still receives two arteries. In another common variation (20%) there are only two bronchial arteries, both arising from the aorta [7].

Another variation related to the blood supply of the esophagus is the artery of Belsey. This is an anastomosis between the left gastric and left inferior phrenic arteries and is found at the inferior part of the esophagus.

Blood from the esophagus is collected into a submucosal venous plexus and then into a periesophageal venous plexus. From the latter plexus the thoracic part of the esophagus drains mainly into the azygos vein and to a lesser extent into the hemiazygos and bronchial veins. The cervical part drains into the inferior thyroid and vertebral veins. In the inferior part of the esophagus there are venous connections to the inferior phrenic veins and the left gastric vein, the latter vein connecting to the portal vein. Due to the low intrathoracic pressure the flow in the upper part of the left gastric vein and its esophageal tributaries is normally directed to the thorax.

2.7 Innervation

The vagus nerves are responsible for the innervation of the esophagus. Since these are mixed nerves, containing somatomotor and visceromotor (parasympathetic) nerve fibers, they supply both striated and smooth muscle components of the esophagus as well as the mucous glands in the mucosa. The vagus nerves also carry sensory fibers which come from the esophagus. Esophageal blood vessels have a sympathetic nerve supply originating in the upper 4–6 thoracic spinal cord segments. Visceral afferent pain fibers use sympathetic routes to reach the upper thoracic spinal cord segments. These segments also receive pain fibers from the heart which explains that it is sometimes difficult to determine the origin of the pain.

The upper part of the esophagus is supplied by branches from the recurrent laryngeal nerves. On the right this nerve arises from the vagus nerve at the level of the subclavian artery, curves backwards and ascends behind this artery to the side of the trachea. On the left the nerve arises at the level of the aortic arch, passes through the aortopulmonary window and also ascends to the side of the trachea. While they ascend each recurrent laryngeal nerve gives off 8–14 branches to the trachea and the esophagus [8]. The ascending parts are embedded in connective tissue around the trachea and the esophagus. When these nerves approach the larynx they are near the groove between the trachea and the esophagus. However, they only tend to lie in this groove just below the entrance into the larynx. Lower, for example 4 cm below the entrance into the larynx, there is a wide variability in position. They may be next to the trachea, next to the esophagus or close to the groove [9]. In its course to the larynx the nerve is crossed by the inferior thyroid artery which may pass anterior or posterior to the nerve, or even may have branches on both sides of the nerve.

At the level of the bifurcation of the trachea and the principal bronchi the vagus nerves form anterior and posterior pulmonary plexuses [10]. Through these nerves many lung functions are controlled, such as the cough reflex, mucus production and bronchus diameter [11]. The right anterior pulmonary plexus is located just above the right pulmonary artery. It is supplied by a median of three vagus nerve branches that arise from the right vagus nerve on its course next to the trachea, containing a small proportion (23%) of the right lung supply. The right posterior pulmonary plexus is located dorsal to the right main bronchus and consists of a median of 13 branches which sequentially arise from the right vagus nerve starting at the level of the superior edge of the main right bronchus (Fig. 2.4). This plexus contains most of the right lung supply (77%). The left anterior pulmonary plexus is located anterosuperior to the left pulmonary artery and is formed by a median of three vagus nerve branches which arise from the vagus nerve as it crosses the aortic arch. As on the right side this plexus has the smallest contribution to the total left lung supply (26%). The large left posterior pulmonary plexus is located dorsal to the left pulmonary artery and left main bronchus, containing 74% of the left lung supply. It consists of a median of 12 branches which sequentially arise from the vagus nerve starting at the superior edge of the left pulmonary artery (Fig. 2.4). Both posterior pulmonary plexuses are

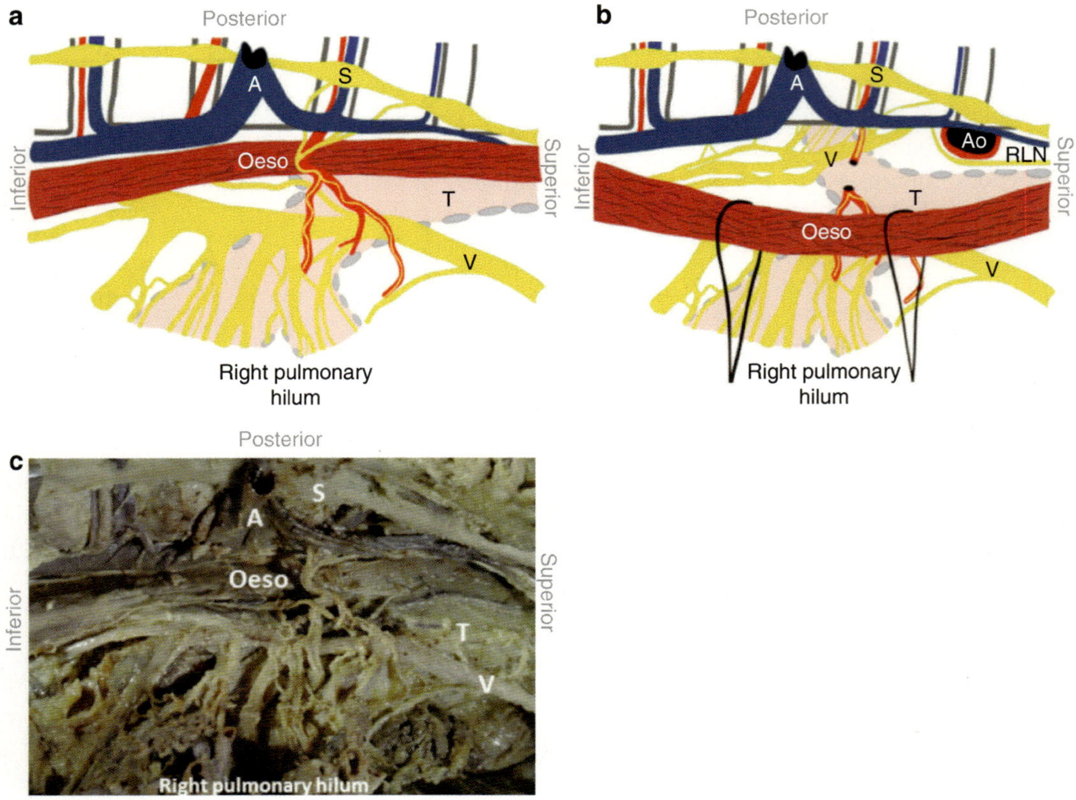

Fig. 2.4 Schematic drawings of the right posterior (**a**) and left posterior (**b**) pulmonary vagus nerve plexuses as encountered during transthoracic esophagectomy from a right lateral approach, including a corresponding photograph (**c**). Abbreviations: *A* azygos vein, *Ao* aorta, *Oeso* oesophagus, *RLN* left recurrent laryngeal nerve, *S* sympathetic trunk, *T* trachea, *V* vagus nerve (From [10])

organized segmentally, the most superior branches innervate the superior and middle lung lobes, and the most inferior innervate the inferior lung lobes.

Caudal to the principal bronchi the vagus nerves form a plexus around the lower part of the esophagus. From here the abdomen is reached as anterior and posterior vagal trunks through the esophageal hiatus of the diaphragm.

2.8 Lymphatic Drainage

The esophageal submucosa contains a network of predominantly longitudinally orientated lymph channels. In general the flow in these vessels is diverted from the tracheal bifurcation. Lymph is collected by deep cervical, mediastinal and left gastric (and from there to coeliac) lymph nodes. The variation in the number of lymph nodes is large, for example the number of mediastinal lymph nodes ranges from 11 up to 54 lymph nodes [12]. The mediastinal lymph nodes are generally grouped using the lymph node map develop by the International Association for the Study of Lung Cancer (Fig. 2.5) [13, 14]. Abdominal lymph nodes are classified using the lymph node map developed by the Japanese society for gastric cancer (Fig. 2.6) [15]. Due to the network of longitudinally orientated lymph channels lymph node metastasis can occur far from the primary tumor and the sentinel node concept does not apply to esophageal cancer [16].

Fig. 2.5 Important mediastinal lymph node stations as seen during thoracolaparoscopic esophagectomy in prone position. Abbreviations: *LN* lymph node, *R* right, *L* left (From [13])

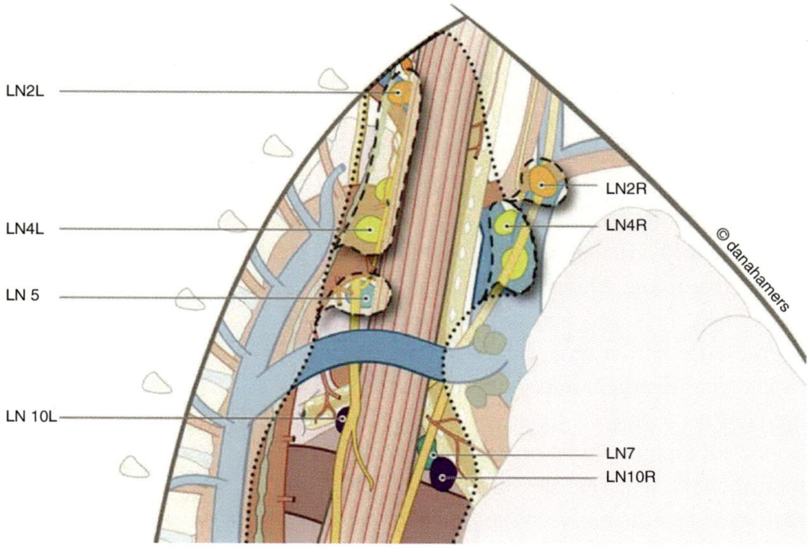

Fig. 2.6 Gastric lymph node map as developed by the Japanese society for gastric cancer. Abbreviations: *APIS* a. phrenica inferior sinistra, *AGES* a. gastroepiploica sinistra, *AGB* aa. gastricae breves, *VGED* v. gastroepiploica dextra, *VCDA* v. colica dextra accessoria, *AGSA* a. gastrica sinistra accessoria, *REGAP* ramus esophagogastricus ascendens posterior, *VCM* v. colica media, *VCD* v. colica dextra, *VPDIA* v. pancreaticoduodenalis inferior anterior; *TGC* truncus gastrocolicus, *VMS* v. mesenterica superior, *VL* v. lienalis, *AHC* a. hepatica communis (From [15])

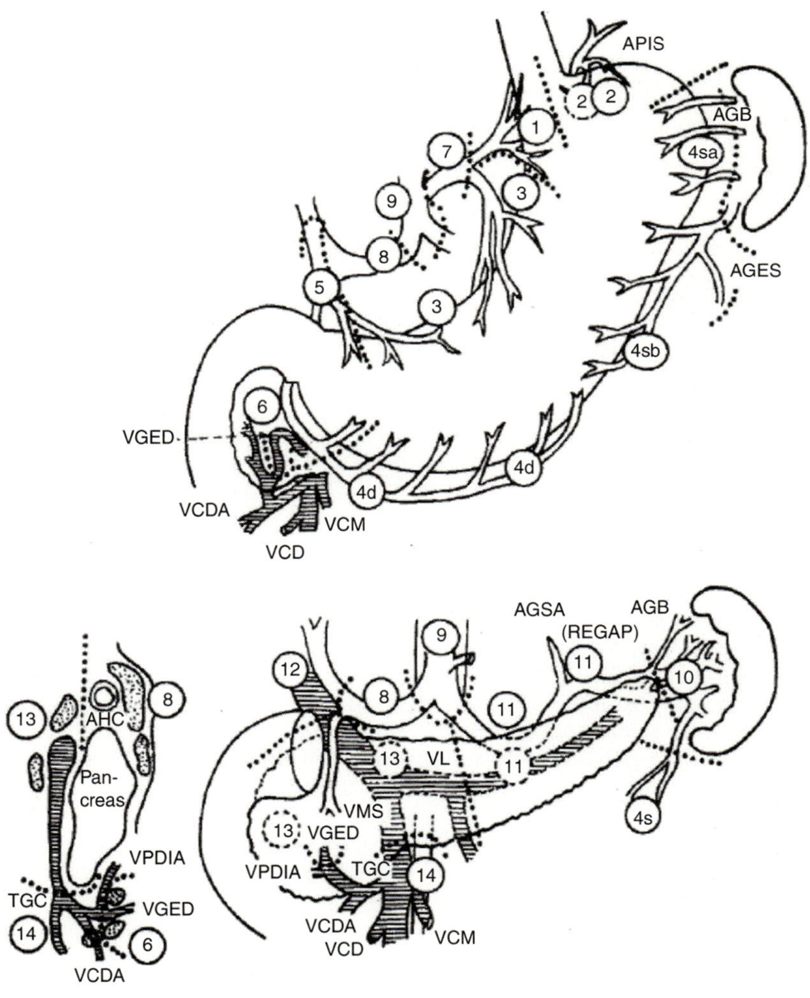

2.9 Concluding Remarks

The function and course of the esophagus set requirements for its construction and attachments. Several sphincters, namely the UES, the LES and the right crus of the diaphragm, keep both ends of the esophagus closed, except during swallowing. The esophagus is embedded in loose connective tissue which allows much freedom of movement. It is attached to the environment by fibro-elastic structures, such as the phrenico-esophageal ligament and by the recently discovered aorto-esophageal ligament. Among the most important topographical relationships are the aortopulmonary window, the azygos vein, the thoracic duct and the recurrent laryngeal nerves. The arterial blood supply is diffuse and consists of shared and proper arteries. Likewise, several vessels are involved in the venous drainage and there is a diffuse lymphatic drainage. The nerve supply is by the vagus nerves which, after contributing to the pulmonary plexuses, form an esophageal plexus from where two vagal trunks reach the abdomen.

References

1. Grodinsky M, Holyoke EA. The fascia and fascial spaces of the head, neck and adjacent regions. Am J Anat. 1938;63:367–408.
2. Guidera AK, Dawes PJ, Fong A, Stringer MD. Head and neck fascia and compartments: no space for spaces. Head Neck. 2014;36:1058–68.
3. Miller L, Vegesna A, Ruggieri M, Braverman A. Normal and abnormal physiology, pharmacology, and anatomy of the gastroesophageal junction high-pressure zone. Ann N Y Acad Sci. 2016; 1380(1):48–57.
4. Cuesta MA, Weijs TJ, Bleys RL, van Hillegersberg R, van Berge Henegouwen MI, Gisbertz SS, Ruurda JP, Straatman J, Osugi H, van der Peet DL. A new concept of the anatomy of the thoracic oesophagus: the meso-oesophagus. Observational study during thoracoscopic esophagectomy. Surg Endosc. 2015; 29:2576–82.
5. Weijs TJ, Goense L, van Rossum PS, Meijer GJ, van Lier AL, Wessels FJ, Braat MN, Lips IM, Ruurda JP, Cuesta MA, van Hillegersberg R, Bleys RL. The peri-esophageal connective tissue layers and related compartments: visualization by histology and magnetic resonance imaging. J Anat. 2017;230(2):262–71.
6. Apaydin N, Uz A, Evirgen O, Loukas M, Tubbs RS, Elhan A. The phrenico-esophageal ligament: an anatomical study. Surg Radiol Anat. 2008;30:29–36.
7. Cauldwell EW, Siekert RG, Lininger RE, Anson BJ. The bronchial arteries; an anatomic study of 150 human cadavers. Surg Gynecol Obstet. 1948;86:395–412.
8. Yalcin B, Tunali S, Ozan H. Extralaryngeal division of the recurrent laryngeal nerve: a new description for the inferior laryngeal nerve. Surg Radiol Anat. 2008;30:215–20.
9. Liebermann-Meffert DM, Walbrun B, Hiebert CA, Siewert JR. Recurrent and superior laryngeal nerves: a new look with implications for the esophageal surgeon. Ann Thorac Surg. 1999;67:217–23.
10. Weijs TJ, Ruurda JP, Luyer MD, Nieuwenhuijzen GA, van Hillegersberg R, Bleys RL. Topography and extent of pulmonary vagus nerve supply with respect to transthoracic oesophagectomy. J Anat. 2015;227:431–9.
11. Mazzone SB, Canning BJ. Autonomic neural control of the airways. Handb Clin Neurol. 2013;117:215–28.
12. Ziyade S, Pinarbasili NB, Ziyade N, Akdemir OC, Sahin F, Soysal Ö, Toker A. Determination of standard number, size and weight of mediastinal lymph nodes in postmortem examinations: reflection on lung cancer surgery. J Cardiothorac Surg. 2013;8:94.
13. Cuesta MA, van der Wielen N, Weijs TJ, Bleys RL, Gisbertz SS, van Duijvendijk P, van Hillegersberg R, Ruurda JP, van Berge Henegouwen MI, Straatman J, Osugi H, van der Peet DL. Surgical anatomy of the supracarinal esophagus based on a minimally invasive approach: vascular and nervous anatomy and technical steps to resection and lymphadenectomy. Surg Endosc. 2017;31:1863–70.
14. Rusch VW, Asamura H, Watanabe H, Giroux DJ, Rami-Porta R, Goldstraw P, Members of IASLC Staging Committee. The IASLC lung cancer staging project: a proposal for a new international lymph node map in the forthcoming seventh edition of the TNM classification for lung cancer. J Thorac Oncol. 2009;4:568–77.
15. Kajitani T. The general rules for the gastric cancer study in surgery and pathology. Part I Clinical classification. Jpn J Surg. 1981;11:127–39.
16. Boone J, Hobbelink MG, Schipper ME, Vleggaar FP, Borel Rinkes IH, de Haas RJ, Ruurda JP, van Hillegersberg R. Sentinel node biopsy during thoracolaparoscopic esophagectomy for advanced esophageal cancer. World J Surg Oncol. 2016;14:117.

Endoscopic Treatment of Early Esophageal Cancer

3

Roos E. Pouw and Bas L.A.M. Weusten

3.1 Introduction

Esophageal cancer limited to the mucosa and low-risk submucosal adenocarcinoma, are associated with a low risk of lymph node and distant metastasis. For these early esophageal cancers, endoscopic treatment has evolved as a minimally invasive and organ preserving alternative to surgery. One of the largest series of 963 patients treated endoscopically for early esophageal adenocarcinoma demonstrated a long-term complete remission rate of 94%, with only two Barrett's cancer related deaths [1]. Endoscopic resection is also well-established for patients with early squamous cell neoplasia of the esophagus, with cause-specific 5-year survival rates exceeding 85% [2]. Endoscopic resection (ER) is the cornerstone of endoscopic therapy. ER not only has a therapeutic goal, by removing neoplastic lesions, it also has important diagnostic value since it provides a substantial tissue specimen enabling accurate histological staging. Whereas surgical resection allows for removal of the affected organ and lymphadenectomy, ER is limited to local removal of neoplasia. Selection of patients suited for curative endoscopic therapy is therefore of the utmost importance and is aimed at identifying patients with a minimal risk of lymph node metastases. For this, accurate histological assessment of infiltration depth, grade of differentiation, presence of lymphovascular invasion and radicality of the resection at the deep resection margins in an ER-specimen are crucial.

ER was pioneered in Japan, where it is still mainly applied in the treatment of early gastric cancer and early squamous neoplasia of the esophagus [3]. During the last decades, endoscopic treatment has also been accepted as the treatment of choice in most Western countries, where it is mainly used in the management of patients with early neoplasia arising against a background of Barrett's esophagus [1, 4].

In patients with Barrett's neoplasia treated by ER, the residual Barrett's mucosa is still at risk for metachronous lesions, which are found in up to 30% of patients during 5-year follow-up [4]. Therefore, additional treatment of residual Barrett's mucosa after focal ER of neoplasia is advisable. For this, different approaches are

Electronic Supplementary Material The online version of this chapter (doi:10.1007/978-3-319-54301-7_3) contains supplementary material, which is available to authorized users. On http://springerlink.com enter the DOI number given above.

R.E. Pouw, M.D., Ph.D. (✉)
Department of Gastroenterology and Hepatology, Academic Medical Center, Amsterdam, The Netherlands
e-mail: r.e.pouw@amc.uva.nl

B.L.A.M. Weusten, M.D., Ph.D.
Department of Gastroenterology and Hepatology, St. Antonius Hospital, Koekoekslaan 1, 3435CM Nieuwegein, The Netherlands
e-mail: b.weusten@antoniusziekenhuis.nl

M.A. Cuesta (ed.), *Minimally Invasive Surgery for Upper Abdominal Cancer*,
DOI 10.1007/978-3-319-54301-7_3

available, of which thermal ablation using radiofrequency ablation (RFA) is currently most widely used [5, 6].

In this book chapter we will give an overview of the indications and principles of endoscopic treatment, different techniques that are available for endoscopic resection, management of the patient after focal removal of early cancer, and future perspectives on the place of endoscopic treatment for early esophageal cancer (Video 3.1).

3.2 Indications for Endoscopic Treatment

3.2.1 Adenocarcinoma Arising in Barrett's Esophagus

Based on multiple high quality, international studies on ER for high-grade dysplasia (HGD) and mucosal adenocarcinoma (T1a), there is solid evidence that ER for mucosal adenocarcinoma is safe and associated with a minimal risk of lymph node metastasis [1, 4]. Therefore, ER has become first choice treatment for this indication in most countries [7].

Traditionally, the risk of lymph node metastasis in submucosal adenocarcinoma (T1b) was considered too high to offer these patients endoscopic follow-up after radical ER. However, this risk of lymph node metastases was mainly based on historical surgical series, from a period when exact depth of infiltration was of little clinical relevance for patient management [8]. Surgical specimens are generally cut in 5 mm slices; consequently, the area with the deepest tumour infiltration may have been missed, resulting in underestimation of the infiltration depth correlated with lymph node metastases if present. Endoscopic resection specimens are smaller and cut in 2 mm slices, resulting in more accurate assessment of tumour infiltration depth. Based on more recent studies in endoscopically treated patients, the risk of lymph node metastasis associated with submucosal cancer appears to be lower than generally assumed [9–13]. For low-risk submucosal adenocarcinoma, defined as radically resected submucosal adenocarcinoma limited to the upper 500 μm of the submucosa (T1sm1), well to moderately differentiated, without lymphovascular invasion, the risk of lymph node metastasis appears to be <2% [9, 10]. This is lower than the 0–4% mortality risk of esophagectomy in expert centres and low-risk submucosal cancer is therefore considered a relative indication for endoscopic treatment [9, 10].

For patients with T1sm1 adenocarcinoma but other high risk histological features (poor differentiation, lymphovascular invasion), or deeper submucosal adenocarcinoma (>500 μm, T1sm2-sm3), the exact risk of lymph node metastasis is unknown, but still considered too high to justify endoscopic therapy. However, a number of recent studies assessing infiltration depth in ER-specimens, suggest a risk of lymph node metastasis of 16–30% in patients with T1sm2-sm3 adenocarcinoma [11–13]. The gold standard in patients with T1sm2-sm3 adenocarcinoma is still surgical treatment, although based on these numbers >70% of these patients will undergo unnecessary esophagectomy. In the future better risk stratification of these patients taking other risk factors for metastatic disease such as differentiation and lymphovascular invasion into account may possibly result in a more tailored approach, only referring high-risk patients for surgery.

In Barrett's esophagus the Paris classification is used to describe the morphological appearance of a lesion, which is related to infiltration depth of a lesion. Protruded lesions (Paris type 0-Is or 0-Ip) are defined as being higher than a closed biopsy forceps (2.5 mm), slightly elevated lesions (Paris type 0-IIa) are less high than a closed biopsy forceps and slightly depressed lesions (Paris type 0-IIc) are less deep than one cup of an open biopsy forceps [14]. In a study evaluating the relation between macroscopic appearance and infiltration depth, protruded lesions and slightly depressed lesions significantly more often infiltrated the submucosa (25–26%), than slightly elevated lesions (9%), or completely flat (Paris type 0-IIb) lesions (0%). None of the Paris type 0-I or type 0-II lesions are associated with a very high risk of submucosal invasion and diagnostic ER therefore appears indicated and safe for these lesions [15]. No good data are available on rate of submucosal invasion in type 0-III lesions, probably since the ulceration present in these lesions prohibits safe and radical ER of these lesions.

3.2.2 Early Squamous Cell Cancer of the Esophagus

Squamous cell cancer invades deeper and spreads to lymph nodes at an earlier stage when compared to esophageal adenocarcinoma, perhaps due to infiltration via the submucosal glandular structures, which are lined with squamous epithelium [16]. The indication for endoscopic treatment in patients with early squamous cell neoplasia is therefore more limited compared to early adenocarcinoma. Patients with high-grade intraepithelial neoplasia (HGIN) have no risk of lymph node metastasis and in case of cancer limited to the lamina propria (T1m1/m2) the risk of lymph node metastasis is minimal (0–5%) [16, 17]. These patients are candidates for curative endoscopic treatment. The risk of lymph node metastasis for squamous cell cancer invading the muscularis mucosae (T1m3) is about 0–12%, and in case of invasion into the superficial submucosa (T1sm1, <200 μm) the risk is about 20% [17]. For patients with T1m3/sm1 disease, endoscopic treatment may be considered if the patient suffers from significant comorbidity. Deeper submucosal invasion (T1sm2/3) is associated with >50% risk of lymph node metastasis and therefore warrants more aggressive therapy such as surgery or chemoradiation [17].

Just as in early esophageal adenocarcinoma, the macroscopic appearance of squamous cell neoplasia is described using the Paris classification, although lesion types are defined using different cut-off levels for elevation and depression. Macroscopic appearance can be used in deciding if a lesion is suited for ER. Excavated lesions (Paris type 0-III, deeper than half the cup of an open biopsy forceps) and more protruding lesions (Paris type 0-I, higher than the cup of an open biopsy forceps) are associated with deep submucosal invasion in >80% and should not be targeted for endoscopic resection. True flat type lesions (Paris type 0-IIb) are limited to the lamina propria in about 69% of cases, slightly depressed lesions (Paris type 0-IIc) in about 39% of cases and slightly elevated lesions (Paris type 0-IIa) are limited to the lamina propria in only 20% of cases [14]. Diagnostic endoscopic resection can therefore be considered for flat type squamous cell neoplasia.

3.3 Endoscopic Treatment Algorithm

After endoscopic detection of an early neoplastic lesion in the esophagus, endoscopic assessment of the morphological appearance of a lesion should guide the decision if ER is feasible, as described above. Biopsies can be obtained to confirm the diagnosis of cancer, but biopsies are not required, since the finding of a macroscopic abnormality warrants diagnostic ER to obtain a definite histological diagnosis. Additional imaging and staging with endoscopic ultrasound (EUS), CAT or PET scan prior to ER is generally not very useful during work-up for early esophageal neoplasia. EUS is not reliable in the differentiation between T1a and T1b cancers, and even discriminating T1 from T2 lesions may be challenging. And given the very low risk of lymph node and distant metastasis associated with early esophageal neoplasia, the yield of finding these with CAT or PET scanning is very low. The most important step during work-up of early esophageal neoplasia is therefore diagnostic ER, which provides a large tissue specimen, enabling accurate histological assessment of risk factors associated with lymph node metastasis. If there are no risk factors, the patient can be managed further endoscopically. If a patient is at high risk for lymph node metastasis based on the outcome of the diagnostic ER, additional staging can still be performed to decide on optimal further treatment. Optimal management for high-risk patients should be discussed during a multidisciplinary team meeting, including a gastroenterologist, surgeon and an oncologist.

After focal ER of early neoplasia arising in Barrett's esophagus, the residual Barrett's mucosa is at risk for recurrence [4]. Therefore additional treatment of the residual Barrett's mucosa is advisable. This can be done by complete ER of the residual Barrett's segment during subsequent ER sessions. This approach has been proven effective in patients with Barrett's esophagus limited to 5 cm in length, however, complete radical ER is associated with a high risk of esophageal stenosis of up to 80% [18]. Thermal ablation of the Barrett's mucosa is an alternative method to eradicate all mucosa at risk. Radiofrequency ablation (RFA) is the most extensively studied technique for this purpose [5, 6, 18].

Despite promising results of radiofrequency ablation (RFA) for true flat early squamous cell neoplasia (MGIN or HGIN) [19], no long-term follow-up data on this approach are available so far, and RFA is therefore not routinely used for this indication. Endoscopic management after focal removal of squamous cell neoplasia mainly consists of endoscopic follow-up at regular intervals to detect recurrences at an early stage.

3.4 Principles of Endoscopic Resection

3.4.1 Delineation and Marking of the Target Lesion

To ensure radical ER of a suspicious lesion with a disease free margin, it is important to delineate the extent of a lesion prior to ER. Advanced imaging techniques, such as virtual chromoendoscopy (e.g. narrow-band imaging, blue-laser imaging), zoom-endoscopy and chromoendoscopy (e.g. Lugol staining in case of early squamous neoplasia), may be helpful to assess the extent of a lesion. Since the endoscopic view during ER is often impaired by the use of distal attachment caps, submucosal lifting and bleeding, the target lesion is delineated by placing coagulation markings around its lateral margins. Especially for lesions that require piecemeal resection, demarcation with markings may be useful to achieve complete resection with a tumour free margin.

3.4.2 En-Bloc Resection Vs. Piecemeal Endoscopic Resection

Most conventional cap-based ER techniques allow for en-bloc resection of lesions with a maximum diameter of 2 cm. Larger lesions require resection in multiple pieces during a so-called "piecemeal" procedure. Piecemeal resections are technically more demanding, time-consuming and have a higher risk of complications. Piecemeal resection is also associated with a higher risk of local recurrence of neoplasia. However, this may be less relevant in patients with early neoplasia arising in Barrett's esophagus, since the majority of these patients will undergo additional thermal ablation of their Barrett's esophagus, minimizing risk of local recurrence [5, 6]. Piecemeal resections result in multiple resection specimens that cannot be easily pieced together and therefore histological evaluation of the radicality of a resection at the lateral resection margins is usually not reliable. Marking the lesion prior to ER and careful endoscopic assessment of the radicality of the resection after ER is therefore pivotal.

3.4.3 Endoscopic Resection Techniques

3.4.3.1 Lift-Suck-Cut Technique

Inoue et al. first described a cap-based ER technique, using a transparent distal attachment cap [3]. For this technique a transparent ER-cap with a distal rim is placed on the tip of an endoscope. The target lesion is lifted from the deeper esophageal wall layers by submucosal injection of saline. A crescent shaped snare is prelooped in the distal rim of the cap. After suctioning the lifted mucosa into the cap, the snare is closed and the captured mucosa can then be resected using electrocautery. ER-cap resections can be performed using a standard gastroscope and one assistant is needed to aid with the submucosal lifting and handling of the snare. A drawback of the ER-cap technique is that it is a technically demanding and time consuming procedure, especially when used for piecemeal resections. Prelooping the snare in the distal rim of the cap can be challenging, and for piecemeal resections submucosal lifting needs to be repeated for every resection.

3.4.3.2 Ligate-and-Cut Technique

The currently most widely used cap-based ER technique in the esophagus is the ligate-and-cut technique (Fig. 3.1). This technique is an easier alternative to the lift-suck-cut technique. For the ligate-and-cut technique a distal attachment cap, holding one or more rubber bands, is attached to the tip of the endoscope. The target lesion is sucked into the cap and by releasing a rubber band the mucosa is captured. This pseudo-polyp can then be resected with a snare. The ligate-and-cut technique can be performed using the multi-band mucosectomy device (Duette®, Wilson Cook, Limerick, Ireland), which has a transparent cap that holds six rubber bands and allows for passage of a snare through the accessory channel of the cranking device alongside the releasing wires, allowing resection after ligation without having to remove the endoscope [20]. The more recently developed Captivator™ Endoscopic Mucosal Resection Device (Boston Scientific Endoscopy, Marlborough, MA, USA) is a comparable device allowing ligate-and-cut ER. An advantage of the ligate-and-cut technique over the

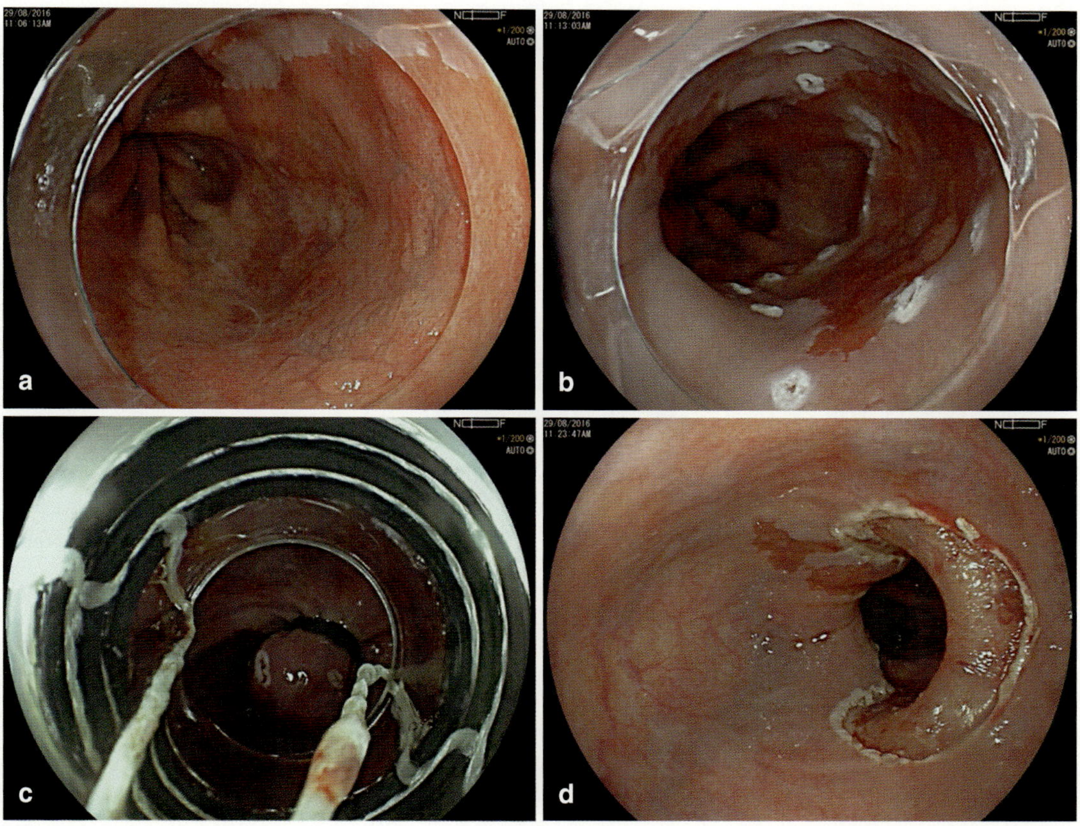

Fig. 3.1 Endoscopic resection of an early cancer in a Barrett's segment using the multiband mucosectomy technique. (**a**) Endoscopic view on a Paris type 0-Ia-IIb lesion. (**b**) The lateral margins of the lesion are marked using electrocoagulation markings. (**c**) View through the cap of the Duette multiband mucosectomy device holding the rubber bands. In the esophagus a pseudopolyp is created by suctioning the mucosa into the cap and releasing a rubber band. This pseudopolyp can subsequently be resected using an electrocautery snare. (**d**) View on the resected area, which shows that all markings have been removed, resulting in an endoscopically radical resection

lift-suck-cut technique is that no submucosal lifting is required, since the rubber bands are not strong enough to hold in the deeper esophageal wall layers. This makes the ligate-and-cut technique easier and quicker to apply, especially when used for piecemeal procedures [20]. Despite the lack of submucosal lifting, the ligate-and-suck technique does not appear to be associated with a higher risk of complications as has been demonstrated in a randomized study comparing both techniques [20], and in a prospective registration of 1060 resections performed with the multiband mucosectomy device [21].

3.4.3.3 Endoscopic Submucosal Dissection

Endoscopic submucosal dissection (ESD) is a technique that overcomes the problem of piecemeal ER for larger neoplastic lesions, and allows for a better-targeted resection of a lesion (Fig. 3.2). The concept of ESD is to incise the mucosa around a lesion, regardless how large, and then remove the lesion by visual submucosal dissection using an electrosurgical knife instead of blind snaring using a snare [22].

After careful delineation of a lesion and placement of coagulation markers around the margins of the lesion, the margins of the lesion are lifted

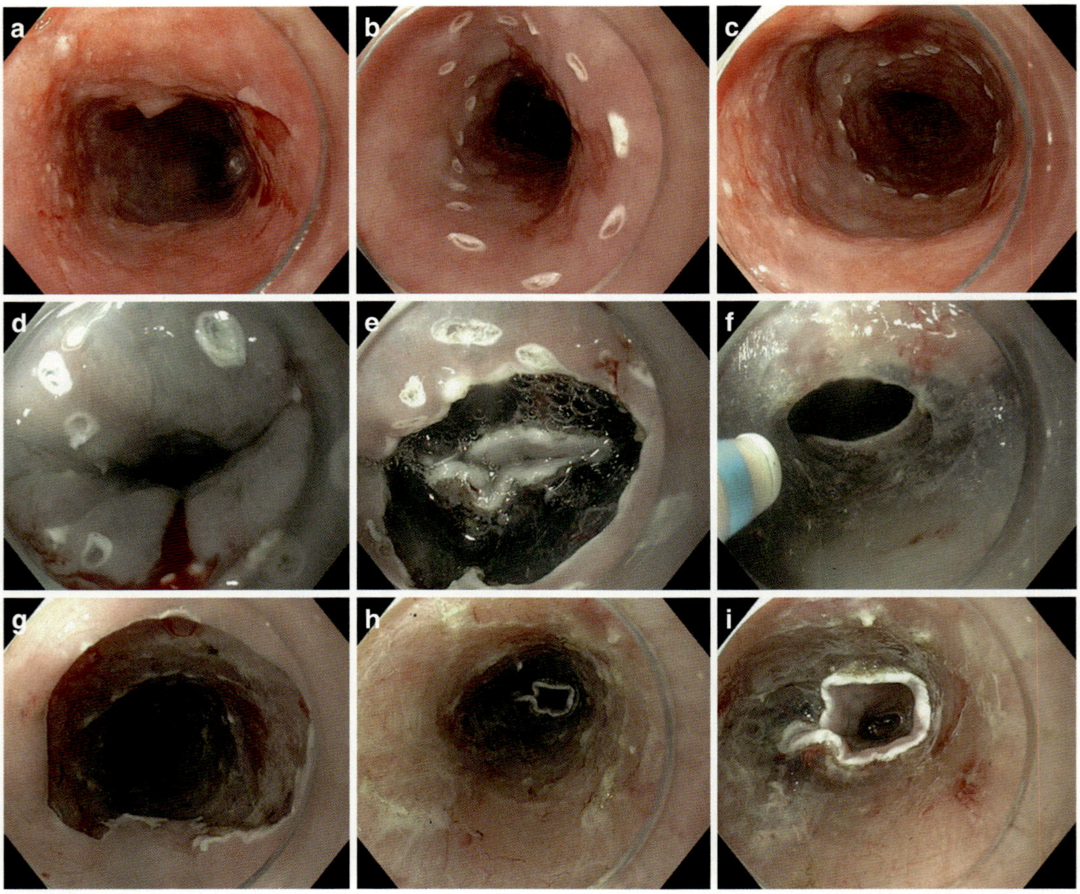

Fig. 3.2 Endoscopic submucosal dissection (ESD) of an early squamous cell cancer. (**a**) Widespread, circumferential early squamous cell cancer. (**b**) Delineation of the most proximal extent of the lesion using electrocoagulation markings. (**c**) Delineation of the most distal extent of the lesion. (**d**) Submucosal lifting of the mucosa. (**e**) Circumferential incision of the proximal delineation margin. (**f**) Submucosal dissection using a dual-knife. (**g–i**) Result after extensive circumferential ESD

by submucosal injection of fluid. Using an electrosurgical knife, the incision line can then be incised circumferentially around the lesion, while constantly repeating submucosal lifting to ensure a safe submucosal fluid cushion. When the incision around the lesion has been completed, the submucosa underneath the lesion can be dissected under constant visualisation, until the target lesion is removed in one piece. A range of different electrosurgical knifes are available for ESD.

Although ESD allows for en-bloc resection of neoplasia, it is technically demanding, time consuming and has a higher risk of complications. Therefore, ESD should only be applied in selected cases by experienced endoscopists with adequate training.

3.4.4 Histological Evaluation of ER Specimens

Endoscopic resection specimens are pinned down on cork or paraffin before fixating them in formalin. After fixation, specimens are routinely cut in 2 mm slices and embedded in paraffin. The tissue blocks are then sectioned, put on glass slides and stained with haematoxylin and eosin. In case of cancer, the pathologist will assess the following criteria:

1. Tissue type (squamous, columnar).
2. Presence of dysplasia or cancer, and in case of dysplasia the degree of dysplasia according to the Vienna classification [23].
3. In case of invasive cancer, infiltration depth should be described as follows: infiltration into the lamina propria (T1m2); infiltration into the muscularis mucosae (T1m3); infiltration into the submucosa measured in microns. In surgical resection specimens, the submucosa is pragmatically divided into three equal parts (T1sm1 to T1sm3). However, ER specimens do not contain the whole thickness of the original submucosal layer. Therefore, the following cut-off levels are defined to describe depth of submucosal invasion in ER specimens: adenocarcinoma limited to the upper 500 μm of the submucosa is considered T1sm1, cancer infiltrating deeper than 500 μm is referred to as T1sm2/3; in squamous cancer the cut-off between T1sm1 and T1sm2/3 infiltration is 200 μm [14].
4. Grade of differentiation (well, moderate, poor, undifferentiated).
5. Presence of lymphovascular invasion.
6. Radicality at the deep (vertical) resection margin.
7. In case of en-bloc resection: worst histology at the lateral resection margins.

3.5 Endoscopic Ablation Techniques

3.5.1 Radiofrequency Ablation

Radiofrequency ablation (RFA) is the most widely studied thermal ablation method for Barrett's esophagus (Fig. 3.3). RFA has demonstrated to result in complete eradication of intestinal metaplasia (89–92%) and neoplasia (95–96%), with or without prior ER of focal neoplastic lesions, with sustained complete remission of neoplasia and intestinal metaplasia in 90% of patients at 5 years [4, 5].

RFA is performed using a catheter with a bipolar electrode. Two main types of devices exist for RFA: a balloon-based ablation system (Barrx360, Medtronic, Minneapolis, MN, USA), which is inserted over a guide-wire and followed by the endoscope in a side-to-side manner. This system allows for circumferential ablation of Barrett's mucosa, but requires a preliminary step of measurement of the esophageal inner diameter using a sizing balloon. A newly designed self-sizing RFA catheter (Barrx 360 Express, Medtronic, Minneapolis, MN, USA) has been developed in order to perform circumferential ablation without the need of the sizing step. For circumferential ablation using the balloon-based systems, the electrode is positioned 1 cm above the proximal extent of the Barrett's mucosa. After inflation of the balloon, radiofrequency ablation is activated via a foot-pedal. One ablation results in a circumferentially

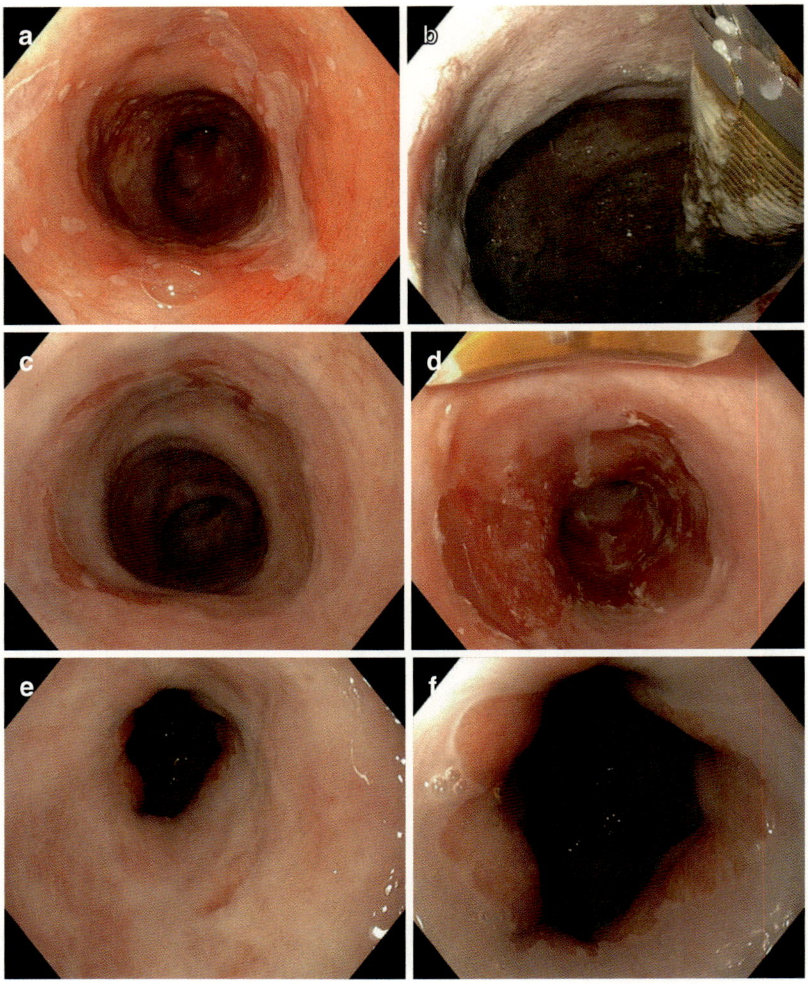

Fig. 3.3 Radiofrequency ablation (RFA) of a long segment Barrett's esophagus with high-grade dysplasia. (**a**) Long segment Barrett's esophagus. (**b**) Circumferential RFA with the balloon-based catheter results in thermal ablation of the Barrett's tissue. (**c**) After 3 months the esophagus has healed with neosquamous epithelium, and only a few small residual islands of Barrett mucosa remain. (**d**) Focal RFA of residual Barrett's mucosa using the cap-based electrode fitted on the tip of the endoscope. (**e**, **f**) Three months after focal RFA, the esophagus is completely lined with normal appearing neosquamous mucosa

treated area of 3–4 cm. By repositioning the ablation catheter in the esophagus, multiple ablations can be performed to treat the whole length of residual Barrett's mucosa.

The second type of ablation system is a focal ablation catheter, attached to the tip of the endoscope, and designed to ablate tongues or islands of BE. Various sizes of focal RFA devices exist, but the Barrx90, allowing for a 90° ablation is the most commonly used. Depending on the length of the Barrett's segment, patients are generally treated once with a circumferential RFA device followed by a median of two focal ablation sessions [4, 5].

3.5.2 Argon Plasma Coagulation

Argon plasma coagulation (APC) uses ionization of a jet of argon gas that is sprayed through a probe that is passed into the esophagus via the endoscope. The advantages of argon plasma coagulation (APC) are its easy availability and low costs. Disadvantages are that it is very operator-dependent, time-consuming and labour intensive approach, especially when used for treatment of a large surface of Barrett's mucosa. Therefore, APC is mainly used to ablate small islands or tongues of Barrett's mucosa. Recently, a modified APC probe called Hybrid APC (Erbe

Elektromedizin, Tübingen, Germany) was introduced. This APC probe has a water-jet channel integrated into the probe, which allows for injection of saline into the submucosal space. By lifting the submucosa prior to thermal ablation, higher energy settings can be used, possibly increasing efficacy, while improving safety [24].

3.5.3 Photodynamic Therapy

Photodynamic therapy (PDT) is an endoscopic ablation technique that was applied to ablate Barrett's mucosa with dysplasia in the past. PDT uses intra-venous administration of a photosensitizing drug that accumulates in the target tissue. Subsequent application of light (usually laser light) of an appropriate wavelength and the presence of oxygen results in a photodynamic reaction, which generates oxygen radicals causing delayed cell death, which usually becomes apparent after 12–24 h. However, due to disappointing efficacy results, high stricture rate and side-effects such as photosensitivity, PDT has become abundant, since better ablative alternatives are available nowadays.

3.5.4 Cryoablation

Cryoablation using either application of compressed CO_2 gas via a cryospray catheter, or application via a balloon-based system, uses application of liquid nitrous oxide to freeze the esophageal mucosa. Deep freezing and slow thawing of the target area causes disruption of cells, vascular ischemia, and thrombosis, resulting in necrosis of the superficial esophageal layers. In contrast to heat-based ablation, cryoablation leaves the tissue architecture intact, and may result in less stricture formation. The balloon-based cryoablation device (C2 Therapeutics, Redwood City, California, USA) has recently proved feasible and safe in a prospective multicentre study in patients with Barrett's esophagus [25].

Currently available data on hybrid-APC ablation and balloon-based cryoablation are still preliminary. Larger, multicentre studies will be required to define the place of these ablation techniques in the future management of patients with esophageal neoplasia.

3.6 Quality of Life

Endoscopic therapy is less invasive than surgery, but little is known about how this organ preserving approach influences quality of life. One study prospectively evaluated the effect of endoscopic treatment for early Barrett's neoplasia on quality of life and fear of cancer (recurrence) and compared this with the effect of Barrett's surveillance and surgery for early Barrett's neoplasia and surgery for advanced esophageal adenocarcinoma [26]. The endoscopic treatment group reported significantly better physical and mental quality of life, and less esophageal cancer related symptoms compared to both surgical groups, as might be expected. However, the endoscopic treatment group reported significant more worry for cancer recurrence compared to the early surgical group. In fact, endoscopically treated patients worried about cancer and recurrence as much as patients treated surgically for advanced esophageal cancer. Further studies in this field are necessary to improve quality of life and counselling of patients undergoing endoscopic treatment.

3.7 Future Prospects of Endoscopic Therapy for Early Esophageal Cancer

The past decades the indication for endoscopic treatment has extended from high-grade dysplasia to mucosal cancer and even low-risk submucosal cancer. Small retrospective studies have shown that the risk of lymph node metastasis in deeper submucosal cancer may be <30%, implying that the majority of these patients will undergo unnecessary additional esophagectomy. Diligent prospective studies on endoscopic treatment in patients with submucosal cancer will hopefully result in better understanding of the true risk of lymph node metastasis associated with submucosal cancer.

Risk stratification based on submucosal infiltration depth and other tumour characteristics may be of future use to select patients who would benefit from adjuvant surgery, and who can safely be kept under endoscopic surveillance.

Another development that may improve management of patients with submucosal cancer is use of a sentinel node procedure. Interesting studies in this field are currently being performed.

ESD will be performed more frequently, when the indication for endoscopic treatment is extended to more high-risk early esophageal cancers, where en-bloc resection should be aimed at. ESD is still technically demanding and should be performed by well-trained and experienced endoscopists. In the future, novel developments may facilitate ESD procedures.

Endoscopic management should be centralized in expert centres. Although ER and ablation benefit from technological developments, making the techniques easier to apply, these are just part of the overall endoscopic management of patients. The most important step is selecting the right patients for endoscopic management, starting with experience in detecting and delineating early esophageal neoplasia. After ER, also adequate histological evaluation of ER specimens is required to allow for adequate selection of low-risk patients. Furthermore, patient management should be discussed in a multidisciplinary team meeting, including gastroenterologists, surgeons and oncologists. Therefore, endoscopic management should be centralized in centres with multidisciplinary expertise in this field.

References

1. Pech O, May A, Manner H, et al. Long-term efficacy and safety of endoscopic resection for patients with mucosal adenocarcinoma of the esophagus. Gastroenterology. 2014;146:652–60.
2. Ono S, Fujishiro M, Niimi K, et al. Long-term outcomes of endoscopic submucosal dissection for superficial esophageal squamous cell neoplasms. Gastrointest Endosc. 2009;70:860–6.
3. Inoue H, Endo M, Takeshita K, et al. A new simplified technique of endoscopic esophageal mucosal resection using a cap-fitted panendoscope (EMRC). Surg Endosc. 1992;6:264–5.
4. Peters FP, Kara MA, Rosmolen WD, et al. Endoscopic treatment of high-grade dysplasia and early stage cancer in Barrett's esophagus. Gastrointest Endosc. 2005;61:506–14.
5. Shaheen NJ, Sharma P, Overholt BF, et al. Radiofrequency ablation in Barrett's esophagus with dysplasia. N Engl J Med. 2009;360:2277–88.
6. Phoa KN, Pouw RE, van Vilsteren FG, et al. Remission of Barrett's esophagus with early neoplasia 5 years after radiofrequency ablation with endoscopic resection: a Netherlands cohort study. Gastroenterology. 2013;145:96–104.
7. Fitzgerald RC, di Pietro M, Ragunath K, et al. British Society of Gastroenterology guidelines on the diagnosis and management of Barrett's oesophagus. Gut. 2014;63:7–42.
8. Westerterp M, Koppert LB, Buskens CJ, et al. Outcome of surgical treatment for early adenocarcinoma of the esophagus or gastro-esophageal junction. Virchows Arch. 2005;446:497–504.
9. Alvarez Herrero L, Pouw RE, van Vilsteren FG, et al. Risk of lymph node metastasis associated with deeper invasion by early adenocarcinoma of the esophagus and cardia: study based on endoscopic resection specimens. Endoscopy. 2010;42:1030–6.
10. Manner H, Pech O, Heldmann Y, et al. The frequency of lymph node metastasis in early-stage adenocarcinoma of the esophagus with incipient submucosal invasion (pT1b sm1) depending on histological risk patterns. Surg Endosc. 2015;29:1888–96.
11. Boys JA, Worrell SG, Chandrasoma P, et al. Can the risk of lymph node metastases be gauged in endoscopically resected submucosal esophageal adenocarcinomas? A multi-center study. J Gastrointest Surg. 2016;20:6–12.
12. Schölvinck DW, Künzli HT, Meijer SL, et al. Management of patients with T1b esophageal adenocarcinoma: a retrospective cohort study on patient management and risk of metastatic disease. Surg Endosc. 2016;30:4102–13.
13. Manner H, Wetzka J, May A, et al. Early-stage adenocarcinoma of the esophagus with mid to deep submucosal invasion (pT1b sm2–3): the frequency of lymph-node metastasis depends on macroscopic and histological risk patterns. Dis Esophagus. 2016 [Epub ahead of print].
14. The Paris endoscopic classification of superficial neoplastic lesions: esophagus, stomach, and colon: November 30 to December 1, 2002. Gastrointest Endosc. 2003;58:S3–43.
15. Peters FP, Brakenhoff KP, Curvers WL, et al. Histologic evaluation of resection specimens obtained at 293 endoscopic resections in Barrett's esophagus. Gastrointest Endosc. 2008;67:604–9.
16. Araki K, Ohno S, Egashira A, et al. Pathologic features of superficial esophageal squamous cell carcinoma with lymph node and distal metastasis. Cancer. 2002;94:570–5.
17. Yoshii T, Ohkawa S, Tamai S, Kameda Y. Clinical outcome of endoscopic mucosal resection for

esophageal squamous cell cancer invading muscularis mucosa and submucosal layer. Dis Esophagus. 2013;26:496–502.
18. Van Vilsteren FG, Pouw RE, Seewald S, et al. Stepwise radical endoscopic resection versus radiofrequency ablation for Barrett's oesophagus with high-grade dysplasia or early cancer: a multicentre randomised trial. Gut. 2011;60:765–73.
19. He S, Bergman J, Zhang Y, et al. Endoscopic radiofrequency ablation for early esophageal squamous cell neoplasia: report of safety and effectiveness from a large prospective trial. Endoscopy. 2015;47:398–408.
20. Pouw RE, van Vilsteren FG, Peters FP, et al. Randomized trial on endoscopic resection-cap versus multiband mucosectomy for piecemeal endoscopic resection of early Barrett's neoplasia. Gastrointest Endosc. 2011;74:35–43.
21. Alvarez Herrero L, Pouw RE, van Vilsteren FG, et al. Safety and efficacy of multiband mucosectomy in 1060 resections in Barrett's esophagus. Endoscopy. 2011;43:177–83.
22. Terheggen G, Horn EM, Vieth M, et al. A randomised trial of endoscopic submucosal dissection versus endoscopic mucosal resection for early Barrett's neoplasia. Gut. 2016 [Epub ahead of print].
23. Schlemper RJ, Riddell RH, Kato Y, et al. The Vienna classification of gastrointestinal epithelial neoplasia. Gut. 2000;47:251–5.
24. Manner H, May A, Kouti I, et al. Efficacy and safety of hybrid-APC for the ablation of Barrett's esophagus. Surg Endosc. 2016;30:1364–70.
25. Schölvinck DW, Künzli HT, Kestens C, et al. Treatment of Barrett's esophagus with a novel focal cryoablation device: a safety and feasibility study. Endoscopy. 2015;47:1106–12.
26. Rosmolen WD, Nieuwkerk PT, Pouw RE, et al. Quality of life and fear of cancer recurrence after endoscopic treatment for early Barrett's neoplasia: a prospective study. Dis Esophagus. 2016 [Epub ahead of print].

Neoadjuvant Treatment of Esophageal and Gastro-Esophageal Cancer

4

Jan Willem van den Berg, Sjoerd M. Lagarde, Bas P.L. Wijnhoven, Ate van der Gaast, and J. Jan B. van Lanschot

4.1 Introduction

The incidence of adenocarcinoma of the esophagus and gastroesophageal (GE) junction has increased rapidly in Western countries, while numbers of squamous cell carcinoma (SCC) have gradually declined. For locally advanced esophageal cancer, surgery remains the mainstay of treatment. However, esophagectomy is historically associated with relatively high rates of irradical resection margins and high numbers of patients presenting with recurrent disease within 2 years after surgery. Therefore, the last decades several multimodality treatment regimens have been developed. Numerous studies evaluated the value of neoadjuvant as well as adjuvant strategies, especially chemotherapy and chemoradiation. In most countries advanced esophageal cancers are treated nowadays by neoadjuvant multimodality treatment regimens. It is thought that neoadjuvant chemotherapy and neoadjuvant chemoradiation eliminate micrometastases and induce locoregional tumor regression which leads to a higher rate of radical esophagectomies due to a reduction in the number of R1 and R2 resections (downstaging). However, its value has been debated for several decades. Up to a few years ago, the majority of the studies did not show any statistically significant benefit for neoadjuvant therapy, but these studies were frequently criticized because of inadequate trial design, limited statistical power (small sample size), and poor outcomes in the surgery alone group. However, in recent years, many different neoadjuvant regimens have been developed and tested. Historically, in the United Kingdom neoadjuvant chemotherapy was advocated while in Continental Europa and the USA neoadjuvant CRT was the preferred treatment. Ultimately the question which modality is superior will hopefully be answered by the Neo-AEGIS study, which compares perioperative chemotherapy (MAGIC) with neoadjuvant chemoradiation (CROSS). This trial design is discussed later on. The present chapter focuses on the different neoadjuvant treatment regimens.

4.2 Neoadjuvant Chemotherapy

Studies in the 80s and 90s of the previous century revealed that patients with esophageal cancer who underwent surgical resection with curative intent had a dismal prognosis, with a 2-year

J.W. van den Berg • S.M. Lagarde • B.P.L. Wijnhoven
J.J.B. van Lanschot (✉)
Department of Surgery, Erasmus Medical Center, Rotterdam, The Netherlands
e-mail: j.vanlanschot@erasmusmc.nl

A. van der Gaast
Department of Medical Oncology, Erasmus Medical Center, Rotterdam, The Netherlands

M.A. Cuesta (ed.), *Minimally Invasive Surgery for Upper Abdominal Cancer*,
DOI 10.1007/978-3-319-54301-7_4

survival rate of only 20–30%. Factors that contributed to these poor outcomes were the presence of locally advanced disease reflected by a high number of irradical resections and (distant) micrometastases at the time of surgery, which could not be detected with the available imaging techniques. To increase survival rates after esophagectomy, there was interest in the combination of chemotherapy and surgical treatment.

Multiple randomized trials have evaluated the benefit of chemotherapy administered prior to resection in patients with esophageal cancer. For example, the European EORTC 40954 trial in which 144 patients with adenocarcinoma of the stomach or GE-junction were randomized to neoadjuvant chemotherapy (5-FU, leucovorin, cisplatin) followed by surgery or surgery alone [1]. This trial was stopped for poor accrual, which limited the power of the study. A significantly increased R0 resection rate was found for patients treated with chemotherapy, however this did not translate into a survival benefit. Other studies such as the OEO2 trial demonstrated a survival benefit compared with resection alone. The OEO2 trial, in which patients (SCC or adenocarcinoma of the esophagus or GE-junction) were randomized to preoperative chemotherapy (cisplatin and fluorouracil) followed by surgery or surgery alone, revealed a survival benefit (HR 0.79, p 0.004) in combination with increased R0 resection rates (60% vs. 54%) [2]. In addition, a 30-day mortality of 10% was observed in both treatment groups. Long-term follow-up revealed a modest improvement in 5-year survival (36% vs. 23%, p = 0.03) [3]. These results can explain why neoadjuvant chemotherapy became standard of care for esophageal cancer in the United Kingdom. For squamous cell carcinoma of the esophagus a Dutch trial randomized patients for preoperative chemotherapy (cisplatin and etoposide) followed by surgery or surgery alone [4]. The 5-year survival was significantly improved after chemotherapy (26% vs. 17%). On the other hand, the USA intergroup 113 trial, which randomly assigned patients with SCC and adenocarcinoma to preoperative chemotherapy (cisplatin and fluorouracil) and surgery or surgery alone, failed to show a survival benefit for patients treated with preoperative chemotherapy [5]. They reported a 2-year survival rate of 35% for patients who received chemotherapy and 37% for those who underwent surgery alone. Postoperative mortality was 6% in both treatment groups. Long term results showed no difference in overall survival for patients receiving preoperative chemotherapy compared with surgery alone [6]. These results can explain why neoadjuvant chemotherapy did not become standard of care for esophageal cancer in the USA. The difference in outcome between the OEO2 trial and the USA intergroup 113 trial is difficult to explain as almost the same chemotherapy regimens have been applied.

The OEO2 trial was followed by the OEO5 trial, which hypothesized that adding a fourth cycle of chemotherapy to the neoadjuvant regimen would lead to better survival rates compared with a short neoadjuvant chemotherapy regimen. The preliminary results of this so called OEO5 trial, which compared prolonged neoadjuvant chemotherapy (4 cycles of epirubicin, cisplatin, capecitabine) with standard chemotherapy (2 cycles of cisplatin and 5-FU) in 895 patients with esophageal or GE-junction cancer have only been published in abstract form at the time of writing this chapter [7]. The OEO5 trial showed that prolonged chemotherapy resulted in increased R0 resection rates, better disease free survival, and progression free survival. The 3-year overall survival rate was 42% after prolonged neoadjuvant chemotherapy versus 39% after the classical OEO2 regimen, i.e. not significantly different, but with a higher toxicity rate in the group receiving 4 cycles of chemotherapy. Survival rates in the OEO5 trial are higher compared with the historical OEO-2 trial data. This may be explained by better patient selection and improved surgical techniques/outcome.

A recent meta-analysis showed a survival benefit for neoadjuvant chemotherapy relative to surgery alone for patients with esophageal or GE-junction cancer (HR all-cause mortality for neoadjuvant chemotherapy (HR 0.88 (95% CI 0.80–0.96), p = 0.003)) [8]. In addition, it was thought that neoadjuvant chemotherapy could result in an increase of surgery related morbidity and mortality, since preoperative therapy might weaken the patient. A recent prospective study in patients with SCC of the esophagus or GEJ indeed showed that neoadjuvant chemotherapy increased the risk of postoperative complications compared with surgery alone [9]. However, a meta-analysis showed that neoadjuvant chemotherapy does not increase the risk of postoperative morbidity and perioperative mortality [10].

4.3 Neoadjuvant Chemoradiation

The role for neoadjuvant chemoradiation has also been debated for many years because of varying results of different studies. The high locoregional and systemic failure after surgery alone urged the need for new treatment options and resulted in combined modality treatment using systemic chemotherapy and locoregional radiotherapy. The goal of combining both neoadjuvant chemotherapy and neoadjuvant chemoradiation is mainly based on the possibility to downstage the primary tumor, resulting in higher R0 resection rates. In addition, neoadjuvant chemotherapy may also eradicate micro-metastatic disease by decreasing cancer-cell dissemination.

Studies on the effect of neoadjuvant chemoradiation for esophageal and GE-junction tumors showed variable results. The French FFCD 9901 trial which randomly assigned 195 patients with stage 1 or 2 esophageal or GE-junction cancer to preoperative chemoradiation (5-FU, cisplatin, and 45 Gy radiation therapy) followed by surgery versus surgery alone did not improve 3-year survival (47.5 vs. 53%) [11]. Chemoradiation prior to surgery did not improve the complete R0 resection rate and was associated with a significantly increased postoperative mortality. However, interpretation of these results is confounded by the fact that the study is underpowered to show a possible survival benefit. A Swedish trial randomized 181 patients with esophageal or GE-junction tumors (SCC and adenocarcinoma) to chemotherapy (cisplatin, FU) with or without radiotherapy (40 Gy) followed by surgical resection (4–6 weeks after completing neoadjuvant treatment) [12]. Chemoradiation significantly increased pathologically complete response (pCR) (28 vs. 9%) and complete R0 resection rate (87 vs. 74%). However, no significant difference in 3-year survival was found (47 vs. 49%). An Australian study randomized 256 patients to chemoradiation (cisplatin, fluorouracil, 35 Gy radiotherapy) followed by surgery or surgery alone [13]. Chemoradiation resulted in a significant increase of R0 resections (80% vs. 59%, $p = 0.0002$). However, no difference in overall survival was shown.

Several other trials and meta-analyses have demonstrated improved survival with preoperative concurrent chemoradiation as compared to surgery alone, for potentially resectable stage II or III localized cancer of the thoracic esophagus. However, the optimal regimen is not established yet. A relatively old Irish trial randomized patients to chemotherapy (fluorouracil and cisplatin) and radiotherapy (40 Gy) followed by surgery or surgery alone. This study in 113 patients revealed 25% complete response and a significantly increased 3-year survival after neoadjuvant chemoradiation followed by surgery (32% vs. 6%) [14]. Postoperative 90-day mortality of both groups combined was 6%. However, this study was criticized because of the unusually low survival rate in the surgery alone group. An American trial (CALGB 9781) randomized patients to chemotherapy (cisplatin and fluorouracil) and radiotherapy (50.4 Gy) followed by surgery or surgery alone. This study, which was closed prematurely after 3 years and only 56 patients (of the planned 475 patients) due to poor accrual, showed an increased 5-year survival (39% vs. 16%), however this did not reach statistical significance [15]. More recently, the Dutch Cross trial randomized 363 patients comparing preoperative chemotherapy consisting of carboplatin (doses titrated to achieve an area under the curve of 2 mg per millilitre per minute) and paclitaxel (50 mg per m^2 body-surface area) and radiotherapy (41.4 Gy in 23 fractions, 5 days per week) followed by surgery with surgery alone in patients with potentially curable esophageal or

GE-junction cancer (SCC and adenocarcinoma) (Fig. 4.1) [16]. This combination of chemotherapy and radiotherapy was well tolerated by the patients and significantly increased the percentage of R0 resections up to 92% compared with 69% in the surgery alone group. In addition, 29% percent of the patients with chemoradiation had a pCR. The median overall survival was also significantly higher in the combined treatment arm than in the surgery arm (49 months vs. 24 months; $P = 0.003$). (Fig. 4.2a, b) The long-term results confirmed the overall survival benefit for neoadjuvant chemoradiation (5-year survival 47 vs. 33%, HR for death 0.67, 95% CI 0.51–0.87) [17]. Due to the overall survival benefit, low toxicity, and high R0 resection rate (91%) of the neoadjuvant chemoradiation, the CROSS regimen is now the preferred multimodality treatment in the Netherlands and several other Western European countries.

The German POET trial suggested a possible superiority of neoadjuvant chemoradiation over chemotherapy. This trial randomized 126 patients with GE-junction tumors to chemotherapy alone (cisplatin, FU, leucovorin) followed by surgery or the same chemotherapy regimen (cisplatin, FU, leucovorin) followed by low-dose RT concurrent with chemotherapy (cisplatin and etoposide) [18]. Induction chemotherapy followed by chemoradiation significantly increased complete pathological response (15.6% vs. 2.0%, $p = 0.03$) and (non-significantly) increased 3-year survival (47 vs. 28%, $p = 0.07$). Recently the long-term results showed a 5 year overall survival of 24.4%

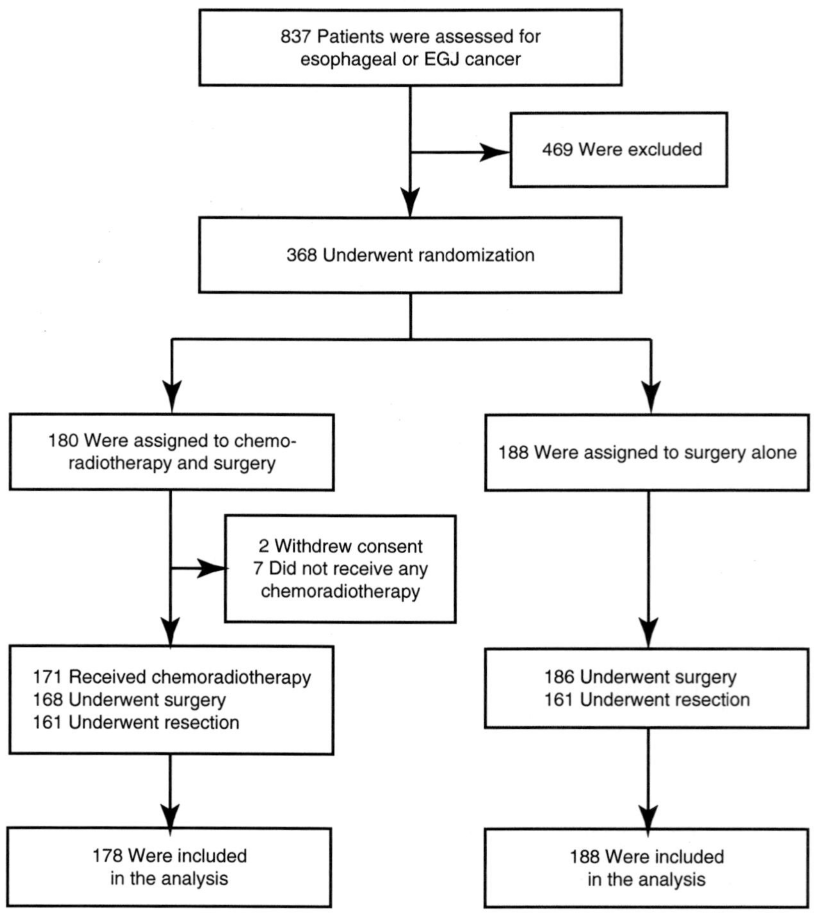

Fig. 4.1 Consort scheme of patients of CROSS trial

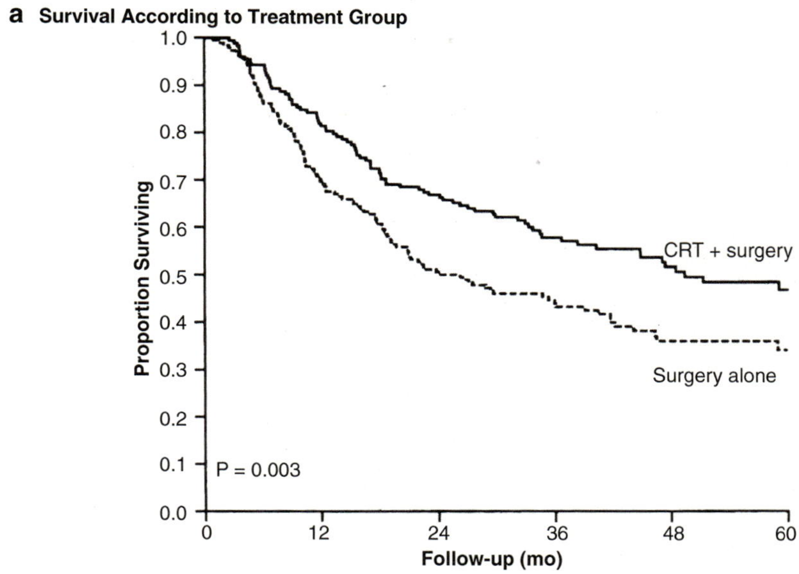

No. at Risk

CRT+surgery	178	145	119	75	49	28
Surgery alone	188	131	94	62	33	17
Total	366	276	213	137	82	45

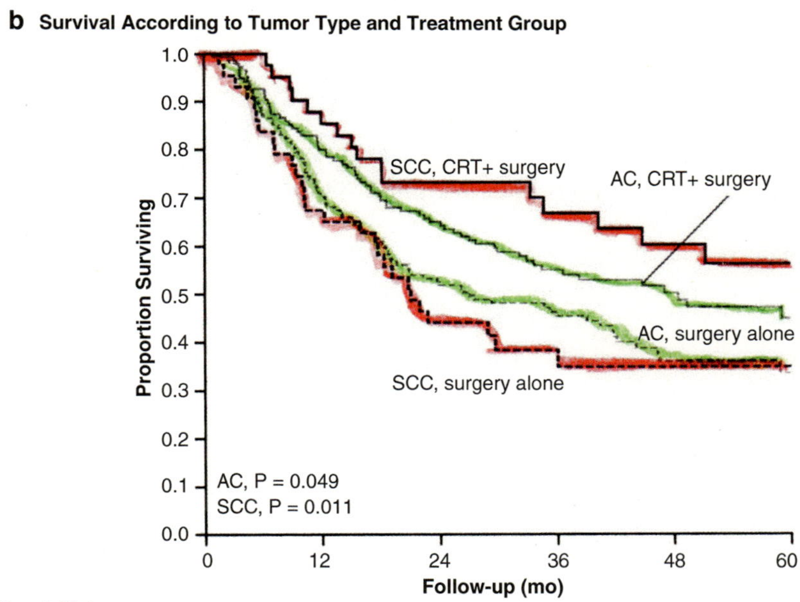

No. at Risk

AC, CRT+surgery	134	107	87	53	34	18
AC, surgery alone	141	99	73	50	25	10
SCC, CRT+surgery	41	35	30	21	15	8
SCC, Surgery alone	43	29	19	11	8	4
Total	359	270	209	135	82	40

Fig. 4.2 (**a**) Estimated overall 5-years survival according to treatment group (CROSS trial); (**b**) estimated overall 5 year survival, according to tumor type and treatment group (CROSS trial)

in the chemotherapy versus 39.5% in the chemoradiation group (p = 0.055) [19]. An Australian trial randomized 75 patients to neoadjuvant chemotherapy (cisplatin and 5-FU) followed by surgery or neoadjuvant chemoradiation (cisplatin and 5-FU in combination with 35 Gy radiation therapy) followed by surgery [20]. After neoadjuvant chemoradiation pCR was significantly increased compared with neoadjuvant chemotherapy, 31 vs. 8% (p = 0.01) respectively. No significant difference in median overall survival was observed, possibly because of the low number of included patients.

Overall, a recent meta-analysis based on 6072 patients found that neoadjuvant chemoradiation followed by surgery compared with surgery alone was the only regimen to significantly improve survival (HR 0.77 (95% CI 0.68–0.87), p < 0.001) [21]. This network meta-analysis states that neoadjuvant chemoradiation followed by surgery is the most effective strategy in improving survival of resectable esophageal cancer. Earlier, a meta-analysis based on 4188 patients included in RCTs (CROSS, FFCD, CALGB 9781) found that neoadjuvant chemotherapy and neoadjuvant chemoradiation reduced overall mortality as compared to surgery alone in patients with T1-3 esophageal adenocarcinoma [22]. In addition, it has been debated that neoadjuvant chemoradiation may enhance the occurrence of postoperative complications, which for example has also been observed after neoadjuvant radiotherapy in rectal surgery. A recent prospective study in patients with SCC of the esophagus or GEJ indeed showed that neoadjuvant chemoradiation increased postoperative mortality compared with surgery alone [9]. However, a meta-analysis showed that neither neoadjuvant chemotherapy nor neoadjuvant chemoradiation increases the risk of postoperative morbidity and mortality [10].

4.4 Perioperative Chemotherapy

For gastric cancer a strategy of perioperative chemotherapy, which is also known as the "sandwich approach", is the predominant approach in Europe. This regimen was based primarily on the United Kingdom Medical Research Council MAGIC trial which randomized 503 patients with adenocarcinoma of the stomach, GE-junction and esophagus, to perioperative ECF (epirubicin/cisplatin/5-FU) and surgery or surgery alone [23]. Perioperative chemotherapy improved 5-year survival rate (36% vs. 23%, p = 0.009). However, only 42% of the patients intentionally treated with chemotherapy completed the full regime. Perioperative mortality (death within 30 days) was similar between both groups (5.6% vs. 5.9%). This study was criticized because of the lack of a standardized surgical procedure as well as the late inclusion of GE-junction and esophageal tumors in the protocol. The initial trial design was for stomach cancer, however due to low accrual, distal esophageal tumors and GE-junction tumors were also included in a later phase. Only one fourth of the patients had esophageal or GE-junction cancers. The inclusion of these last subgroups may have biased the results. Moreover, no clear evidence has been given about the additional value of the adjuvant phase of the study, and long term results have never been published.

The French FNCLCC-FFCD trial randomized 224 patients with adenocarcinoma of the esophagus, GE-junction, or stomach to perioperative chemotherapy (cisplatin and fluorouracil) and surgery or surgery alone [24]. Perioperative chemotherapy significantly improved 5-year survival (38% vs. 24%, p = 0.02), curative resection rate, disease-free survival (5-year rate: 34% vs. 19%, P = 0.003), while there was no difference in 30-day mortality (4.5% vs. 4.6%). In this study 75% of the patients had esophageal or GE-junction tumor.

4.5 Neoadjuvant Versus Adjuvant Strategies

Relatively few studies focused on postoperative strategies. In general, the data suggest that postoperative regimens fail to improve survival. There are only a few randomized trials of adjuvant chemotherapy for resected esophageal adenocarcinoma and only a few Japanese studies in resected esophageal squamous cell carcinoma that showed no survival benefit [25, 26]. Recently, the superiority of neoadjuvant as compared to adjuvant chemotherapy was shown in the Japanese JCOG9907 trial [27]. Patients (n = 330) with SCC of the esophagus were randomly assigned to surgery preceded or followed by chemotherapy (cisplatin and 5-FU). Five-year overall survival was significantly higher after preoperative chemotherapy (55% vs. 43%, p = 0.04). One of the reasons that neoadjuvant chemotherapy may lead to better results is the fact that many patients do not tolerate adjuvant chemotherapy after an esophagectomy.

4.6 Future Perspectives

Over the last decades multiple trials have indicated that multimodality treatment of patients with esophageal and GE-junction cancer is necessary to obtain optimal results. At the moment several phase 3 trials are ongoing to further determine the optimal (neo)-adjuvant treatment regimen. The NeoAegis trial is recruiting patients to evaluate survival of patients treated with perioperative chemotherapy plus surgery versus neoadjuvant chemoradiation plus surgery (MAGIC vs. CROSS) in esophageal and junctional adenocarcinoma. The French PROTECT trial, investigates the effect of preoperative radiotherapy (41.4 Gy) in combination with two different chemotherapy regimens, namely FOLFOX (folinic acid, fluorouracil, oxalipatin) versus paclitaxel and carboplatin [28].

The recurrence patterns after CROSS followed by surgery for esophageal or GE-junction cancer reveal that isolated infield locoregional recurrence is very rare [29]. This indicates that increase of the dosis of radiotherapy is reasonless. Isolated outfield lymphatic recurrence is also very rare which counters a possible positive effect of enlargement of the radiation field. The occurrence of distant metastases, whether or not in combination with locoregional recurrence, is the major problem. Therefore, a more effective systemic therapy is needed to improve long-term survival. However, it is unlikely that much can be expected from new combinations or adjusted doses of the classical chemotherapeutic agents.

Several studies investigate the possible beneficial effects of monoclonal antibodies as neoadjuvant treatment for different types of cancer. For example in metastatic colorectal cancer and metastatic breast cancer the addition of monoclonal antibodies to standard chemotherapy regimens has improved survival [30, 31]. However, up to now, for esophageal cancer no beneficial effects of monoclonal antibodies have been reported. A recent study added bevacizumab and erlotinib to neoadjuvant chemoradiation for patients with esophageal or GE-junction cancer [32]. The addition of bevacizumab and erlotinib did not demonstrate any survival benefit. Another phase 2 trial showed that for patients with gastric or GE-junction adenocarcinoma the addition of bevacizumab to perioperative epirubicin, cisplatin, and capecitabine is feasible [33]. However, the phase-3 part of this STO3 trial is still ongoing. Also other monoclonal antibodies, for example against the vascular endothelial growth factor receptor 2 (ramucirumab), are promising additions to the standard of care for gastric or gastro-oesophageal cancer.

The success of immunotherapy for other tumors gives high expectations for a possible beneficial effect in esophageal and GE-junction tumors. Just as e.g. melanoma, esophageal cancer has a relatively high burden of genetic mutations which probably act as "neoantigens" and could be tested as potential targets for immunotherapy [34, 35].

The CROSS trial revealed that following chemoradiation, 49% of patients with SCC and 23% of patients with an adenocarcinoma had a pCR in the resection specimen. Also other studies described the effect of neoadjuvant chemoradiation on the occurrence of pCR. Several trials showed that this "sterilizing" effect is increased after chemoradiation compared with chemotherapy alone [12, 18, 20]. The occurrence of pathologically complete response opens the possibility for new (organ sparing) treatment options. It can be hypothesized that patients with pCR do not benefit from esophagectomy. Those patients could undergo an organ sparing approach if identified correctly. Such approach would consist of active surveillance if clinically complete response (cCR) has been accomplished by chemoradiation. These effects of neoadjuvant chemoradiation on the occurrence of pCR raises questions about the timing and necessity of esophagectomy after application of the CROSS regimen. Therefore, a prospective trial (preSANO) is ongoing in the Netherlands which analyzes the optimal diagnostic set for determining the presence or absence of residual disease after chemoradiation [36]. If the preSANO trial shows that the presence or absence of residual tumor can be predicted reasonably after chemoradiation, a subsequent randomized controlled trial will compare chemoradiation plus standard surgery with chemoradiation plus surgery as needed (SANO trial). In this active surveillance group surgery will only be performed after CROSS if residual disease has been proven or is highly suspected. A comparable randomized trial (Esostrate trial) has recently been initiated in France.

In conclusion, the use of preoperative chemoradiation or chemotherapy followed by surgery is currently the prevailing treatment for most patients selected for curatively intended treatment. However, up to now none of these two regimens has been proven superior. Possibly a treatment more individualized for each patient will further improve the results of neoadjuvant therapy in combination with surgery. Recently, three subtypes of esophageal adenocarcinoma have been described [37]. This subclassification may have therapeutic relevance and could result in individualized treatment regimens for patients with esophageal or GE-junction tumors to obtain the optimal results from neoadjuvant therapy and surgery.

References

1. Schuhmacher C, Gretschel S, Lordick F, Reichardt P, Hohenberger W, Eisenberger CF, et al. Neoadjuvant chemotherapy compared with surgery alone for locally advanced cancer of the stomach and cardia: European Organisation for research and treatment of cancer randomized trial 40954. J Clin Oncol. 2010;28(35):5210–8. Epub 2010/11/10.
2. Group MRCOCW. Surgical resection with or without preoperative chemotherapy in oesophageal cancer: a randomised controlled trial. Lancet. 2002;359(9319):1727–33. Epub 2002/06/07.
3. Allum WH, Stenning SP, Bancewicz J, Clark PI, Langley RE. Long-term results of a randomized trial of surgery with or without preoperative chemotherapy in esophageal cancer. J Clin Oncol. 2009;27(30):5062–7. Epub 2009/09/23.
4. Boonstra JJ, Kok TC, Wijnhoven BP, van Heijl M, van Berge Henegouwen MI, Ten Kate FJ, et al. Chemotherapy followed by surgery versus surgery alone in patients with resectable oesophageal squamous cell carcinoma: long-term results of a randomized controlled trial. BMC Cancer. 2011;11:181. Epub 2011/05/21.
5. Kelsen DP, Ginsberg R, Pajak TF, Sheahan DG, Gunderson L, Mortimer J, et al. Chemotherapy followed by surgery compared with surgery alone for localized esophageal cancer. N Engl J Med. 1998;339(27):1979–84. Epub 1998/12/31.
6. Kelsen DP, Winter KA, Gunderson LL, Mortimer J, Estes NC, Haller DG, et al. Long-term results of RTOG trial 8911 (USA intergroup 113): a random assignment trial comparison of chemotherapy followed by surgery compared with surgery alone for esophageal cancer. J Clin Oncol. 2007;25(24):3719–25. Epub 2007/08/21.
7. Cunningham D, Langley RE, Nankivell M, Blazeby J, Griffin M, Crelin A, et al. Neoadjuvant chemotherapy for resectable oesophageal and junctional adenocarcinoma: results from the UK Medical Research Council randomised OEO5 trial (ISRCTN 01852072). Ann Oncol. 2015;26(Suppl 4):iv117–iv21.
8. Kidane B, Coughlin S, Vogt K, Malthaner R. Preoperative chemotherapy for resectable thoracic esophageal cancer. Cochrane Database Syst Rev. 2015;5:CD001556. Epub 2015/05/20.
9. Klevebro F, Lindblad M, Johansson J, Lundell L, Nilsson M. Outcome of neoadjuvant therapies for cancer of the oesophagus or gastro-oesophageal junction based on a national data registry. Br J Surg. 2016;103(13):1864–73. Epub 2016/10/01.
10. Kumagai K, Rouvelas I, Tsai JA, Mariosa D, Klevebro F, Lindblad M, et al. Meta-analysis of postoperative morbidity and perioperative mortality in patients receiving neoadjuvant chemotherapy or chemoradiotherapy for resectable oesophageal and gastro-oesophageal junctional cancers. Br J Surg. 2014;101(4):321–38. Epub 2014/02/05.
11. Mariette C, Dahan L, Mornex F, Maillard E, Thomas PA, Meunier B, et al. Surgery alone versus chemoradiotherapy followed by surgery for stage I and II esophageal cancer: final analysis of randomized controlled phase III trial FFCD 9901. J Clin Oncol. 2014;32(23):2416–22. Epub 2014/07/02.
12. Klevebro F, Alexandersson von Döbeln G, Wang N, Johnsen G, Jacobsen AB, Friesland S, et al. A randomized clinical trial of neoadjuvant chemotherapy versus neoadjuvant chemoradiotherapy for cancer of

the oesophagus or gastro-oesophageal junction. Ann Oncol. 2016;27(4):660–7. Epub 2016/01/20.
13. Burmeister BH, Smithers BM, Gebski V, Fitzgerald L, Simes RJ, Devitt P, et al. Surgery alone versus chemoradiotherapy followed by surgery for resectable cancer of the oesophagus: a randomised controlled phase III trial. Lancet Oncol. 2005;6(9):659–68. Epub 2005/09/01.
14. Walsh TN, Noonan N, Hollywood D, Kelly A, Keeling N, Hennessy TP. A comparison of multimodal therapy and surgery for esophageal adenocarcinoma. N Engl J Med. 1996;335(7):462–7. Epub 1996/08/15.
15. Tepper J, Krasna MJ, Niedzwiecki D, Hollis D, Reed CE, Goldberg R, et al. Phase III trial of trimodality therapy with cisplatin, fluorouracil, radiotherapy, and surgery compared with surgery alone for esophageal cancer: CALGB 9781. J Clin Oncol. 2008;26(7):1086–92. Epub 2008/03/04.
16. van Hagen P, Hulshof MC, van Lanschot JJ, Steyerberg EW, van Berge Henegouwen MI, Wijnhoven BP, et al. Preoperative chemoradiotherapy for esophageal or junctional cancer. N Engl J Med. 2012;366(22):2074–84. Epub 2012/06/01.
17. Shapiro J, van Lanschot JJ, Hulshof MC, van Hagen P, van Berge Henegouwen MI, Wijnhoven BP, et al. Neoadjuvant chemoradiotherapy plus surgery versus surgery alone for oesophageal or junctional cancer (CROSS): long-term results of a randomised controlled trial. Lancet Oncol. 2015;16(9):1090–8. Epub 2015/08/10.
18. Stahl M, Walz MK, Stuschke M, Lehmann N, Meyer HJ, Riera-Knorrenschild J, et al. Phase III comparison of preoperative chemotherapy compared with chemoradiotherapy in patients with locally advanced adenocarcinoma of the esophagogastric junction. J Clin Oncol. 2009;27(6):851–6. Epub 2009/01/14.
19. Stahl M, Riera-Knorrenschild J, Stuschke M, Engenhart-Cabillic R, Bitzer M, Budach W, et al. Preoperative chemoradiotherapy and the long-term run in curative treatment of locally advanced oesophagogastric junction adenocarcinoma: update of the POET phase III study. J Clin Oncol. 2016;34(suppl; abstr 4031).
20. Burmeister BH, Thomas JM, Burmeister EA, Walpole ET, Harvey JA, Thomson DB, et al. Is concurrent radiation therapy required in patients receiving preoperative chemotherapy for adenocarcinoma of the oesophagus? A randomised phase II trial. Eur J Cancer. 2011;47(3):354–60. Epub 2010/11/19.
21. Pasquali S, Yim G, Vohra RS, Mocellin S, Nyanhongo D, Marriott P, et al. Survival after neoadjuvant and adjuvant treatments compared to surgery alone for resectable esophageal carcinoma: a network meta-analysis. Ann Surg. 2017;265(3):481–91.
22. Sjoquist KM, Burmeister BH, Smithers BM, Zalcberg JR, Simes RJ, Barbour A, et al. Survival after neoadjuvant chemotherapy or chemoradiotherapy for resectable oesophageal carcinoma: an updated meta-analysis. Lancet Oncol. 2011;12(7):681–92. Epub 2011/06/21.
23. Cunningham D, Allum WH, Stenning SP, Thompson JN, Van de Velde CJ, Nicolson M, et al. Perioperative chemotherapy versus surgery alone for resectable gastroesophageal cancer. N Engl J Med. 2006;355(1):11–20. Epub 2006/07/11.
24. Ychou M, Boige V, Pignon JP, Conroy T, Bouche O, Lebreton G, et al. Perioperative chemotherapy compared with surgery alone for resectable gastroesophageal adenocarcinoma: an FNCLCC and FFCD multicenter phase III trial. J Clin Oncol. 2011;29(13):1715–21. Epub 2011/03/30.
25. Ando N, Iizuka T, Kakegawa T, Isono K, Watanabe H, Ide H, et al. A randomized trial of surgery with and without chemotherapy for localized squamous carcinoma of the thoracic esophagus: the Japan Clinical Oncology Group Study. J Thorac Cardiovasc Surg. 1997;114(2):205–9. Epub 1997/08/01.
26. Ando N, Iizuka T, Ide H, Ishida K, Shinoda M, Nishimaki T, et al. Surgery plus chemotherapy compared with surgery alone for localized squamous cell carcinoma of the thoracic esophagus: a Japan Clinical Oncology Group Study—JCOG9204. J Clin Oncol. 2003;21(24):4592–6. Epub 2003/12/16.
27. Ando N, Kato H, Igaki H, Shinoda M, Ozawa S, Shimizu H, et al. A randomized trial comparing postoperative adjuvant chemotherapy with cisplatin and 5-fluorouracil versus preoperative chemotherapy for localized advanced squamous cell carcinoma of the thoracic esophagus (JCOG9907). Ann Surg Oncol. 2012;19(1):68–74. Epub 2011/09/01.
28. Messager M, Mirabel X, Tresch E, Paumier A, Vendrely V, Dahan L, et al. Preoperative chemoradiation with paclitaxel-carboplatin or with fluorouracil-oxaliplatin-folinic acid (FOLFOX) for resectable esophageal and junctional cancer: the PROTECT-1402, randomized phase 2 trial. BMC Cancer. 2016;16:318. Epub 2016/05/20.
29. Oppedijk V, van der Gaast A, van Lanschot JJ, van Hagen P, van Os R, van Rij CM, et al. Patterns of recurrence after surgery alone versus preoperative chemoradiotherapy and surgery in the CROSS trials. J Clin Oncol. 2014;32(5):385–91. Epub 2014/01/15.
30. Slamon DJ, Leyland-Jones B, Shak S, Fuchs H, Paton V, Bajamonde A, et al. Use of chemotherapy plus a monoclonal antibody against HER2 for metastatic breast cancer that overexpresses HER2. N Engl J Med. 2001;344(11):783–92. Epub 2001/03/15.
31. Hurwitz H, Fehrenbacher L, Novotny W, Cartwright T, Hainsworth J, Heim W, et al. Bevacizumab plus irinotecan, fluorouracil, and leucovorin for metastatic colorectal cancer. N Engl J Med. 2004;350(23):2335–42. Epub 2004/06/04.
32. Bendell JC, Meluch A, Peyton J, Rubin M, Waterhouse D, Webb C, et al. A phase II trial of preoperative concurrent chemotherapy/radiation therapy plus bevacizumab/erlotinib in the treatment of localized esophageal cancer. Clin Adv Hematol Oncol. 2012;10(7):430–7. Epub 2012/08/17.
33. Okines AF, Langley RE, Thompson LC, Stenning SP, Stevenson L, Falk S, et al. Bevacizumab with

peri-operative epirubicin, cisplatin and capecitabine (ECX) in localised gastro-oesophageal adenocarcinoma: a safety report. Ann Oncol. 2013;24(3):702–9. Epub 2012/10/31.

34. Alexandrov LB, Nik-Zainal S, Wedge DC, Aparicio SA, Behjati S, Biankin AV, et al. Signatures of mutational processes in human cancer. Nature. 2013;500(7463):415–21. Epub 2013/08/16.
35. Mellman I, Coukos G, Dranoff G. Cancer immunotherapy comes of age. Nature. 2011;480(7378):480–9. Epub 2011/12/24.
36. Noordman BJ, Shapiro J, Spaander MC, Krishnadath KK, van Laarhoven HW, van Berge Henegouwen MI, et al. Accuracy of detecting residual disease after cross neoadjuvant chemoradiotherapy for esophageal cancer (preSANO Trial): rationale and protocol. JMIR Res Protoc. 2015;4(2):e79. Epub 2015/06/30.
37. Secrier M, Li X, de Silva N, Eldridge MD, Contino G, Bornschein J, et al. Mutational signatures in esophageal adenocarcinoma define etiologically distinct subgroups with therapeutic relevance. Nat Genet. 2016;48(10):1131–41. Epub 2016/09/07.

Transhiatal or Transthoracic Esophagectomy

5

Leonie R. van der Werf and Bas P.L. Wijnhoven

5.1 Introduction

A surgical resection remains the most important treatment modality for the cure of non-metastasized esophageal cancer. For many years, open esophagectomy was performed worldwide through two approaches: the transhiatal esophagectomy (THE) and transthoracic esophagectomy (TTE). Pertaining in-hospital mortality rates were between 3 and 10%, and the 5-year survival rate after surgery was 20–30%. Resulting contributions to improved patient-care and selection were the improvement of perioperative care, the introduction of neoadjuvant treatments, the centralization of surgery in high volume centres and the better imaging modalities. Hence, short and long-term outcomes of surgical resection have improved substantially.

Minimally invasive esophagectomy (MIE) was pioneered in the early nineties and popularized in the last decades by many surgeons. Three meta-analyses support the concept that MIE may be associated with less respiratory complications, a reduction of morbidity and a faster postoperative recovery [1–3]. At the same time, the procedure is technically demanding and programs to safely introduce these techniques are warranted. Two randomized trials compared open esophagectomy with MIE: the total (thoraco-laparoscopic) MIE in the TIME-trial and the hybrid (laparoscopy and thoracotomy) esophagectomy in the MIRO-trial. Both studies show the short-term advantages of MIE: less blood loss, a lower rate of respiratory infection, a shorter hospital stay and a better quality of life in favour of the MIE. The quality of the specimen resected is similar to the open technique (radicality and number of lymph nodes). Long-term oncological outcome of the TIME trial at 1-year and 3-year showed no differences between the two groups concerning overall and disease-free survival [4].

In this chapter we review the transhiatal and transthoracic esophagectomy and discuss the comparison of the outcomes of these two open approaches by a randomized controlled study, the HIVEX trial.

5.2 Comparing THE with TTE: The HIVEX Trial

5.2.1 Transhiatal Esophagectomy

Via an upper abdominal incision, the distal esophagus and locoregional lymph nodes in the posterior mediastinum are dissected en bloc through a widened hiatus. The upper abdominal

L.R. van der Werf • B.P.L. Wijnhoven (✉)
Department of Surgery, Erasmus University Medical Center, Rotterdam, The Netherlands
e-mail: L.vanderWerf@dica.nl; b.wijnhoven@erasmusmc.nl

M.A. Cuesta (ed.), *Minimally Invasive Surgery for Upper Abdominal Cancer*,
DOI 10.1007/978-3-319-54301-7_5

lymph nodes are dissected including the paracardial lymph nodes, the nodes along the lesser curvature and the nodes at the left gastric artery. A standard D1 plus or D2 lymphadenectomy of the celiac trunk is performed. The cervical esophagus is dissected via a left (or right) cervical incision and the intrathoracic esophagus dissected bluntly and stripped with the aid of a vein stripper. Creation of gastric tube and resection of the specimen is then followed by positioning the gastric tube in the prevertebral plane to the neck where the anastomosis is made [5].

5.2.2 Transthoracic Esophageal Resection

Several techniques are used: Ivor Lewis procedure (right thoracotomy and laparotomy), Mc Keown (three-stage with neck incision) and the Sweet procedure (left thoraco-abdominal incision). The three-stage and the two-stage open esophagectomy involves an esophageal resection, creation of a gastric tube, a two-field lymphadenectomy (celiac trunk and mediastinal lymphadenectomy) followed by a cervical anastomosis in the three-stage procedure and an intrathoracic anastomosis in the case of an Ivor Lewis procedure. The extent of the mediastinal lymphadenectomy is still debated, but the majority of the patients undergoes a total mediastinal lymphadenectomy.

5.2.3 Differences Between Open TTE and THE

In 2001, Hulscher et al. published a meta-analysis on transthoracic and transhiatal esophagectomy [6]. Six prospective comparative studies including three control-randomized studies (RCT) and 18 retrospective comparative studies were included (all published between 1990 and 1999). The three RCTs in this meta-analysis were all underpowered and focused on squamous cell carcinoma [7–9]. In 2002, Hulscher et al. published the Dutch HIVEX trial, a RCT comparing TTE with THE [10]. In 2007, Omloo et al. published a long-term follow-up of this trial (5 years) [11].

The HIVEX trial included 220 patients with adenocarcinoma type I of the distal esophagus or adenocarcinoma type II of the gastric cardia involving the distal esophagus. Patients were randomized to THE or TTE with extended en bloc lymphadenectomy. Primary endpoints of this study were overall survival and disease-free survival. Secondary endpoints were the perioperative data and other parameters such as postoperative morbidity and mortality, the quality of the resected specimen, the number of lymph nodes involved and the number of quality-adjusted life-years gained.

Perioperative morbidity was higher after TTE, but there was no statistically significant difference between the groups THE and TTE regarding in-hospital mortality (2% in the transhiatal group and 4% in the transthoracic group, $p = 0.45$). In the TTE group, 57% of patients had pulmonary complications vs. 27% in the THE group ($p = <0.001$). Chyle leakage occurred more in the TTE group, 10% vs. 2% ($p = 0.02$). In the THE group, vocal-cord paralysis was more common but this difference was not significant (21% vs. 13%, $p = 0.15$). Mechanical ventilation time, ICU stay and hospital stay were significantly higher in the TTE group (postoperative ventilation time: 2 days vs. 1 day, $p = <0.001$; ICU stay: 6 days vs. 2 days, $p = <0.001$; and postoperative hospital stay: 19 days vs. 15 days, $p = <0.001$).

After a median follow-up of 4.7 years, 142 patients had died: 74 (70%) after THE and 68 (60%) after TTE ($p = 0.12$). Although the difference in survival was not statistically significant, there was at 5 years a trend toward a survival benefit holding for the extended approach. Disease-free survival was 27% in the THE group, as compared with 39% in the TTE group, whereas overall survival was 29% as compared with 39% (Figs. 5.1 and 5.2).

The conclusion of this HIVEX trial was that THE was associated with a lower morbidity rate than TTE with its extended en bloc lymphadenectomy. Although median overall, disease-free, and quality-adjusted survival did not differ statistically between the groups, there was at 5 years a

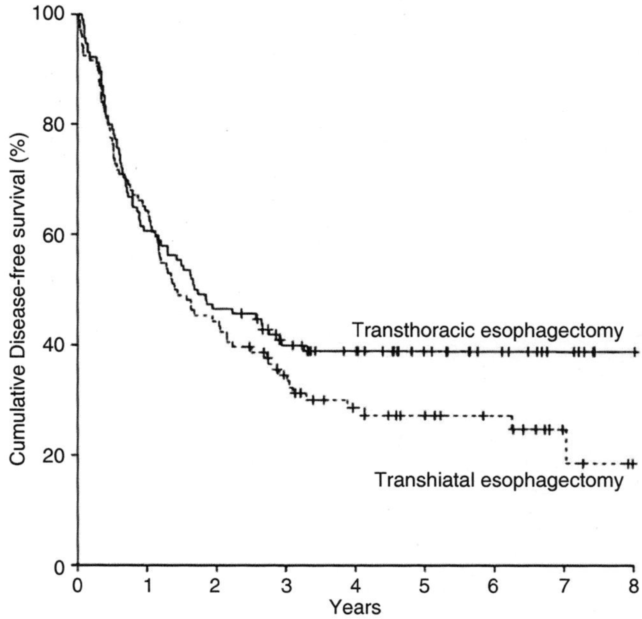

No. At Risk

Transhiatal esophagectomy	106	68	47	32	20	15	11	4
Transthoracic esophagectomy	114	69	53	39	31	20	13	7

Fig. 5.1 Kaplan Meier curves showing disease free survival among patients randomly assigned to transhiatal esophagectomy or transthoracic esophagectomy with extended en bloc lymphadenectomy. From Extended transthoracic resection compared with limited transhiatal resection for adenocarcinoma of the esophagus, Hulscher JB, van Sandick JW, de Boer AGEM et al., 347. Massachusetts Medical Society. Reprinted with permission

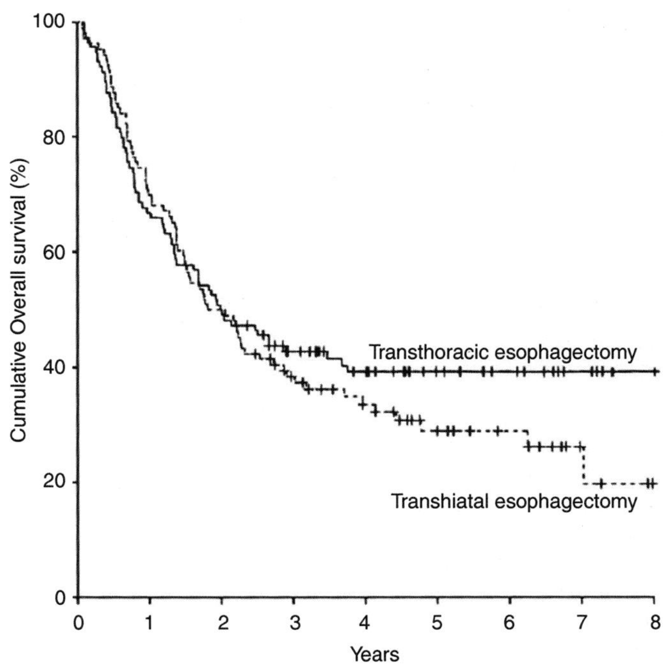

No. At Risk

Transhiatal esophagectomy	106	74	53	35	25	16	11	4
Transthoracic esophagectomy	114	76	57	42	31	20	14	7

Fig. 5.2 Kaplan Meier curves showing overall survival among patients randomly assigned to transhiatal esophagectomy or transthoracic esophagectomy with extended en bloc lymphadenectomy. From Extended transthoracic resection compared with limited transhiatal resection for adenocarcinoma of the esophagus, Hulscher JB, van Sandick JW, de Boer AGEM et al., 347. Massachusetts Medical Society. Reprinted with permission

trend toward improved long-term survival holding for the extended transthoracic approach.

The long-term follow-up of this randomized trial was published in 2007. Omloo et al., analysed a total of 95 patients who underwent a THE and 110 patients who underwent a TTE. After transhiatal and transthoracic resection, 5-years survival was 34% and 36%, respectively (p = 0.71).

5.2.3.1 Who May Benefit from TTE or THE?

In a subgroup analysis, based on the location of the primary tumour (classified after pathological examination of the resection specimen), no overall survival benefit for either surgical approach was seen in 115 patients with a type II tumour (p = 0.81). In 90 patients with a type I tumour, an absolute survival benefit of 14% was observed with the transthoracic approach (51% vs. 37%, p = 0.33). Moreover, there was evidence that depending on the number of positive lymph nodes in the resection specimen, the effect of treatment differed. In patients (n = 55) without positive nodes, the locoregional disease-free survival after THE was comparable to that of TTE (86% and 89%, respectively). A poor outcome was found for patients (n = 46) with more than eight positive lymph nodes in the resection specimen: the survival was 0% in both groups. Regarding patients (n = 104) with one to eight positive lymph nodes in the resection specimen, a 5-year locoregional disease-free survival advantage was seen for those patients operated via the transthoracic approach (64% vs. 23%, p = 0.02). The authors concluded that there is no significant overall survival benefit for either approach. However, when compared with THE, a TTE for type I esophageal cancer shows an ongoing trend towards a better 5-year survival rate. Moreover, patients with a limited number of positive lymph nodes (between one and eight) in their resection specimen also seem to benefit from TTE. In patients with a limited nodal burden, a more extensive nodal dissection may indeed cure the patient. However, when the number of positive nodes is very high, this reflects systemic disease and then more extensive surgery can not cure the patient. Moreover, in patients with a very limited nodal spread, the locoregional nodes can be removed by a THE as well as a TTE.

5.2.3.2 Post-Operative Morbidity

Most studies showed more complications for the TTE as compared to the THE. The meta-analysis of Hulscher et al. [2] showed more perioperative blood loss, pulmonary complications, chyle leakage, and wound infections in the transthoracic group. More anastomotic leakage and vocal cord paralysis were found in the transhiatal group. The in-hospital mortality rates for transthoracic resection in comparison with transhiatal were higher (9.2% vs. 5.7%, RR: 1.60, 95% confidence interval: 1.89–1.35). The question arises whether these differences still are representative because in recent years we see better patient selection, improvement of perioperative care and refinement of surgical techniques. Lacking recent RCTs we note a cohort study in 2014 by Davies et al. including 680 patients operated between 2000 and 2010, showing a shorter median hospital stay for transhiatal surgery (14 days vs. 17 days, p < 0.001). The in-hospital mortality rate also favoured THE (1.1% vs. 3.2% for THE and TTE respectively, p = 0.110). The results show a median of 20 nodes in the transthoracic group vs. 13 in the transhiatal group (p < 0.001) [12].

5.3 Minimally Invasive Esophagectomy (MIE)

Over the last decades, the safe and oncological-proficient operation termed MIE emerged. Ideally, minimally invasive techniques should be as radical as open approaches and not compromise oncological outcome [13]. It may be fair to say that during the early developmental phase of MIE a somewhat different oncological operation was performed—attributable to the enormous technical challenges and search for optimal techniques. More recent studies show, however, that indices of the number of lymph nodes dissected and surgical margins for MIE are similar or perhaps superior to open approaches. Two RCTs have been performed, one total MIE (TIME trial) and the other hybrid, in which laparoscopy and right posterolateral thoracotomy are performed with intrathoracic anastomosis (MIRO trial) [14, 15]. The long-term follow-up of the TIME trial up to 3 years posits similar survival-outcomes for the open and the MIE groups [16].

Minimally invasive esophagectomy may harbour several advantages for the surgeons as well. The developments of high definition and 3D cameras with robotic platforms offer an excellent and detailed view of the operation field. This facilitates a careful dissection along the tissue planes enabling an increased radical nodal dissection with less blood loss. Also, ergonomics of the instruments has improved and the surgeon may feel more comfortable during MIE than at open surgery. The possible advantages of robotic surgery including esophageal cancer resections seems clear but this has yet to be evidenced by the ROBOT trial, which compares the open esophageal resection vs. the laparoscopy and thoracoscopy as assisted by robot [17].

Minimally invasive surgery—especially in prone position—is technically challenging and needs careful introduction using a structured program.

5.4 Influence of Neoadjuvant Therapy

The extended use of neoadjuvant therapy changed the prognosis of the resectable esophageal cancer cure. According to the long-term outcome of the CROSS trial, a better survival after neoadjuvant chemoradiotherapy is seen for both adenocarcinoma and squamous cell cancer (Carboplatin and Paclitaxel for 5 weeks with concurrent radiotherapy, 41.4 Gy given in 23 fractions, 5 days a week). Five-year overall and progression-free survival rates were 47 and 44% in the neo-adjuvant chemoradiotherapy-plus-surgery group while in the surgery-alone group 33% and 27%, respectively. Holding for the squamous cell cancer, it was 61% vs. 30% and 58% vs. 28%; whereas in the adenocarcinomas case it was 43% vs. 33% and 41% vs. 27%, respectively [18, 19].

The dissection of lymph nodes is important for the staging of esophageal cancer and the number of dissected lymph nodes is an important predictor of survival in patients with esophageal cancer.

Based on data from the CROSS study, Talsma et al. found that in the group of patients treated by surgery alone, the number of resected lymph nodes indeed had a prognostic impact on the survival rate [20]. But the therapeutic value of lymphadenectomy is still controversial in this study after CRT because the number of resected nodes was not associated with survival. Also, a cohort study by Lagergren et al. showed no significant influence of the number of resected nodes on the 5-year survival rates (disease specific and overall) in patients with the surgery-alone group [21].

As described above, an important distinction between the outcomes of transthoracic and of transhiatal esophagectomies concerns the differences in lymph-node yield and the possible influence on locoregional recurrent disease. Moreover, given the data on the association between the number of nodes dissected after neoadjuvant chemoradiotherapy, the question arises what the best surgical approach is for Gastro-esophageal junction tumours: either the transhiatal approach with limiting morbidity and inability to dissect the nodes from the middle and upper mediastinum, or the transthoracic MIE with extended mediastinal nodal dissection. The trend in the Netherlands is to operate distal oesophageal tumours (type I) totally minimally invasive by use of thoracoscopy and laparoscopy after neoadjuvant therapy. For type II tumours (cardia cancers) many Dutch surgeons prefer a thoracoscopic or transhiatal approach by laparoscopy after neoadjuvant therapy.

Discussions concern whether to organize a new trial, one comparable with the HIVEX trial, in which patients will be treated by neoadjuvant therapy and by minimally invasive surgery. This trial is yet to be accomplished.

Conclusion

Evidence concerning which approach is the best for distal esophageal and GEJ cancers was produced by the HIVEX trial that compared the

Transhiatal vs. Transthoracic approach without neoadjuvant therapy. Given the current use of neoadjuvant therapy, there is no comparison of cohorts or of randomized studies that compare MIE THE with MIE TTE for distal or GEJ types 1 and 2 tumours after neoadjuvant therapy. Such a study is crucial for improving the treatment of the distal and GEJ cancers.

References

1. Biere SS, Cuesta MA, van der Peet DL. Minimally invasive versus open esophagectomy for cancer: a systematic review and meta-analysis. Minerva Chir. 2009;64:121–33.
2. Sgourakis G, Gockel I, Radtke A, et al. Minimally invasive versus open esophagectomy: meta-analysis of outcomes. Dig Dis Sci. 2010;55:3031–40.
3. Nagpal K, Ahmed K, Vats A, et al. Is minimally invasive surgery beneficial in the management of esophageal cancer? A meta-analysis. Surg Endosc. 2010;24:1621–9.
4. Maas KW, Biere SS, Scheepers JJ, et al. Laparoscopic versus open transhiatal esophagectomy for distal and junction cancer. Rev Esp Enferm Dig. 2012;104: 197–202.
5. Orringer MB, Marshall B, Chang AC, Lee J, Pickens A, Lau CL. Two thousand transhiatal esophagectomies: changing trends, lessons learned. Ann Surg. 2007;246:363–74.
6. Hulscher JB, Tijssen JG, Obertop H, van Lanschot JJ. Transthoracic versus transhiatal resection for carcinoma of the esophagus: a meta-analysis. Ann Thorac Surg. 2001;72:306–13.
7. Chu KM, Law SY, Fok M, Wong J. A prospective randomized comparison of transhiatal and transthoracic resection for lower-third esophageal carcinoma. Am J Surg. 1997;174:320–4.
8. Goldminc M, Maddern G, Le Prise E, et al. Oesophagectomy by a transhiatal approach or thoracotomy: a prospective randomized trial. Br J Surg. 1993;80:367–70.
9. Jacobi CA, Zieren HU, Muller JM, Pichlmaier H. Surgical therapy of esophageal carcinoma: the influence of surgical approach and esophageal resection on cardiopulmonary function. Eur J Cardiothorac Surg. 1997;11:32–7.
10. Hulscher JB, van Sandick JW, de Boer AG, et al. Extended transthoracic resection compared with limited transhiatal resection for adenocarcinoma of the esophagus. N Engl J Med. 2002;347:1662–9.
11. Omloo JMT, Lagarde SM, Hulscher JBF, et al. Extended tranthoracic resection compared with limited transhiatal resection for adenocarcinoma of the mid/distal esophagus. Ann Surg. 2007;246:992–1001.
12. Davies AR, Sandhu H, Pillai A, et al. Surgical resection strategy and the influence of radicality on outcomes in oesophageal cancer. Br J Surg. 2014;101:511–7.
13. Luketich JD, Pennathur A, Awais O, et al. Outcomes after minimally invasive esophagectomy. Review of over 1000 patients. Ann Surg. 2012;256:95–103.
14. Biere SS, van Berge Henegouwen MI, Maas KW, et al. Minimally invasive versus open oesophagectomy for patients with oesophageal cancer: a multicentre, open-label, randomised controlled trial. Lancet. 2012;379:1887–92.
15. Mariette C, Meunier B, Pezet D. Hybrid mini-invasive versus open oesophagectomy for patients with oesophageal cancer: a multicentre openlabel randomized phase III controlled trial, the MIRO trial. J Clin Oncol. 2015;33(supplement 2, abstract 5).
16. Maas KW, Cuesta MA, van Berge Henegouwen MI, et al. Quality of life and late complications after minimally invasive compared to open esophagectomy: results of a randomized trial. World J Surg. 2015;39:1986–93.
17. van der Sluis PC, Ruurda JP, van der Horst S, et al. Robot-assisted minimally invasive thoraco-laparoscopic esophagectomy versus open transthoracic esophagectomy for resectable esophageal cancer, a randomized controlled trial (ROBOT trial). Trials. 2012;13:230.
18. van Hagen P, Huslhof MC, van Lanschot JJ, et al. Preoperative chemoradiotherapy for esophageal or junctional cancer. N Engl J Med. 2012;366:2074–84.
19. Shapiro J, van Lanschot JJB, Huslhof MCCM, et al. Long-term results of a randomised controlled trial comparing neoadjuvant chemoradiotherapy plus surgery with surgery alone for oesophageal or junctional cancer (CROSS trial). Lancet Oncol. 2015;16: 1090–8.
20. Talsma KA, Shapiro J, Looman CW, et al. Lymph node retrieval during esophagectomy with and without neoadjuvant chemoradiotherapy: prognostic and therapeutic impact on survival. Ann Surg. 2014; 260:786–92.
21. Lagergren J, Mattsson F, Zylstra J, et al. Extent of lymphadenectomy and prognosis after esophageal cancer surgery. JAMA Surg. 2016;151:32–9.

6 Open or Minimally Invasive Esophagectomy After Neoadjuvant Therapy

Donald L. van der Peet, Jennifer Straatman, Nicole I. van der Wielen, and Miguel A. Cuesta

In 1991, Dallemagne introduced the right thoracoscopic approach in lateral position for esophageal cancer with total lung block, thereby mimicking the conventional approach [1]. Initial reports showed a high conversion rate to thoracotomy and a high respiratory morbidity rate. Searching for reduction of the conversion rate and the respiratory infection rate, Cuschieri et al. redesigned the thoracoscopic approach in prone decubitus position so that a total collapse of the lung was no longer necessary for dissecting the esophagus and thereby possibly reducing the rate of respiratory infections [2].

After a feasibility period, Minimally Invasive Esophagectomy (MIE) by thoracoscopy in prone or lateral decubitus position or by transhiatal approach is being widely implemented and increasingly performed all over the world for patients with resectable esophageal cancer (EC) to reduce postoperative respiratory complications and to enhance the quality of life by avoiding a right thoracotomy and laparotomy [3–5]. Other important, recent developments in esophageal surgery concern the systematic use of neoadjuvant treatment, such as the use of chemotherapy (MAGIC scheme), or chemoradiotherapy (CROSS scheme) [6, 7]. Neoadjuvant therapy for tumor stages 2 and 3 significantly increases 5-year survival of patients with esophageal cancer in both squamous cell cancer (SCC) as well as adenocarcinomas (ADC).

Current topic of discussion in the West is the extent of mediastinal lymphadenectomy. In 1994, the ISDE had defined four types of mediastinal lymphadenectomy in treating esophageal cancer (SCC) according to extent: the standard, the extended, the total mediastinal and the three-field lymphadenectomy [8]. The implementation of neoadjuvant treatment and the subsequent effects on survival rates, regardless of lymph node yield, requires a new look at mediastinal lymphadenectomy.

Minimally Invasive Esophagectomy should entail the same operation as the standard open esophageal resection with the only difference being the approach: thoraco*scopy* instead of thoraco*tomy* and laparo*scopy* instead of laparo*tomy*.

Six issues will be discussed concerning the implementation of MIE for cancer:

(1) choice of the extent of esophageal resection, and use of neoadjuvant therapy; (2) reasons to approach esophageal cancer by MIE; (3)

Electronic Supplementary Material The online version of this chapter (doi:10.1007/978-3-319-54301-7_6) contains supplementary material, which is available to authorized users. On http://springerlink.com enter the DOI number given above.

D.L. van der Peet • J. Straatman • N.I. van der Wielen
M.A. Cuesta (✉)
Department of Gastrointestinal Surgery,
VU University Medical Center,
De Boelelaan 1117, 1018 HV Amsterdam,
The Netherlands
e-mail: dl.vanderpeet@vumc.nl; ma.cuesta@vumc.nl

M.A. Cuesta (ed.), *Minimally Invasive Surgery for Upper Abdominal Cancer*,
DOI 10.1007/978-3-319-54301-7_6

determining the best Minimally Invasive approach for Gastro-Esophageal Junction (GEJ) cancers; (4) implementation of Evidence based MIE; (5) future lines of research of MIE; and (6) learning curve and teaching process [9].

6.1 The Choice of the Extent of MI Esophageal Resection and Use of Neoadjuvant Therapy

Based on information gathered in Japan about the frequency and localization of lymph node metastases according to tumor location [10] and the evidence obtained by Randomized Controlled Trials (RCT) [11], middle and upper esophageal cancers should be approached by a three-stage McKeown operation with total mediastinal lymphadenectomy (LN) with a cervical anastomosis after neoadjuvant therapy. In cases of lower esophageal and GEJ, Siewert 1 and 2, a transhiatal approach or a two-stage Ivor Lewis operation is performed, with standard LN with intrathoracic anastomosis after neoadjuvant therapy [12]. If there is suspicion of enlarged lymph nodes by PET CT-scan in the paratracheal area in these distal tumors, mostly ADC, lymphadenectomy of these areas is also added. In high-risk patients with distal or GEJ cancers, the transhiatal approach might be opted for (Video 6.1).

6.2 Reasons to Approach the Esophageal Cancer by MIE

Minimally invasive esophagectomy is associated with less operative trauma and consequently less morbidity. Performing a thoracoscopy avoids a thoracotomy. Fewer pulmonary complications are reported in comparison to an open procedure, possibly even less pulmonary complications are seen if complete lung block is omitted, as done in thoracoscopy in prone position. In laparoscopic transhiatal dissection, the operation is performed under direct vision and probably with less manipulation and retraction of the mediastinum (heart) and therefore less hemodynamic complications. It will add to a better quality of life and perhaps a better survival in the era of neoadjuvant treatment [13–18].

All surgical approaches used for open esophagectomy have been implemented for MIE. The transhiatal approach, the three-stage esophageal resection (McKeown procedure), the two stage Ivor Lewis operation, the thoracoscopy in prone position and the esophageal resection facilitated by robot (RAMIE) [1–5, 19–22].

6.3 Determining the Best Minimally Invasive Approach for Gastro-Esophageal Junction (GEJ) Cancers

Gastroesophageal junction adenocarcinomas account for 30–40% of all esophageal cancers in the West. The Siewert classification—accepting its limitations—is used to locate these tumors [12]. Based on localization neoadjuvant treatment regimens and surgical strategies are determined, with most oncologists prescribing neoadjuvant chemotherapy instead of chemoradiotherapy for type 2 and 3 tumors. Type 1 is located mainly on the side of the esophagus, type 3 on the subcardial side of the stomach and type 2 at the gastric cardia. Siewert type 3 tumors are treated with a laparoscopic total gastrectomy. Siewert type 2 tumors, may be treated by an MIE Ivor Lewis procedure or a laparoscopic total gastrectomy, extended to the distal esophagus, in order to achieve a R0 resection, followed by an esophagogastrotomy. Anastomosis between distal esophagus and jejunum may be performed with the Orvil® or a linear stapler anastomosis through the transhiatal approach. Some surgeons prefer a laparoscopic transhiatal esophageal resection with gastric conduit anastomosis in cervical area. In the case of extensive growth of the tumor along the lesser curvature an open esophageal and gastric resection is performed followed by a colon interposition. Finally for Siewert type 1 tumors, a MIE Ivor Lewis procedure is advised.

The Ivor Lewis approach with intrathoracic anastomosis is a perfect operation for many infracarinal esophageal cancers [23, 24]. Whilst textbook, it is an operation with a high difficulty grade because of the intrathoracic anastomosis. The operation commences with laparoscopy (celiac trunk lymphadenectomy, gastric dissection, creation of a gastric conduit and hiatal dissection) followed by right thoracoscopy (esophageal resection and lymphadenectomy) and intrathoracic anastomosis through thoracoscopy. While there are different types of intrathoracic anastomosis, nonetheless no evidence posits one as graded superior to the other.

In overview, we have the manual anastomosis or an end-to-side anastomosis with a conventional circular stapler (21, 25 or 28 mm after a pursestring suture on the esophageal stump or a prepared Orvil device®). A side-to-side anastomosis can be performed using a linear stapler, closing the anterior defect by a transversal suture using conventional suture material or the prepared V-Lock® suture [25]. Finally the robot-assisted anastomosis is increasingly used permitting a manual high anastomosis in the apex of the thorax because of the ergonomy obtained by the robot [26].

In the Netherlands, anastomotic leaks after MIE Ivor Lewis had initially been reported as high as 14%, subsequently reduced to current rates holding between 5 and 10% with a 30-days mortality of 2.1%. Surgeons must adhere to a proper algorithm for treating these postoperative anastomotic leaks as early as possible, thereby following the maxim that: "Patients who do not progress every day should be studied immediately by CT-scan and endoscopy for assessment of the anastomosis".

6.4 Implementation of Evidence Based MIE

Minimally invasive techniques for esophagectomy have been implemented all over the world. In 2015, using the Medline database we located 748 papers on MIE esophagectomy and 478 for specifically thoracoscopic esophagectomy. There are four meta-analyses and one randomized controlled trial, being the TIME trial, which compared the total MIE by thoracoscopy in prone and laparoscopy versus the total open approach [13, 27–31]. The outcome of the hybrid MIRO hybrid trial comparing laparoscopy and thoracotomy with intrathoracic anastomosis versus open approach will be extensively presented elsewhere in this book. The most important outcome of this randomized trial, that compares patients to hybrid MIE (laparoscopy with right thoracotomy) or open intervention followed by intrathoracic anastomosis showed a significant reduction in major morbidity and pulmonary complications in favor of the hybrid group. Mortality was found the same in both studied groups [32].

Until 2006, the two most important large series of MIE (the Luketich's series published in 2003 with patients operated by thoracoscopy in lateral position (222 patients), and the Palanivelu's series of 130 patients operated in thoracoscopic prone position) were compared with Hulscher's series of patients who underwent open esophagectomy via a transthoracic approach in lateral decubitus (114 patients). Comparing these series, overall survival rates are reported at 3 years of 34%, 42% and 40% respectively. Moreover, the comparative rates of pulmonary complications were 20%, 2,3% and 57% respectively; while the comparative rates of median Intensive Care stay were 1 day, 1 day and 6 days respectively; and a hospital stay of 7, 8 and 19 days respectively [3, 4, 11].

These striking differences called for evidence-based analysis of effectiveness. Therefore, from 2010 to 2012 the TIME trial was performed in our department. This was a multicentre, open-label randomized controlled trial [31] comparing thoracoscopy in prone position plus laparoscopy versus right posterolateral thoracotomy and laparotomy followed by intrathoracic or cervical anastomosis after neoadjuvant therapy. Characteristics of patients are depicted in Table 6.1. Primary end point of the trial was determining the rates of respiratory infections in the first 2 weeks and in-hospital stay, while the secondary end points were the quality of the specimen and Quality of life (QoL). Alongside analysis was conducted for hospital stay, operative data, postoperative data, complication rate, mortality rates and survival rates.

Table 6.1 Baseline demographic and clinical characteristics in the intention-to-treat groups

	MI esophagectomy	Open esophagectomy	
	N = 59	N = 56	p-value
Age (years), mean ± SD	61.8 ± 8.4	62.3 ± 8.4	0.772
Gender, N (%)			0.270
Male	43 (72.9%)	46 (82.1%)	
Female	16 (27.1%)	10 (17.9%)	
ASA classification (N)			0.454
I	10	15	
II	34	32	
III	14	8	
IV	1	1	
BMI (kg/m^2), mean ± SD	24.5 ± 3.6	24 ± 3.8	0.463
Previous surgery	31 (53%)	29 (52%)	0.588
Type of carcinoma			0.468
Adenocarcinoma	35 (59%)	36 (64%)	
Squamous cell carcinoma	24 (41%)	19 (34%)	
Other	0 (0%)	1 (2%)	
Location of tumour			0.529
Upper third	1 (2%)	3 (5%)	
Middle third	26 (44%)	22 (39%)	
Lower third or gastro-esophageal junction	32 (54%)	31 (55%)	
Neoadjuvant treatment			0.533
Chemoradiotherapy	52 (93%)	54 (92%)	
Chemotherapy alone	4 (7%)	5 (8%)	

Concerning the primary outcome, a statistical difference in incidence of postoperative pulmonary infections within 2 weeks and in hospital was found of 9% and 12% versus 29% and 34% respectively in favor of the MIE group. Concerning the secondary outcomes, hospital stay was statistically different (11 and 14 days) in favor of the MIE; but also differences were observed in the QoL questionnaires (the SF-36 physical component), EORTC C30 (global health) and OES 18 (taking and pain) were found at 2 weeks after operation in favor of MIE. Moreover other outcomes such as the total of retrieved lymph nodes, the rate of R0 resection (98% and 90%), and the in-hospital mortality rates (3.4% and 1.8%) were not statistically different between the two groups. Other outcomes, such as operative time, were shorter in the open group whereas blood loss and the VAS score were less in MIE group. Importantly, the outcomes of technical complications such as anastomotic leakage and thoracic complications were not different between the groups, whilst the only exception being incidence of vocal cord palsy that showed an initial difference of 2% versus 14% in favor of the MIE group (Table 6.2). Explanation for this outcome is difficult but has to be sought in the spreading of CO_2 from the thorax in the cervical area creating a better plane for dissection. The rates of reoperations (14 and 10%, respectively) were no different between the two groups. Moreover, at 1-year follow up there were no differences in overall and disease-free survival rates between the two groups (around 75%) (Fig. 6.1), yet the QoL questionnaires point out some differences at the 1-year follow up. The global health, the pain and the physical component of the SF-36 were still statistically different after 1 year in favor of the MIE intervention (Table 6.3)). Explanation for this is obtained by the advantage of avoidance of the thoracotomy with prevention of the postthoracotomy syndrome

[33]. Analysis of 3 year overall and disease free survival show no differences between the two groups (Fig. 6.2).

Different MIE definitions and approaches are available: (a) the lateral thoracoscopic position, the prone position and the semiprone position [1, 2]; (b) the Hybrid MIE type 1 in which a laparoscopy is combined with a right thoracotomy as seen in the MIRO trial [32], (c) the hybrid MIE 2 that combines a thoracoscopy and the laparotomy [14], and (d) the robot-assisted (RAMIE) thoracoscopy with standard laparoscopy [22].

Important study has been done in USA where Luketich et al. has published a prospective phase II multicenter trial by the Eastern cooperative oncology group [34]. The aim of the study has been to assess the feasibility of MIE in a multi-institutional setting. Seventeen credential sites

Table 6.2 Short term results of open versus minimally invasive esophagectomy as recorded in the TIME trial

	MI esophagectomy N = 59	Open esophagectomy N = 56	p-value
Duration of surgery (min), mean ± SD	326 ± 70	295 ± 75	0.023
Abdominal phase	148 ± 57	129 ± 81	0.172
Thoracic phase	127 ± 41	97 ± 48	0.001
Blood loss (mL), median (IQR)*	200 (100–300)	475 (300–588)	<0.001
Conversion (N)	8		
Morbidity			
Pulmonary complications	7	19	0.005
Anastomotic leak	7	4	0.39
Reoperations	8	6	0.641
30-day mortality	1	0	0.329

*Interquartile range

Table 6.3 One year results comparing minimally invasive and open esophagectomy, as performed in the randomized clinical trial: the TIME trial

	MI esophagectomy	Open esophagectomy	P-value
Mortality	76%	68%	0.167
EORTC C30			
Overall score			
Preop	66 (22; 60–72)	63 (23; 56–70)	0.631
6 weeks	61 (18; 56–67)	51 (21; 44–58)	0.020
1 year	79 (10; 76–83)	67 (21; 60–75)	0.004
EORTC OES 18			
Talking			
Preop	5 (12; 1–9)	13 (26; 4–21)	0.745
6 weeks	18 (26; 10–26)	37 (39; 25–49)	0.008
1 year	5 (14; 0–11)	10 (21; 3–18)	0.288
Pain			
Preop	15 (23; 8–23)	22 (23; 15–30)	0.189
6 weeks	8 (11; 5–11)	19 (21; 13–26)	0.002
1 year	6 (9; 2–8)	16 (16; 10–22)	0.001

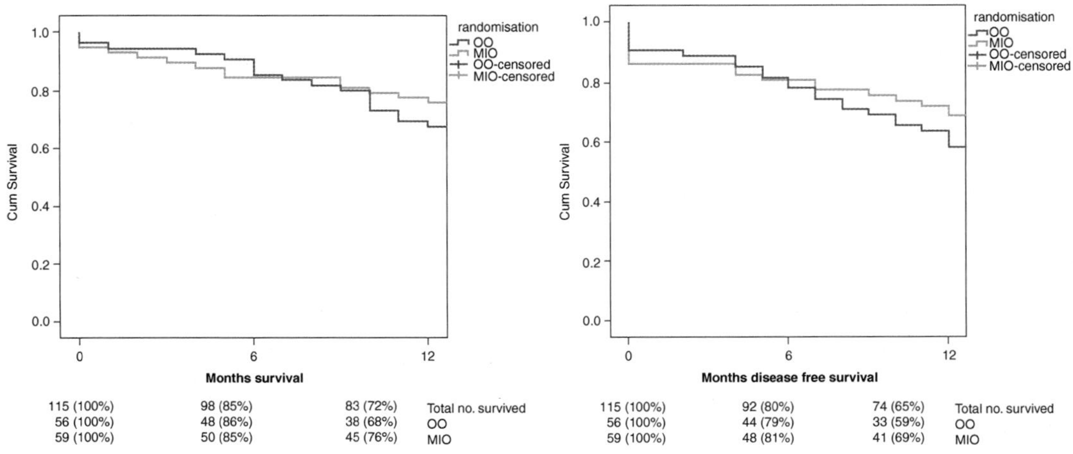

Fig. 6.1 Overall and disease free survival after 1 year

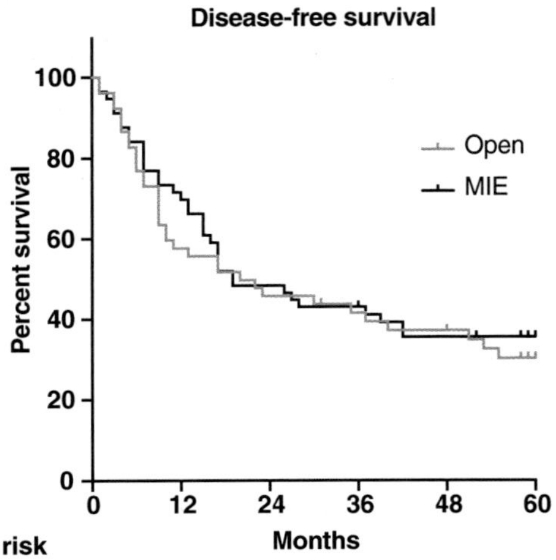

No at risk						
Open	54	30	24	20	17	9
MIE	57	40	29	24	21	16
Total	111	70	53	44	38	25

Fig. 6.2 Disease free survival after 3 years

have enrolled 95 patients for stage 3 or 2 MIE. Thirty day and perioperative mortality has been 2.1% and 2.9% respectively, whereas the IC and hospital stay were 2 and 9 days respectively. Concerning the complications, anastomotic leak was found in 8.6% and respiratory complications in 9.5% (ARDS in 5.7% and pneumonitis in 3.8%). At a median follow up of 35.8 months the estimated 3 year overall survival was 58.4% with a locoregional recurrence of 6.7%. They concluded that this multicenter study has demonstrated that MIE is feasible and safe with good oncological results. This approach can be adopted by other centers with appropriate expertise in open esophagectomy and minimally invasive surgery.

A large controlled cohort study from China compared 735 patients with squamous cell esophageal cancer treated with MIE with 652 propensity-matched patients treated with open esophagectomy. They showed that short term outcome such as postoperative complications, median hospital stay and readmission rate to Intensive Care was significantly lower in favor of the MIE group. Moreover lymph nodes retrieved and perioperative mortality (1.1% versus 2%) were not different between the two groups [35].

Concerning the semiprone position as proposed in Japan, this seems an important addition to the standard prone approach. This includes the possibility to balance the patient from prone to right semi lateral position in order to better visualize the supracarinal area and do a better lymphadenectomy along both recurrent laryngeal nerves [36]. Concerning the thoracoscopy in prone approach there are some differences in the position of trocars between Asian and Western world surgeons. The first positions the trocars anteriorly of the scapula adding mostly a small thoracotomy for retraction, whereas the second positions the trocars posteriorly, between the scapula and the spine, adding only a small thoracotomy at the end of the procedure for retrieval of the specimen and introduction of the circular stapler in the case of Ivor Lewis operation.

Differences between the lateral and prone position show that, while in the prone position single intubation with two lung ventilation is appropriate in the case of cervical anastomosis (we use an insufflation of 7–8 mmHg CO_2 for helping retraction of the lung), in the lateral position a double lumen selective intubation (one lung ventilation) is usually used. Question arise if prone position is good enough whether a urgent conversion to thoracotomy is needed because of bleeding. Sufficient experience assures that conversion may be effectively performed equally in both positions.

Differences between surgery in prone and lateral position have been studied by Kubo et al. with two cohorts of 28 patients in lateral and 30 in prone position. Blood loss and duration of systemic inflammatory response were significantly better in the prone group, with a tendency of the respiratory complications to be also lower in the prone group. Their conclusion was that while thoracoscopy in lateral position was safe and feasible, the prone position might be a potentially less invasive procedure than the lateral position [37].

The FREGAT French group compared the 30-day postoperative mortality (POM) between two important cohorts of patients (663 MIE and 2346 open esophagectomy patients) of the French register. Thirty-day postoperative mortality was 3.3% versus 5.7%, the in-hospital mortality 5.6% versus 8.1% and at 90-day mortality 6.9% and 10%. This study suggests that POM is significantly reduced after MIE for EC. This is highly valuable evidence for aiding in decision-making regarding an optimal (hybrid 1 MIE) approach [38].

Concerning long-term survival, the above-mentioned TIME trial 3 year outcome showed no differences in survival between the MIE and the open esophagectomy indicate that the MIE approach is oncological safe.

6.5 Future Lines of Research of MIE

There are some ongoing RCT's such as the ROBOT trial that compares the open esophagectomy with the thoracoscopic approach assisted by the robot [39], but also RCT's that will compare the MIE with the open and hybrid approaches. In the UK and in Japan surgeons still harbor doubts about the advantages of MIE, therefore three new trials have been started. In the UK, the ROMIO trial with three arms: the MIE, the hybrid 1 and the open [40]. In Japan surgeons are comparing the prone position with the open esophagectomy [41] and in China an RCT is currently being initiated to compare lateral MIE with the open approach.

Looking for safety and evidence of MIE Ivor Lewis the ICAN trial has started in the Netherlands comparing the MIE followed by intrathoracic or cervical anastomosis for esophageal cancer. Two-hundred patients will be included in which the primary outcome is the anastomotic leakage requiring intervention or reoperation and the secondary outcomes the peroperative data including QoL and cost-effectiveness [42].

6.6 Learning Process

To initiate teaching of the MIE approach, surgeons of a designated proctored Upper GI group will need to have access to an adequate volume of patients with EC and have gained enough experience in open esophagectomy and minimally invasive surgery. Moreover, with the approval of the direction of the hospital and the department they have to organize a dedicated team (at least with two surgeons, a dedicated anesthesiologist and scrub nurses) and visit a center of excellence to learn how this type of intervention has to be performed. Consequently, apprentice surgeons, will under the guidance of an authorized mentor need to be monitored while carrying out several MIE procedures in their own hospital. Furthermore, centralization policy is mandatory in order to stimulate a better care of patients with esophageal cancer, and at the same time to improve the surgeon's expertise. In the Netherlands a Surgical Department has to perform every year at least 20 esophageal resections (and 20 gastric resections) in order to continue with this surgical program. This centralization policy has increased the expertise, and the quality of surgery but also the quality of esophageal studies. A cooperative Upper GI group is organized in order to care for patients and quality of surgery [43].

Conclusion

Minimally invasive esophagectomy in the era of neoadjuvant therapy has resulted in important advantages, such as a lower incidence of pulmonary infections, whilst maintaining similar results for completeness of resection. Quality of life scores are improved following minimally invasive esophagectomy, from the early postoperative phase up to 1 year after surgery. Survival rates are similar for open and MIE, with a follow-up up to 3 years.

Current research and randomized clinical trials focus on determining the optimal surgical strategy in established practice. Further studies will determine significant improvements in reducing morbidity and increasing the benefits of the intrathoracic anastomosis.

In the time of imaging-integrated surgery it is clear that the MIE approach should be increasingly implemented in all centers worldwide having an adequate volume of patients and expertise.

References

1. Dallemagne B, Weerts JM, Jehaes C. Thoracoscopic esophageal resection. In: Cuesta MA, Nagy AG, editors. Minimally invasive surgery in gastrointestinal cancer. Edingburgh: Churchill Livingstone; 1993. p. 59–68.
2. Cuschieri A. Thoracoscopic subtotal esophagectomy. Endosc Surg Allied Technol. 1994;2:21–5.
3. Luketich JD, Alvelo-Rivera M, Buenaventura PO, et al. Minimally invasive esophagectomy: outcomes in 222 patients. Ann Surg. 2003;238:486–94.
4. Palanivelu C, Prakash A, Senthilkumar R, et al. Minimally invasive esophagectomy: thoracoscopic mobilization of the esophagus and mediastinal lymphadenectomy in prone position-experience of 130 patients. J Am Coll Surg. 2006;2013:7–16.
5. Scheepers JJ, Veenhof XA, van der Peet DL, et al. Laparoscopic transhiatal resection for malignancies of the distal esophagus: outcome of the first 50 resected patients. Surgery. 2008;143:278–85.
6. Cunningham D, Allum WH, Stenning SP, et al. Perioperative chemotherapy versus surgery alone for resectable gastroesophageal cancer. N Engl J Med. 2006;355:11–20.
7. Van Hagen P, Huslhof MC, van Lanschot JJ, et al. Preoperative chemoradiotherapy for esophageal or junctional cancer. N Engl J Med. 2012;366:2074–84.
8. Bumm R, Wong J. More or less surgery for esophageal cancer: extent of lymphadenectomy for squamous cell carcinoma-how much is necessary? Dis Esophagus. 1994;7:151–5.
9. Cuesta MA, van der Wielen N, Straatman J, van der Peet DL. Video-assisted thoracoscopic esophagectomy: keynote lecture. Gen Thorac Cardiovasc Surg. 2016;64:380–5.
10. Akiyama H, Tsurumaru M, Ono Y, et al. Background of lymph node dissection for squamous cell carcinoma of the esophagus. In: Sato T, Lizukan T, editors. Color atlas of surgical anatomy for esophageal cancer. Tokyo: Springer; 1992. p. 9–24.
11. Hulscher JBF, van Sandick JW, de Boer AGEM, et al. Extended transthoracic resection compared with limited transhiatal resection for adenocarcinoma of the esophagus. N Engl J Med. 2002;347:1662–9.
12. Siewert JR, Stein HJ. Carcinoma of the cardia: carcinoma of the gastroesophageal junction. Classification, pathology and extent of resection. Dis Esophagus. 1996;9:173–82.
13. Biere SSAY, Cuesta MA, van der Peet DL. Minimally invasive versus open esophagectomy for cancer: a systematic review and meta-analysis. Minerva Chir. 2009;64:121–33.
14. Osugi H, Takemura M, Higashino M, et al. A comparison of video-assisted thoracoscopic oesophagectomy and radical lymph node dissection for squamous cell cancer of the oesophagus with open operation. Br J Surg. 2003;90:108–13.
15. Taguchi S, Osugi H, Hirashino M, et al. Comparison of three-field esophagectomy for esophageal cancer incorporating open or thoracoscopic thoracotomy. Surg Endosc. 2003;17:1445–50.
16. Gemmill EH, McCulloch P. Systematic review of minimally invasive resection for gastro-oesophageal cancer. Br J Surg. 2007;94:1461–7.
17. Smithers BM, Gotley DC, Martin I, Thomas JM. Comparison of the outcomes between open and minimally invasive esophagectomy. Ann Surg. 2007;245:232–40.
18. Maas KW, Biere SS, van Hoogstraten IM, et al. Immunological changes after minimally invasive or conventional esophageal resection for cancer: a randomized trial. World J Surg. 2014;38:131–7.
19. Cuesta MA, van der Peet DL, Biere SSAY, Scheepers JJG, Heijnen BHM. Laparoscopic transhiatal esophagectomy. In: Puntambeker S, Cuesta MA, editors. Atlas of minimally invasive surgery in esophageal carcinoma. London: Springer; 2010. p. 171–89.
20. Cuesta MA, Scheepers JJG, Oosterhuis W, Biere SSAY, van der Peet DL, Heijnen BHM. Thoracoscopic esophageal resection for cancer in prone decubitus position: operative technique. In: Puntambeker S, Cuesta MA, editors. Atlas of minimally invasive surgery in esophageal carcinoma. London: Springer; 2010. p. 149–69.
21. Cadiere GB, Dapri G, Himpens J, et al. Ivor |Lewis esophagectomy with manual esofagogastric anastomosis by thoracoscopic in prone position and laparoscopy. Surg Endosc. 2010;24:1482–5.
22. Van der Sluis PC, Ruurda JP, Verhage RJ, et al. Oncologic long-term results of robotic assisted minimally invasive thoraco-laparoscopic esophagectomy with two field lymphadenectomy for esophageal cancer. Ann Surg Oncol. 2015;22(Suppl 3):1350–6.
23. Lewis I. The surgical treatment of carcinoma of the oesophagus with special reference to a new operation for growths of the middle third. Br J Surg. 1946;34:18–31.
24. Luketich JD, Pennathur A, Awais O, et al. Outcomes after minimally invasive esophagectomy. Review of over 1000 patients. Ann Surg. 2012;256:95–103.
25. Maas KW, Biere SSAY, Scheepers JJG, et al. Minimally invasive intrathoracic anastomosis after Ivor Lewis esophagectomy for cancer. A review of transoral or transthoracic use of staplers. Surg Endosc. 2012;26:1795–802.
26. Diez del Val I, Loureiro C, McCulloch P. The IDEAL prospective development study format for reporting surgical innovations. An illustrative case study of robotic oesophagectomy. Int J Surg. 2015;19:104–11.
27. Verhage RJ, Hazebroek EJ, Boone J, et al. Minimally invasive surgery compared to open procedures in esophagectomy for cancer: a systematic review of the literature. Minerva Chir. 2009;64:135–46.
28. Sgourakis G, Gockel I, Radtke A, et al. Minimally invasive versus open esophagectomy: meta-analysis of outcomes. Dig Dis Sci. 2010;55:3031–40.

29. Nagpal K, Ahmed K, Vats A, et al. Is minimally invasive surgery beneficial in the management of esophageal cancer ? A meta-analysis. Surg Endosc. 2010;24:1621–9.
30. Biere SSAY, Maas KW, Cuesta MA, van der Peet DL. Cervical or thoracic anastomosis after esophagectomy for cancer: a systematic review and meta-analysis. Dig Surg. 2011;28:29–35.
31. SSAY B, van Berge Henegouwen MI, Maas KW, et al. Minimally invasive versus open esophagectomy for patients with esophageal cancer: a multicentre, open –label, randomised controlled trial. Lancet. 2012;379:1887–92.
32. Mariette C, Meunier B, Pezet D, et al. Hybrid mini-invasive versus open oesophagectomy for patients with oesophageal cancer: a multicentre open label randomized phase III controlled trial, the MIRO trial. J Clin Oncol. 2015;33(suppl 2, abstract 5).
33. Maas KW, Cuesta MA, van Berge Henegouwen MI, et al. Quality of life and late complications after minimally invasive compared to open esophagectomy: results of a randomized trial. World J Surg. 2015;39:1986–93.
34. Luketich JD, Pennathur A, Franchetti Y, et al. Minimally invasive esophagectomy: results of prospective phase II multicenter trial-the eastern cooperative oncology group (E2202) study. Ann Surg. 2015;261:702–7.
35. Wang H, Shen Y, Feng M, et al. Outcomes, quality of life, and survival after esophagectomy for squamous cell carcinoma: a propensity score-matched comparison of operative approaches. J Thorac Cardiovasc Surg. 2015;149:1006–14.
36. Kawakubo H, Takeuchi H, Kitagawa Y. Current status and future perspectives on minimally invasive esophagectomy. Korean J Thorac Cardiovasc Surg. 2013;46:241–8.
37. Kubo N, Ohira M, Yamashita Y, et al. Thoracoscopic esophagectomy in the prone position versus in the lateral position for patients with esophageal cancer: a comparison of short term surgical results. Surg Laparosc Endosc Percutan Tech. 2014;24:158–63.
38. Messager M, Pasquer A, Duhamel A, et al. Laparoscopic gastric mobilization reduces postoperative mortality after esophageal cancer surgery: A French Nationwide Study. Ann Surg. 2015;262:817–23.
39. van der Sluis PC, Ruurda JP, van der Horst S, et al. Robot-assisted minimally invasive thoraco-laparoscopic esophagectomy versus open transthoracic esophagectomy for resectable esophageal cancer, a randomized controlled trial (ROBOT trial). Trials. 2012;13:230. doi:10.1186/1745-6215-13-230.
40. Avery KN, Metcalfe C, Berrisford R, et al. The feasibility of a randomized controlled trial of esophagectomy for esophageal cancer- the Romio (Randomized Oesophagectomy: Minimally Invasive or Open) study: protocol for a randomized controlled trial. Trials. 2014;15:200.
41. Kataoka K, Takeuchi H, Mizusawa J, et al. A randomized phase III trial of thoracoscopic versus open esophagectomy for thoracic esophageal cancer: Japan Clinical Oncology Group Study JCOG 1409. Jpn J Clin Oncol. 2016;46:174–7.
42. Van Workum F, Bouwense SA, Luyer MD, et al. Intrathoracic versus cervical anastomosis after minimally invasive esophagectomy for esophageal cancer: study protocol of the ICAN randomized controlled trial. Trials. 2016;17(1):505.
43. Cuesta MA, van der Wielen N, Straatman J, van der Peet DL. Mastering minimally invasive esophagectomy requires a mentor; experience of a personal mentorship. Ann Med Surg. 2016;13:38–41.

7 Thoracoscopic Radical Esophagectomy for Cancer

Harushi Osugi, Kousuke Narumiya, and Kenji Kudou

Since the first report by Dallemagne regarding the left lateral position in 1991 and by Cuschieri regarding the prone position in 1992, the minimally invasive oesphagectomy treatment for cancer has gradually become popular and now is being performed widely. For oesophageal cancer, the same quality of mediastinal dissection as evidenced by open surgery should be achievable through thoracoscopy. Upon learning the technique, the previously undescribed fine anatomy called microanatomy could lead to a magnified view through the camera at close vicinity to the dissection; hence, the thoracoscopic surgeon's knowledge of the layer structure in the mediastinum became profounder. The proper dissection along the anatomical layer minimizes the tissue damage, bleeding and duration of the procedure, without oncological compromise. Reducing surgical damage in the mediastinum by the rational dissection along the anatomical layers has become the important factor in minimally invasive surgery together with reducing the thoracic wound.

Three field lymphadenectomy has been performed routinely since mid-1980s in Japan [1], but the extent of lymph node dissection is still issue of discussion, regarding the variations of the extended, the total mediastinal or the three-field lymphadenectomy is still in discussion. However, the precision of the dissection has not been established because of difficulties in its scientific evaluation. According to the Efficacy Index [the incidence of metastasis to a region (%), multiplied by the 5-year survival rate (%) of patients with metastasis to that region and divided by 100] [2], the bilateral recurrent nodes and tracheobronchial nodes should be dissected precisely, although dissection of these nodes will require substantial effort by surgeons and associated with the risk of postoperative complications. The sensitivity for diagnosing the presence of metastasis in each lymph node station is low [3]. Therefore when retrieving only nodes likely being metastasized, is no excuse for omitting dissection of these nodes. Moreover neoadjuvant therapy is widely used to improve patient survival. The Japanese guideline recom-

Electronic Supplementary Material The online version of this chapter (doi:10.1007/978-3-319-54301-7_7) contains supplementary material, which is available to authorized users. On http://springerlink.com enter the DOI number given above.

H. Osugi (✉) • K. Narumiya • K. Kudou
Department of Surgery, Institute of Gastroenterology, Tokyo Women's Medical University,
8-1 Kawada-Cho, Sinju-ku 162-8666, Japan
e-mail: osugi.harushi@twmu.ac.jp

M.A. Cuesta (ed.), *Minimally Invasive Surgery for Upper Abdominal Cancer*,
DOI 10.1007/978-3-319-54301-7_7

mending neoadjuvant chemotherapy for the patients with resectable tumor and nodal involvement constitutes a response to the result of JCOG9907 study [4, 5]. Therefore, Japanese surgeons are privileged to perform oesphagectomy in patients without radiotherapy treatment. In this chapter, microanatomy, which is essential for precise dissection through thoracoscopy, will be demonstrated in patients without mediastinal fibrosis as caused by neoadjuvant treatment, especially radiation. As the left-lateral position has been the preferred approach since introduction of thoracoscopy in 1995 at our institute [6], the figures are obtained for the left-lateral patients (the upper and left is the ventral and cranial, respectively). So, in order to adapt to the monitor image in the prone position of the patients, the figures should be rotated 90° to the right.

7.1 Thoracoscopic Mediastinal Dissection

7.1.1 Layer Structures and Principle of Dissection in the Mediastinum

Figure 7.1 demonstrates the layer structure of the mediastinum cranial to the aortic arch. The most outer structures under the mediastinal pleura forms the neural branches. The sympathetic branches from the right trunk dominate over the left and surround the oesophagus and thoracic duct. Thick black arrows indicate our dissecting layer for total mobilization in the upper mediastinum. Figure 7.2 demonstrates the layer

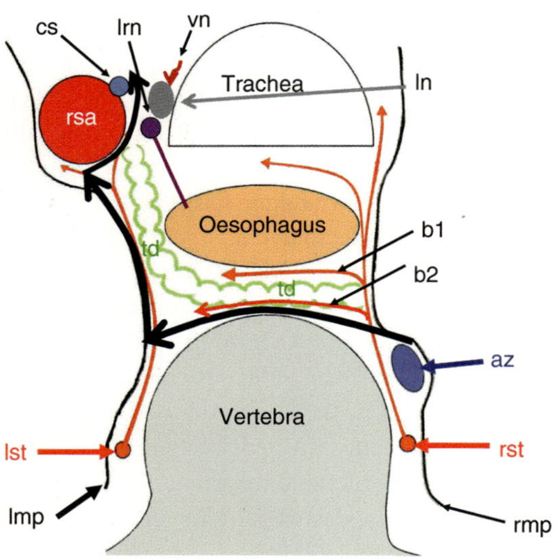

Fig. 7.1 Illustration of the anatomy, cranial to the aortic arch. *Black heavy arrows* indicate dissecting layers for the total mobilization in the upper mediastinum. The sympathetic branches from the right trunk dominate over the left and surround the thoracic duct. *rmp* right mediastinal pleura, *lmp* left mediastinal pleura, *rst* right trunk of the sympathetic nerve (b1 is the branch between the oesophagus and thoracic duct and the landmark of dissection when the thoracic duct is preserved; b2 are the branches that surround the thoracic duct and are divided for total mediastinal mobilization), *lst* left trunk of the sympathetic nerve, *az* azygos vein, *td* thoracic duct, *rsa* right subclavian artery, *cs* cardiac branches of the sympathetic nerve from the cervical ganglion, *lrn* left recurrent nerve, *ln* nodes along the left recurrent nerve, *vn* vessels of the left recurrent nodes (commonly present in front of the node)

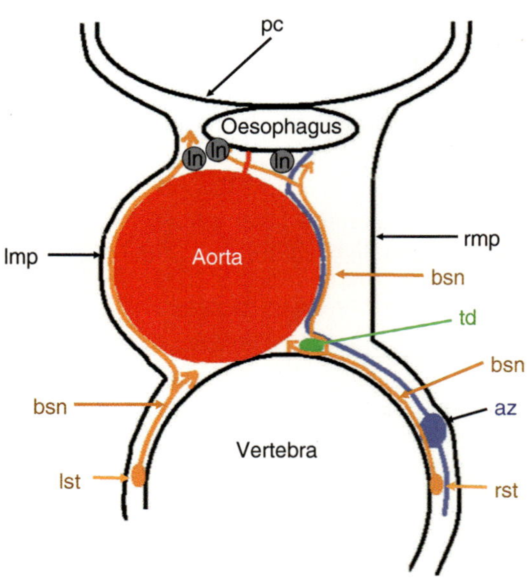

Fig. 7.2 Illustration of the anatomy, caudal to the pulmonary hilum. *rst* right trunk of sympathetic nerve, *lst* left trunk of sympathetic nerve, *bsn* branches from trunk of sympathetic nerve, *td* thoracic duct, *rmp* right mediastinal pleura, *lmp* left mediastinal pleura, *pc* pericardium, *ln* lymp nodes along the aorta and oesophagus (the most left nodes, can be dissected through right transthoracic approach, present at the angle between the fibrous membrane on the aorta and left mediastinal pleura)

structure of the mediastinum caudal to the pulmonary hilum. The most outer structure under the mediastinal pleura forms the neural branches from the sympathetic trunks and the right branches dominantly encase the oesophagus. Almost all structures divided during the mediastinal dissection run transversally—except the oesophagus, vagal nerves, and thoracic duct. Therefore, mobilization should be done transversally or orthogonally to the aorta and the tracheobronchus. After identifying structures under magnified view, the neural branches are then divided without sealing in order to avoid overuse of energy devices and unnecessary tissue damage. Under magnified view, the epineurium of the recurrent and vagal nerves can be identified easily as part of a shiny fine membrane with fine vessels running longitudinally (Fig. 7.3). As no vessel penetrates the epineurium in the dissection field, hence exposing the epineurium is the ideal layer of dissection. Under the magnified view, the structure of lymph node becomes obvious. Histologically, the lymph node has only the afferent lymphatics on the convex capsule (Fig. 7.4), and only at the hilum receives the artery and the vasoacting unmyelinated nerve and gives off the vein and efferent lymphatic vessel (Fig. 7.5). These hilar structures fix the lymph nodes. In another words each node has its own direction of hilar fixing. Understanding the direction of the fixation does facilitate nodal dissection (Figs. 7.6 and 7.7).

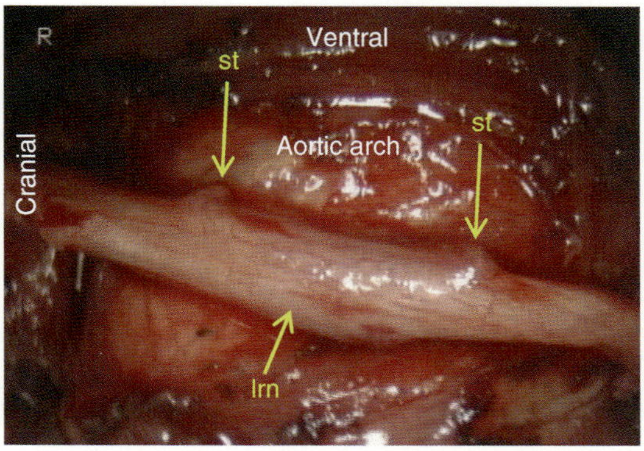

Fig. 7.3 Epineurium of the left recurrent nerve. Under magnified view, the glossy appearance with the fine vessels running longitudinally can be recognized. No vessel penetrates the epineurium in the dissection field. *lrn* left recurrent nerve, *st* stump of nerve's branches

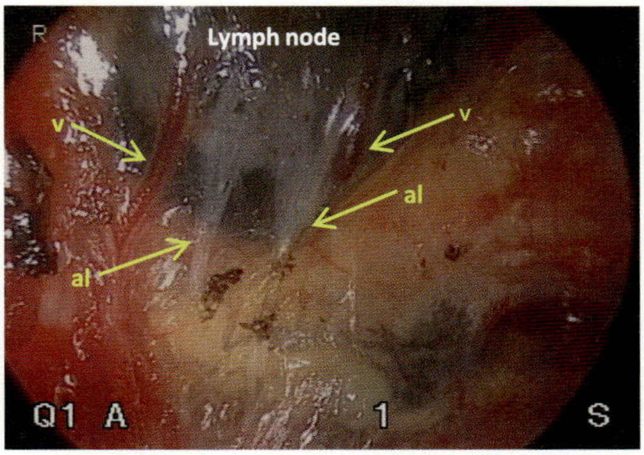

Fig. 7.4 Magnified view of lymph nodes with anthracosis and its vessels. *v* fine vein of the lymph node, *al* afferent lymphatic of the lymph node. Under magnified view, even the thickness of the vein and lymphatic can be comparable

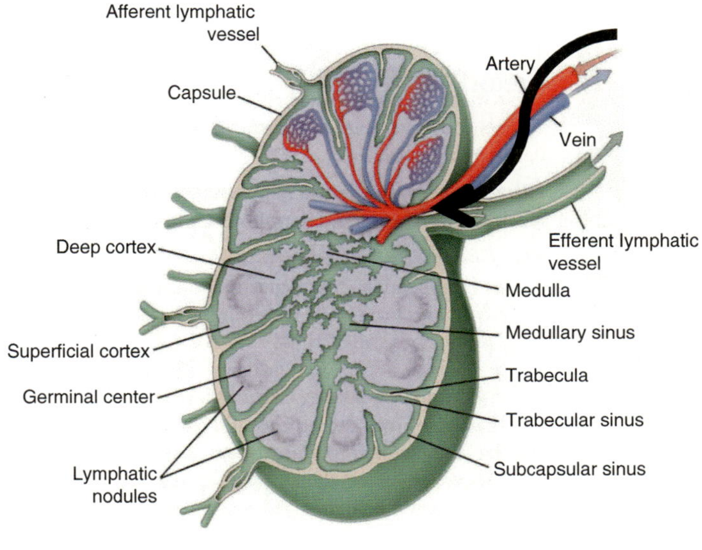

Fig. 7.5 Illustration of histology of the lymph node. A *black arrow* indicates the vasoacting unmyelinated nerve. The hilar structures fix the node

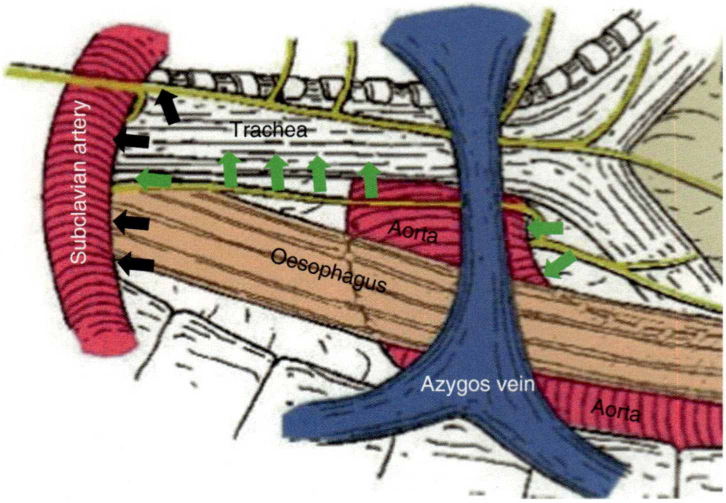

Fig. 7.6 Illustration of direction of hilum of the lymph node in the upper mediastinum. *Arrows* indicate direction of hilum. *Black arrows* and *green arrows* indicate right recurrent nodes and left recurrent nodes respectively

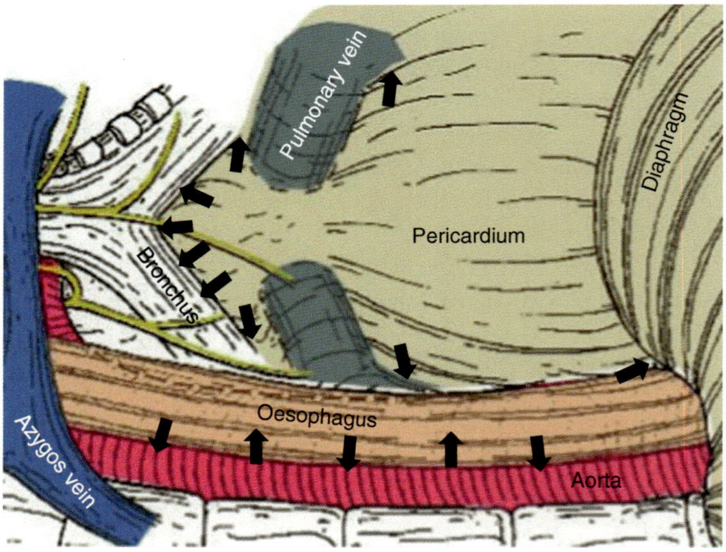

Fig. 7.7 Illustration of direction of the hilum of the lymph node in the middle and lower mediastinum. *Arrows* indicate direction of hilum. There are two kinds of lymph nodes determinable by the direction of the hilum along the oesophagus and aorta. One is when its hilum faces to the aorta (para-aortic node) and the other is when it faces to the oesophagus (para-oesophageal node)

7.2 Dissection of the Right Recurrent Nodes

Firstly, the mediastinal pleura is incised along the right vagal nerve, the right subclavian artery, and ventral margin of the vertebra. Dividing the tracheoesophageal artery, arising from the right subclavian artery and running on the right side of the oesophagus to the anterior aspect of the trachea at the anterior edge of vertebra, the fatty tissue consisting of the recurrent nodes becomes mobile. Then the epineurium of the vagal nerve is exposed and the right recurrent nerve is identified at its recurring point (just caudal to the right subclavian artery). The dissection along the recurrent nerve is carried out by exposing its epineurium and dividing the oesophageal branches (commonly four or five are divided) up to the caudal border of the right lobe of the thyroid gland. The nodes present dorsal to the recurrent nerve. The recurrent nerve should be carefully differentiated from the sympathetic nerve and from the cervical ganglion (Fig. 7.8). The sympathetic nerve runs along the right subclavian artery through the arch of the recurrent nerve, and to the frontal aspect of the trachea, and forms a V shape together with the vagal nerve in contrast to the recurrent nerves that forms a U shape. In some

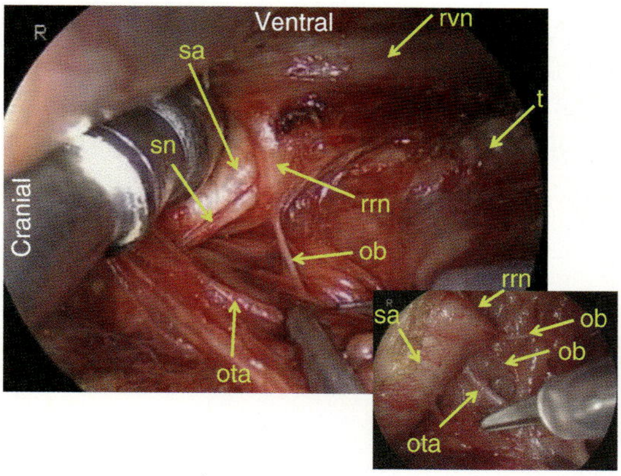

Fig. 7.8 Dissection along the right recurrent nerve. *t* trachea, *rvn* right vagal nerve, *sa* subclavian artery, *sn* sympathetic nerve from the cervical ganglion (The nerve runs on the subclavian artery, through the arch of recurrent nerve to the frontal aspect of the trachea), *rrn* right recurrent nerve, *ob* oesophageal branch of the recurrent nerve, *ota* oesophagotracheal artery (Left upper shows the common site of the artery and right lower shows the artery branches proximally as very close to the recurrent nerve)

patients, the tracheoesophageal artery divides at proximal site of the subclavian artery, near the recurrent nerve (Fig. 7.8). In these patients, care should be taken not to injure the artery, so to avoid incurring palsy of the nerve (Videos 7.1, 7.2, 7.3, 7.4 and 7.5).

7.3 Mobilization of the Dorsal Aspect of the Oesophagus

Cranial to the aortic arch, the dorsal aspect of the oesophagus is rather avascular and anatomically simple. However, there can be three planes of dissection according to the right sympathetic branches. When the thoracic duct is preserved, dissection should be performed along b1 (Fig. 7.1). For the total mediastinal mobilization, along b2 (Fig. 7.1), the thoracic duct is excised and the branches of the left sympathetic trunk are cut, and then the left mediastinal pleura is exposed (Fig. 7.9). The azygos vein arch is mobilized and divided following double ligation. The ligated ends are retracted through the chest wall ventrally and dorsally to enhance mediastinal exposure. The pleura is then incised along the anterior edge of the vertebral column dorsally and the right bronchial artery is doubly

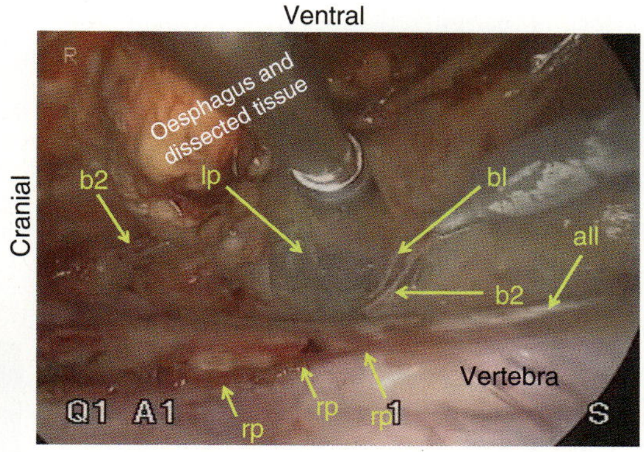

Fig. 7.9 Mobilization of the dorsal aspect of the oesophagus. *rp* cut edge of the right mediastinal pleura, *all* anterior longitudinal ligament of vertebra, *b2* branches of the right trunk of sympathetic nerve, surrounding the thoracic duct (indicating b2 in the Fig. 7.1), *bl* branches of the left trunk of sympathetic nerve, *lp* left mediastinal pleura. After dividing the most left branches of the right trunk, the left mediastinal pleura can be exposed properly

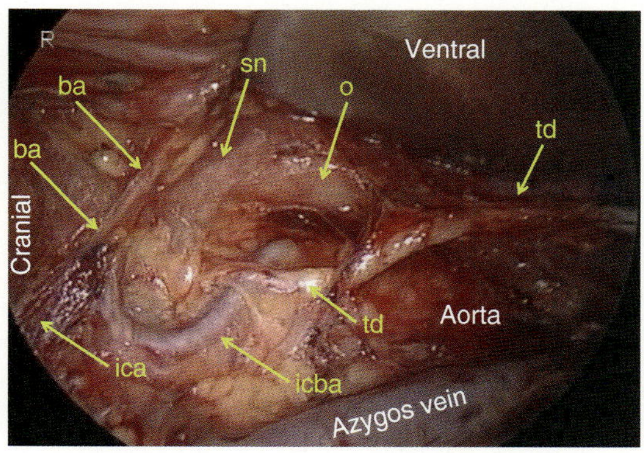

Fig. 7.10 Intercostobrachial artery (third intercostal artery) and thoracic duct. *td* thoracic duct (the thoracic duct runs most dorsally at the root of the intercostobrachial artery and is surrounded with the sympathetic nerves), *o* oesophagus, *icba* intercostobrachial artery, *ica* third intercostal artery, *ba* right bronchial artery (The fine sympathetic nerve is seen running along the artery), *sn* band of sympathetic nerve from the right thoracic trunk (this case, the band is very thick)

clipped and divided at its root as it bifurcates from the intercostobrachial artery (third intercostal artery) (Fig. 7.10). Dissection is continued exposing the ventral aspect of the intercostobrachial artery as far as to the right wall of the aortic arch. Then the intrathoracic descending aorta is exposed. Cranial to the aortic arch, dissection is carried out ventrally, exposing the left mediastinal pleura until pulsation of the left subclavian artery is recognized. The fine fibrous membrane consisting of sympathetic branches, covers the vascular sheath of the aorta (Fig. 7.11). Because there is no lymph node under this membrane, dissection exposing this membrane seems to be ideal. The dissection progresses to the left so that the sympathetic branches from the left trunk are recognized and divided and the left mediastinal pleura exposed (Fig. 7.2). After this, the proper oesophageal arteries are divided at the root by penetrating the fibrous membrane (Fig. 7.11), and then the lymph nodes, even located at the

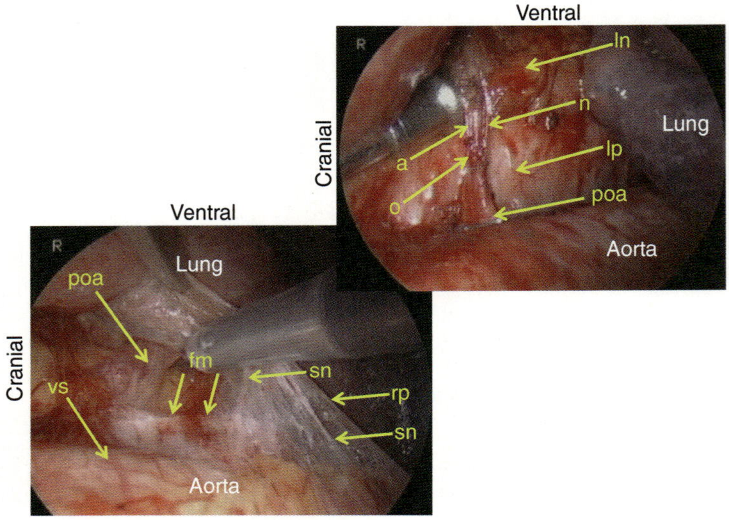

Fig. 7.11 Fibrous membrane of the aorta and proper oesophageal artery. *sn* fine branches of the right trunk of sympathetic nerve, *rp* right mediastinal pleura, *fm* fibrous membrane covering the aorta (The tip of the membrane turning up and down by the retraction of the oesophagus), *vs* aortic vascular sheath under the membrane, *poa* proper oesophageal artery (In right upper, the artery is clipped together with fine sheath at its root), *o* the fine sheath is opened, *a* the proper oesophageal artery is exposed, *n* the fine nerve runs parallel with the artery and fixes the lymph node, *ln* lymph node, *lp* left mediastinal pleura

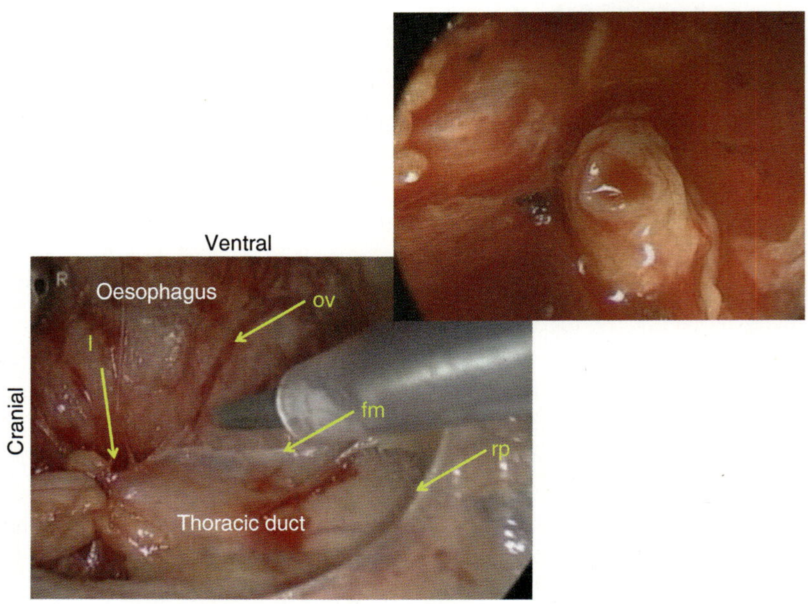

Fig. 7.12 Thoracic duct. *rp* cut edge of right mediastinal pleura, *fm* fibrous membrane (encases thoracic duct together with the aorta), *l* ligation on the thoracic duct, *ov* fine vessel on the oesophagus, right upper shows the particular appearance of the stump of the thoracic duct because of its intramural smooth muscle

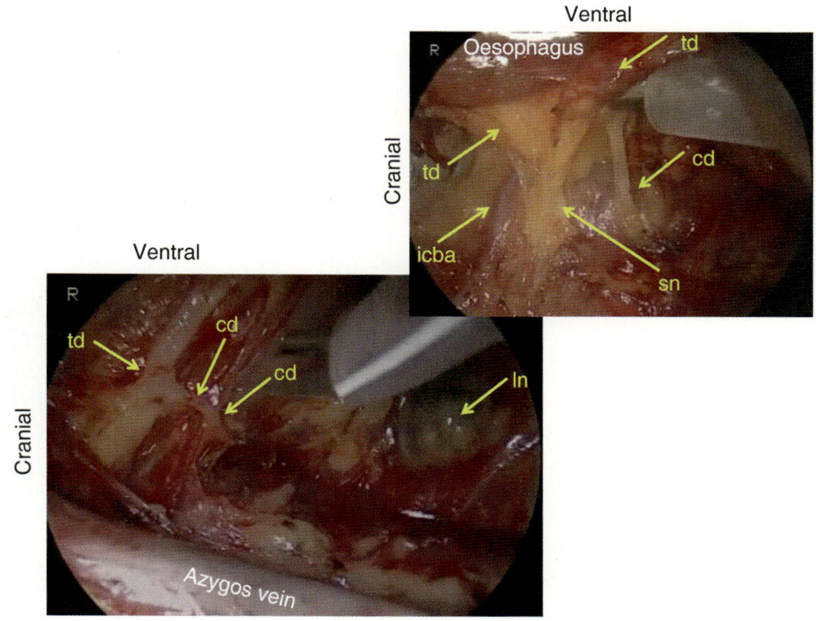

Fig. 7.13 Lymphatic collecting duct. *td* thoracic duct, *cd* collecting duct, *icba* intracostobrachial artery, *sn* branches of the right trunk of sympathetic nerve, *ln* lymph node. Right upper shows the collecting duct from the thoracic wall and left lower shows the collecting duct from the mediastinum. The collecting duct is as seen thicker than the afferent lymphatic (Fig. 7.4) because of its intramural smooth muscle

left side of the aorta, are dissected. This maneuver enables total mobilization of the mesoesophagus, which Cuesta et al. has demonstrated [7]. Because the thoracic duct is covered with this fibrous membrane, this fibrous membrane should be divided for combined resection of the duct (Fig. 7.12). At the level of the pulmonary hilum, the lymphatic collecting ducts from the chest wall and the mediastinum, draining into the thoracic duct as depicted (Fig. 7.13).

7.4 Mobilization of the Ventral Aspect of the Oesophagus

The right mediastinal pleura is divided along the ventral aspect of the oesophagus to the oesophageal hiatus. The right vagal nerve is divided at the level of tracheal bifurcation, just caudal to the pulmonary branches. The oesophagus is mobilized from trachea by dividing the neural and vascular communications between bilateral edges of tracheal cartilage and oesophagus. There is no vascular communications between membranous part of the trachea and the oesophagus. As anatomy of the frontal aspect of the oesophagus is very simple caudal to the carina, dissection exposing the pericardium can be performed easily—without bleeding requiring hemostasis. At the level of the tracheal bifurcation, the oesophagus contacts with membranous part of the left main bronchus and is fixed to the left vagal nerve and branches of the bronchial artery coming from the left side of the oesophagus. By using the magnified view, the oesophagus is found to be fixed with muscular structures. A bundle of the longitudinal muscle of the oesophagus separates from the wall, runs cranially and inserts on the left edge of the cartilage of the tracheobronchus (the oesophagotracheal muscle), the left mediastinal pleura (the oesophagopleural muscle), and the pericardium (no anatomical terminology yet, namely the oesophagopericardial muscle) (Fig. 7.14). The embryological development of the oesophagus is completed by a union between the prolonged pharyngeal bud and the stomach bud at the level of the tracheal bifurcation. It is a likelihood that in this process a part of the outer muscle may separate from the oesophagus, runs cranially and inserts on the mediastinal structures. This fact indicates that the ventral aspect of the oesophagus should be mobilized caudo-cranially, otherwise the oesophageal wall is torn.

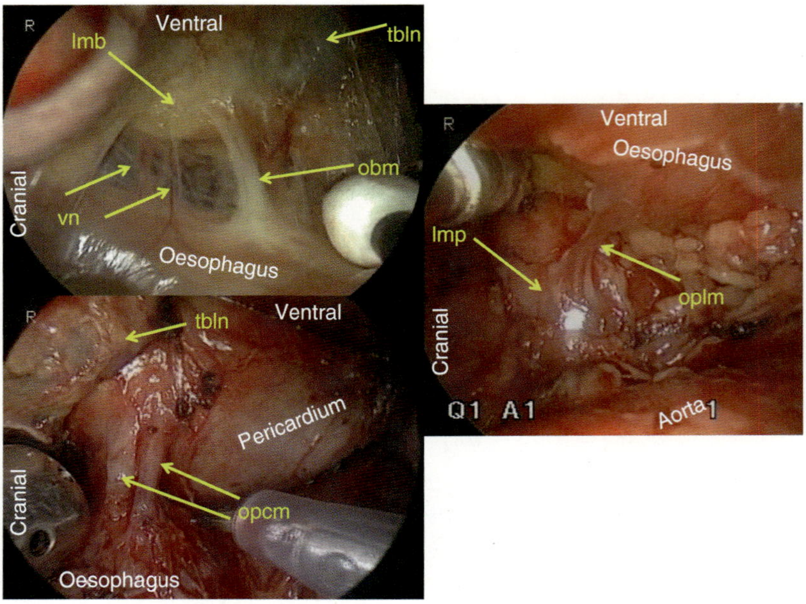

Fig. 7.14 Muscular fixation of the oesophagus. *lmb* left main bronchus, *tbln* tracheobronchial lymph node, *obm* oesophagobronchial muscle, *vn* fine vessels and nerves between oesophagus and bronchus, *lmp* left mediastinal pleura, *oplm* oesophagopleural muscle, *opcm* oesophagopericardial muscle (In this case, band of the muscle is very thick). These muscles were confirmed as smooth muscle histologically

7.5 Dissection of the Left Recurrent Nodes

Following mobilization of the dorsal and left aspects of the esophagus, the tracheobronchus is retracted ventrally to separate from the now dorsally retracted oesophagus. The right oesophagotracheal fibrous band is excised (Fig. 7.15) and the trachea is gradually retracted ventrally and rotated to the left applying the retractor on the right edge of the tracheal cartilage in order to expose the left side. When the left oesophagotracheal fibrous band is excised, and with the aid of the angulated camera and progressive dorsal retraction of the oesophagus, the dissection is continued on the left side of the cartilage part of the trachea where the fine pretracheal branches of the left recurrent laryngeal nerve are cut. As a result of this, the sympathetic cardiac branches from the cervical ganglion are recognized under the fine membrane (Figs. 7.1 and 7.16). Because there is no vessel penetrating this fine membrane, mobilization of the tissue from this membrane can be performed bluntly without any bleeding. Following this mobilization, the left recurrent laryngeal nerve together with its surrounding lymph nodes can be retracted dorsally by retracting the oesophagus and applying traction on the oesophageal branches of the nerve (Fig. 7.16). This improves the exposure which facilitates further cranial dissection. Superiorly in the neck, several fine branches arising from the left recurrent laryngeal nerve give this area a characteristic appearance like a rake signifying the upper limit of the thoracic dissection. Finally, the left recurrent nerve is separated from the tissue including the lymph nodes and the oesophagus by dividing 5–10 of its oesophageal branches. For safe and complete isolation of the nerve, its epineurium (Figs. 7.3 and 7.17), which appears glossy with fine vessels running longitudinally should be exposed. After total isolation of the left recurrent laryngeal nerve, the left side of the lymphatic tissue is dissected by exposing the left subclavian artery and dividing the thoracic duct as it approaches the left subclavian artery. Overall, anatomical boundaries for the dissection of the left recurrent laryngeal lymph nodes include the left side of the cartilage part of the trachea, cardiac branches of sympathetic nerve, the left subclavian artery and the left mediastinal pleura where en-bloc resection without direct traction on the recurrent laryngeal nerve forms the main surgical principle.

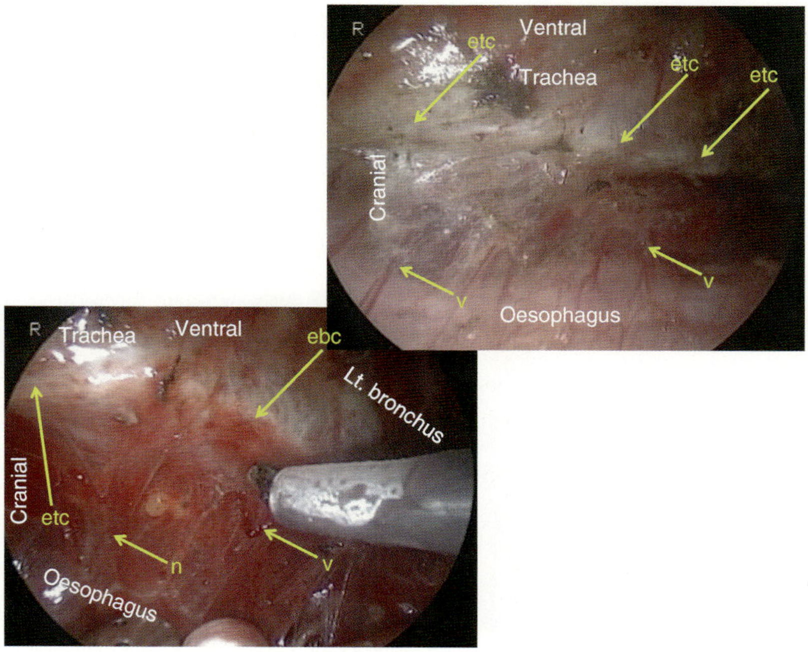

Fig. 7.15 Mobilization of the oesophagus from left side of the trachea. *etc*. edge of the tracheal cartilage, *ebc* edge of the bronchial cartilage, *v* fine vessels in the oesophagotracheal fibrous band, *n* fine nerves in the oesophagotracheal fibrous band

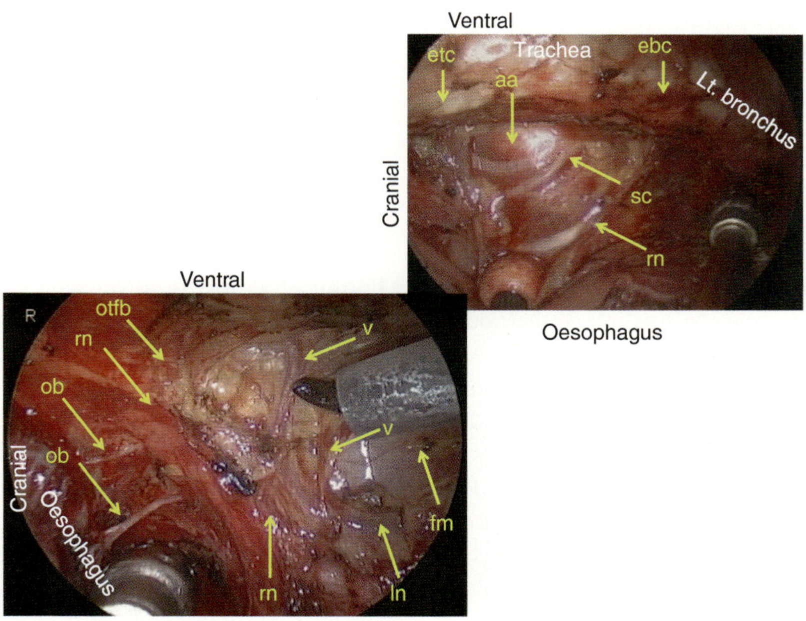

Fig. 7.16 Dissection along the left recurrent nerve. *etc* edge of the tracheal cartilage, *ebc* edge of the bronchial cartilage, *aa* right wall of the aortic arch, *rn* left recurrent verve, *sc* sympathetic cardiac nerve from the cervical ganglion (This nerve presents in front of the recurrent nerve and is covered with the fine fibrous membrane. There is no vessel penetrating this membrane), *fm* fine fibrous membrane covering sympathetic cardiac nerve, *v* vessels of lymph node (commonly seen in front of the nodes. cf. Fig 7.1, vn), *ln* lymph node, *otfb* cut edge of the oesophagotracheal fibrous band, *ob* oesophageal branch of the left recurrent nerve

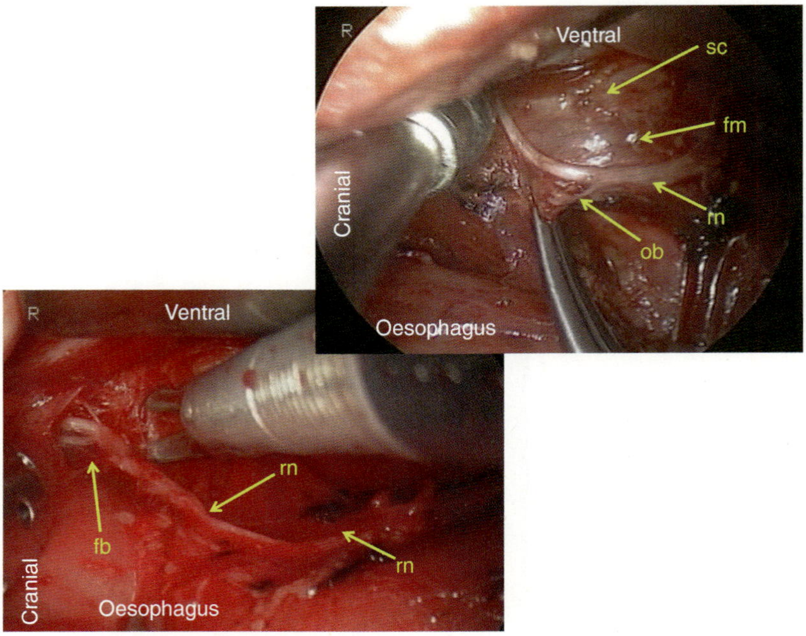

Fig. 7.17 Isolation of the left recurrent nerve. *sc* sympathetic cardiac nerve from the cervical ganglion, *fm* fine fibrous membrane covering sympathetic cardiac nerve, *rn* left recurrent nerve, *ob* oesophageal branch of the recurrent nerve, *fb* fine oesophageal and tracheal branches of the recurrent nerve (Rake appearance signifies the upper limit of the thoracic dissection)

7.6 Dissection of the Tracheobronchial Nodes

For dissection of the infracarinal nodes—as the most lateral nodes are fixed toward the pulmonary hilum (Fig. 7.7)—the fixation of the most right lateral node is divided with energy devices first. The avascular frontal aspect of the nodes is mobilized from the pericardium. Then the nodes are retracted contra-laterally to the right main bronchus and the fixation of the nodes is divided from the right main bronchus. At the tracheal bifurcation, the branch of bronchial artery enters the nodes ventrally and the branches of the vagal nerve fix the nodes dorsally. After getting the mobility of the nodes by dividing these fixations, the nodes are retracted contra-laterally to the left main bronchus, and then are dissected by dividing the fixation to the left main bronchus. It can be reported that the anomaly of right pulmonary vein is observed in 0.3–9% of the patients. The anomaly of V2 (the vein from pulmonary segment 2) is the most frequent and V6 (the vein from pulmonary segment 6) is the second [8]. The anomaly vein runs on the membranous part of the right main bronchus and among the subcarinal nodes, and penetrates the pericardium to the left atrium (Fig. 7.18). Careful observation by CT scan enables the surgeon to avoid the injury of the anomaly vein during the dissection. Fortunately for oesophageal surgeons, this anomaly is seldom seen on the left side.

In the aortobronchial window, the left side of the cartilage part of tracheobronchus is exposed first. Then the nodes are retracted contra-laterally to the posterior aspect of the pulmonary artery, and dissected by dividing the branch of the bronchial artery and the nerve coming from the lesser curvature of the aortic arch (Fig. 7.19). Particular care must be taken not to pull out the left bronchial arteries from the lesser curvature of the aortic arch because bleeding here can be fatal.

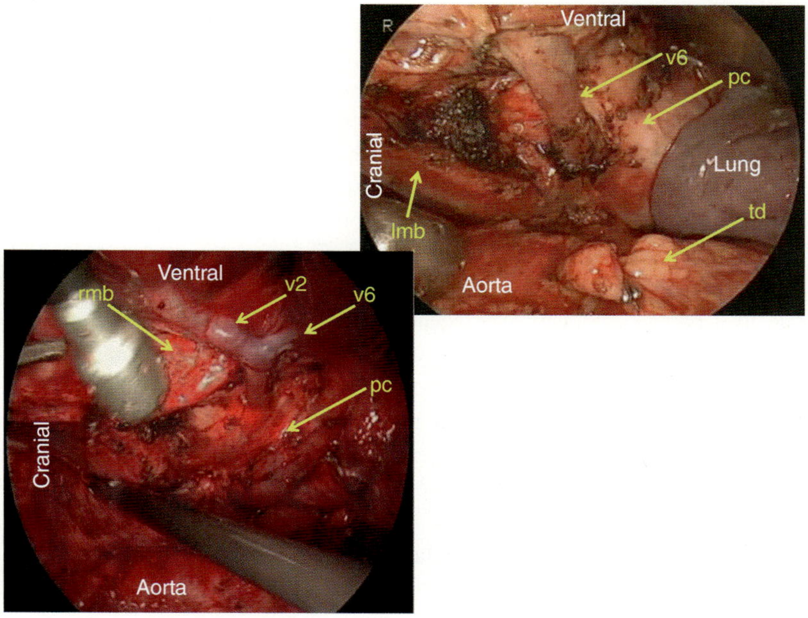

Fig. 7.18 Anomaly of the pulmonary vein. *td* thoracic duct, *pc* pericardium, *v6* anomaly vein from the pulmonary segment 6, *V2* anomaly vein from the pulmonary segment 2, *lmb* left main bronchus, *rmb* right main bronchus

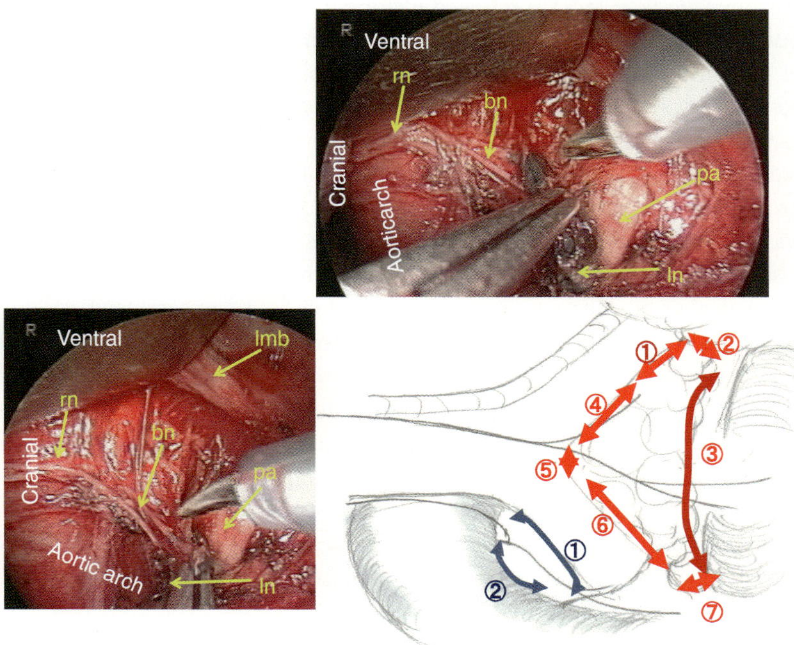

Fig. 7.19 Dissection in the aorto-bronchial window. *rn* left recurrent nerve, *bn* branches of recurrent nerve, *pa* posterior aspect of pulmonary artery, *ln* lymph nodes to be dissected, *lmb* left main bronchus. Illustration shows the order of dissection (*Red* and *blue* figures in *circle* indicate the order of dissection of nodes at tracheal bifurcation and aorto-bronchial window, respectively)

7.7 Efficacy of Thoracoscopic Approach

Originally, the thoracoscopic approach tended to be indicated initially for pre-invasive cases. Then the indication became similar to that of open surgery, excepting where extensive pleural adhesion prevented camera insertion, suspicion of contiguous tumor spreading to the adjacent vital organs, and due to a patient's choice. The recent population-based analyses revealed that a bit more than 30% of oesophagectomy treatments for cancer are being performed thoracoscopically and the percentage of use is still increasing [9–11]. However, the high level evidence vindicating thoracoscopic approach is not sufficient, because of plethoric heterogeneity in choosing an approach, such as either Ivor Lewis or Mckeown, either transthoracic or transhiatal, prone position or left lateral position, and either laparotomy or laparoscopy (hybrid type of interventions), etc. Only one prospective randomized control trial [12] and five meta-analyses [13–17] evaluating the benefits of thoracoscopy over open surgery are available. The peer-randomized trial done by Cuesta et al. [12] revealed that the minimally invasive group patients had lower incidence of pulmonary infection and higher quality of life postoperatively without any adverse effects comparing open surgery. Although the duration of procedure was significantly longer in the minimally invasive group than in the open group, blood loss was less significantly. Following feasibility tests, case-studies and cohort-studies have reported that the benefits of thoracoscopic oesophagectomy compared to open surgery are very similar. Also the five meta-analyses [13–17] and the recent reviews [18, 19] revealed the superiority of thoracoscopic surgery in reducing postoperative pulmonary complication, blood loss, the length of hospitalization, and the deterioration of the postoperative quality of life. One retrospective study on thoracoscopy showed how it preserved the pulmonary function better than open surgery [20]. Notwithstanding, among the three population-based analyses, two did report thoracoscopic oesophagectomy negatively. The British study demonstrated there was no significant difference in the outcome between the minimally invasive group and open group, excepting the former having a significant higher risk of reintervention with increasing odds ratio coming about at each progressive study year [9]. The other study from Japan revealed that, comparing with open surgery, minimally invasive oesophagectomy was associated with higher incidence of overall morbidities (40.8% vs. 44.3%), anastomotic leakage (12.5% vs. 14.9%), and reintervention (5.6% vs. 8.0%) [10].

Our conjecture is that cause of variance with the other studies is that thoracoscopic oesophagectomies done by surgeons in their learning phase inevitably influenced these population-based analyses. The operative and in-hospital mortality after oesophagectomy is conversely related with hospital volume [21] and the same outcome is seen after thoracoscopic oesophagectomy. The outcome of oesophagectomy strongly depends on a surgeon's experience. When it is performed thoracoscopically, surgeons require additional experience and skills. We note that only well-trained surgeons were involved in the case-studies and cohort-studies, as well as in the randomized control study. Studying our own experience, we can say that the learning curve was not steep so that the basic skills for thoracoscopic oesophagectomy could be acquired during the first 17 cases; to which we add that the most significant event in the learning curve came between the first 36 cases and the rest [22]. Our reflection is that by after proper learning, thoracoscopy will become effective. Also, we note that the surgeons experience was the only independent factor reducing postoperative pulmonary complication (risk of pulmonary infection % = 31.1 – 0.4 × number of experienced cases) [22]. However, with the proper instruction by the expert surgeon the learning curve could steepen safely [23]. In order to perform thoracoscopic oesophagectomy effectively and safely, the dedicated team (of at least with two surgeons, whom learned well how to perform the minimally invasive surgery at a center of excellence) has to be organized [24]. Oncologic adverse effect were not observed by meta-analyses. Thoracoscopic approach did not spoil the quality of mediastinal dissection, retrieval of mediastinal nodes, and the survival. Our patient survival rate after thoracoscopic oesophagectomy was 92, 88, 69, 52, and 24% at 5-years for pStage 0, 1, 2, 3, and 4, respectively. The indication was the same as with open surgery and the perioperative treatment was neoadjuvant and/or adjuvant chemotherapy. Although the data are retrospective, the survival is favorably compared with open oesophagectomy and is similar to that of gastric cancer. A retrospective study reported the thoracoscopic approach as an independent factor for better survival together with less T-factor and node negative [25]. However, the evidence of oncologic superiority of thoracoscopy over open surgery is still being evaluated with pragmatic-randomized control trials.

Apart from quantitative evaluation of thoracoscopy, the quality of dissection has been improving by understanding the mediastinal anatomy in vivo under the magnified view. The novel anatomical knowledge as enhanced through thoracoscopy can be valuable feedback in open surgery in order to improve the quality of mediastinal dissection. In this chapter, the focus has been on the microanatomy usually recognized in patients not previously radiated. It is supposed that in those patients with neoadjuvant treatment, especially involving radiation, fine anatomy may become obscure because of mediastinal fibrosis. Nevertheless, understanding the innate microanatomy is essential for performing an ideal oesophagectomy, even in those patients with different grades of mediastinal fibrosis caused by neoadjuvant therapy.

References

1. Fijita H. The history of lymphadenectomy for esophageal cancer and the future prospects for esophageal cancer surgery. Surg Today. 2015;45:140–9.
2. Udagawa H, Ueno M, Shinohara H, et al. The importance of grouping of lymph node stations and rationale of three-field lymphadenectomy for thoracic esophageal cancer. J Surg Oncol. 2012;106:742–7.
3. Funai T, Osugi H, Higashino M, et al. Estimation of lymph node metastasis by size in patients with intrathoracic oesophageal cancer. Br J Surg. 2000;87:1234–9.
4. Ando N, Kato H, Igaki H, et al. A randomized trial comparing postoperative adjuvant chemotherapy with cisplatin and 5-fluorouracil versus preoperative chemotherapy for localized advanced squamous cell carcinoma of the thoracic esophagus (JCOG9907). Ann Surg Oncol. 2012;19:68–74.
5. Tachimori Y, Ozawa S, Numasaki H, et al. Comprehensive registry of esophageal cancer in Japan 2009. Esophagus. 2016;13:110–37.
6. Osugi H, Takemura M, Higashsino M, et al. Video-assisted thoracoscopic esophagectomy and radical lymph node dissection for esophageal cancer. Surg Endosc. 2002;16:1588–93.
7. Cuesta MA, Weijs TJ, Bleys RLAW, et al. A new concept of the anatomy of the thoracic oesophagus: the meso-oesophagus. Observational study during thoracoscopic esophagectomy. Surg Endosc. 2015;29:2576–82.
8. Akiba T, Morikawa T, Inagaki T, et al. A new classification for right top pulmonary vein. Ann Thorac Surg. 2013;95:1227–30.
9. Mamidanna R, Bottle A, Aylin P, et al. Short-term outcomes following open versus minimally invasive esophagectomy for cancer in England. A population-based national study. Ann Surg. 2012;255:197–203.
10. Takeuchi H, Miyata H, Gotoh M, et al. A risk model for esophagectomy using data of 5354 patients included in a Japanese National Web-Based database. Ann Surg. 2014;260:259–66.
11. Yerokun BA, Sun Z, Yang CFJ, et al. Minimally invasive versus open esophagectomy for esophageal cancer: a population-based analysis. Ann Thorac Surg. 2016;102:416–23.
12. Biere SS, van Berge Henegouwen M, Maas K, et al. Minimally invasive versus open oesophagectomy for patients with oesophageal cancer: a multicentre, open-label, randomised controlled trial. Lancet. 2012;379:1887–92.
13. Biere SS, Cuesta MA, van der Peet DL. Minimally invasive versus open esophagectomy for cancer: a systematic review and meta-analysis. Minerva Chir. 2009;64:121–33.
14. Nagpal K, Ahmed K, Vats A, et al. Is minimally invasive surgery beneficial in the management of esophageal cancer? A meta-analysis. Surg Endosc. 2010;24:1621–9.
15. Sgourakis G, Gockel I, Radtke A, et al. Minimally invasive versus open esophagectomy: meta-analysis of outcomes. Dig Dis Sci. 2010;55:3031–40.
16. Dantoc M, Cox MR, Eslick GD. Evidence to support the use of minimally invasive esophagectomy for esophageal cancer: a meta-analysis. Arch Surg. 2012;147:768–76.
17. Gou W, Ma X, Yan S, et al. Combined thoracoscopic-laparoscopic esophagectomy versus open esophagectomy: a meta-analysis of outcomes. Surg Endosc. 2016;30:3873–81.
18. Giugliano DN, Berger AC, Rosato EL, et al. Total minimally invasive esophagectomy for esophageal cancer: approaches and outcomes. Langenbeck's Arch Surg. 2016;401:747–56.
19. Rodham P, Batty JA, McElnay PJ, et al. Dose minimally invasive oesophagectomy provide a benefit in hospital length of stay when compared with open oesophagectomy? Interact Cardiovasc Thorac Surg. 2016;22:360–7.
20. Taguchi S, Osugi H, Higashino M, et al. Comparison of three-field esophagectomy for esophageal cancer incorporating open or thoracoscopic thoracotomy. Surg Endosc. 2003;17:1445–50.
21. Fujita H, Ozawa S, Kuwano H, et al. Esophagectomy for cancer: clinical concerns support centralizing operations within the larger hospitals. Dis Esophagus. 2010;23:145–52.

22. Osugi H, Takemura M, Higashino M, et al. Learning curve of video-assisted thoracoscopic esophagectomy and extensive lymphadenectomy for squamous cell cancer of the thoracic esophagus and results. Surg Endosc. 2003;17:515–9.
23. Ninomiya I, Osugi H, Tomizawa N, et al. Learning of thoracoscopic radical esophagectomy: how can the learning curve be made short and flat? Dis Esophagus. 2010;23:618–26.
24. Cuesta MA, Wielen NI, Straatman J, et al. Video-assisted thoracoscopic esophagectomy: keynote lecture. Gen Thorac Cardiovasc Surg. 2016;64:380–5.
25. Burdall OC, Boddy AP, Fullick J, et al. A comparative study of survival after minimally invasive and open oesophagectomy. Surg Endosc. 2015;29:431–7.

8 Total or Hybrid Minimally Invasive Esophagectomy?

Christophe Mariette

8.1 Introduction

Oesophageal cancer's global incidence continues to increase rapidly. In Western society this is reflected by an increasing incidence of oesophageal adenocarcinomas, with the epidemiological shift felt to be related to increased obesity, gastro-oesophageal reflux disease, and Barrett's oesophagus—the dominant risk factors for the development of this tumour. Surgical resection with radical lymphadenectomy, usually after the administration of neoadjuvant chemotherapy or chemoradiotherapy, remains the key component in the multimodality treatment of oesophageal cancer. Oesophagectomy is a complex surgical procedure for which the mortality rates have historically been significant [1]. In the modern practice of high volume centres with appropriate multidisciplinary teams, the mortality rate after oesophageal resection has been reduced significantly [2]. Despite this boon, it remains an operation associated with substantial rates of morbidity. Hence, minimally invasive surgery has been championed in the previous three decades as a means of reducing postoperative morbidity for a variety of oncological gastrointestinal resections. Concerning oesophageal resection, it has been hoped that the application of minimally invasive surgery may similarly reduce postoperative morbidity and mortality. By the early 1990s, some surgeons had developed and used protocols for thoracoscopic oesophagectomy, initially restricting its use to T1 and T2 oesophageal cancer without neoadjuvant chemoradiation [3, 4]. Subsequently, indications for minimally invasive oesophagectomy (MIO) have been expanded to include more advanced disease, irrespective of the whether patients have received neoadjuvant treatments.

The techniques representing minimally invasive approaches to oesophageal resection vary widely. Many authors have described totally minimally invasive approaches (thoracoscopy and laparoscopy) whilst others describe hybrid procedures where one stage of the operation is performed either by thoracoscopy or laparoscopy and the other by conventional open surgery.

Why, unlike other minimally invasive procedures, has MIO not been broadly adopted? Regardless what approach is used, MIO remains a very complex operation with many questions remaining unanswered as to the real advantages of applying a minimally invasive technique for resection of a disease that often is advanced at the time of surgery. Whereas the feasibility and safety

C. Mariette, M.D., Ph.D.
Department of Digestive and Oncological Surgery, Claude Huriez University Hospital, Univ. Lille, F-59000 Lille, France

UMR-S 1172, JPARC—Centre de Recherche Jean-Pierre AUBERT Neurosciences et Cancer, Univ. Lille, F-59000 Lille, France

Inserm, UMR-S 1172, F-59000 Lille, France

SIRIC ONCOLille, Lille, France
e-mail: christophe.mariette@chru-lille.fr

M.A. Cuesta (ed.), *Minimally Invasive Surgery for Upper Abdominal Cancer*,
DOI 10.1007/978-3-319-54301-7_8

of MIO have been assessed in a prospective phase II multicenter study [5], yet the mortality, morbidity, oncological radicality, reproducibility and the cost of the procedure remain topics under debate for implementing MIO. Many retrospective and comparative non-randomized studies, as included in some recent meta-analyses focusing on the role of MIO [6–10], have been conducted. Given only two randomized trials have been reported to date, uncertainty remains about the advantages of MIO compared to open oesophagectomy.

In the absence of meta-analyses of randomized controlled studies, this chapter appraises the available literature regarding the short-term perioperative and long-term oncological outcomes for patients undergoing MIO for cancer, with a focus on the total versus hybrid approaches.

8.2 MIO Techniques

As there has never been a consensus regarding the superiority of any of the various open oesophagectomy techniques, it comes as no surprise that agreeing on what constitutes the best minimally invasive approach is difficult.

Totally minimally invasive approaches to oesophageal resection attempt to replicate established open procedures. A minimally invasive transhiatal technique utilizes laparoscopic abdominal dissection and preparation of the gastric conduit followed by a cervical anastomosis created via a traditional open approach in the neck. Mediastinal dissection of perioesophageal lymph nodes, including those in the subcarinal station, can be assessed through the hiatus using the lighting and magnification afforded by the laparoscopic camera. The oesophageal specimen can be removed through the neck incision. Some surgeons prefer to combine the laparoscopic transhiatal approach with a mini-laparotomy to facilitate gastric tube creation as well as to remove the specimen. Finally, the oesophagus can also be removed from the mediastinum via an inversion technique with or without division of the vagus nerve. As with open surgery, many surgeons prefer a thoracoscopic approach, typically performed through the right chest, with patients positioned in lateral decubitus or prone positions. Thoracoscopy can be used as a part of a three-stage MIO, where the procedure begins in the chest and ends with laparoscopy and a cervical anastomosis, or as part of the two-stage Ivor Lewis oesophagectomy where the oesophagogastric anastomosis resides in the chest. In this procedure, the specimen is removed through a mini-thoracotomy, and the anastomosis is created at the apex of the chest.

Combinations of open and minimally invasive techniques (hybrid techniques) are perhaps more widely utilized, such as laparoscopy with thoracotomy or thoracoscopy with laparotomy. These hybrid techniques are applied for a variety of reasons and may be necessitated by oncological considerations, prior surgery in either cavity, surgeon experience and surgeon preference.

Although the goal of MIO is to perform an equivalent operation to the open procedure without omitting any critical steps, some aspects considered as routine for open oesophagectomy have fallen out of favour with many surgeons, such as performance of a pyloroplasty and jejunostomy placement.

8.3 MIO Postoperative Outcomes

The primary goal of MIO is to decrease surgical morbidity associated with the open approach. Except sparse data coming from randomized controlled trials to be further detailed [11–13], most data derives from retrospective or prospective non-randomized series. These suggest that mortality rates appear equivalent or even lower in large comparative cohorts, with some evidence of a reduced postoperative complication rate favouring the minimally invasive approach (Tables 8.1 and 8.2). It is likely that the benefits of MIO may be overshadowed by the persistent rate of significant morbidity, which continues to occur independent of surgical approach. It seems conceivable that in the absence of such complications, patients with a minimal-access approach enjoy quicker recovery, a quicker return to normal activities and decreased long-term pain when compared to patients with similarly uncomplicated open procedures. This, however, has yet to be proven.

Table 8.1 Mortality and overall morbidity of minimally invasive and open oesophagectomy

Authors	n	Approaches	Mortality n (%)	Overall morbidity n (%)
Law et al. [14]	22	MIO (TSO)	0	18 (81.8)
	63	Open	0	63 (100)
Nguyen et al. [15]	18	MIO (TLSO)	0	7 (38.9)
	36	Open	0	19 (52.8)
Osugi et al. [16]	77	MIO (VATS)	0	31 (40.3)
	72	Open	0	32 (44.4)
Kunisaki et al. [17]	15	MIO (VATS + HALS)	0	NS
	30	Open	0	NS
Van den Broek et al. [18]	25	MIO (THO)	0	14 (70)
	20	Open	0	18 (72)
Bresadola et al. [19]	14	MIO (THO and TLSO)	0	8 (57.1)
	14	Open	0	6 (42.9)
Bernabe et al. [20]	17	MIO (THO)	0	NS
	14	Open	0	NS
Shiraishi et al. [21]	116	MIO (TLSO)	3 (2.6)	NS
	37	Open	3 (8.1)	NS
Braghetto et al. [22]	47	MIO (VATS/LSO)	3 (6.3)	18 (38.2)
	119	Open	13 (10.9)	72 (60.5)
Smithers et al. [23]	332	MIO (TLSO)	7 (2.1)	207 (62.3)
	114	Open	3 (2.6)	76 (66.7)
Fabian et al. [24]	22	MIO (TLSE)	1 (4.5)	15 (68.2)
	43	Open	4 (9.8)	31 (72.1)
Zingg et al. [25]	56	MIO (TLSO)	2 (3.6)	19 (34.5)
	98	Open	6 (6.1)	20 (23.5)
Perry et al. [26]	21	MIO (LIO)	0	13 (62)
	21	Open	1 (5)	17 (81)
Parameswaran et al. [27]	50	MIO (TLSO)	1 (2)	24 (48)
	30	Open	1 (3)	15 (50)
Pham et al. [28]	44	MIO (TLSO)	3 (6.8)	NS
	46	Open	2 (4.3)	NS
Schoppman et al. [29]	31	MIO (TLSO)	0	11 (35.5)
	31	Open	0	23 (74.2)
Singh et al. [30]	33	MIO (TLSO)	Values NS	Values NS
	31	Open	p = 0.34	P = 0.06
Mamidanna et al. [31]	1155	MIO (TLSO, HMIO)	46 (4.0)	NS
	6347	Open	274 (4.3)	NS
Ben-David et al. [32]	100	MIO (TLSO)	1 (1)	NS
	32	Open	2 (5)	NS
Briez et al. [33]	140	MIO (HMIO)	2.1	35.7
	140	Open	12.9	59.3
Xie et al. [34]	106	MIO (TLSO)	2 (1.9)	28 (26.4)
	163	Open	4 (2.5)	56 (34.4)
Hsu et al. [35]	66	MIO (TLSO)	5 (7.6)	NS
	63	Open	5 (7.9)	NS

MIO minimally invasive oesophagectomy, *VATS* video-assisted thoracoscopic oesophagectomy, *HMIO* hybrid MIO, *HALS* hand-assited laparoscopic oesophagectomy, *TSO* thoracoscopic-assisted oesophagectomy, *TLSO* thoracolaparoscopic oesophagectomy, *LIO* laparoscopic inversion oesophagectomy, *LSO* laparoscopic oesophagectomy, *NS* not stated

Table 8.2 Comparison of rates of morbidities for MIO and open oesophagectomy

Authors	n	Approaches	Pneumonia n (%)	Cardiac arrhythmia n (%)	Anastomotic leak n (%)	Gastric conduit ischemia n (%)	Chylothorax n (%)	Length of stay (days)	Operative blood loss (mls)	Operative time (min)
Law et al. [14]	22	MIO (TSO)	3 (13.6)	3 (13.6)	0	NS	NS	NS	450 (200–800)	240 (160–350)
	63	Open	11 (17.5)	14 (22.2)	2 (3.2)	NS	NS	NS	700 (300–2500)	250 (190–420)
Nguyen et al. [15]	18	MIO (TLSO)	2 (11.1)	NS	2 (11.1)	0	0	11.3±14.2	297±233	364±73
	36	Open	6 (16.7)	NS	4 (11.1)	1 (2.8)	1 (2.8)	22.8±18.0	1108±790	411±93
Osugi et al. [16]	77	MIO (VATS)	12 (15.6)	1 (1.3)	1 (1.3)	0	3 (3.9)	NS	284 (330)	227 (90)
	72	Open	14 (19.4)	3 (4.2)	2 (2.8)	0	0	NS	310 (170)	186 (35)
Kunisaki et al. [17]	15	MIO (VATS + HALS)	0	NS	2 (13.3)	NS	NS	29.6±12.9	447.9 (±214.8)	544.4 (±64.5)
	30	Open	1 (3.3)	NS	1 (3.3)	NS	NS	32.7±14.0	674.7 (±445.6)	487.8 (±97.8)
Van den Broek et al. [18]	25	MIO (THO)	2 (8)	NS	2 (8)	0	2 (8)	16	NS	NS
	20	Open	2 (10)	NS	3 (15)	0	0	16	NS	NS
Bresadola et al. [19]	14	MIO (THO and TLSO)	1 (7.1)	NS	1 (7.1)	NS	0	16.4 (±8.4)	NS	469.0 (±42.6)
	14	Open	2 (14.2)	NS	2 (14.2)	NS	0	22.3 (±10.6)	NS	370.8 (±16.7)
Bernabe et al. [20]	17	MIO (THO)	NS	NS	NS	NS	NS	9.1 (±3.2)	331 (±220)	336 (±53)
	14	Open	NS	NS	NS	NS	NS	11.6 (±2.9)	542 (±212)	388 (±102)
Shiraishi et al. [21]	116	MIO (TLSO)	25 (21.6)	3 (2.6)	13 (11.2)	NS	NS	NS	670.2 (±561.1)	426.0 (±87.1)
	37	Open	12 (32.4)	4 (10.8)	9 (24.3)	NS	NS	NS	487.4 (±110.5)	487.4 (±110.5)
Braghetto et al. [22]	47	MIO (VATS/ LSO)	7 (14.8)	NS	3 (6.4)	0	1 (2.1)	NS	NS	NS
	119	Open	22 (18.5)	NS	17 (14.3)	1 (0.8)	0	NS	NS	NS
Smithers et al. [23]	332	MIO (TLSO)	87 (26.2)	55 (16.6)	18 (5.4)	5 (1.5)	17 (5.1)	11 (7–49)	300 (15–1000)	330 (270–540)
	114	Open	35 (27.8)	21 (18.4)	10 (8.7)	2 (1.7)	7 (6.1)	14 (8–44)	600 (0–3000)	300 (150–480)
Fabian et al. [24]	22	MIO (TLSE)	1 (4.5)	4 (18.2)	3 (13.6)	1 (4.5)	0	9.5	178 (±96)	333 (±72)
	43	Open	10 (23.3)	8 (18.6)	3 (7.0)	0	2 (4.7)	11	356 (±136)	270 (±87)
Zingg et al. [25]	56	MIO (TLSO)	17 (30.9)	NS	NS	NS	NS	19.7 (±2.0)	320 (±49)	250 (±7.2)
	98	Open	33 (38.8)	NS	NS	NS	NS	21.9 (±2.0)	857 (±82)	209 (±7.8)
Perry et al. [26]	21	MIO (LIO)	1 (5)	4 (19)	4 (19)	NS	NS	10 (8–14)	168 (149)	399 (86)
	21	Open	2 (10)	7 (33)	6 (29)	NS	NS	14 (10–19)	526 (289)	408 (127)

Table 8.2 (continued)

Authors	n	Approaches	Pneumonia n (%)	Cardiac arrhythmia n (%)	Anastomotic leak n (%)	Gastric conduit ischemia n (%)	Chylothorax n (%)	Length of stay (days)	Operative blood loss (mls)	Operative time (min)
Parameswaran et al. [27]	50	MIO (TLSO)	4 (8)	NS	4 (8)	5 (16)	3 (6)	12 (8–86)	NS	442 (305–580)
	30	Open	2 (7)	NS	1 (3)	2 (10)	1 (3)	10 (6–56)	NS	266 (219–390)
Pham et al. [28]	44	MIO (TLSO)	11 (25)	NS	4 (9)	1 (2)	NS	15 (12–20)	407 (±267)	543 (72.6)
	46	Open	7 (15)	NS	5 (11)	1 (2)	NS	14 (11–23)	780 (± 610)	437 (97.0)
Schoppman et al. [29]	31	MIO (TLSO)	2 (6.2)	NS	1 (3.2)	0	2 (6.4)	NS	NS	411 (270–600)
	31	Open	11 (35.5)	NS	8 (25.8)	1 (3.2)	1 (3.2)	NS	NS	400 (240–550)
Singh et al. [30]	33	MIO (TLSO)	NS	NS	NS	NS	NS	No difference	Reduced after MIO	Longer for MIO
	31	Open	NS	NS	NS	NS	NS	($p = 0.17$)	($p < 0.01$)	($p < 0.01$)
Mamidanna et al. [31]	1155	MIO (TLSO, HMIO)	230 (19.9)	102 (8.8)	NS	NS	NS	15 (12–23)	NS	NS
	6347	Open	1181 (18.6)	611 (9.6)	NS	NS	NS	15 (12–22)	NS	NS
Ben-David et al. [32]	100	MIO (TLSO)	9 (9)	8 (8)	5 (5)	NS	3 (3)	7.5 (6–49)	125 (100–300)	330 (270–480)
	32	Open	5 (15.6)	NS	4 (12.5)	NS	NS	14 (10–98)	NS	NS
Briez et al. [33]	140	MIO (HMIO)	15.7	NS	5.7	0.7	NS	12 (8–80)	NS	NS
	140	Open	42.9	NS	4.3	0.0	NS	16 (8–180)	NS	NS
Xie et al. [34]	106	MIO (TLSO)	2 (1.9)	NS	5 (4.7)	NS	4 (3.8)	11.8 (±6.7)	187.2 (±37.8)	249.6 (±41.7)
	163	Open	8 (4.9)	NS	6 (3.7)	NS	5 (3.1)	13.9 (±7.3)	198.5 (±46.5)	256.3 (±41.7)
Hsu et al. [35]	66	MIO (TLSO)	7 (10.6)	NS	18 (27.3)	NS	4 (6.1)	NS	462.4 (±467.8)	510.9 (±121.3)
	63	Open	16 (25.4)	NS	19 (30.2)	NS	3 (4.8)	NS	615.5 (±591.6)	460.5 (±92.4)

MIO minimally invasive oesophagectomy, *VATS* video-assisted thoracoscopic oesophagectomy, *HMIO* hybrid MIO, *HALS* hand-assited laparoscopic oesophagectomy, *TSO* thoracoscopic –assisted oesophagectomy, *TLSO* thoracolaparoscopic oesophagectomy; *LIO* laparoscopic inversion oesophagectomy, *LSO* laparoscopic oesophagectomy, *NS* not stated

Results coming from five published meta-analyses, based on non-randomized comparative data, are contradictory. Two did not find significant differences between the MIO and the open approaches [36, 37] whereas three suggest that patients undergoing MIO had better postoperative outcomes with no compromise in oncological outcomes [8–10]. Patients undergoing MIO had significantly lower blood loss, and shorter postoperative ICU and hospital stay. There was a 30–50% decrease in overall morbidity in the MIO group. Subgroup analyses demonstrated significantly lower incidence of medical related complications, especially respiratory complications after MIO. However, surgical related postoperative outcomes such as anastomotic leak, anastomotic stricture, gastric conduit ischemia, chyle leak, and vocal cord palsy were globally comparable between the two techniques. Regarding postoperative mortality, the largest meta-analysis having included 48 studies and 14,311 patients, identified a reduced incidence of intra-hospital postoperative mortality (OR 0.69, 95% CI 0.55–0.89) [10]. This has been confirmed by a large French study that exhibited a reduction of 30-day (5.9% vs. 3.3%, p = 0.029) and 90-day (10.1% vs. 6.9%, p = 0.018) postoperative mortality favouring the MIO approach [38].

8.4 MIO Oncological Outcomes

If MIO is to become the approach of choice, then it must demonstrate not to compromise oncological outcomes. Improved lighting and visibility, along with the magnification afforded by minimally invasive equipment, may prove superior for meticulous dissection and lymph node harvest. However, not until large series report long-term survival by stage and pending published results of large randomized trials, the true oncologic value of MIO will remain controversial. Table 8.3 reflects the fact that no study to date has shown conclusive evidence of improved overall survival favouring a minimally invasive resection. Whilst several studies have suggested a benefit in terms of lymph node harvest, yet many have failed to meet the broadly accepted recommendations of the number of lymph nodes that should be retrieved for optimum staging and prognosis (Table 8.3). This puts into some question the quality of resection in several studies and makes oncological comparisons difficult. In a meta-analysis comparing oncological outcomes of MIO versus open group, the median (range) number of lymph nodes found was higher in the MIO group (16 (5.7–33.9)) compared to the open group (10 (3.0–32.8), p = 0.04); whereas no statistical difference was found for survival within respective time interval, although the difference favoured the MIO group [9]. More data on oncological data outcomes is needed, especially from future randomized controlled trials.

Table 8.3 Long-term oncological outcomes for MIO and open oesophagectomy

Authors	N	Approaches	Number of lymph nodes retrieved (median)	RO resection rate n (%)	3-year survival
Law et al. [14]	22	MIO (TSO)	7 [2–13]	10	62% (2 years)
	63	Open	13 [5–34]	NS	63% (2 years)
Nguyen et al. [15]	18	MIO (TLSO)	10.8±8.4	18	NS
	36	Open	6.6±5.8	NS	NS
Osugi et al. [16]	77	MIO (VATS)	33.9±12	NS	70%
	72	Open	32.8±14	NS	60%
Kunisaki et al. [17]	15	MIO (VATS + HALS)	24.5±10	NS	NS
	30	Open	26.6±10.4	NS	NS
Van den Broek et al. [18]	25	MIO (THO)	7±4.9	21 (84)	60% (f/u 17±11 months)
	20	Open	6.5±4.9	18 (90)	50% (f/u 54±16 months)
Bresadola et al. [19]	14	MIO (THO/TLSO)	22.2±12	NS	NS
	14	Open	18.6±13.4	NS	NS
Bernabe et al. [20]	17	MIO (THO)	9.8 (NS)	NS	NS
	14	Open	8.7 (NS)	NS	NS
Shiraishi et al. [21]	116	MIO (TLSO)	31.8 (NS)	NS	NS
	37	Open	30.1 (NS)	NS	NS
Braghetto et al. [22]	47	MIO (VATS/LSO)	NS	NS	45.5%
	119	Open	NS	NS	32.5%
Smithers et al. [23]	332	MIO (TLSO)	17 [9–33]	263	42%
	114	Open	16 [1–44]	90	30%
Fabian et al. [24]	22	MIO (TLSE)	15±6	22 (100)	NS
	43	Open	8±7	NS	NS

Table 8.3 (continued)

Authors	N	Approaches	Number of lymph nodes retrieved (median)	RO resection rate n (%)	3-year survival
Zingg et al. [25]	56	MIO (TLSO)	5.7±0.4	NS	Median survival – 35 months MIO 29 months Open
	98	Open	6.7±0.5	NS	
Perry et al. [26]	21	MIO (LIO)	10 [4–12]	NS	NS
	21	Open	3 [0–7]	NS	NS
Parameswaran et al. [27]	50	MIO (TLSO)	23 [7–49]	NS	74% (2 year survival)
	30	Open	10 [2–23]	NS	58% (2 year survival)
Pham et al. [28]	44	MIO (TLSO)	13 [9–15]	NS	NS
	46	Open	8 [3–14]	NS	NS
Schoppman et al. [29]	31	MIO (TLSO)	17.9±7.7	29 (93.5)	64%
	31	Open	20.5±12.6	30 (96.8)	46%
Singh et al. [30]	33	MIO (TLSO)	14 (6–16)	30	55% (2 year survival)
	31	Open	8 (3–14)	30	32% (2 year survival)
Mamidanna et al. [31]	1155	MIO (TLSO/HMIO)	NS	NS	NS
	6347	Open	NS	NS	NS
Ben-David et al. [32]	100	MIO (TLSO)	NS	99 (99)	NS
	32	Open	NS	32 (100)	NS
Briez et al. [33]	140	MIO (HMIO)	22 [8–53]	85.7	58% (2 year survival)
	140	Open	22 [6–56]	87.9	57% (2 year survival)
Xie et al. [34]	106	MIO (TLSO)	30.4 (±5.4)	NS	NS
	163	Open	30.2 (±5.0)	NS	NS
Hsu et al. [35]	66	MIO (TLSO)	28.3 (±16.6)	64 (97.0)	70.9%
	63	Open	25.9 (±15.3)	61 (96.8)	47.6%

MIO minimally invasive oesophagectomy, *VATS* video-assisted thoracoscopic oesophagectomy, *HMIO* hybrid MIO, *HALS* hand-assited laparoscopic oesophagectomy, *TSO* thoracoscopic-assisted oesophagectomy, *TLSO* thoracolaparoscopic oesophagectomy, *LIO* laparoscopic inversion oesophagectomy, *LSO* laparoscopic oesophagectomy, *NS* not stated

8.5 Results from Two Randomized Controlled Trials

Up till now, results of two multicentre randomised controlled trials have been reported comparing the results of minimally invasive and open oesophagectomy [11–13]: the TIME trial and the MIRO trial.

The TIME trial randomly assigned 56 patients to open oesophagectomy and 59 to a minimally invasive operation with all patients receiving equivalent neoadjuvant chemotherapy or chemoradiotherapy regimes. Both minimally invasive and open surgical groups had a mixture of two-stage and three-stage operations with the majority of patients having a cervical anastomosis. The primary outcome measure chosen was pulmonary infection within 2 weeks of surgery defined by clinical manifestation of pneumonia confirmed by radiological imaging and a positive sputum sample. Sixteen patients (29%) in the open surgical group and five (9%) patients in the minimally invasive group (p = 0.005) developed pneumonia in the first two postoperative weeks. These results suggest a significant benefit in terms of respiratory complications in favour of the minimally invasive approach, even if some qualifications could be made [39]. Mid-term 1-year results were recently reported with a high rate of symptomatic anastomotic stenosis, which was similar between the MIO and the open group (44% vs. 39%), and a better quality of life in favor of MIO for the physical component summary of the SF 36 questionnaire, EORTC C30 global health domain and OES18 pain domain [40].

The French multicenter phase III MIRO trial [12, 13] has randomised patients to either hybrid oesophagectomy (laparoscopic gastric mobilisation and open right thoracotomy) or open oesophagectomy. The MIRO trial tested the impact of laparoscopic gastric conduit creation with open thoracotomy (hybrid procedure) on major 30-day postoperative morbidity, especially on pulmonary complications. It hypothesised that hybrid MIO may decrease major postoperative morbidity without compromising oncological outcomes through an easily reproducible surgical procedure. Secondary objectives assessed the overall 30-day morbidity, 30-day mortality, disease-free and overall survival, quality of life and medico-economic analysis. The trial randomly assigned 104 patients to open oesophagectomy and 103 to a hybrid approach group. Sixty-seven (64.4%) patients in the open group had major postoperative morbidity compared with 37 (35.9%) in the hybrid group (OR 0·31, 95% CI 0·18–0·55; p = 0·0001). Thirty-one (30.1%) patients after an open operation had major pulmonary complications compared with 18 (17.7%) after a hybrid approach (p = 0·037), whereas the 30-day mortality rate was 1.9% vs. 1.0%, respectively. Medical related postoperative complications were significantly lower in the hybrid approach (19.6% vs. 39.8%), whereas the surgical related complications were not different between the groups even if favouring the hybrid group (14.7% vs. 20.4%). Regarding oncological outcomes, the 2-year overall survival rate (76.7% vs. 63.2%, p = 0.127) and disease-free survival rate (63.1% vs. 54.5%, p = 0.224) had not significantly improved in the MIO group. The MIRO results provide further evidence that a hybrid minimally invasive approach reduces the short-term insult of oesophagectomy without a negative impact on long-term oncological outcomes.

8.6 Total Versus Hybrid Oesophagectomy

Many authors reporting total minimally invasive approaches describe most as modifying the technique for avoiding the complexity of an intrathoracic anastomosis and consequently performing systematically the anastomosis in the neck. Others describe hybrid procedures where one stage of the operation is performed—either by thoracoscopy or laparoscopy and the other by conventional open surgery. The thoracoscopic approach is the widely-used hybrid procedure reported, being based on the hypothesis that thoracic-incision-related pain is the prominent factor responsible for postoperative pulmonary complications. However, the hybrid thoracoscopic approach calls for a three-stage procedure with a cervical anastomosis and subsequent morbidity. Others have reported a hybrid approach with laparoscopic gastric mobilization and open thoracotomy. This being based on the hypothesis that the high rate of postoperative complications after oesophagectomy—especially respiratory complications—is more related to the combination of two surgical incisions on both sides of the diaphragm than to the thorax opening, and hence is responsible for deterioration of the ventilatory mechanisms [33].

Even with only one phase of the operation being minimally invasive, yet blood loss, overall morbidity and respiratory complications were still found to be lower in retrospective comparative studies comparing open versus Hybrid MIO (HMIO) [8, 41]. This is consistent with open versus totally MIO analysis, and highlights the purported advantages of applying a minimally invasive approach to oesophagectomy. Postoperative mortality was also found to be significantly reduced with laparoscopic gastric mobilization [33, 38], offering similar oncological outcomes.

Looking at the two randomized trials reported to date, the TIME trial comparing totally MIO versus open [11] and the MIRO trial comparing HMIO and open oesophagectomy [12, 13], similar conclusions can be drawn. We see comparable odd ratios reported for decreasing postoperative complications that were 0.30 [0.12–0.76] in the TIME trial versus 0.31 [0.18–0.55] in the MIRO trial. Regarding oncological results, only the MIRO trial reported long-term outcomes that were not significantly different between groups, slightly favouring HMIO [12, 13].

HMIO—especially laparoscopic gastric mobilization—appears easy, reproducible, and not requiring modification of the surgical technique; It appears feasible despite the tumour or patients' characteristics or the centre experience, and does not compromise carcinologic resection, necessitating probably a little learning curve.

Totally MIO increases complexity and consequently brings a higher potential for error, requires according most reports modifications of the surgical technique with the need for a cervical anastomosis and its proper morbidity, needs very experienced hands, is time-demanding and probably is less easily reproducible. In addition, oncological safety of totally MIO is still a concern at present time, with few data on long-term oncological outcomes reported, especially for locally advanced tumours.

Scientific comparison between MIO and HMIO is of huge scientific interest. However, considering the limited results of randomized trials published, we can expect small differences while requiring a very large number of patients to be enrolled. More than placing MIO and HMIO in opposition, probably the more interesting course could be to choose one or the other approach according to the patient's profile, the tumour extension and the centre/surgeon expertise.

Conclusions

MIO has been gaining in popularity but—as seen with open surgery—no consensus has been reached regarding the superiority of any particular MIO adaptation. Even if some large comparative studies show a significantly better postoperative course following MIO harbouring no compromise of oncological outcomes, yet more data from randomized trials is needed. Randomized trials, however, have drawbacks due to the wide variety of techniques available, the heterogeneity in surgeons' preferences, the relative low number of procedures performed, the complexity of such surgery, and the variety and definition of postoperative complications after oesophagectomy. Certainly, the positive results of the TIME and the soon to be published MIRO trial add credence to what many surgeons find intuitive—that a less invasive approach could reduce morbidity after oesophagectomy. As the rates of postoperative mortality have fallen in specialist centres, our focus must turn to minimising the traditionally high level of morbidity associated with this operation.

To date, the data coming from non-randomized studies do suggest MIO is safe, and at least is comparable to open resection for both surgical and oncological outcomes. Data from meta-analyses suggest that MIO may have advantages in terms of less blood loss, less time in intensive care, fewer pulmonary complications and shorter hospital stay. However, the effect of MIO on quality of life and return to normal activity needs to be confirmed and medico-economic analyses need to be performed. Hence, requiring more large randomized controlled trials of oesophagectomy.

References

1. Birkmeyer JD, Siewers AE, Finlayson EV, et al. Hospital volume and surgical mortality in the United States. N Engl J Med. 2002;346:1128–37.
2. Pasquer A, Renaud F, Hec F, et al. FREGAT Working Group-FRENCH. Is centralization needed for esophageal and gastric cancer patients with low operative risk?: a nationwide study. Ann Surg. 2016;264:823–30.
3. Akaishi T, Kaneda I, Higuchi N, et al. Thoracoscopic en bloc total esophagectomy with radical mediastinal lymphadenectomy. J Thorac Cardiovasc Surg. 1996; 112:1533–40.
4. Gossot D, Fourquier P, Celerier M. Thoracoscopic esophagectomy: technique and initial results. Ann Thorac Surg. 1993;56:667–70.
5. Luketich JD, Pennathur A, Franchetti Y, et al. Minimally invasive esophagectomy: results of a prospective phase II multicenter trial-the eastern cooperative oncology group (E2202) study. Ann Surg. 2015;261:702–7.
6. Gemmill EH, McCulloch P. Systematic review of minimally invasive resection for gastro-oesophageal cancer. Br J Surg. 2007;94:1461–7.
7. Mariette C, Robb WB. Open or minimally invasive resection for oesophageal cancer? Recent Results Cancer Res. 2012;196:155–67.
8. Nagpal K, Ahmed K, Vats A, et al. Is minimally invasive surgery beneficial in the management of esophageal cancer? A meta-analysis. Surg Endosc. 2010; 24:1621–9.
9. Dantoc M, Cox MR, Eslick GD. Evidence to support the use of minimally invasive esophagectomy for esophageal cancer: a meta-analysis. Arch Surg. 2012; 147:768–76.

10. Zhou C, Zhang L, Wang H, et al. Superiority of minimally invasive oesophagectomy in reducing in-hospital mortality of patients with resectable oesophageal cancer: a meta-analysis. PLoS One. 2015;10:e0132889.
11. Biere SS, van Berge Henegouwen MI, Maas KW, et al. Minimally invasive versus open oesophagectomy for patients with oesophageal cancer: a multicentre, open-label, randomised controlled trial. Lancet. 2012;379:1887–92.
12. Briez N, Piessen G, Bonnetain F, et al. Open versus laparoscopically-assisted oesophagectomy for cancer: a multicentre randomised controlled phase III trial—the MIRO trial. BMC Cancer. 2011;11:310.
13. Mariette C, Meunier B, Pezet D, et al. Hybrid minimally invasive versus open oesophagectomy for patients with oesophageal cancer: a multicentre, open-label, randomised phase III controlled trial, the MIRO trial. Paper presented at the American society of clinical oncology gastrointestinal cancers symposium, San Francisco, 15–17 January 2015.
14. Law S, Fok M, Chu KM, et al. Thoracoscopic esophagectomy for esophageal cancer. Surgery. 1997;122:8–14.
15. Nguyen NT, Follette DM, Wolfe BM, et al. Comparison of minimally invasive esophagectomy with transthoracic and transhiatal esophagectomy. Arch Surg. 2000;135:920–5.
16. Osugi H, Takemura M, Higashino M, et al. A comparison of video-assisted thoracoscopic oesophagectomy and radical lymph node dissection for squamous cell cancer of the oesophagus with open operation. Br J Surg. 2003;90:108–13.
17. Kunisaki C, Hatori S, Imada T, et al. Video-assisted thoracoscopic esophagectomy with a voice-controlled robot: the AESOP system. Surg Laparosc Endosc Percutan Tech. 2004;14:323–7.
18. Van den Broek WT, Makay O, Berends FJ, et al. Laparoscopically assisted transhiatal resection for malignancies of the distal esophagus. Surg Endosc. 2004;18:812–7.
19. Bresadola V, Terrosu G, Cojutti A, et al. Laparoscopic versus open gastroplasty in esophagectomy for esophageal cancer: a comparative study. Surg Laparosc Endosc Percutan Tech. 2006;16:63–7.
20. Bernabe KQ, Bolton JS, Richardson WS. Laparoscopic hand-assisted versus open transhiatal esophagectomy: a case-control study. Surg Endosc. 2005;19:334–7.
21. Shiraishi T, Kawahara K, Shirakusa T, et al. Risk analysis in resection of thoracic esophageal cancer in the era of endoscopic surgery. Ann Thorac Surg. 2006;81:1083–9.
22. Braghetto I, Csendes A, Cardemil G, et al. Open transthoracic or transhiatal esophagectomy versus minimally invasive esophagectomy in terms of morbidity, mortality and survival. Surg Endosc. 2006;20:1681–6.
23. Smithers BM, Gotley DC, Martin I, et al. Comparison of the outcomes between open and minimally invasive esophagectomy. Ann Surg. 2007;245:232–40.
24. Fabian T, Martin JT, McKelvey AA, et al. Minimally invasive oesophagectomy : a teaching hospital's first experience. Dis Esophagus. 2008;21:220–5.
25. Zingg U, McQuinn A, DiValentino D, et al. Minimally invasive versus open esophagectomy for patients with esophageal cancer. Ann Thorac Surg. 2009;87:911–9.
26. Perry KA, Enestvedt CK, Pham T, et al. Comparison of laparoscopic inversion esophagectomy and open transhiatal esophagectomy for high-grade dysplasia and stage I esophageal adenocarcinoma. Arch Surg. 2009;144:679–84.
27. Parameswaran R, Veeramootoo D, Krishnadas R, et al. Comparative experience of open and minimally invasive esophagogastric resection. World J Surg. 2009;33:1868–75.
28. Pham TH, Perry KA, Dolan JP, et al. Comparison of perioperative outcomes after combined thoracoscopic-laparoscopic esophagectomy and open Ivor-Lewis esophagectomy. Am J Surg. 2010;199:594–8.
29. Schoppmann SF, Prager G, Langer FB, et al. Open versus minimally invasive esophagectomy: a single-center case controlled study. Surg Endosc. 2010;24:3044–53.
30. Singh RK, Pham TH, Diggs BS, et al. Minimally invasive esophagectomy provides equivalent oncologic outcomes to open esophagectomy for locally advanced (stage II or III) esophageal carcinoma. Arch Surg. 2010;146:711–4.
31. Mamidanna R, Bottle A, Aylin P, et al. Short-term outcomes following open versus minimally invasive esophagectomy for cancer in England: a population-based national study. Ann Surg. 2012;255:197–203.
32. Ben-David K, Sarosi GA, Cendan JC, et al. Decreasing morbidity and mortality in 100 consecutive minimally invasive esophagectomies. Surg Endosc. 2012;26:162–7.
33. Briez N, Piessen G, Torres F, et al. Effects of hybrid minimally invasive oesophagectomy on major postoperative pulmonary complications. Br J Surg. 2012;99:1547–53.
34. Xie MR, Liu CQ, Guo MF, et al. Short-term outcomes of minimally invasive Ivor-Lewis esophagectomy for esophageal cancer. Ann Thorac Surg. 2014;97:1721–7.
35. Hsu PK, Huang CS, Wu YC, et al. Open versus thoracoscopic esophagectomy in patients with esophageal squamous cell carcinoma. World J Surg. 2014;38:402–9.
36. Biere SS, Cuesta MA, van der Peet DL. Minimally invasive versus open esophagectomy for cancer: a systematic review and meta-analysis. Minerva Chir. 2009;64:121–33.
37. Sgourakis G, Gockel I, Radtke A, et al. Minimally invasive versus open esophagectomy: meta-analysis of outcomes. Dig Dis Sci. 2010;55:3031–40.
38. Messager M, Pasquer A, Duhamel A, et al. FREGAT working group-FRENCH. Laparoscopic gastric mobilization reduces postoperative mortality after esophageal cancer surgery: a French nationwide study. Ann Surg. 2015;262:817–22.

39. Mariette C, Robb WB. Minimally invasive versus open oesophagectomy for oesophageal cancer. Lancet. 2012;380:885–6.
40. Maas KW, Cuesta MA, van Berge Henegouwen MI, et al. Quality of life and late complications after minimally invasive compared to open esophagectomy: results of a randomized trial. World J Surg. 2015;39:1986–93.
41. Lee JM, Cheng JW, Lin MT, et al. Is there any benefit to incorporating a laparoscopic procedure into minimally invasive esophagectomy? The impact on perioperative results in patients with esophageal cancer. World J Surg. 2011;35:790–7.

9 Transthoracic Esophagectomy Approach by Thoracoscopy: 3 or 2 Stage?

James D. Luketich and M.N. Jaimes Vanegas

Esophageal cancer is the eighth most common cancer worldwide and the sixth leading cause of cancer-related deaths [1]. The incidence of esophageal cancer has been increasing dramatically over the last few decades, and esophageal cancer affects more than 450,000 people worldwide. Although squamous cell carcinoma predominates worldwide, in the western world this pronounced rise has been due to an increase in the incidence of adenocarcinoma of the esophagus [2]. The number of new cases in the United States in 2016 is estimated to be 16,910 [3]. Esophagectomy is an important, potentially curative treatment for localized esophageal cancer, however it is a complex operation and the morbidity and mortality are significant.

In a systematic review of literature, including more than 1100 patients, comparing minimally invasive esophagectomy (MIE) and open esophagectomy, MIE was associated with decreased morbidity and a shorter hospital stay compared with open esophagectomy [4]. Regarding the location for the anastomosis, both cervical and intrathoracic anastomosis have potential benefits. With a cervical anastomosis the surgeon is able to reach a more proximal resection margin and, even though there is a higher cervical anastomotic leak rate, it has lower associated morbidity. On the other hand, with an intrathoracic anastomosis, there tends to be a slightly higher rate of anastomotic leak, but also a lower incidence of recurrent laryngeal nerve (RLN) injury, and the ability to remove some of the potentially ischemic gastric tip as has been described in prior publications [5].

In an attempt to lower the morbidity related to esophagectomy, in 1996 we adopted at University of Pittsburgh Medical Center (UPMC) a minimally invasive approach to esophagectomy.

Since 1996, we have performed over 2000 minimally invasive esophagectomies. We have made several refinements to the MIE procedure that we believe significantly improved our surgical outcomes. It included the minimal handling of the final gastric conduit (no touch technique), keeping the width of the gastric conduit no smaller than 3 cm, selective application of an omental flap, and conversion from routine use of minimally invasive, three-hole esophagectomy to our new routine of minimally invasive Ivor Lewis esophagectomy. The Ivor Lewis, 2 stage MIE remains the mainstay in the surgical treatment of esophageal adenocarcinoma at UPMC [6].

J.D. Luketich (✉) • M.N. Jaimes Vanegas
Department of Cardiothoracic Surgery
University of Pittsburgh Medical Center (UPMC), Health System, Pittsburgh, PA, USA
e-mail: luketichjd@upmc.edu

M.A. Cuesta (ed.), *Minimally Invasive Surgery for Upper Abdominal Cancer*,
DOI 10.1007/978-3-319-54301-7_9

9.1 Gastric Conduit Concerns

Early in the UPMC experience, a very narrow gastric tube (2–2.5 cm in diameter) was trialed and was noted to be associated with an increase in gastric tip necrosis and anastomotic leaks. By increasing the diameter of the gastric conduit to a minimum of 3 cm, a decrease in anastomotic complications has been observed. It should be noted that this finding was somewhat anecdotal relatively early in our experience and was not part of a controlled trial of observations.

9.2 Omental Flap

Regarding the details of our omental flap, we create a 3-cm wide, 8–10 cm long omental pedicle, originating from the upper greater curvature of the stomach, laparoscopically. Key steps of the laparoscopic technique are, (1) identifying 2–3 arcades that branch off at right angles from the main gastroepiploic arcade, (2) preserving these branches as they traverse away from the greater curve out onto the omentum, (3) dissecting the fine adhesions between the undersurface of this omental flap and the transverse colon, (4) preventing a colonic enterotomy and avoiding damage to the blood supply of the omental flap, (5) tacking the distal tip of your new omental flap to the proximal gastric conduit, which will be pass into the chest via the hiatal opening with the newly created conduit. The primary disadvantage of laparoscopic harvest of an omental flap is that it can be time consuming (20–30 min), especially in obese patients or those with adhesions from multiple prior surgeries. Currently, the omental flap technique is utilized selectively, most commonly in high-risk patients who have undergone neo-adjuvant chemoradiation.

9.3 Three Hole Considerations

A neck dissection and subsequent creation of a cervical anastomosis has been associated with a higher rate of complications such as anastomotic leak, stricture, and injury to the RLN. This is particularly of concern in the setting of injury to RLN, which may have a profound impact on the risk of aspiration pneumonia due to poor clearance of pulmonary secretions. Another disadvantage of the neck anastomosis is the additional length of conduit needed to reach this area resulting in a potential increase in anastomotic tension, a marginal blood supply to the gastric tip and subsequent ischemia at the tip of the gastric conduit, resulting in a higher incidence of anastomotic leaks.

9.4 Ivor Lewis Considerations

Due to the concerns enumerated above, and the fact that we were seeing an increase in tumors of the lower third of the esophagus, we began to perform minimally invasive, Ivor Lewis esophagectomy more frequently in 2002, and reported our initial experience of 50 patients in 2006. In that report, we showed that a minimally invasive Ivor Lewis esophagectomy was feasible and that the technique was reproducible.

In an attempt to lower the morbidity related to the three hole esophagectomy, we adopted at our institution a minimally invasive Ivor Lewis approach. When we reviewed our experience with MIE in 2012, we reported on over 1000 patients. We evaluated the general outcomes after MIE, and also were able to compare the modified McKeown minimally invasive approach to the MIE Ivor Lewis. At that time our McKeown approach included thoracoscopic esophageal mobilization and dissection, laparoscopic abdominal portion and a neck anastomosis [MIE-neck]. Our Ivor Lewis approach included a laparoscopic approach first followed by thoracoscopic surgery, and a chest anastomosis [MIE-chest]. The MIE-neck was performed in 481 patients (48%) and MIE-Ivor Lewis in 530 patients (52%). The operative mortality was 1.68%. The median length of stay (8 days) and ICU stay (2 days) were similar between the two approaches. Mortality rate was 0.9%, and recurrent nerve injury was less frequent (1%) in the Ivor Lewis MIE group ($P < 0.001$).

Both approaches to MIE allowed an adequate lymph node resection (greater than 20), good postoperative outcomes, and low mortality regardless of the site of the anastomosis.

However, the MIE Ivor Lewis approach was associated with a reduced RLN injury and slight decrease in mortality to 0.9% [7].

9.5 Open Support of the Ivor Lewis Approach

One meta-analysis of more than 5000 patients comparing open Transhiatal versus open Ivor Lewis esophagectomy also found an increase in RLN injuries and anastomotic leak with a transhiatal approach with a neck anastomosis [8]. Initially, while starting our institutional MIE experience, we performed the MIE with a transhiatal approach but given the fact that complete mediastinal lymph node dissection was not possible in our hands, we rapidly adopted the addition of the VATS approach to a minimally invasive McKeown-type approach to perform the MIE [9]. However, as our experience grew, we were able to reduce the morbidity associated with RLN dysfunction by avoiding the neck dissection, and also noted the need for less length of our new gastric conduit and evolved to the minimally invasive Ivor Lewis approach.

9.6 Transhiatal Limitations

Orringer et al., in an important study of transhiatal esophagectomy (THE), reported the results in more than 2000 patients with an operative mortality rate that had steadily decreased with increasing hospital volume and surgeon experience, from 10 to 1%. Similarly, he demonstrated that complications, such as RLN injury, decreased with increased volume from 32% in the period of 1978 to 1982 to 1% to 2% in current era. These data point to the steep learning curve that many surgeons may experience if the neck approach is chosen [10]. Another factor to take into account in the current era of surgical training, is that many residents get minimal neck surgery experience during their general surgical and thoracic surgical training. All of these factors have led us to a greater degree of comfort in performing and teaching esophagectomy as an Ivor Lewis MIE at UPMC [7].

9.7 Epidemiology of Esophageal Cancer

Now a days, the vast majority of esophageal tumors that we encounter in the U.S.A and the Western world, are located in the distal esophagus and gastroesophageal junction, which makes high intrathoracic anastomosis usually adequate in regards to the proximal esophageal resection margin. For the purpose of this chapter, we will review in detail the surgical technique for MIE-neck anastomosis and MIE-thoracic anastomosis at UPMC, since on occasion a higher anastomosis is required depending on the nature of the esophageal tumor or proximal extent of Barrett's mucosa.

9.8 Operative Technique for MIE-Neck as Described in 2003 Outcomes Report of 222 Patients at Our Institution [9]

9.8.1 VATS Steps

The surgery starts with an esophagogastroduodenoscopy (EGD) to make a final assessment of the tumor's location and the gastric conduit's suitability for reconstruction. If the EGD, endoscopic ultrasound (EUS), or computerized tomography (CT) scan findings suggest gastric extension, T4 local extension or possible metastases, we perform a staging laparoscopy or a thoracoscopy or both. Patients are then intubated with a double-lumen tube and positioned in the left lateral decubitus position. The surgeon stands on the right and the assistant on the left. Four to Five thoracoscopic ports are used (Fig. 9.1). A 10-mm camera port is placed at the seventh to eighth intercostal space, just anterior to the midaxillary line. A 5-mm port is placed at the eighth or nineth intercostal space, posterior to the posterior axillary line, for the ultrasonic coagulating shears. A 10-mm port is placed in the anterior axillary line at the fourth intercostal space; this port is used to pass a fan shaped retractor to retract the lung anteriorly and allow exposure of the esophagus. The last 5-mm port is placed just posterior to

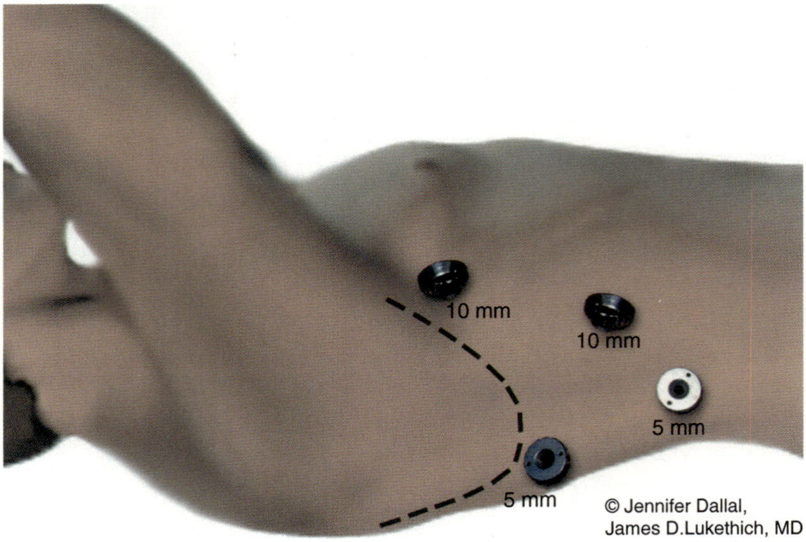

Fig. 9.1 Video-assisted thoracoscopic surgical port sites. Reproduced with permission from the UPMC Heart, Lung and Esophageal Surgery Institute, University of Pittsburgh Medical Center, Pittsburgh, PA

the scapula tip; it is used to place instruments for retraction and counter-traction. In most patients a single retracting suture (0-Endostitch) is placed near the central tendon of the diaphragm and brought out through the inferior anterior chest wall through a 1-mm skin incision. Doing so provides downward traction on the diaphragm, allowing good exposure of the distal esophagus.

Next, the inferior pulmonary ligament is divided. The mediastinal pleura overlying the esophagus is divided up to the level of the azygos vein to expose the thoracic esophagus. An endoscopic stapler (Endo-GIA vascular load) is used to divide the azygos vein. Care is taken to preserve the mediastinal pleura above the azygos vein, leaving some degree of a mediastinal seal around the gastric tube near the thoracic inlet, thereby minimizing the downward extension of a cervical leak into the chest. Circumferential mobilization of the esophagus is performed up to the level of 1–2 cm above the carina, including all surrounding lymph nodes, periesophageal tissue and fat; the plane along the pericardium, aorta and contralateral mediastinal pleura up to but not including the thoracic duct and azygos vein laterally. Care is taken to clip any aortoesophageal vessels and to clip any lymphatic branches from the thoracic duct. A Penrose drain is placed around the esophagus to facilitate traction and exposure. The entire intrathoracic esophagus is mobilized from the thoracic inlet to the diaphragmatic reflection. As the dissection proceeds toward the thoracic inlet, care is taken to stay near the esophagus to avoid trauma to the posterior membranous trachea and the recurrent laryngeal nerves. Care is also taken to avoid extending the distal dissection too low into the peritoneal cavity to avoid difficulty in maintaining pneumoperitoneum during the abdominal dissection. Each intercostal space is injected with 1–2 mL of 0.5% bupivacaine with epinephrine. The lung is then inflated to search for any air leaks from the trachea, proximal bronchus, and re-expanded lung. We then, place a 28-F chest tube, close the thoracic ports, and turn the patient to the supine position.

9.8.2 Laparoscopic Steps

Prior to beginning the laparoscopic and neck phases of the McKeown approach, the double lumen tube must be switched to a single lumen tube to avoid excessive stiffness of the trachea during the neck dissection.

The surgeon remains on the patient's right; the patient is positioned in steep reverse Trendelenburg. The arms are on arm boards approximately 30° away from the midline. Five abdominal ports (four 5-mm and one 11-mm) are used (Fig. 9.2). The gastrohepatic ligament is divided; the right and left crura of the diaphragm are dissected. The stomach

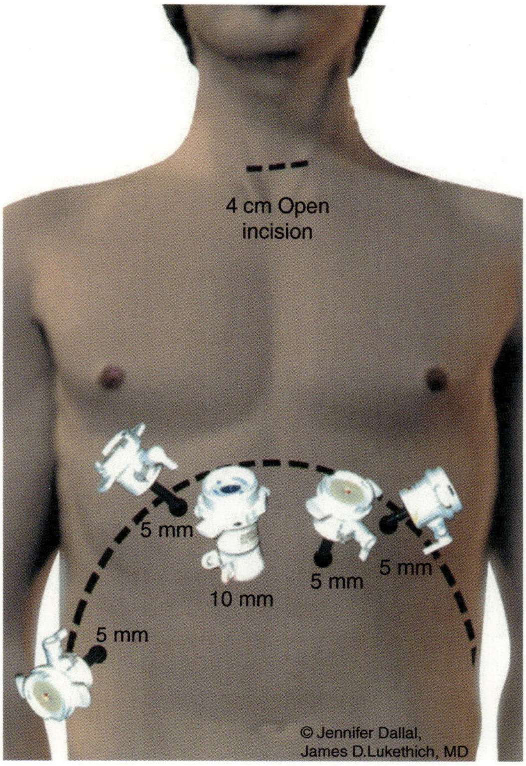

Fig. 9.2 Abdominal port sites for laparoscopy. Cervical incision. Reproduced with permission from the UPMC Heart, Lung and Esophageal Surgery Institute, University of Pittsburgh Medical Center, Pittsburgh, PA

is mobilized by dividing the short gastric vessels using the harmonic scalpel. The gastrocolic omentum is divided with care taken to preserve the right gastroepiploic arcade. The stomach is retracted superiorly, and the left gastric vessels are identified. The left gastric artery and vein can be divided from the retrogastric or lesser curve view, depending on the anatomy, using the Endo-GIA stapler (vascular load). We perform pyloroplasty in all cases. The harmonic scalpel is used to open the pylorus, and the Endo-stitch (2.0) is used to close the pylorus transversely. A gastric tube is then constructed by dividing the stomach starting at the lesser curve and preserving the right gastric vessels with the Endo-GI stapler. The initial staple load is fired approximately 5-6 cm superior to the pylorus, preserving the right gastric artery. There may be some variability in the construction of the gastric tube based on the characteristics of the tumor. It may be necessary to construct a slightly more narrow tube or to resect some of the proximal stomach in tumors with significant gastric extension. If gastric extension of the tumor is significant on pre-op EGD or Laparoscopic staging procedure, we generally prefer to resect more stomach and to make an intrathoracic anastomosis. For most patients in the 2003 report, there was minimal gastric involvement. If extensive gastric cardia extension is present, it may be necessary to perform a colon interposition. If so, we prefer to do this via open laparotomy.

Currently, we prefer a gastric tube of 3 cm in diameter (Fig. 9.3). Extreme caution must be used when manipulating the gastric tube during mobilization and stapling to avoid trauma. The most cephalad portion of the gastric tube is then attached to the esophageal and gastric specimen using two 2.0 Endo-sutures. An additional superficial stitch may be placed on the anterior proximal gastric tube to facilitate orientation and prevent twisting as the tube is brought up into the neck. We also place a marking stitch at the point where the diameter of the conduit enlarges somewhat near the lower antral reservoir. If performing an Ivor Lewis, when we retrieve the gastric conduit into the chest, we look for this transition stitch and try to maintain the antral reservoir completely within the abdomen. An omental flap is used only as part of the Ivor-Lewis approach.

A feeding jejunostomy tube is placed laparoscopically by first attaching a limb of proximal jejunum (35–40 cm distal to the ligament of Treitz) to the anterior abdominal wall in the left lateral mid-quadrant with the Endo-stitch (2.0). We add an additional 10-mm port in the right lower quadrant to facilitate suturing of the jejunum to the anterior abdominal wall. A laparoscopic j-tube kit is used (MIC jejunal feeding tube. HALYARD, Alpharetta, GA). Under direct laparoscopic vision, a large needle and the guide wire and catheter are directed into the loop of jejunum that has been tacked to the anterior abdominal wall. The entry site into the jejunum is carefully witzeled using 2-0 endo-stitches. The entry site of the needle catheter j-tube is tacked completely to the anterior abdominal wall for a distance of several centimeters to seal the area and to prevent torsion.

The last step in the abdominal operation is the dissection of the phrenoesophageal membrane.

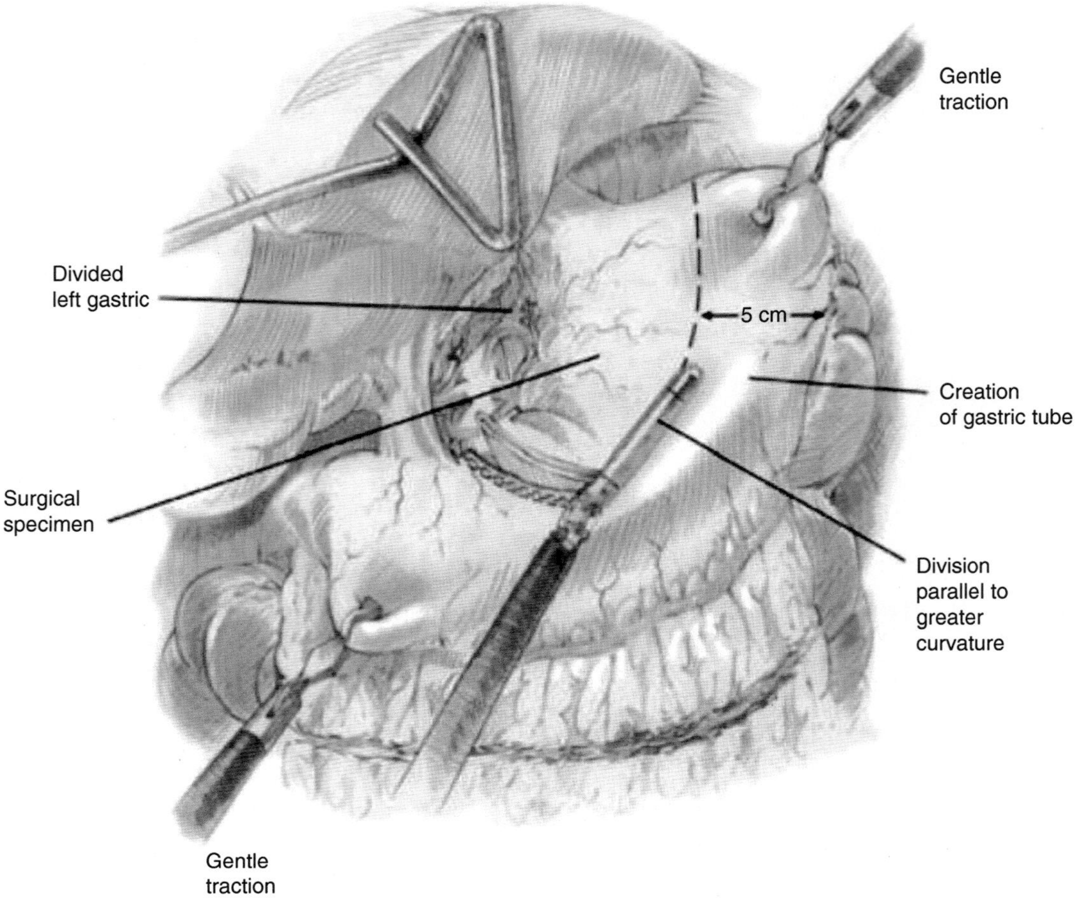

Fig. 9.3 Construction of gastric conduit. Reproduced with permission from the UPMC Heart, Lung and Esophageal Surgery Institute, University of Pittsburgh Medical Center, Pittsburgh, PA

Doing so at this stage helps to minimize the loss of pneumoperitoneum into the mediastinum during the earlier parts of the laparoscopic procedure. In some cases, it may be necessary to partially divide the right and left crura to allow easy passage of the gastric specimen and tube through the hiatus and to prevent later gastric outlet obstruction. However, in the current era, more frequently, we are dealing with a larger hiatal opening due to an associated hiatal hernia and it actually may be necessary to close this opening to some degree.

9.8.3 Neck Steps

Next, a 4- to 6-cm horizontal neck incision is made. The omohyoid muscle is visualized and divided. Deep to the omohyoid dissection we switch to bipolar electrocautery to minimize risk to the recurrent laryngeal nerve. The cervical esophagus is exposed. Careful dissection is performed down until the thoracic dissection plane is encountered, generally quite easily since the video-assisted thoracoscopic surgery (VATS) dissection is continued well into the thoracic inlet. In addition, we leave a penrose drain around the esophagus during the thoracic dissection and push the drain into the peri-esophageal plane at the thoracic inlet, so that it is easily visualized during the neck dissection and actually allows the surgeon to pull the penrose out through the neck to facilitate the neck dissection. The esophagogastric specimen is pulled out of the neck incision and the cervical esophagus divided high (2–3 cm below the cricopharyngeal muscle). The specimen is removed from the field. An anastomosis is performed between the cervical esophagus and gastric tube using standard techniques. In most patients, we prefer using a 25–28-mm EEA stapler. Alternatively, if length is somewhat of a concern, we perform a hand-sewn esophagogastric anastomosis, with a single layer of interrupted stitches of nonabsorbable 3-0 Silk or PDS sutures.

Next, the surgeon returns to the laparoscopic view and gently pulls downward on the pyloroantral area to retrieve any excess gastric tube that may have been pulled up into the chest during the neck anastomosis and mobilization. The laparoscopic pull is performed gently, and only until the assistant at the neck observes the tube and the anastomosis beginning to be pulled down at the level of the anastomosis. We strive to achieve a very high anastomosis just below the level of the cricopharyngeus to ensure adequate removal of any islands of Barrett's and to ensure that any anastomotic leak, will be more likely to drain out via the neck.

The last step of the laparoscopic approach is to place tacking sutures between the gastric tube and the diaphragm to prevent hiatal herniation. Care must be taken during this step to maintain orientation of the greater curve vessels towards the left crus and to avoid compromise of these vessels during suturing. We usually place three tacking sutures; one between the left crus and stomach just anterior to the greater curve arcade; the second on the right side of the gastric tube just above the right gastric vessels to the right crus; the third suture is placed anteriorly between the stomach and the diaphragm [9].

9.9 Operative Technique for Ivor Lewis MIE

With any esophagectomy, we always start the case with an on-table endoscopy that allows for assessment of the proximal and distal extent of the tumor as well as to plan the surgical resection margins and also determine the optimal site of anastomosis. For example, a tumor with more gastric cardia extension may require a more extensive resection of stomach in the abdomen and will necessitate the anastomosis to be performed in the chest, rather than the neck. On the other hand, in a patient with a tumor extending proximally to the high thoracic esophagus, a more proximal resection margin and anastomosis in the neck may be required. It is key to limit insufflation with air while performing the EGD, as this may interfere with subsequent laparoscopic surgery. We always decompress the stomach before removal of the endoscope. Patients with a mid on upper esophageal tumor require a bronchoscopy to evaluate the airway and exclude its involvement. The endotracheal tube is then changed to a double-lumen endotracheal tube [11].

9.10 Laparoscopic Phase

9.10.1 Port Placement and Exploration

Proper port placement is important to optimize exposure and the conduct of the operation (Fig. 9.2). Port placement can be modified to suit the body habitus of the patient or in patients with prior surgery. The patient is positioned in a steep reverse Trendelenburg position. A total of five abdominal ports (four 5-mm and one 10–12-mm) are used. The first port placed is a 10–12-mm port, which is placed with a cut down technique. Subsequent ports are placed under direct visualization of the laparoscope. A liver retractor is placed, and the left lobe of the liver is retracted. After placement of the ports, the first step is an exploration of the abdomen to rule out advanced disease before starting the gastric mobilization.

9.10.2 Gastric Mobilization

The mobilization of the stomach is started with the division of the gastrohepatic ligament. Subsequently, the right crus is visualized and dissected, followed by dissection of the left crura of the diaphragm. It is important to avoid dividing the phrenoesophageal membrane at this point, which may lead to loss of pneumoperitoneum. It is important to handle the stomach gently during the mobilization using a no-touch technique of our planned gastric conduit. The greater curvature of the stomach is mobilized by dividing the short gastric vessels using the ultrasonic coagulating shears. We leave 3–4 cm of fat margin with the arcade to help separate the conduit from its ultimate position near the posterior membranous airway. The gastrocolic omentum is then divided, with care taken to preserve the right gastroepiploic arcade. During this portion of the dissection, we selectively mobilize and preserve a well-vascularized omental flap which later would be used as a buttress after construction of the intrathoracic anastomosis. The omental flap is used only if chemo and radiation have been used preoperatively. The posterior attachments of the stomach are then divided after retraction of the stomach anteriorly. A complete celiac node dissection is performed before division of the left gastric vessels with a vascular stapler. On a rare occasion, during gastric mobilization, we may encounter a hepatic branch originating from the left gastric artery. If there is a concern that this branch is a significant major replaced left hepatic artery, we apply a removable clip and observe the left lobe of the liver. If there is concern about ischemia, we remove the clip and preserve this replaced left hepatic artery.

9.10.3 Pyloroplasty

The next step is the performance of the pyloroplasty. The pylorus is mobilized, and its mobility is verified by lifting the pylorus gently up to the caudate lobe of the liver without any tension. A Kocher maneuver is performed to achieve adequate mobilization. An additional 5/11 port is placed in the mid right lower quadrant of the abdomen to facilitate the construction of the pyloroplasty, construction of the gastric tube, and placement of the feeding jejunostomy tube. Then we place two traction sutures at the edges of the pylorus with the Endostitch (2.0). A Heineke-Mikulicz type pyloroplasty is then performed. The pylorus is incised longitudinally with the harmonic scalpel and then closed transversely with interrupted sutures using the Endostitch device. The pyloroplasty is buttressed with an omental patch.

9.10.4 Construction of the Gastric Tube

This is a critical component of the procedure. We create a gastric tube approximately 3 cm in diameter, starting at the lesser curve (Fig. 9.3). The right gastric vessels are preserved. We start with a stapling device (Endo-GIA) beginning in the lesser curve, about 5 cm proximal to the pylorus. It is important to avoid excessive manipulation and trauma to the gastric conduit during this step. To facilitate exposure and protect our planned conduit with a no-touch technique, we have one assistant gently retracting the fundic tip of the stomach (which will subsequently be resected) superiorly and another assistant simultaneously gently retracting the pyloroantral area inferiorly. This retraction facilitates proper alignment and the construction of a gastric tube with uniform diameter of 3 cm. In rare instances, if it is thought that the gastric margin may be a concern, the gastric staple line on the specimen side is sent for a frozen section before the thoracic portion of the operation.

We then routinely place a jejunostomy tube using Seldinger technique, at about 40 cm from the ligament of Treitz. The jejunum is secured to the anterior abdominal wall at the jejunostomy site after doing a Witzel tunnel, then we place an anti-torsion stitch about 3 cm distal to the jejunostomy tube site, using a 2-0 Endo-stitch. The final step is the division of the phrenoesophageal membrane. At this time a careful 360° dissection is performed and the gastric resected specimen is carefully pushed up into the hiatus to facilitate later VATS retrieval. The abdomen is inspected to make sure that hemostasis is adequate and the incisions are closed.

9.11 Thoracoscopic Phase

9.11.1 Thoracoscopic Port Placement

The patient is placed in a left lateral decubitus position. The position of the double-lumen tube is verified with flexible bronchoscopy, and single-lung ventilation is used. Typically, we use five thoracoscopic ports. The fifth, 5-mm port, placed anteriorly is used by the first assistant intermittently for suction. Similar to the ports in the abdomen, optimal port placement is important. A 10-mm port is placed at the seventh to eighth intercostal space, just anterior to the mid-axillary line, for the camera. Another 10-mm port is placed at the eighth or ninth intercostal space, posterior to the posterior axillary line, for the dissection instrument (ultrasonic coagulating shears). A 10-mm port is placed in the anterior axillary line, at the fourth intercostal space, and this is used to pass a fan-shaped retractor to retract the lung anteriorly and allow exposure of the esophagus. A 5-mm port is placed just posterior to the scapula tip, which is used to place instruments for retraction and counter traction. After thoracoscopic exploration, we place a retracting suture near the central tendon of the diaphragm (Endostitch 0), and this suture is brought out through the chest wall through a 1-mm skin incision several centimeters below the camera port. This allows us to provide downward traction on the diaphragm and aids with exposure of the distal esophagus. Later in the case, we make a 5 cm access incision to enable passage of the end-to-end stapler (EEA) and, for removal of the specimen.

9.11.2 Esophageal Mobilization and Lymph Node Dissection

We then proceed with the division of the inferior pulmonary ligament. The mediastinal pleura overlying the esophagus is divided and opened up to the level of the azygos vein to expose the thoracic esophagus. The azygos vein is then dissected and divided with an endoscopic vascular stapler. The esophagus, along with the periesophageal tissue and lymph nodes, is circumferentially mobilized from the diaphragm to the level about 2 cm above the carina. A Penrose drain is placed around the esophagus to facilitate traction and exposure. We use an ultrasonic coagulating instrument for the dissection, and endoscopic clips are applied generously for larger vessels and any lymphatics. Above the azygos vein, it is important to keep the plane of dissection directly on the esophagus to prevent injury to the airway and the recurrent laryngeal nerve. Mediastinal lymph node dissection, including a complete dissection of the subcarinal lymph nodes, is performed. With the most common location of tumors being distal esophageal or gastroesophageal junction tumors, we do not perform aggressive nodal dissection near the thoracic inlet to decrease the chance of recurrent laryngeal nerve injury. In addition, the vagi are divided at the level of the azygos vein to minimize traction injury to the recurrent laryngeal nerves. During the thoracoscopic mobilization of the esophagus, it is important to avoid thermal or ultrasonic injury to the airway and the pericardium. The distal esophagus and the gastric conduit are brought up in the chest. It is important to maintain the proper orientation of the gastric conduit, with care taken not to twist the conduit. We prefer a high intrathoracic anastomosis near the thoracic inlet; however, one should be cautious not to divide the esophagus too proximally because this makes construction of the intrathoracic anastomosis technically difficult. In some patients, when there is a concern about the proximal extent of the tumor, repeat endoscopy may be required at this point to determine the site of transection. A 5 cm access incision is made at approximately the 6th intercostal space, we then apply a wound protector; the specimen is removed through this access and sent for frozen-section analysis of margins.

9.11.3 Construction of Anastomosis

We then perform a stapled EEA intrathoracic anastomosis. The first step of the stapled anastomosis is the placement of a 28-mm EEA anvil in the proximal esophagus. The anvil is secured with a purse string suture (Endostitch 2-0). We have found that it is difficult to place this first suture perfectly, as the anvil tends to move and migrate out of the open esophagus. Therefore, we add a second purse string suture to secure the anvil. Because the fundus of the stomach is the most ischemic portion of the conduit, we plan the anastomosis so as to discard the fundic tip. The tip of the fundus is opened, the conduit is flushed with warm antibiotic saline to minimize soilage. Next, the EEA stapler is advanced into the gastrostomy just created in the tip of the fundus. A stapled anastomosis between the gastric conduit and the esophagus, high above the azygos vein, is then performed (Fig. 9.4). The redundant portion of the fundus is excised with a reticulating endo GIA staple, purple load (Fig. 9.5). A nasogastric tube is placed across the anastomosis, under direct visualization, and secured. The anastomosis is checked for any leaks. Avoiding use of the tip of the fundus helps minimize leaks. In some patients (those who have received pre op chemo-radiation), we buttress the anastomosis with an omental flap, which was earlier mobilized during the abdominal phase of the dissection. During the conclusion of the abdominal portion of the operation, the hiatus, if enlarged, is closed posteriorly, and typically one suture is required (Endostitch 0). This is decided based on the size of the hiatal opening, and tailored to avoid narrowing of the conduit and prevent herniation. In addition, at the conclusion of the chest portion of the operation, the conduit is

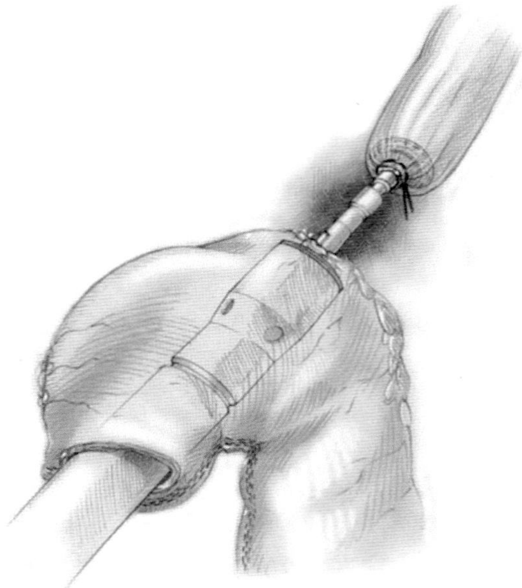

Fig. 9.4 Construction of minimally invasive Ivor Lewis anastomosis. Reproduced with permission from the UPMC Heart, Lung and Esophageal Surgery Institute, University of Pittsburgh Medical Center, Pittsburgh, PA

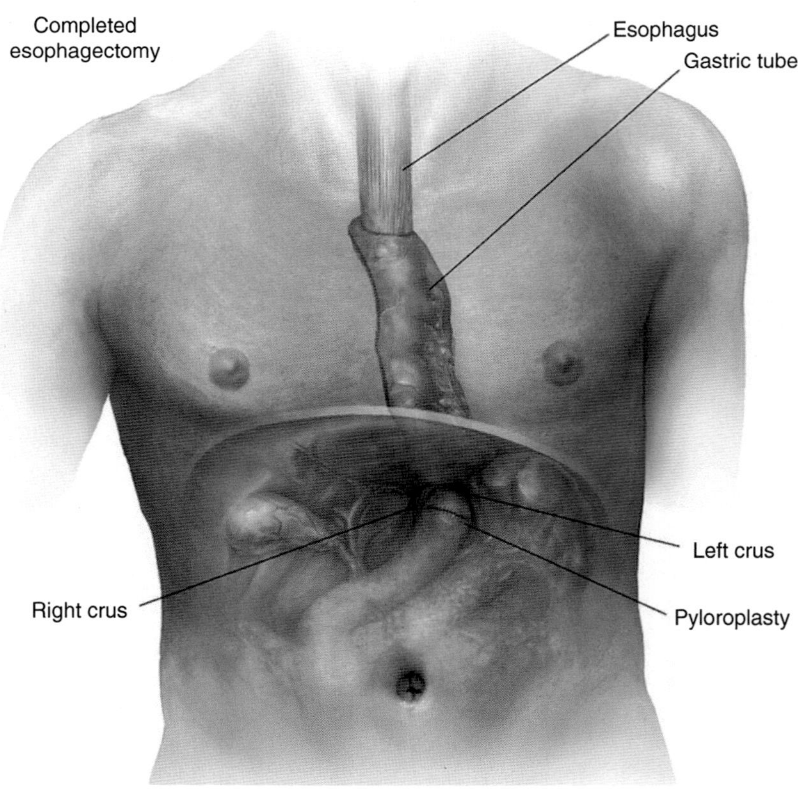

Fig. 9.5 Final aspect of the gastric conduit and anastomosis. Reproduced with permission from the UPMC Heart, Lung and Esophageal Surgery Institute, University of Pittsburgh Medical Center, Pittsburgh, PA

anchored to the right crus with an endostitch. This approach is used to minimize herniation of abdominal organs into the chest.

The chest is inspected closely, and hemostasis is verified. The conduit should be straight and free of redundancy. It is important to drain the chest well and place drains strategically in the chest. This is critical because a well-drained small leak, should it occur, is easy to manage. We place a 28F chest tube posteriorly in the pleural space, and a second No. 10 Jackson-Pratt drain posterior to the anastomosis, tracking behind the gastric conduit to the diaphragm, exiting at the costophrenic angle. It is also important to secure these drains well. We also perform a multilevel intercostal block at the conclusion of the procedure, and close all thoracic incisions in usual fashion. The chest tube is placed on suction, and the patient is turned to a supine position. The double-lumen endotracheal tube is then changed to a single-lumen endotracheal tube. A flexible bronchoscopy is performed, and any secretions in the bronchial tree are aspirated. We also perform an exhaustive aspiration of all oropharyngeal secretions at the end of the case, prior to exchange of the double lumen tube to avoid aspiration of oropharyngeal and/or esophageal debris and secretions.

9.12 Discussion of Thoracic Anastomotic Techniques

Campos et al. published in 2010 their preliminary results on 37 patients of a standardized 25 mm/4.8 mm circular-stapled anastomosis using a trans-orally placed anvil. The esophagogastric anastomosis was created using a 25-mm anvil passed trans-orally, in a tilted position, and connected to a 90-cm long polyvinyl chloride delivery tube through an opening in the esophageal stump. The anastomosis was completed by joining the anvil to a circular stapler (end-to-end anastomosis stapler (EEA XL) 25 mm with 4.8-mm staples) inserted into the gastric conduit. There were no intra-operative technical failures of the anastomosis or deaths. Five patients had strictures (13.5%) and all were successfully treated with endoscopic dilations. One patient had an anastomotic leak (2.7%) that was successfully treated by re-operation and endoscopic stenting of the anastomosis. They concluded that the circular-stapled anastomosis with the transoral anvil allowed for an efficient, safe and reproducible anastomosis [12].

A literature search on the current techniques and approaches for intrathoracic anastomosis was published in 2012 by Maas et al. Twelve studies were evaluated on leakage and stenosis rate of the anastomosis. The most frequent applied technique was the stapled anastomosis. Stapled EEA anastomoses can be divided into a transthoracic or a transoral introduction. This stapled approach can be performed with a circular or linear stapler. The reported anastomotic leakage rate ranges from 0 to 10%. The reported anastomotic stenosis rate ranges from 0 to 27.5%. The review found no important differences between the two most frequently used stapled anastomoses: the transoral introduction of the anvil and the transthoracic [13].

A large meta-analysis published in 2015 comprising 15 studies, total of 3.203 patients, compared the main clinical outcomes following linear stapler (LS) and hand-sewn (HS) esophagogastric anastomosis, including the rates of anastomotic leakage and stricture. Compared with HS, LS esophagogastric anastomosis has a lower rate of anastomosis leakage for several possible reasons: (1) the stapled anastomoses are considered to be more expedient and less traumatic to tissues; (2) the lateral stay sutures allow for reduced tension on the anastomosis without compromising gastric conduit microcirculation; and (3) LS provides triple-layered staple construction that is less traumatic and more watertight than HS.

A significantly reduced rate of anastomotic stricture associated with LS was also found. Performing a subgroup analysis, although there was no significant difference in the decrease in thoracic anastomotic leakage, there was a significant decrease in cervical anastomotic leakage associated with LS. The meta-analysis concluded that the LS technique contributes to a reduced rate of leakage and stricture compared with the HS method [14].

On the other hand, a meta-analysis published in 2013 showed no significant difference in the incidence of esophageal anastomotic leak (EAL) for the following technical factors: hand-sewn versus stapled esophagogastric anastomosis (EGA), minimally invasive versus open esophagectomy, anterior versus posterior route of reconstruction, and ischemic conditioning of the gastric conduit. However, the only technical factor associated with an increased incidence of EAL was a cervical location of the anastomosis, most likely due to a greater stretch placed upon the gastric conduit and impaired conduit microcirculation, as demonstrated on four randomized, controlled trials comprising 298 patients, included in the report, that compared cervical and thoracic EGA. Anastomotic leak was seen more commonly in the cervical group (13.64%) than in the thoracic group (2.96%) [15].

Despite this, some highly experienced surgeons have demonstrated a very low rate of anastomotic leak while performing cervical esophagogastric anastomosis [10].

In a recently published French large multicenter database study, the incidence of severe esophageal anastomotic leak (SEAL) after esophagectomy for esophageal cancer, in their large study population (2439 patients), was 8.5%. The results of the study suggest that SEAL was significantly associated with an adverse impact upon overall and disease-free survivals, and it was also associated with an increase in the incidence of overall, loco-regional, and mixed cancer recurrences. Clinically significant differences in survival were seen in all stages, but statistically significant only for stage 0 and stage III. The incidence of SEAL was independently associated with low hospital procedural volume, cervical anastomosis, upper third tumor location, and ASA score III/IV in multivariable analysis. The findings of this study call attention to the long-term consequences of failure during the anastomotic formation in esophagectomy, and further advise about short- and long-term benefits to the centralization of esophagectomy to high-volume centers [16].

In our experience, we have performed all types of intrathoracic anastomosis including hand sewn, EEA and linear stapled. We currently prefer the EEA technique, when possible with a 28-mm stapler.

9.13 MIE at Other Centers in the United States

We conducted a multi-center, phase II, prospective cooperative group study (coordinated by ECOG) to assess the feasibility of MIE in a multi-institutional setting. Patients with biopsy-proven high-grade-dysplasia or esophageal cancer were enrolled at 17 credentialed sites. Protocol surgery consisted of either 3-stage MIE or Ivor Lewis MIE. MIE was completed in 95 of the 104 patients eligible for the primary analysis (91.3%). The 30-day mortality in eligible patients who underwent MIE was 2.1%; perioperative mortality in all registered patients eligible for primary analysis was 2.9%. Median intensive care unit and hospital stay were 2 and 9 days, respectively. Grade 3 or higher adverse events included anastomotic leak (8.6%), acute respiratory distress syndrome (5.7%), pneumonitis (3.8%), and atrial fibrillation (2.9%). At a median follow-up of 35.8 months, the estimated 3-year overall survival was 58.4% (95% confidence interval: 47.7%–67.6%). Locoregional recurrence occurred in only seven patients (6.7%). We demonstrated that MIE is feasible and safe with low peri-operative morbidity and mortality and good oncological results in centers with significant open and minimally invasive esophageal surgical experience. The MIE approach can be adopted by other centers with appropriate expertise in open esophagectomy and minimally invasive procedures involving the foregut [17].

Conclusion

Surgical resection is a primary curative modality in patients with resectable esophageal cancer. One of the main concerns for recommendation of esophagectomy is the associated risks of surgery. In an effort to decrease the morbidity of esophagectomy, we have adopted a minimally invasive strategy. We have described our current technique of minimally invasive Ivor Lewis esophagectomy, as well as the minimally invasive McKeown esophagectomy technique in detail. Esophageal surgeons should decide on every individual case about the need for a cervical versus an intrathoracic anastomosis, based mainly on the location and extension of the tumor, but also on the surgical expertise required to perform every single step of a minimally invasive esophagectomy.

References

1. Di Pardo BJ, et al. The global burden of esophageal cancer: a disability-adjusted life-year approach. World J Surg. 2016;40(2):395–401.
2. Pennathur A, Gibson MK, Jobe BA, et al. Oesophageal carcinoma. Lancet. 2013;381:400–12.
3. Siegel RL, Miller KD, Jemal A. Cancer statistics, 2016. CA Cancer J Clin. 2016;66(1):7–30.
4. Verhage RJ, Hazebroek EJ, Boone J, et al. Minimally invasive surgery compared to open procedures in esophagectomy for cancer: a systematic review of the literature. Minerva Chir. 2009;64:135–46.
5. Pennathur A, Zhang J, Chen H, et al. The "best operation" for esophageal cancer? Ann Thorac Surg. 2010;89:S2163–7.
6. Zhang J, et al. Refinement of minimally invasive esophagectomy techniques after 15 years of experience. J Gastrointest Surg. 2012;16:1768–74.
7. Luketich JD, Pennathur A, Awais O, et al. Outcomes after minimally invasive esophagectomy: review of over 1000 patients. Ann Surg. 2012;256:95–103.
8. Rindani R, Martin CJ, Cox MR. Transhiatal versus Ivor-Lewis oesophagectomy: is there a difference? Aust N Z J Surg. 1999;69:187–94.
9. Luketich JD, Alvelo-Rivera M, Buenaventura PO, et al. Minimally invasive esophagectomy: outcomes in 222 patients. Ann Surg. 2003;238:486–94; discussion 494–5.
10. Orringer MB, Marshall B, Chang AC, et al. Two thousand transhiatal esophagectomies: changing trends, lessons learned. Ann Surg. 2007;246:363–72; discussion 372–4.
11. Pennathur A, Awais O, Luketich JD. Technique of minimally invasive Ivor Lewis esophagectomy. Ann Thorac Surg. 2010;89:S2159–62.
12. Campos GM, et al. A safe and reproducible anastomotic technique for minimally invasive Ivor Lewis esophagectomy: the circular stapled anastomosis with the transoral anvil. Eur J Cardiothorac Surg. 2010;37:1421–6.
13. Maas KW, et al. Minimally invasive intrathoracic anastomosis after Ivor Lewis esophagectomy for cancer: a review of transoral or transthoracic use of staplers. Surg Endosc. 2012;26:1795–802.
14. Deng X-F, et al. Hand-sewn vs linearly stapled esophagogastric anastomosis for esophageal cancer: a meta-analysis. World J Gastroenterol. 2015;21(15):4757–64.
15. Markar S, et al. Technical factors that affect anastomotic integrity following esophagectomy: systematic review and meta-analysis. Ann Surg Oncol. 2013;20:4271–81.
16. Markar S, et al. The impact of severe anastomotic leak on long-term survival and cancer recurrence after surgical resection for esophageal malignancy. Ann Surg. 2015;262:972–80.
17. Luketich JD, Pennathur A, et al. Minimally invasive esophagectomy: results of a prospective phase II multicenter trial-the Eastern Cooperative Oncology Group (E2202) Study. Ann Surg. 2015;261:702–7.

10 Minimally Invasive Approach of Gastro-Esophageal Junction Cancer

Annelijn E. Slaman, Suzanne S. Gisbertz, Mark I. van Berge Henegouwen, and Miguel A. Cuesta

10.1 Introduction

Esophageal cancer is the sixth most-common cause of death from cancer worldwide with over 450.000 new cases annually [1]. In Northern and Western Europe, the USA, Canada and Oceania the predominant histologic subtype of esophageal cancer is an adenocarcinoma and the prevalence of this subtype is increasing rapidly in these countries, particularly for males [2]. Risk factors for developing an adenocarcinoma are symptomatic gastro-esophageal reflux disease (GERD), Barrett's esophagus, obesity and a combination of alcohol and smoking. Mainly, adenocarcinomas develop in the distal third of the esophagus or in the gastro-esophageal junction (GEJ). The main symptoms of patients with esophageal cancer are dysphagia, weight loss, pain in the stomach or symptoms of anemia [3]. When patients present with symptoms, a variety of diagnostic instruments is available to assess the location and spread of the tumor and to check for local or distant metastases. To assess the precise location of the tumor and to confirm the diagnosis, an endoscopy with biopsy has to be performed. For the treatment of GEJ tumours in particular it is important to assess the spread of the tumor into the esophagus and the gastric cardia. Lymphatic dissemination and the possibility of distant metastases are further investigated by endoscopic ultrasound (EUS), computed tomography scan (CT-scan) of the neck, thorax and abdomen, and a PET-CT-scan. If local tumor ingrowth and/or distant metastases are suspected, biopsies can confirm this. Esophageal carcinomas are staged according to the seventh edition of the American Joint Committee on Cancer staging system [4]. This classification predicts the overall survival (OS) rates per stage groupings for adenocarcinomas and squamous cell carcinomas separately. It shows a risk-adjusted 5-years OS ranging from 15 to 85% for adenocarcinomas and ranging from 15 to 75% for squamous cell carcinomas, depending on the stage group. Moreover, if tumors are staged with T1a or lower it should be treated by endomucosal resection and above stage T1a patients will undergo an esophageal resection. For the surgical classification of GEJ adenocarcinomas, the Siewert classification is used despite its limitations. This classification divides tumors in type I–III based on anatomical criteria [5]:

Electronic Supplementary Material The online version of this chapter (doi:10.1007/978-3-319-54301-7_10) contains supplementary material, which is available to authorized users. On http://springerlink.com enter the DOI number given above.

A.E. Slaman • S.S. Gisbertz (✉)
M.I. van Berge Henegouwen
Department of Surgery, Academic Medical Center, Amsterdam, The Netherlands
e-mail: a.e.slaman@amc.uva.nl; s.s.gisbertz@amc.uva.nl; m.i.vanbergehenegouwen@amc.uva.nl

M.A. Cuesta
Department of Surgery, VU University, Amsterdam, The Netherlands

M.A. Cuesta (ed.), *Minimally Invasive Surgery for Upper Abdominal Cancer*, DOI 10.1007/978-3-319-54301-7_10

- **Type I:** Adenocarcinoma is located mainly on the side of the esophagus.
- **Type II:** True cardia carcinoma infiltrating from 1 cm on the side of the esophagus up to 2 cm in the stomach.
- **Type III:** Subcardial gastric carcinoma that grows from 2 to 5 cm distal of the Z-line.

An esophageal resection has always been the main curative treatment of esophageal cancer. Since the promising results of a randomized controlled trial that introduced neoadjuvant chemoradiotherapy (nCRTx) as an important additional treatment to surgery for esophageal cancer, survival rates have been improved importantly, with the increase in the 5-year-overall survival rate from 33 to 47% [6, 7]. However, esophagectomies are still associated with high morbidity and mortality rates. To reduce the morbidity and to increase the quality of life (QoL), a minimally invasive esophagectomy approach (MIE) was introduced in the early 90s. Looking for evidence, the outcomes of the TIME trial showed advantages of MIE when compared to open esophagectomy (OE), such as a decreasing incidence of postoperative pulmonary infections, a shorter length of hospital stay and better QoL scores, indicating an improved patient recovery [8]. Concerning oncological safety, no differences were found in OS and disease-free survival after one and 3 years follow-up, with a better Quality of Life (QoL) of physical components at 1 year follow-up [9]. Therefore, MIE is currently considered to be a safe surgical procedure and the majority of patients with a resectable esophageal or GEJ-tumor should be approached by a minimally invasive approach. Yet, several factors influence the surgeon's discretion in that choice and this chapter treats these (Videos 10.1, 10.2, 10.3 and 10.4).

10.1.1 Treatment Possibilities for GEJ Tumors

Discussion exists about what type of neoadjuvant treatment is indicated for GEJ cancer. Most oncologists will recommend neoadjuvant chemotherapy for GEJ tumors with Siewert type 2 and 3, whereas they will choose for Chemoradiotherapy (nCRTx) for Siewert type 1 tumors. After neoadjuvant therapy, there are two main surgical approaches for resection of GEJ tumors: the transthoracic (the 2-staged Ivor-Lewis esophagectomy or 3-staged McKeown esophagectomy) or the transhiatal esophagectomy (THE). The decision for the surgical approach is based on the surgeon's discretion, since there is no evidence about the best surgical approach in terms of morbidity and oncological outcomes yet.

Generally, a laparoscopic gastrectomy is performed for Siewert type III. For type II, a MIE Ivor-Lewis procedure is the main choice and as an alternative procedure a laparoscopic total gastrectomy with a high esophagogastrostomy anastomosis using the Orvil Circular Stapler (®Medtronic Inc., Minneapolis, MN, USA [10]) can be performed. Some surgeons indicate a laparoscopic THE with an anastomosis in the cervical area and in the case of extensive growth of the tumor along the lesser curvature an open esophageal and gastric resection followed by a colon interposition is indicated. Finally, a laparoscopic two-staged Ivor-Lewis or a three-staged McKeown approach will be the choice for a Siewert type I tumor.

10.1.2 Preparation for Operation

Along with the use of neoadjuvant treatment, patients have to be optimally prepared for operation. This includes improvements of the general condition by optimal nutrition, physiotherapy and psychotherapy. Moreover, concerning the operative planning, it is important to study the radiotherapy charts (radiation field) to see if the proximal esophagus or parts of the stomach have been exposed to radiotherapy. If the intrathoracic anastomosis is the preferred location of reconstruction, then the anastomosis could be created in a non-radiated area in order to reduce the leakage rate.

10.2 Surgical Techniques

10.2.1 Two-Staged Minimally Invasive Ivor-Lewis Procedure

The Ivor-Lewis esophagectomy with intrathoracic anastomosis is a perfect operation for many infracarinal esophageal cancers, but has a high difficulty grade due to the creation of the intrathoracic anastomosis. The patient is intubated by selective intubation, which is only used for the anastomotic phase during thoracoscopy. The operation commences with a laparoscopy (extensive celiac trunk type D1+ lymphadenectomy, gastric dissection along greater curvature with preservation of gastroepiploic vessels, creation of a gastric conduit by staplers and hiatal dissection) followed by right thoracoscopy in prone position of the patient (including dissection and mobilization of the esophagus, a mediastinal lymphadenectomy and division of the esophagus in the area between the carina and the azygos vein).

The gastric tube and the esophageal specimen are pulled into the thorax through a wide hiatus, followed by creation of an intrathoracic anastomosis. Although there are different types of intrathoracic anastomoses, no evidence posits one type of anastomosis as superior to another. As options, we can create a manual anastomosis or an end-to-side anastomosis using a conventional circular stapler (21, 25 or 28 mm) after a pursestring suture on the esophageal stump or we can use a prepared Orvil device (®Medtronic Inc. Minneapolis, MN, USA [10]). Additionally, the side-to-side anastomosis can be performed using a linear stapler, closing the anterior defect by a transversal suture using conventional suture material or the prepared V-loc Wound Closure™ (®Medtronic Inc. Minneapolis, MN, USA [11]). Furthermore, the robot-assisted anastomosis (RAMIE) is increasingly used thereby permitting a high manual anastomosis in the apex of the thorax because of the ergonomy obtained by the robot [12].

Initiating the formation of a stapled anastomosis, a small thoracotomy is necessary to position the circular stapler into the gastric tube, whilst this is not required if a manual or linear stapler anastomosis is created. However, at the end of the procedure the specimen needs to be retrieved through the abdomen (patient must be repositioned again) or by a small thoracotomy incision if thoracoscopy was performed.

Concerning the type of intubation needed during the anastomosis phase, only a single-lumen intubation with two-lung ventilation (no collapse of the right lung is necessary) is required for the manual, RAMIE and the linear anastomosis. Holding to an anastomosis that is performed by a circular stapler, a total collapse of the right lung during anastomosis is essential, either by (a) selective intubation (one-lung ventilation), by (b) placing a Fogarty balloon catheter in the right bronchus to be inflated (during the anastomotic phase) or by (c) applying to the wound a protection device with a glove or a gel cap system along with maintaining a thoracic insufflation at 7–8 mmHg.

General principles for the anastomosis have to be assured, such as good vascular irrigation, no tension on the anastomosis and a watertight anastomosis. To get better outcomes of the anastomosis in which the esophagus is not covered by peritoneum, a new technique has been developed at our Department. This new technique contains an anastomosis that is covered by a pleural flap followed by a wrap of omentum around the anastomosis (the 'Flap and Wrap Technique') and might be considered as an important improvement.

This technique can be performed after the esophagus is divided by the mini thoracotomy (Fig. 10.1). The anvil is introduced and stitched in the proximal esophagus by the Endo Stitch device (®Medtronic Inc. Minneapolis, MN, USA [13]) (Figs. 10.2, 10.3, 10.4, 10.5, and 10.6) and the gastric tube is stapled end-to-side by the circular stapler (Figs. 10.7, 10.8, 10.9, 10.10, and 10.11). Performing the Flap and Wrap technique, a single stich is used to fix the created gastric tube behind the pleural flap (Fig. 10.12). Therefore, the weight of the gastric tube is shifted to the pleural flap while this flap covers the gastric tube to prevent traction on the anastomosis and to protect it against the negative pressure in the thorax. The final part of the "Flap and Wrap" technique consists of wrapping the omentum around the anastomosis to ensure that it is fully covered (Fig. 10.13).

10.2.2 Three-Staged Minimally Invasive McKeown Procedure

The three-staged minimally invasive McKeown esophagectomy with cervical anastomosis is preferably used if there is mediastinal lymphadenopathy, or if intrathoracic anastomosis cannot be performed if tumor growth in proximal direc-

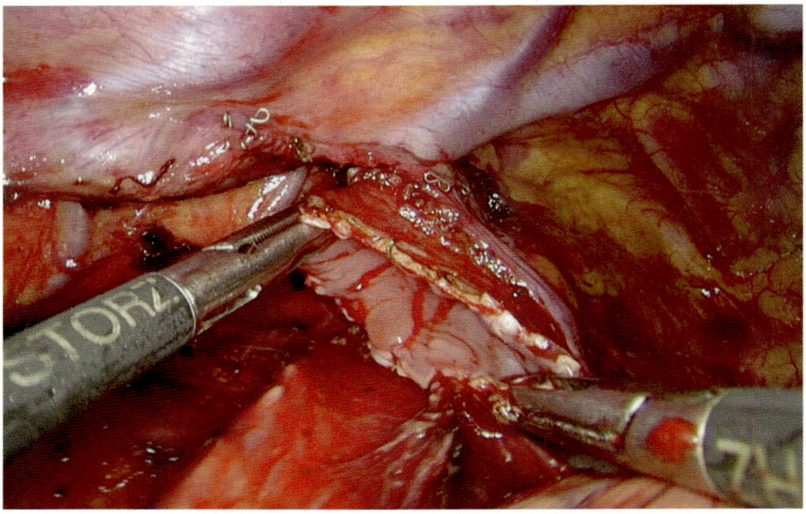

Fig. 10.1 Intrathoracic division of the esophagus

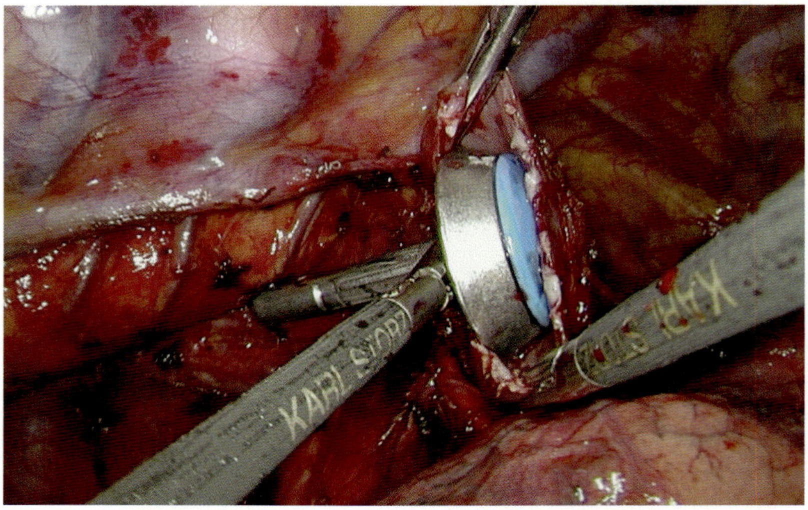

Fig. 10.2 Introduction of 29 mm anvil in the esophagus

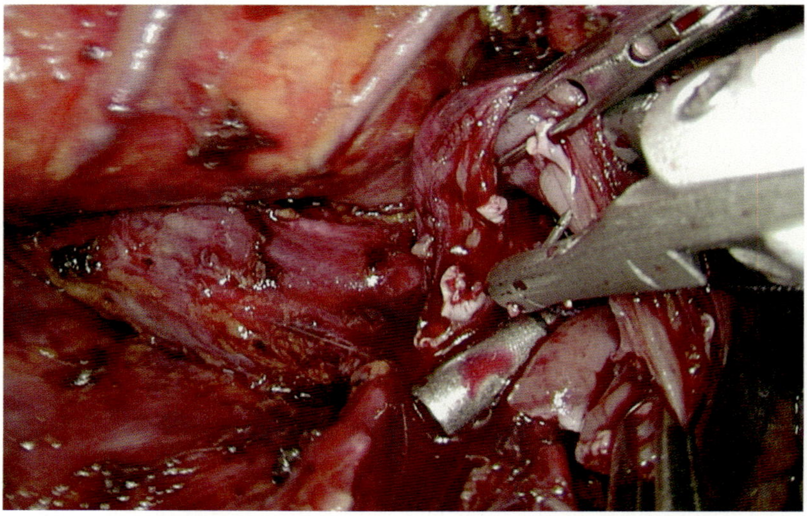

Fig. 10.3 Starting the purse string suture around the anvil

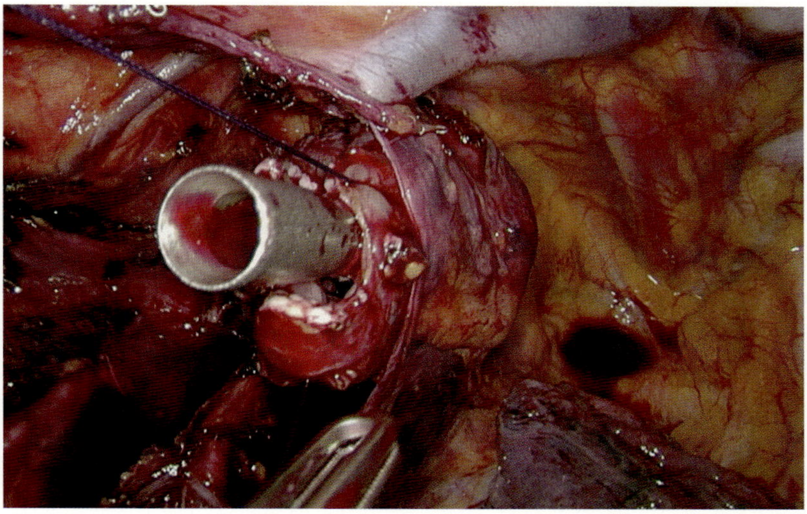

Fig. 10.4 Closure of the esophagus by means of purse string

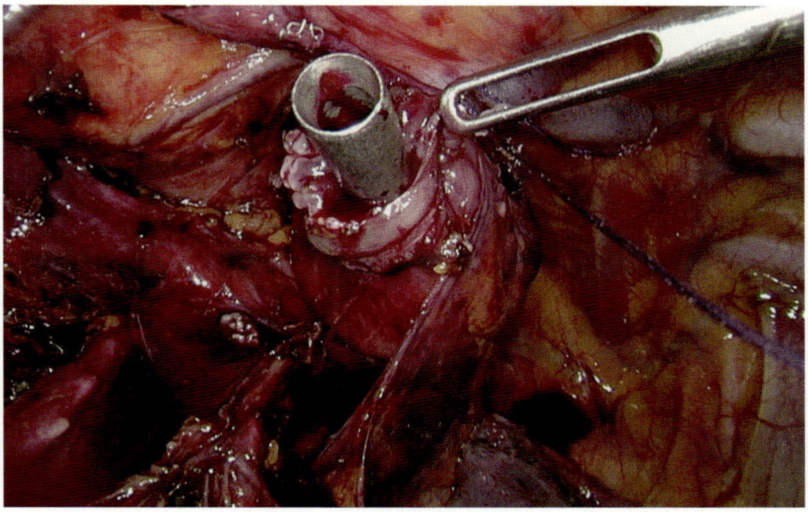

Fig. 10.5 Closure of the esophagus by means of purse string

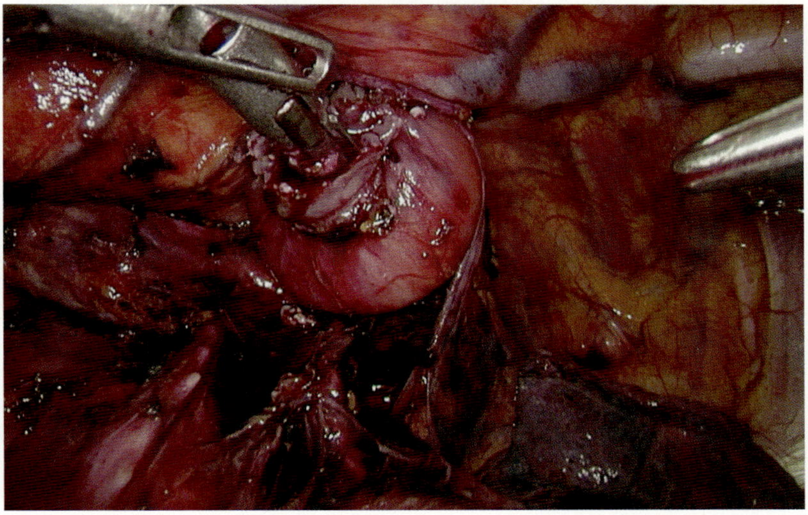

Fig. 10.6 Closure of the esophagus by means of purse string

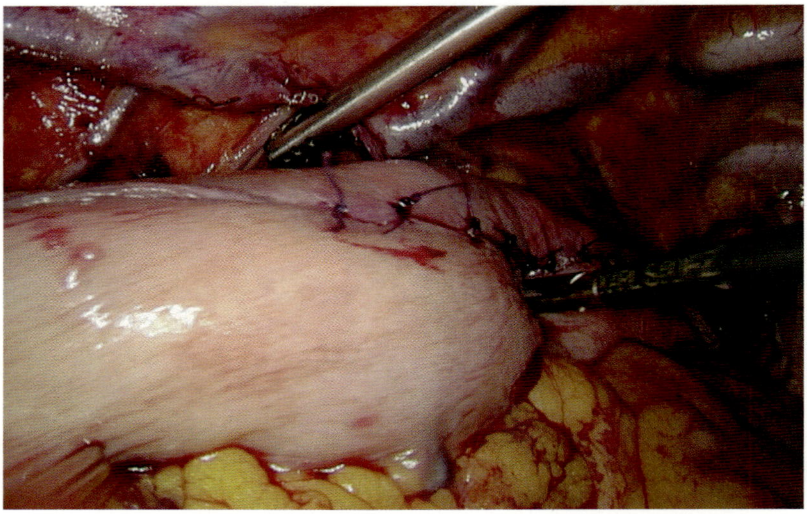

Fig. 10.7 Gastric tube in thorax

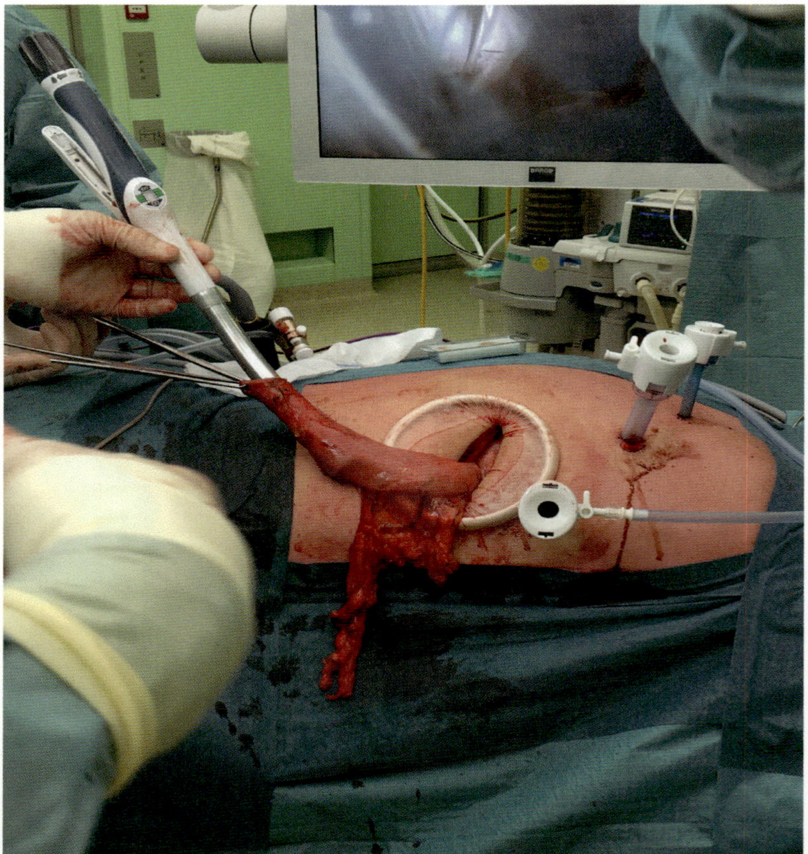

Fig. 10.8 Circular stapler positioned in the gastric tube through a small thoracotomy

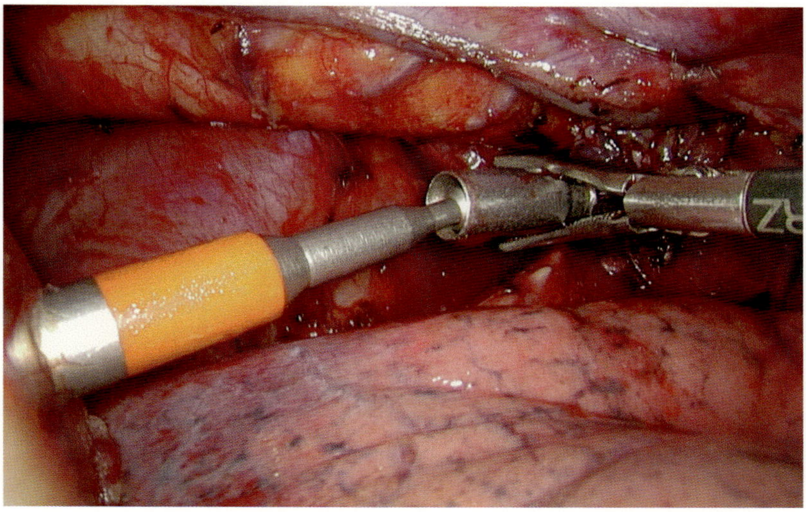

Fig. 10.9 Creation of end to side anastomosis

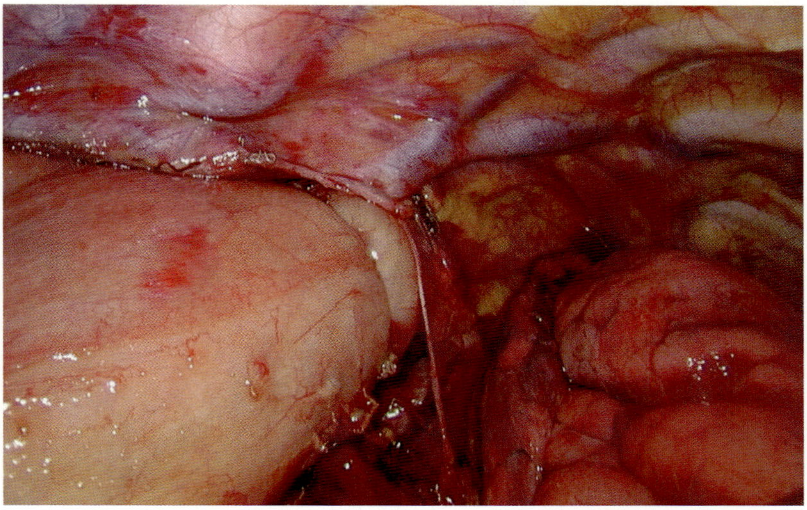

Fig. 10.10 Creation of end to side anastomosis

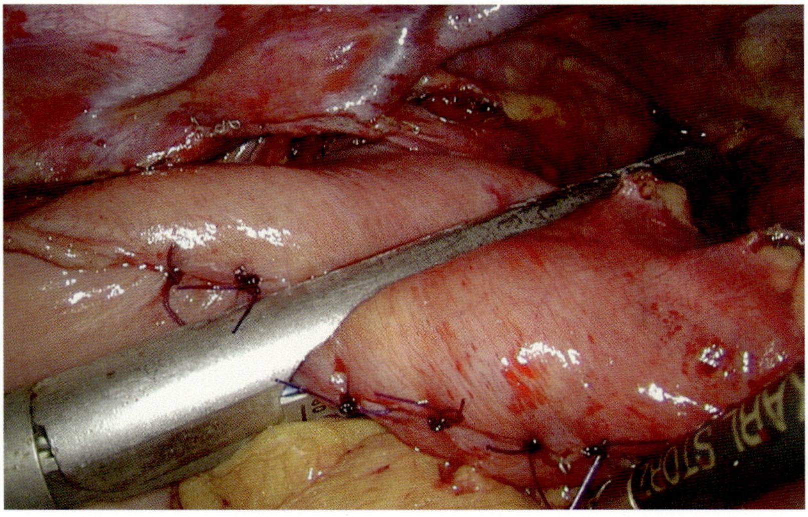

Fig. 10.11 Resection of the lateral loop

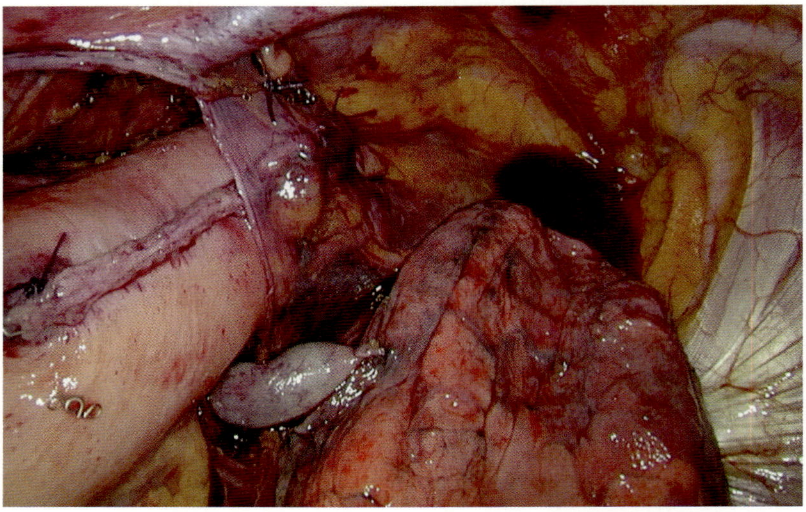

Fig. 10.12 Anastomosis covered by pleural flap

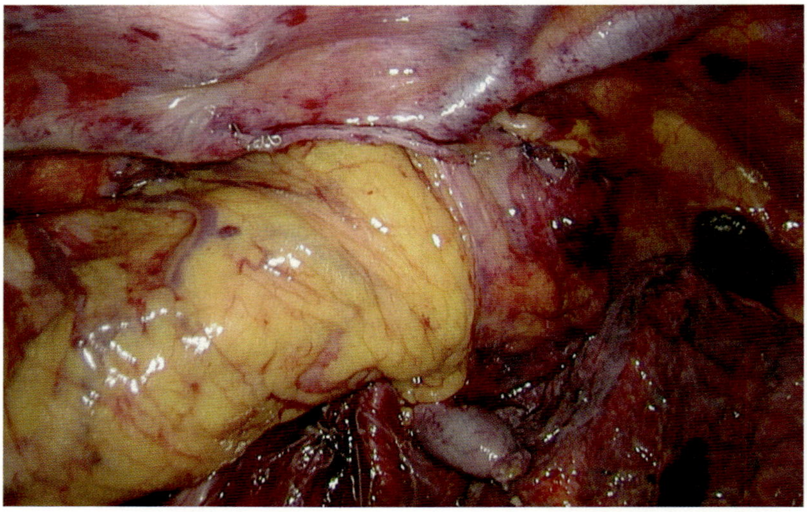

Fig. 10.13 Anastomosis covered by omental wrap

tion is too extended and the proximal residual esophagus is too short for an intrathoracic anastomosis.

This procedure is started through a right thoracoscopy in prone position with a single-lumen tracheal intubation, followed by upper laparoscopy and left cervical incision. To maintain a partial collapse of the right lung during thoracoscopy, the thoracic cavity must be insufflated with carbon dioxide at 7–8 mmHg. During thoracoscopy the esophagus is dissected and a mediastinal lymphadenectomy is performed as comparable to the previous described in the Ivor Lewis esophagectomy section. No Kocher maneuver or intervention to the pylorus is performed.

After thoracoscopy, the patient is repositioned in French position to perform a laparoscopy with formation of the gastric conduit as comparable with the Ivor-Lewis procedure. Subsequently, a cervical anastomosis can be created starting with left cervical incision to decrease the risk of bilateral recurrent laryngeal nerve injury. The esophagus is divided and the gastric tube is pulled into the cervical region via the prevertebral route. A cervical end-to-end anastomosis is the created manually. The advantages of a cervical anastomosis is compared to an intrathoracic anastomosis (Ivor-Lewis procedure) are better clinical management of leakages (e.g. by bedside opening of the wound) and a larger proximal resection margin.

10.2.3 Transhiatal Esophagectomy

This procedure is performed by laparoscopy and left cervical incision. Starting with transhiatal dissection of the esophagus (and tumor) from the pericardial sac and aortic planes up to the carina, it is followed by an extended celiac trunk lymphadenectomy and gastric dissection. After dissection of the cervical esophagus, a small-assisting-protected laparotomy is performed to retrieve the whole specimen by stripping. Extracorporeal creation of gastric tube and resection of the specimen is then followed by pulling the gastric tube into the cervical wound where the anastomosis is made. Due to the transhiatal approach, the mediastinal lymphadenectomy is limited [14]. Details of the surgical techniques have been published elsewhere [15, 16].

10.3 Postoperative Care

Two policies of postoperative care are found among surgeons. Surgeons may try to consolidate the use of some form of fast-track treatment that includes no nasogastric tube at all and the start of oral liquid feeding on the first postoperative day. Many surgeons—including those in our center—may follow a more conservative tendency to leave the nasogastric tube in situ. This is based on the hypothesis that if the gastric tube will obtain all oral liquids on the first postoperative day and the pylorus does not open sufficiently, a traction on the anastomosis due to weight is expected, which will lead to some form of leakage. Correspondingly, at our center we adopted the more conservative approach to leave the nasogastric tube in situ for more than four to five 5 days with active suction at the tube. An X-ray is performed on the fifth day to check the width of the gastric tube. Only if these factors are optimal the nasogastric tube is removed and patients initiate the progressive oral feeding. In some centers standard Swallow X-ray is performed within the first few days after surgery to assess passage through pylorus.

10.4 Evidence for Surgical Techniques

In the era before the systematic use of neoadjuvant therapy, the Dutch HIVEX-trial compared the transhiatal approach versus the transthoracic approach for esophageal carcinoma [17]. The trial revealed no differences in survival rates between the two approaches for GEJ tumors type 2, whereas for type 1 and other tumor locations the survival rates after TTE were higher. In order to update this comparison in the current era of nCRTx and MIE, a comparable trial should be performed. The so-called IVORY-trial is currently in preparation and will compare minimally invasive transhiatal versus the transthoracic approach after nCRTx for distal and GEJ tumors type 1 and 2 according to the Siewert classification. The advantages of the transthoracic approach are an extensive esophageal dissection, a more complete mediastinal lymphadenectomy and possibly a better anastomosis. Because the thoracic anastomosis is more distally created than the cervical anastomosis, it is possible to perform a more extended gastric resection that will help to achieve free resection margins in type 2 tumors. What is more, the gastric tube may be shorter, but is better vascularized and consequently may result in less morbidity, especially with less anastomotic leakages. Moreover, it seems that Siewert type 1 tumors will metastasize to the paratracheal lymph nodes in 10% of the patients after neoadjuvant therapy, whilst this is less than 2% for type 2 tumors after neoadjuvant therapy [18]. The role and extension of mediastinal lymphadenectomy is still controversial after the use of the nCRTx according to the CROSS-study [19].

Currently, after esophagectomy for cancer both cervical and intrathoracic esophagogastric anastomoses are used. Although a cervical anastomosis seems to be the best option for proximal and mid-esophageal tumors, yet a cervical anastomosis is followed by a higher frequency of anastomotic leakages—probably due to the worse irrigation at the top of the gastric tube [16]. Additionally, after MIE with cervical anastomoses for distal or GEJ tumors, patients do have more complaints of dysphagia, dumping and regurgitation [20]. This might be attributable to the higher incidence of strictures in these patients [21, 22]. A recent study showed that there seems to be a trend to create more Ivor-Lewis esophageal resections for GEJ-tumors than McKeown esophagectomies, involving an increase from 15 to 46% of intrathoracic anastomoses [23] in the period from 2007 to 2014. In contrast, in the same period the incidence of three-stage McKeown esophagectomy decreased from 85 into 54%. To reach consensus about this ongoing topic the multicenter ICAN-trial has been launched to compare the short-term outcomes of transthoracic resections between patients with a cervical anastomosis (McKeown procedure) versus patients with an intrathoracic anastomosis (Ivor-Lewis procedure). The first patients have been recently included [20].

Concerning the surgical techniques, another important improvement with the aim to decrease the anastomotic leakage rate is the covering of the intrathoracic anastomosis by wrapping the omentum around it. A systematic review not only showed a significant decrease in the anastomotic leakages rate, but also in the length of hospital stay [24].

Another point of discussion is the position of patients, lateral or in prone position during Ivor-Lewis or McKeown esophagectomy. Initially, the lateral decubitus position with selective intubation and ventilation of one lung was preferred. However, the introduction of the prone position by Cuschieri in 1994 described many advantages of this position over the lateral decubitus position, such as no necessity for a complete lung block and a better visualization of the esophageal area [25]. A recently published systematic review from Markar et al., suggests that the prone position is associated with less pulmonary complications, less blood loss, and a higher number of resected lymph nodes [26]. It must be noted that there was some evidence of heterogeneity for the analysis of pulmonary complications and blood loss in this review.

Thus, not only the proper approach or the extension of lymphadenectomy, but also the ideal thoracoscopic position of the patient will be important items for future studies in patients who undergo MIE.

10.5 Our Own Experience

In the Netherlands since the last few years most esophageal resections have been centralized in high-volume centers. Along with the increased use of minimally invasive surgery, the morbidity and mortality rates in patients have since decreased [8, 23, 27]. Moreover, neoadjuvant therapies such as nCRTx and chemotherapy are now extensively used. Data from the National Dutch Register (DUCA) show that the use of the thoracic esophagectomy increased from 47% in 2011 to 69% in 2015; that the use of the Ivor-Lewis approach increased from 11 to 47%; that the implementation of total MIE increased from 32 to 71%; and that neoadjuvant therapy was administered in 91% of the registered 846 patients in 2015 [28].

Responding to the increase of distal esophageal and GEJ adenocarcinomas to more than 80% of all esophageal cancers in the Netherlands, our Department has increased the use of MIE Ivor-Lewis approach—a comparable development found at the other upper GI centers in The Netherlands. The first multicenter study about MIE Ivor-Lewis esophagectomy included more than 282 patients from six centers, performing different types of anastomoses, and showed a leakages in more than 15% of the patients with a 30-days mortality of 2.1% [29]. This high-leakage rate obliged the surgeons to analyze these numbers, the learning curve and the cause of this rate. The result of this analysis in our department produced a change in the used anastomosis technique, resulting in the "flap and wrap" technique as described in the intrathoracic anastomosis paragraph of this chapter. This anastomosis technique is increasingly used in our Department, rising from 24.2% of the total esophageal resections in 2014 up to 72% of the resections in 2016. With this anastomosis technique we have obtained an important decrease of anastomotic leakages to less than 5% for intrathoracic anastomosis with the Flap and Wrap technique, whereas leakages are still found in 20% of the patients with a cervical anastomosis without Flap and Wrap technique (unpublished data). Moreover, an important decrease of overall morbidity, reoperation rate, readmissions to the ICU and in ICU length of stay have been found (LOS). It seems that a lower incidence of the morbidity rates is associated to a higher frequency of transthoracic resections.

10.6 Outcome of Published Series

Data about morbidity and mortality rates following a minimally invasive esophagectomy after neoadjuvant therapy for GEJ tumors specifically is scarce. The largest prospective study described the morbidity and mortality rates of a series of more than 1000 patients in whom minimally invasive Ivor-Lewis esophagectomy and McKeown esophagectomy is performed [30]. They did not find any differences in the frequency of anastomotic leakages requiring surgery (4% versus 5%, respectively). However, there were significant differences in the occurrence of vocal cord paralyses, with a higher incidence among McKeown esophagectomies than Ivor-Lewis procedures (8% versus 1%, respectively). Moreover, no difference in 30-days mortality was reported (0.9% versus 2.5%, respectively). In general, there seems to be a trend towards lower morbidity rates among MIE Ivor-Lewis resections as compared to MIE McKeown resections and THE, but results of evidence based studies comparing these different approaches are lacking [20, 30]. Therefore, the outcomes for each modality are described separately in the following sections.

10.6.1 Outcomes for Minimally Invasive TTE: Ivor-Lewis Esophagectomy

Two studies that reported short-term outcomes of MIE Ivor-Lewis resections for GEJ tumors specifically are recently reported.

One study reported a multicentric series of patients with a distal or a GEJ tumor of the esophagus treated by MIE Ivor Lewis and the other study compared two cohorts, MIE Ivor Lewis and MIE McKeown procedure.

Straatman et al. (2016) investigated the short-term outcomes of 282 patients among six different European centers who underwent minimally invasive Ivor-Lewis esophagectomy for only distal and GEJ tumors and showed a morbidity rate of 44% [29]. The most frequent complications were anastomotic leakages (15.2%), pulmonary complications (13.1%), and cardiac complications (4.3%). Perioperative outcomes were: a median operative time of 333 min, 242 mL blood loss (median) and 1.8% conversions to open Ivor-Lewis esophagectomy. Radical resections (R0) were performed in 93% of the patients. Further postoperative outcomes were a median length of stay of 12 days, and a median length of ICU stay of 2 days and the 30-day morbidity was 2.1%.

The second retrospective study compared 356 patients who underwent Ivor-Lewis MIE (intrathoracic anastomosis, n = 210) with patients who underwent McKeown or Orringer MIE (cervical anastomosis, n = 146) [20]. The incidence of recurrent laryngeal nerve palsy was 14.4% after a cervical anastomosis and 0% after an intrathoracic anastomosis. Dysphagia, dumping, and regurgitation were reported less frequently after creation of an intrathoracic anastomosis. Dilatation of benign strictures occurred in 43.8% of the cervical anastomoses versus in 6.2% of the intrathoracic anastomoses. If a benign stricture was identified, it was dilated for a median of four times in the cervical group and only once in the intrathoracic group. Anastomotic leakage for which reoperation was required occurred in 8.2% after cervical anastomosis and in 11.4% after intrathoracic anastomosis (not significant). Median ICU stay, hospital stay, in-hospital mortality, 30-day mortality, and 90-day mortality were similar between the groups (not significant). They conclude that MIE with an intrathoracic anastomosis is associated with better functional results with less dysphagia, less benign anastomotic strictures requiring fewer dilatations, and a lower incidence of recurrent laryngeal nerve palsy as compared to MIE with cervical anastomoses. Other postoperative morbidity and mortality did not differ between the groups.

10.6.2 Diagnosis and Treatment of Anastomotic Leakages

Surgeons must adhere to a proper algorithm as early as possible in the treatment for the postoperative anastomotic leaks, thereby following the maxim that: "Patients who do not progress every day should be studied immediately by CT-scan and endoscopy for assessment of the anastomosis". The incidence of postoperative anastomotic leakages varies from 1 to 20%. Most patients with anastomotic leakages show very unspecific symptoms, such as fever, subcutaneous emphysema, sepsis, respiratory or circulatory distress. For cervical anastomotic leakages, a cervical wound infection is a more specific symptom that indicates an underlying anastomotic leakage.

The severity of anastomotic leakages is classified following the classification proposed by The Esophageal Complications Consensus Group, which is based on the treatment of the anastomotic leakage [31]. Type I anastomotic leakage is described as 'a local defect that requires no change in treatment or treated with dietary modification or medically'. Type II is treated with an intervention, but no surgical treatment is necessary (for example if the anastomotic leakage is treated with stent placing), type III is the worst type of anastomotic leakage and requires a surgical operation. As this classification already suggests, the consequences of an anastomotic leakage can be hazardous and can develop to mediastinitis or empyema, leading to sepsis, ICU admission or even death of a patient. Hence, adequate postoperative follow-up is required, especially in the first 7 days. If there is clinical suspicion of anastomotic leakage a CT scan and endoscopic examination of the gastric tube should be performed in order to diagnose the complication properly. Immediate start with antibiotics is required, with addition of placement of a nasogastric tube in order to decompress the gastric tube. If cervical anastomotic leakage occurs, opening of the skin can easily treat it. Descending mediastinitis after cervical anastomosis is difficult to treat and should be treated by adequate drainage of the abscess and eventually the placement of a stent. Intrathoracic anastomotic leakages are strongly associated with mediastinitis and/or empyema and should be diagnosed in an early stage to prevent severe development to one of these complications. The first step in treatment of these complications is immediate addition of antibiotics and placement of a nasogastric probe. If patients show systemic symptoms, placement of a stent by an endoscopist is required. If the leakage worseness into a connection with the pleural cavity and/or the gastric tube becomes ischemic, a thoracotomy with removal of the anastomosis and drainage of the pleural cavity is recommended, sometimes with addition of a surgical plasty. If there is enough length of the gastric tube left, a new anastomosis can be performed.

10.7 Oncological Outcomes

The randomized controlled TIME-trial analyzed the survivors of esophageal cancer after MIE and OE after a 1-year and 3-year follow-up [9]. All patients received neoadjuvant therapy. The overall survival rates (68% and 76%, resp.) and the disease-free survival rates (59% and 69%, resp.) after 1 year were not significantly different between the open and MIE group, whereas outcomes of QoL questionnaires remained in favor of MIE. Unpublished data from this trial showed that the data of overall survival, disease-free survival and oncological data after 3 years of follow-up was not different between the two groups, indicating that the MIE is an oncologically safe procedure.

A prospective multicenter study showed an 3-year overall survival rate of 58.4% in patients who underwent MIE [32]. Neoadjuvant therapy was received by 34% of these patients. The recurrence rate after a median follow-up of 35.8 months was 28.4%, including locoregional recurrences in 6.7% of the patients.

Higher ypT or ypN, extracapsular lymph node invasion and R1-resections are other predictive factors to negatively influence the disease-free survival for patients with distal- or GEJ-tumors who underwent neoadjuvant therapy followed by open or minimally invasive TTE with an extended en bloc two-field lymphadenectomy [18].

Conclusion

The incidence of cancer of the distal esophagus and GEJ is increasing, whereby adenocarcinomas are dominating in the Western World (up to 80% of all esophageal carcinomas). The advantages of MIE as a treatment of esophageal or a GEJ cancer in comparison with OE are important improvements in the short-term outcomes, such as less blood loss, less respiratory infections, a better postoperative quality of life, with similar 1-year and 3-years survival rates. Tumors of the GEJ are classified by the Siewert classification, despite all its limitations. For Siewert types 1 and 2, the Ivor-Lewis esophagectomy is an ideal operation following neoadjuvant therapy. There is an important increase in the use of this approach per year with 41% of all esophageal resections in the Netherlands in 2015. This approach includes an intrathoracic anastomosis after laparoscopic preparation of the gastric tube and thoracoscopic esophageal resection and intrathoracic anastomosis in prone position. Other surgical options for an esophageal resection include a transhiatal esophagectomy or the (transthoracic) McKeown resection, in which a cervical anastomosis is performed. The transhiatal approach has its limitations due to the incapacity to perform a mediastinal lymphadenectomy and is reserved to frail patients with a distal or GEJ tumour who cannot undergo thoracoscopy. In a non-randomized study, patients with intrathoracic anastomoses showed a better functional outcome than the group with cervical anastomoses along with less dysphagia, less benign strictures and lower incidence than recurrent nerve palsy. The proposed ICAN study will help to solve this question, comparing cervical with intrathoracic anastomoses. Our experience with intrathoracic anastomoses accompanied by the Flap and Wrap technique limited the postoperative leakage rate to approximately 5% whereas the leakage rate in patients with cervical anastomoses remains up to 20%.

There is still no consensus about the ideal type of intrathoracic anastomosis. Different types of anastomoses are used, including manual, linear stapler, circular stapler and robot manual-assisted anastomoses. There is no evidence that one technique is better than the other, but general principles for anastomoses such as the need of a well-vascularised gastric tube, no tension or traction on the anastomosis and adequate patency are important factors to respect. In our experience, the Flap and Wrap anastomosis technique in which the anastomosis is covered behind a flap of pleura, fixed with stitches and having wrapped the entire anastomosis in omentum, hence accounts for a relative low leakage rate. Moreover, a total mediastinal lymphadenectomy is highly recommended after neoadjuvant therapy to increase survival rates, since having located lymph node metastases predicts the lowest disease-free survival of all lymph node fields.

References

1. Ferlay J, Steliarova-Foucher E, Lortet-Tieulent J, Rosso S, Coebergh JWW, Comber H, Forman D, Bray F. Cancer incidence and mortality patterns in Europe: estimates for 40 countries in 2012. Eur J Cancer. 2013;49:1374–403.
2. Arnold M, Soerjomataram I, Ferlay J, Forman D. Global incidence of oesophageal cancer by histological subtype in 2012. Gut. 2015;64:381–7.
3. Pennathur A, Gibson MK, Jobe BA, Luketich JD. Oesophageal carcinoma. Lancet. 2013;381:400–12.
4. Rice TW, Blackstone EH, Rusch VW. 7th Edition of the AJCC cancer staging manual: esophagus and esophagogastric junction. Ann Surg Oncol. 2010;17: 1721–4.
5. Rüdiger Siewert J, Feith M, Werner M, Stein HJ. Adenocarcinoma of the esophagogastric junction: results of surgical therapy based on anatomical/topographic classification in 1,002 consecutive patients. Ann Surg. 2000;232:353–61.
6. Shapiro J, van Lanschot JJB, Hulshof MCCM, et al. Neoadjuvant chemoradiotherapy plus surgery versus surgery alone for oesophageal or junctional cancer (CROSS): long-term results of a randomised controlled trial. Lancet Oncol. 2015;16:1090–8.
7. van Hagen P, Hulshof MCCM, van Lanschot JJB, et al. Preoperative chemoradiotherapy for esophageal or junctional cancer. N Engl J Med. 2012;366:2074–84.
8. Biere SSAY, Van Berge Henegouwen MI, Maas KW, et al. Minimally invasive versus open oesophagectomy for patients with oesophageal cancer: a multicentre, open-label, randomised controlled trial. Lancet. 2012;379:1887–92.
9. Maas KW, Cuesta MA, Van Berge Henegouwen MI, Roig J, Bonavina L, Rosman C, Gisbertz SS, Biere SSAY, Van Der Peet DL. Quality of life and late complications after minimally invasive compared to open esophagectomy: results of a randomized trial. World J Surg. 2015;39:1986–93.

10. Medtronic Inc. Orvil circular stapler. 2013.
11. Medtronic Inc. V-loc wound closure. 2015.
12. van Hillegersberg R, Seesing MFJ, Brenkman HJF, Ruurda JP. Robot-assisted minimally invasive esophagectomy. Chirurg. 2016;87:635–42.
13. Medtronic Inc. Endo Stitch device. 2008.
14. Parry K, Ruurda JP, van der Sluis PC, van Hillegersberg R. Current status of laparoscopic transhiatal esophagectomy for esophageal cancer patients: a systematic review of the literature. Dis Esophagus. 2017; 30(1):1–7.
15. Orringer M. Transhiatal esophagectomy without thoracotomy for carcinoma of the thoracic esophagus. Ann Surg. 1984;200:282–8.
16. Scheepers JJG, Veenhof XAFA, van der Peet DL, van Groeningen C, Mulder C, Meijer S, Cuesta MA. Laparoscopic transhiatal resection for malignancies of the distal esophagus: outcome of the first 50 resected patients. Surgery. 2008;143:278–85.
17. Omloo JMT, Lagarde SM, Hulscher JBF, Reitsma JB, Fockens P, van Dekken H, Ten Kate FJW, Obertop H, Tilanus HW, van Lanschot JJB. Extended transthoracic resection compared with limited transhiatal resection for adenocarcinoma of the mid/distal esophagus: five-year survival of a randomized clinical trial. Ann Surg. 2007;246:992–1000.
18. Anderegg MCJ, Lagarde SM, Jagadesham VP, et al. Prognostic significance of the location of lymph node metastases in patients with adenocarcinoma of the distal esophagus or gastroesophageal junction. Ann Surg. 2016;264:847–53.
19. Koen Talsma A, Shapiro J, Looman CWN, van Hagen P, Steyerberg EW, van der Gaast A, van Berge Henegouwen MI, Wijnhoven BPL, van Lanschot JJB. Lymph node retrieval during esophagectomy with and without neoadjuvant chemoradiotherapy. Ann Surg. 2014;260:786–93.
20. van Workum F, van der Maas J, van den Wildenberg F, Polat F, Kouwenhoven EA, van Det MJ, Nieuwenhuijzen G, Luyer MD, Rosman C. Improved functional results after minimally invasive esophagectomy: intrathoracic versus cervical anastomosis. Ann Thorac Surg. 2016;103(1):267–73.
21. Biere SSAY, Maas KW, Cuesta MA, Van Der Peet DL. Cervical or thoracic anastomosis after esophagectomy for cancer: a systematic review and meta-analysis. Dig Surg. 2011;28:29–35.
22. Markar SR, Arya S, Karthikesalingam A, Hanna GB. Technical factors that affect anastomotic integrity following esophagectomy: systematic review and meta-analysis. Ann Surg Oncol. 2013;20:4274–81.
23. Haverkamp L, Seesing MFJ, Ruurda JP, Boone J, Hillegersberg RV. Worldwide trends in surgical techniques in the treatment of esophageal and gastroesophageal junction cancer. Dis Esophagus. 2017; 30(1):1–7.
24. Yuan Y, Zeng X, Hu Y, Xie T, Zhao Y. Omentoplasty for oesophagogastrostomy after oesophagectomy. Cochrane Database Syst Rev. 2014;11:CD008446.
25. Cuschieri A. Thoracoscopic subtotal oesophagectomy. Endosc Surg Allied Technol. 1994;2(1):21–5.
26. Markar SR, Wiggins T, Antonowicz S, Zacharakis E, Hanna GB. Minimally invasive esophagectomy: lateral decubitus vs. prone positioning; systematic review and pooled analysis. Surg Oncol. 2015;24: 212–9.
27. Wouters MWJM, Karim-Kos HE, le Cessie S, Wijnhoven BPL, Stassen LPS, Steup WH, Tilanus HW, Tollenaar RAEM. Centralization of esophageal cancer surgery: does it improve clinical outcome? Ann Surg Oncol. 2009;16:1789–98.
28. Dutch Upper GI Cancer Audit. 2015.
29. Straatman J, van der Wielen N, Nieuwenhuijzen GAP, et al. Techniques and short-term outcomes for total minimally invasive Ivor Lewis esophageal resection in distal esophageal and gastroesophageal junction cancers: pooled data from six European centers. Surg Endosc. 2017;31(1):119–26.
30. Luketich JD, Pennathur A, Awais O, et al. Outcomes after minimaly invasive esophagectomy: review over 1000 patients. Ann Surg. 2012;256:95–103.
31. Low D, Alderson D, Cecconello I, et al. International consensus on standardization of data collection for complications associated with esophagectomy: Esophagectomy Complications Consensus Group (ECCG). Ann Surg. 2015;262:286–94.
32. Luketich JD, Pennathur A, Franchetti Y, et al. Minimally invasive esophagectomy. Results of a prospective phase II multicenter trial. Ann Surg. 2015;261:702–7.

Robot Assisted Minimally Invasive Esophagectomy (RAMIE)

11

Pieter C. van der Sluis, Jelle P.H. Ruurda,
Sylvia van der Horst, and Richard van Hillegersberg

11.1 Background

Esophageal cancer is the sixth most common cause of cancer death worldwide, with occurrence rates varying greatly by geographic location [1]. The standard treatment for locally advanced esophageal cancer with curative intent is multimodality treatment containing either preoperative chemoradiation or perioperative chemotherapy followed by open esophagectomy [2, 3]. However, the open transthoracic esophagectomy is associated with high morbidity and mortality [4, 5].

Minimally invasive esophagectomy (MIE) was designed to improve the outcome of esophagectomy. Systematic reviews and results from a randomized controlled trial, comparing MIE to open transthoracic esophagectomy, showed decreased blood loss, fewer postoperative complications and shorter hospital stays, with comparable short-term oncologic results [6–9].

However, MIE is not widely applied yet. Technical limitations and concerns about oncologic efficacy have been the main reasons for a limited application of this technique. Hence, the open procedure remains the preferred approach in most centers worldwide [10].

Robot-assisted minimally invasive thoraco-laparoscopic esophagectomy (RAMIE) was developed in 2003 in the University Medical Center Utrecht (UMC Utrecht) to overcome the technical limitations of conventional MIE with the availability of three-dimensional vision and the use of more sophisticated precision instruments [11–13] (Video 11.1). RAMIE was shown to be feasible and safe in a cohort of Western European patients with advanced esophageal cancer in both literature and our own results [13, 14]. Furthermore RAMIE was oncologically effective, with a high percentage of R0 radical resections (95%) and adequate lymphadenectomy. RAMIE provided good local control with a low percentage of local recurrence at long-term follow up [15].

Electronic Supplementary Material The online version of this chapter (doi:10.1007/978-3-319-54301-7_11) contains supplementary material, which is available to authorized users. On http://springerlink.com enter the DOI number given above.

P.C. van der Sluis, M.D., M.Sc.
R. van Hillegersberg, M.D., Ph.D. (✉)
J.P.H. Ruurda, M.D., Ph.D. • S. van der Horst, M.Sc
Department of Surgical Oncology, University Medical Center Utrecht, Utrecht, The Netherlands

Department of Surgery, University Medical Center Utrecht, Heidelberglaan 100, 3508 GA Utrecht, The Netherlands
e-mail: p.c.vandersluis-2@umcutrecht.nl; r.vanhillegersberg@umcutrecht.nl

M.A. Cuesta (ed.), *Minimally Invasive Surgery for Upper Abdominal Cancer*,
DOI 10.1007/978-3-319-54301-7_11

11.2 Robot-Assisted Minimally Invasive Thoraco-Laparoscopic Esophagectomy (RAMIE) at UMC Utrecht

11.2.1 Preparation and Positioning

General and thoracic epidural anesthetics are combined to ensure sufficient intraoperative and postoperative analgesia. Recently we started using single-dose and bilateral paravertebral block combined with sufentanil in the context of our enhanced recovery after esophagectomy program. This may provide similar postoperative analgesia and early discharge avoiding the disadvantages of epidural anesthesia such as catheter malposition and hypotension [16].

The patient is intubated with a left-side double-lumen tube. During the thoracoscopic phase of the operation (first stage), patients are positioned in the left lateral decubitus position, tilted 45° towards the prone position to keep the collapsed lung from the operating field. The operating table is flexed, lowering the legs and upper thorax (the patient is positioned with the xyphoid above the pivoting point of the table). This extends the thorax maximally and widens the intercostal space for introduction of the trocars. The trocars positions are marked relatively from the scapula (Fig. 11.1). The robotic system (DaVinci Si system, Intuitive Surgical Inc., Sunnyvale CA, USA) is placed at the dorsocranial side of the patient (Fig. 11.2).

Before incision, the right lung is collapsed. A 10-mm camera port is placed at the sixth intercostal space, posterior to the posterior axillary line. Two 8-mm ports are placed under direct sight anterior to the scapular rim in the fourth intercostal space and more towards posterior in the ninth intercostal space. Two conventional 10 mm disposable trocars are used in the fifth and seventh intercostal spaces just posterior to the posterior axillary line. These ports are used for thoracoscopic assistance such as suction, traction, clipping and insertion of additional surgical needs. CO_2 insufflation of the thoracic cavity permits excellent vision, without the need for retracting the lung from the operative field. In case of a none-compliant lung, a retractor can be used.

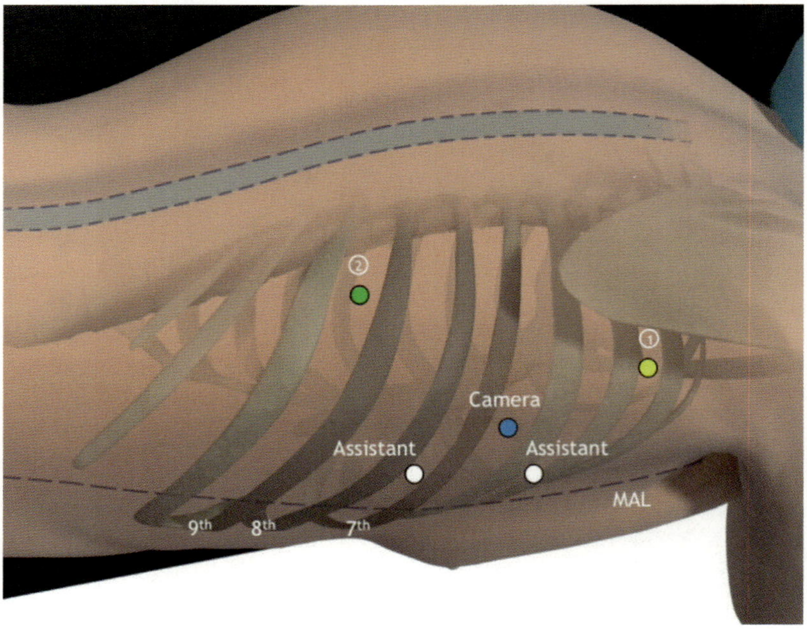

Fig. 11.1 Trocar placement in the thoracic phase. Robotic arms *1* (*yellow*) and *2* (*green*), camera (*blue*), and two assisting ports (*white*). *MAL* (*midaxillary line*) (©2014 Intuitive Surgical Inc., used with permission)

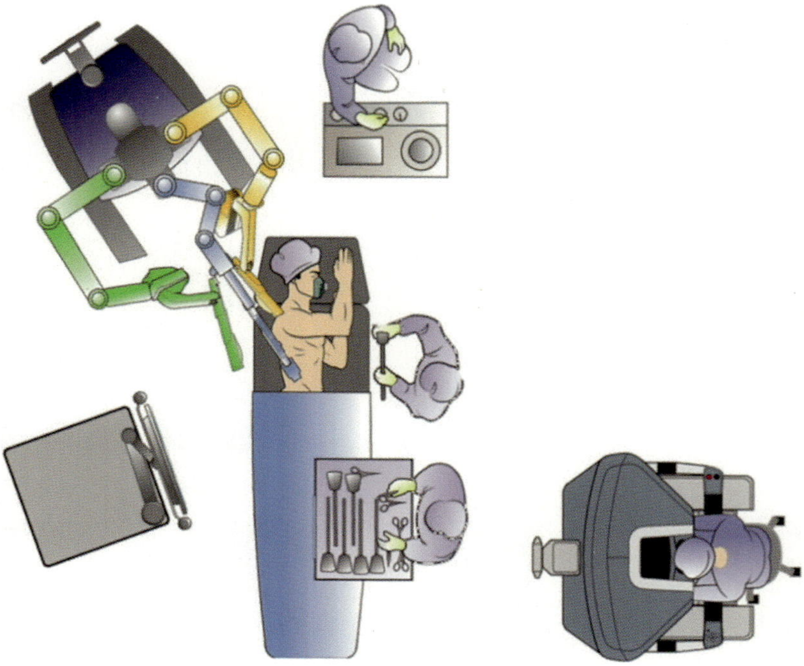

Fig. 11.2 Operating room set-up. (© 2014 Intuitive Surgical Inc., used with permission)

11.3 Thoracoscopic Phase: Operative Procedure

After introduction of the trocars, possible pulmonary adhesions are divided to obtain a clear sight of the operating field. The pulmonary ligament is divided, the parietal pleura is dissected at the anterior side of the esophagus from the diaphragm up to the azygos arch. The azygos vein is ligated using robotically applied Hem-o-lok® clips (size Large, Teleflex Medical, Limerick, PA, USA). These clips are endowristed facilitating precise positioning. Dissection of the parietal pleura is continued above the arch for a right paratracheal lymph node dissection. The right vagal nerve is dissected below the level of the carina to preserve its pulmonary branches and serves as lateral boundary of the paratracheal lymph node dissection [17, 18]. Subsequently, the parietal pleura is dissected at the posterior side along the azygos vein. Paratracheally left, the left recurrent nerve is identified and carefully protected. Lymph node dissection is performed en bloc with the esophagus from the aorta (Fig. 11.3) and along the avascular plain over the pericardium. At the level of the diaphragm, the thoracic duct is clipped with a 10-mm endoscopic clipping device (Endoclip™ II; Covidien, Mansfield, Massachusetts, USA). At this level, a Penrose drain is placed around the esophagus and retracted by the assistant to facilitate esophageal mobilization. In this way, the esophagus can be resected en bloc with the surrounding mediastinal lymph nodes and the thoracic duct from the diaphragm up to the thoracic inlet. Lymphadenectomy will include the paratracheal (lymph node station 2R and 2L), tracheobronchial (lymph node station 4), aortopulmonary window (station 5), carina (station 7, Fig. 11.4) and periesophageal (station 8) lymph nodes [19]. Aortoesophageal vessels are clipped and divided by the assisting surgeon. A thoracic tube is left in place and the thoracic wounds closed in two layers.

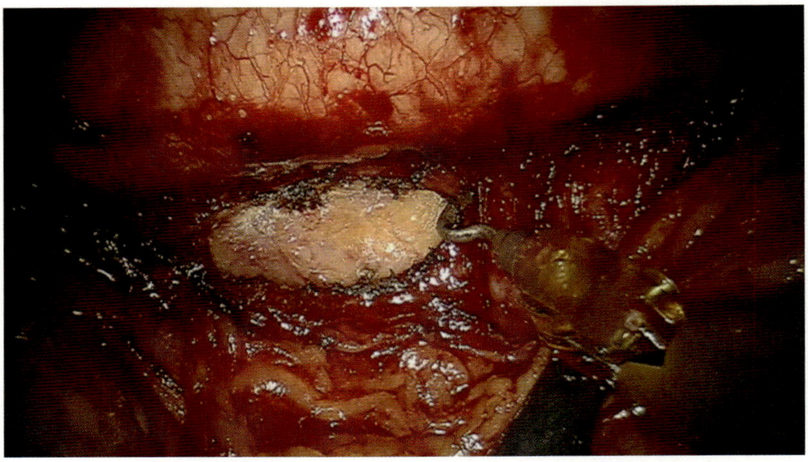

Fig. 11.3 Aortic dissection, demonstrating the peri-esophageal fascia

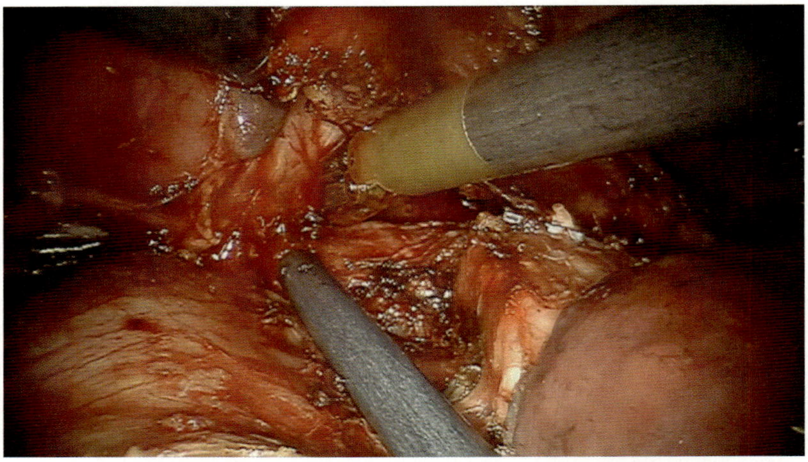

Fig. 11.4 Carinal lymph node dissection

11.4 Laparoscopic Phase: Positioning

After completion of the thoracoscopic phase the patient is put in supine position for the abdominal phase (second stage). A laparoscopic approach is used without the robotic system. The camera is inserted through the 12-mm left paraumbilical trocar port. All other ports are created under direct vision. A 12-mm working port is placed at the right midclavicular line at the umbilical level for introduction of the harmonic scalpel. Two 5-mm assisting trocars ports are used as working ports places subcostally and a 12 mm trocar is placed right in the flank for the liver retractor.

11.5 Laparoscopic Phase: Operative Procedure

Pneumoperitoneum is created with CO_2 insufflation of 12 mmHg. First, the abdominal cavity and the liver are inspected for possible metastases followed by opening of the hepatogastric ligament. The greater and lesser curvatures are dissected with ultrasonic harmonic scalpel (Ultracision, Ethicon Endosurgery, Johnson & Johnson, New Brunswick, New Jersey, USA) with careful sparing of the right gastroepiploic vessels. Abdominal lymphadenectomy includes lymph nodes surrounding the left gastric artery, the splenic artery, common hepatic artery and the lesser omental lymph nodes The left gastric artery is ligated with Hem-o-lok (Teleflex Medical, Weck Driv, NC) and transected at its origin.

Thereafter, the distal esophagus is dissected from the right and left crus by opening of the hiatus. The intra-abdominal CO_2 level is reduced to 6 mmHg to avoid excessive intrathoracic pressure and a chest tube is placed in the left pleural sinus to prevent a pressure pneumothorax.

Through a left-sided vertical incision along the sternocleidoid muscle, the cervical phase (third stage) of esophagectomy is initiated to facilitate mobilization of the cervical esophagus. The inferior thyroid artery is ligated. The esophagus is dissected and a cord is sutured to the proximal part of the specimen to enable pull-up of the gastric conduit along the anatomical tract of the esophagus through the mediastinum under laparoscopic view. No formal cervical lymph node dissection is carried out, but a cervical lymphadenectomy is performed if lymph node metastases are suspected macroscopically during the cervical phase of esophagectomy.

Pneumoperitoneum is installed and the esophagus and surrounding lymph nodes are pulled through the hiatus into the abdomen under direct laparoscopic vision. The left paraumbilical port is widened to a 7-cm transverse transabdominal incision for removal of the resection specimen and stomach using a wound protector. A gastric conduit 5 cm wide is created with GIA linear staplers (GIATM 80, 3_8mm; Medtronic, Minneapolis, Minnesota). The staples are oversewn with 3–0 polydioxanone [20]. The esophagus and cardia resection specimen is sent for pathological examination and the paratracheal, subcarinal, peri-esophageal and left gastric artery were marked in the resection specimen [21].

The gastric conduit is pulled up through the mediastinum along the original anatomic tract of the esophagus with the aid of a laparoscopic camera bag used as protector. A cervical end-to-side anastomosis is created between the gastric tube and the cervical oesophagus using 3/0 polydioxanone single-layer running sutures [22]. The excess gastric tubing is removed using a GIA linear stapler and sent in for pathological analysis.

A jejunostomy feeding tube (Freka® FCJ-Set, Fresenius Kabi AG, Bad Homburg vd H., Germany) is placed at the level of the transverse incision and cervical and abdominal wounds are closed. The abdomen is closed in layers with PDS loop for the fascia and skin intracutaneously with monocryl. Patients are transferred to the intensive care unit (ICU) after the surgical procedure.

11.6 Future Directions

Since the introduction of RAMIE we have gained considerable experience with the use of the da Vinci robot in over 300 cases. However, we are continuously trying to improve RAMIE and pushing the limits by technical modifications and trying to operate more advanced cases. Recent progress, such as the hand sewn intrathoracic anastomosis, RAMIE for upper esophageal cancer with paratracheal lymph node metastases and cT4b tumors are described here.

11.7 Hand Sewn Intrathoracic Anastomosis and Upper Esophageal Cancer

Until recently we performed a three stage esophagectomy (McKeown procedure) with a cervical hand-sewn end-to-side esophagogastric anastomosis without the use of robot. The incidence of anastomotic leakage after RAMIE with cervical esophagogastrostomy was reported to be relatively high (15–30%) [13, 15]. Furthermore, intrathoracic manifestations of anastomotic leakage occur in more than half of patients with cervical anastomotic leakage [23, 24]. The incidence of leakage from intrathoracic anastomosis was reported to be lower [25, 26]. Therefore, we started performing a two stage (Ivor-Lewis) procedure with a robotic-handsewn end-to-side intrathoracic anastomosis for distal esophageal tumors. Constructing an intrathoracic anastomosis in the upper thoracic aperture during conventional thoracoscopy might be technically challenging [27]. The robot overcomes these technical problems due to the endowristed intracorporeal instruments, tremor filtering and its three-dimensional view of the surgical field. Therefore, in our opinion the robot contributes to a high quality hand sewn intrathoracic anastomosis, which is confirmed by the outcomes of our first experiences with the robotic-handsewn intrathoracic anastomosis.

Aforementioned technical advantages were also beneficial in esophagectomy for upper esophageal cancer. The upper mediastinum and thoracic aperture can be reached with an excellent 3D view and magnified observation of the operative field [28]. In this way, we were able to achieve an R0 resection in 28 out of 29 patients (97%) with upper esophageal tumors and paratracheal lymph node involvement (unpublished data).

11.8 cT4b Esophageal Cancer

Until recently patients with cT4b tumors were considered inoperable and guidelines recommend definitive chemoradiotherapy (dCRT) as the treatment of choice [29]. Definitive chemoradiotherapy is associated with a high rate of esophageal stenosis and esophageal perforation [30] Furthermore functional results are poor and recurrence occurs frequently in up to 41% [31]. Therefore, we started salvage surgery in patients with cT4b esophageal tumors after long-course chemoradiotherapy.

After long course chemoradiotherapy. Patients are restaged with positron emission tomography–computed tomography and endobronchial ultrasound. Patients are selected for salvage surgery if tumor ingrowth in the surrounding organs was reduced. We believe that the enlarged 3D image allows for very precise dissection of the irradiated tumor tissue from the trachea, bronchi, and aorta. The level of precision makes dissection in downstaged T4b tumors feasible. We are awaiting the long-term oncologic and functional results with this approach for cT4b patients before it can be recommended for all patients.

Conclusion

Robot assisted surgical procedures may overcome the technical limitations of standard laparoscopic and thoracoscopic procedures. The surgeon, who controls the console of the Da Vinci Robot, has a tenfold magnified 3D view of the surgical field. The articulated arms and instruments allow for more degrees of freedom of movement and the tremor of the surgeon is filtered out. These combined factors facilitate a precise radical dissection of the esophagus and peri-esophageal tissue along vital structures, such as the aorta, trachea, pulmonary vein and laryngeal recurrent nerve [12, 13]. Furthermore, a proper and accurate lymph node dissection can be performed, which may result in lower tumor recurrence [15].

Robot-assisted esophagectomy was shown to be a feasible and safe technique. In 2009 our initial results with this technique were reported. In a prospective cohort study, 47 patients with esophageal cancer underwent robot-assisted thoraco-laparoscopic esophagectomy using the Da Vinci® robot. The esophagus was dissected en-bloc with surrounding lymph nodes, which includes a paratracheal, subcarinal and para-esophageal lymph node dissection [13].

In 2015 we reported that RAMIE was oncologically effective, with a high percentage of R0 radical resections and adequate lymphadenectomy. RAMIE provided good local control with a low percentage of local recurrence at long-term follow up [15].

However, until now, the level of evidence for robot-assisted minimally invasive thoraco-laparoscopic esophagectomy is based on case series or expert opinions only (Level 4 or 5). This emphasizes the need for well conducted randomized controlled trials and long-term survival studies within a framework of measured and comparable outcomes to prove the superiority of robot-assisted minimally invasive thoraco-laparoscopic esophagectomy over the worldwide current standard open transthoracic esophagectomy. Therefore we started the ROBOT-trial (NCT01544790) to compare robot-assisted minimally invasive thoraco-laparoscopic esophagectomy with open transthoracic esophagectomy as surgical treatment for resectable esophageal cancer. The inclusion of this randomized controlled trial is closed and results are awaited soon.

References

1. Jemal A, Bray F, Center MM, et al. Global cancer statistics. CA Cancer J Clin. 2011;61(2):69–90.
2. Mariette C, Piessen G, Triboulet JP. Therapeutic strategies in oesophageal carcinoma: role of surgery and other modalities. Lancet Oncol. 2007;8(6):545–53.
3. Boone J, Livestro DP, Elias SG, et al. International survey on esophageal cancer: part I surgical techniques. Dis Esophagus. 2009;22(3):195–202.
4. Hulscher JB, van Sandick JW, de Boer AG, et al. Extended transthoracic resection compared with limited transhiatal resection for adenocarcinoma of the esophagus. N Engl J Med. 2002;347(21):1662–9.
5. Omloo JMT, Lagarde SM, Hulscher JBF, et al. Extended transthoracic resection compared with limited transhiatal resection for adenocarcinoma of the mid/distal esophagus. Ann Surg. 2007;246(6): 992–1001.
6. Verhage RJ, Hazebroek EJ, Boone J, et al. Minimally invasive surgery compared to open procedures in esophagectomy for cancer: a systematic review of the literature. Minerva Chir. 2009;64:135–46.
7. Safranek PM, Cubitt J, Booth MI, et al. Review of open and minimal access approaches to oesophagectomy for cancer. Br J Surg. 2010;97(12):1845–53.
8. Gemmill EH, McCulloch P. Systematic review of minimally invasive resection for gastro-oesophageal cancer. Br J Surg. 2007;94(12):1461–7.
9. Biere SS, van Berge Henegouwen MI, Maas KW, et al. Minimally invasive versus open oesophagectomy for patients with oesophageal cancer: a multicentre, open-label, randomised controlled trial. Lancet. 2012;379(9829):1887–92.
10. Mamidanna R, Bottle A, Aylin P, et al. Short-term outcomes following open versus minimally invasive esophagectomy for cancer in England: a population-based national study. Ann Surg. 2012;255(2): 197–203.
11. Ruurda JP, van Vroonhoven TJ, Broeders IA. Robot-assisted surgical systems: a new era in laparoscopic surgery. Ann R Coll Surg Engl. 2002;84:223–6.
12. van Hillegersberg R, Boone J, Draaisma WA, et al. First experience with robot-assisted thoracoscopic esophagolymphadenectomy for esophageal cancer. Surg Endosc. 2006;20(9):1435–9.
13. Boone J, Schipper ME, Moojen WA, et al. Robot-assisted thoracoscopic oesophagectomy for cancer. Br J Surg. 2009;96(8):878–86.
14. Ruurda JP, van der Sluis PC, van der Horst S, van Hilllegersberg R. Robot-assisted minimally invasive esophagectomy for esophageal cancer: a systematic review. J Surg Oncol. 2015;112:257–65.
15. van der Sluis PC, Ruurda JP, Verhage RJ, van der Horst S, Haverkamp L, Siersema PD, Borel Rinkes IH, Ten Kate FJ, van Hillegersberg R. Oncologic long-term results of robot-assisted minimally invasive thoraco-laparoscopic esophagectomy with two-field lymphadenectomy for esophageal cancer. Ann Surg Oncol. 2015;22:1350–6.
16. Zhang W, Fang C, Li J, Geng QT, Wang S, Kang F, et al. Single-dose, bilateral paravertebral block plus intravenous sufentanil analgesia in patients with esophageal cancer undergoing combined thoracoscopic-laparoscopic esophagectomy: a safe and effective alternative. J Cardiothorac Vasc Anesth. 2014;28(4): 966–72.
17. Weijs TJ, Ruurda JP, Luyer MD, Nieuwenhuijzen GA, van Hillegersberg R, Bleys RL. Topography and extent of pulmonary vagus nerve supply with respect to transthoracic oesophagectomy. J Anat. 2015;227(4):431–9.
18. Weijs TJ, Ruurda JP, Luyer MD, Nieuwenhuijzen GA, van der Horst S, Bleys RL, et al. Preserving the pulmonary vagus nerve branches during thoracoscopic esophagectomy. Surg Endosc. 2016;30(9):3816–22. doi:10.1007/s00464-015-4683-y. [Epub ahead of print].
19. Naruke T, Tsuchiya R, Kondo H, et al. Lymph node sampling in lung cancer: how should it be done? Eur J Cardiothorac Surg. 1999;16(Suppl 1):S17–24.
20. Boone J, Rinkes IH, van Hillegersberg R. Gastric conduit staple line after esophagectomy: to oversew or not? J Thorac Cardiovasc Surg. 2006;132:1491–2.
21. Verhage RJ, Zandvoort HJ, ten Kate FJ, et al. How to define a positive circumferential resection margin in T3 adenocarcinoma of the esophagus. Am J Surg Pathol. 2011;35(6):919–26.
22. Haverkamp L, van der Sluis PC, Verhage RJ, Siersema PD, Ruurda JP, van Hillegersberg R. End-to-end cervical esophagogastric anastomoses are associated with a higher number of strictures compared with end-to-side anastomoses. J Gastrointest Surg. 2013;17:872–6.
23. van Rossum PS, Haverkamp L, Carvello M, Ruurda JP, van Hillegersberg R. Management and outcome of cervical versus intrathoracic manifestation of cervical anastomotic leakage after transthoracic esophagectomy for cancer. Dis Esophagus. 2017;30:1–8.
24. Biere SS, Maas KW, Cuesta MA, van der Peet DL. Cervical or thoracic anastomosis after esophagectomy for cancer: a systematic review and meta-analysis. Dig Surg. 2011;28:29–35.
25. van Workum F, van den Wildenberg FJ, Polat F, de Wilt JH, Rosman C. Minimally invasive oesophagectomy: preliminary results after introduction of an intrathoracic anastomosis. Dig Surg. 2014;31:95–10.
26. Straatman J, van der Wielen N, Nieuwenhuijzen GA, Rosman C, Roig J, Scheepers JJ, Cuesta MA, Luyer MD, van Berge Henegouwen MI, van Workum F, Gisbertz SS, van der Peet DL. Techniques and short-term outcomes for total minimally invasive Ivor Lewis esophageal resection in distal esophageal and gastro-esophageal junction cancers: pooled data from six European centers. Surg Endosc. 2017;31(1):119–26. [Epub ahead of print].
27. Cerfolio RJ, Bryant AS, Hawn MT. Technical aspects and early results of robotic esophagectomy with chest anastomosis. J Thorac Cardiovasc Surg. 2013;145(1):90–6.

28. Suda K, Ishida Y, Kawamura Y, Inaba K, Kanaya S, Teramukai S, et al. Robot-assisted thoracoscopic lymphadenectomy along the left recurrent laryngeal nerve for esophageal squamous cell carcinoma in the prone position: technical report and short-term outcomes. World J Surg. 2012;36(7):1608–16.
29. Ajani JA, D'Amico TA, Almhanna K, Bentrem DJ, Besh S, Chao J, et al. Esophageal and esophagogastric junction cancers, version 1.2015. J Natl Compr Cancer Netw. 2015;13(2):194–227.
30. Versteijne E, van Laarhoven HW, van Hooft JE, van Os RM, Geijsen ED, van Berge Henegouwen MI, et al. Definitive chemoradiation for patients with inoperable and/or unresectable esophageal cancer: locoregional recurrence pattern. Dis Esophagus. 2015;28(5):453–9.
31. Gkika E, Gauler T, Eberhardt W, Stahl M, Stuschke M, Pöttgen CI. Long-term results of definitive radiochemotherapy in locally advanced cancers of the cervical esophagus. Dis Esophagus. 2014;27(7):678–84.

Minimally Invasive Esophagectomy Step by Step: How I Do It

12

Miguel A. Cuesta, Joris J. Scheepers, Jan Willem Dekker, and Donald L. van der Peet

12.1 3 Stage McKeown MIE Procedure (see the Video 12.1)

There are three different thoracoscopic approaches: the prone position, the lateral position and the semiprone position.

The advantages of the prone position are: (a) the attainable range of thoracic cage and diaphragmatic excursion is greater than in the side position; (b) the amplitude of mediastinal swing or displacement is less; (c) exposure of the esophageal area is facilitated; (d) the weight of the lung itself allows it to fall forward; and (e) in the event of bleeding the blood flows away from its source, thus permitting its control with greater ease.

Electronic Supplementary Material The online version of this chapter (doi:10.1007/978-3-319-54301-7_12) contains supplementary material, which is available to authorized users. On http://springerlink.com enter the DOI number given above.

M.A. Cuesta (✉)
Department of Surgery, VU University Medical Centre, Amsterdam, The Netherlands

Department of Surgery, Reinier de Graaf Ziekenhuis, Delft, The Netherlands
e-mail: ma.cuesta@vumc.nl

J.J. Scheepers • J.W. Dekker
Department of Surgery, Reinier de Graaf Ziekenhuis, Delft, The Netherlands

D.L. van der Peet
Department of Surgery, VU University Medical Centre, Amsterdam, The Netherlands

This approach was not commonly used until its introduction for Minimally Invasive Esophagectomy.

12.1.1 Thoracoscopy in Prone Position

1. After induction of general anaesthesia, standard intratracheal intubation follows.

   Patient is then positioned in prone decubitus position on a standard device in order to support on the head, upper thorax and pelvis. Abdomen is maintained free for breathing excursions. Position of the arms is very important in order to get abduction of the scapula. The arms are positioned on a support device in flexion of the shoulders and ellebows (Fig. 12.1a).

   In this way the area between the spine and the inner edge of the scapula is broadened.
2. Surgeon stands on the right side of patient with the first assistant on his/her right side looking to the monitor in front of them. Scrub nurse stand on the left side of the surgeon (Fig. 12.1b).
3. Four trocars are placed along the inner edge of the right scapula (Fig. 12.1c). The first at the level of the lowest point of the scapula, a 10 mm for the 30° thoracoscope. The second, at the level of fourth intercostal space, 5 mm; the third, at the level of eighth intercostal space, 12 mm and the last, at the level of third as work trocar for assistant (suction, lung retraction etc.). The first trocar is introduced open in the thoracic cavity, after

M.A. Cuesta (ed.), *Minimally Invasive Surgery for Upper Abdominal Cancer*,
DOI 10.1007/978-3-319-54301-7_12

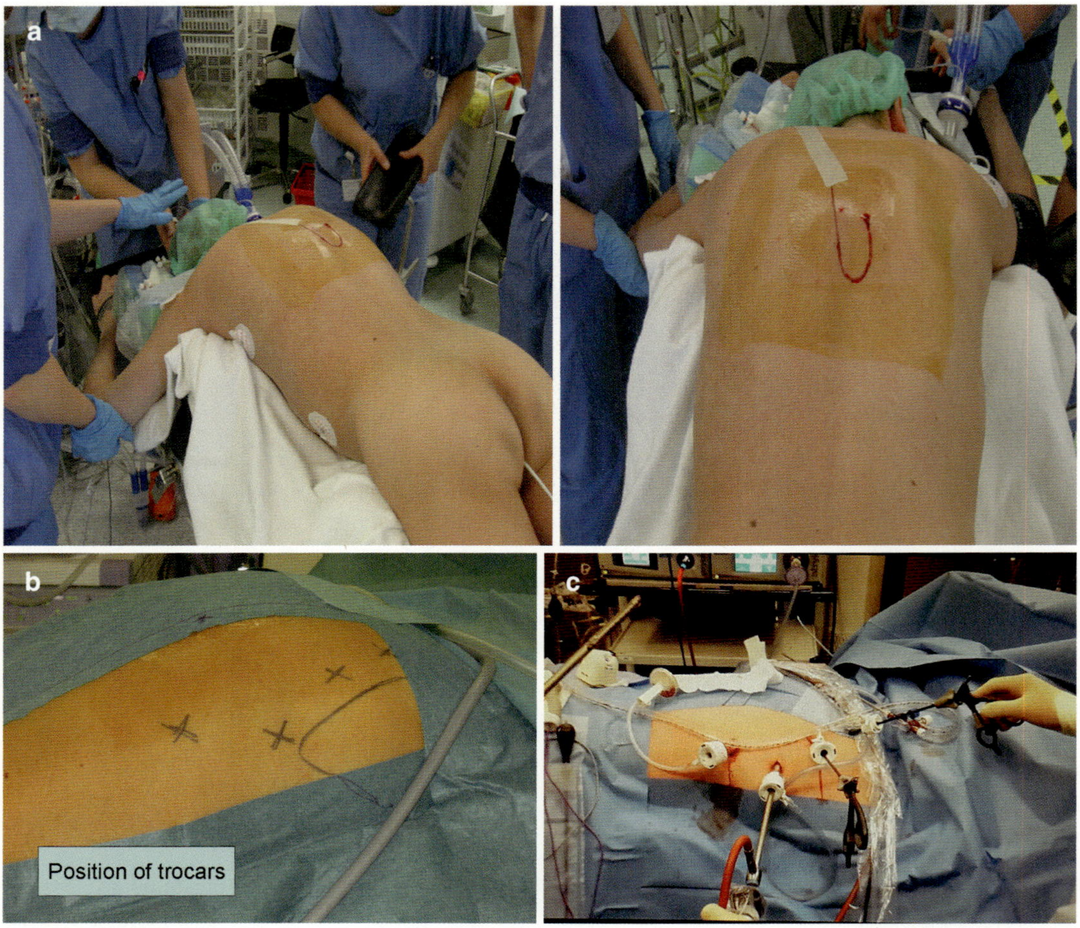

Fig. 12.1 (**a–c**) Placement of patient in the prone position. Operating room setting during operation. Position of trocars along the medial aspect of the scapula

control by finger palpation that the thoracic space is free of adhesions. After introduction of the first trocar a positive insufflation of 7–8 mmHg is initiated in order to retract enough the right lung for an adequate visualization of the posterior mediastinum.

4. Inspection is performed of the pleural cavity and the esophageal area in order to assess if resection is possible (Fig. 12.2a, b).

   Dissection starts anteriorly by cutting the pulmonary ligament, following the cutting line along the lung, along of the right pulmonary vein, the right bronchus up to the azygos vein.

5. Dissection is performed as much as possible from this right side. The esophagus is dissected as far to the left from the hiatus and pericard sac. Dissection and lymphadenectomy of the right bronchus and carina is performed. Lymphadenectomy is not picking of lymph nodes but 'en bloc', the lymph nodes remain attached to the specimen. The right vagal nerve is dissected and divided at the lower edge of the right bronchus. The left bronchus and the distal trachea are now dissected. Dissection takes place by means of the hook and sealing device taking care do not touch the trachea or bronchi.
6. Furthermore the azygos vein is dissected free and divided by means of vascular endo-stapler.
7. On the posterior side, the mediastinal pleura is cut longitudinally along the azygos vein

from the aorta arch to the costo-phrenic angle. In this way a broad piece of pleura is resected with the esophagus.

8. Along the plane of the descending aorta, the thoracic duct (between the aorta and azygos vein) is dissected free and clipped at distal and proximal level. Other surgeons prefer to preserve the thoracic duct. With retraction of the esophagus to the right, the tissue (fascia) from the aorta to the esophagus (mesoesophagus) is divided by means of sealing device (Fig. 12.3a–d). In this way the posterior plane of the pericard, left pulmonary vein and contralateral pleura is reached. Gentle traction of esophagus is needed by the first assistant.
9. Dissection continues in proximal direction between esophagus and trachea (pars membranacea) to stop at the apex of the thoracic cavity (Fig. 12.4a–e).
10. If a total mediastinal lymphadenectomy is indicated the paratracheal lymphadenectomy starts at the right side. After stripping the pleura to reach the superior vena cava, from there the lymphadenectomy is performed up

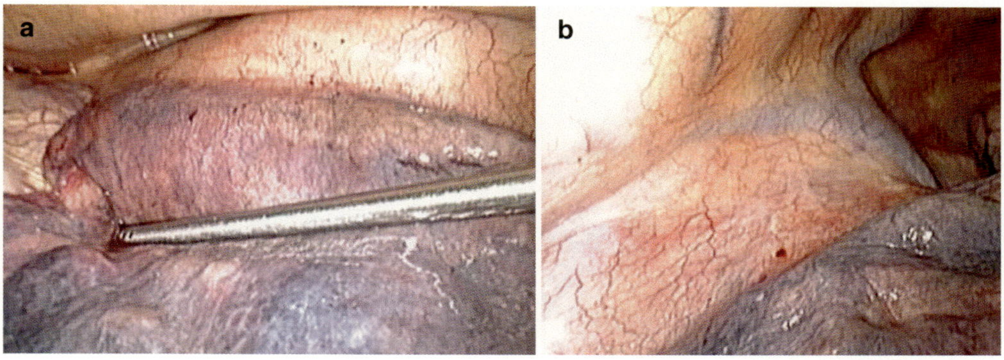

Fig. 12.2 (**a**, **b**) Inspection of the thorax

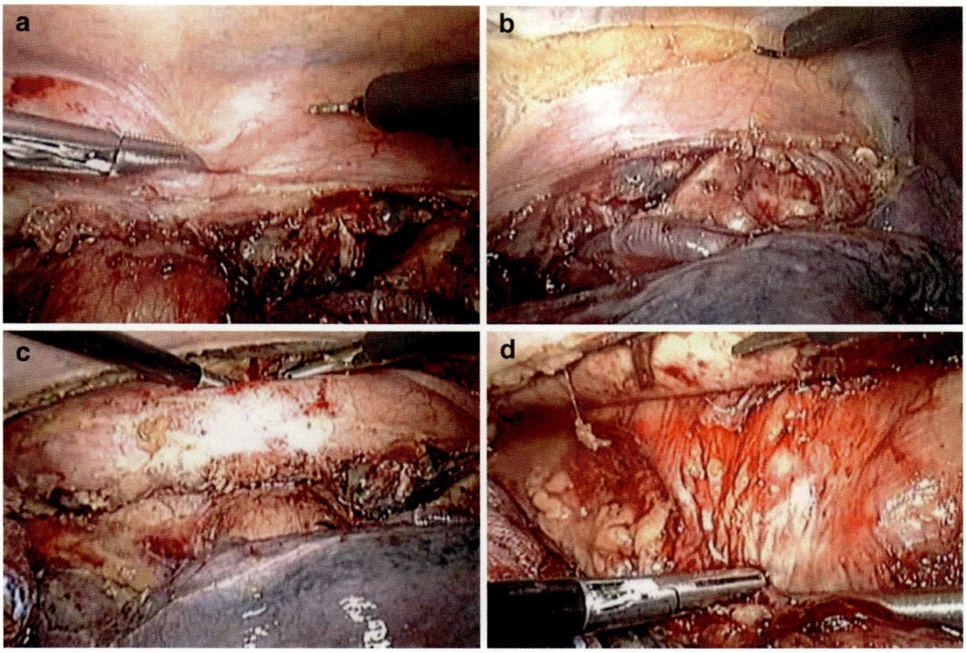

Fig. 12.3 (**a–c**) Opening the pleura on both sides of the esophagus. (**d**) View of the mesoesophagus

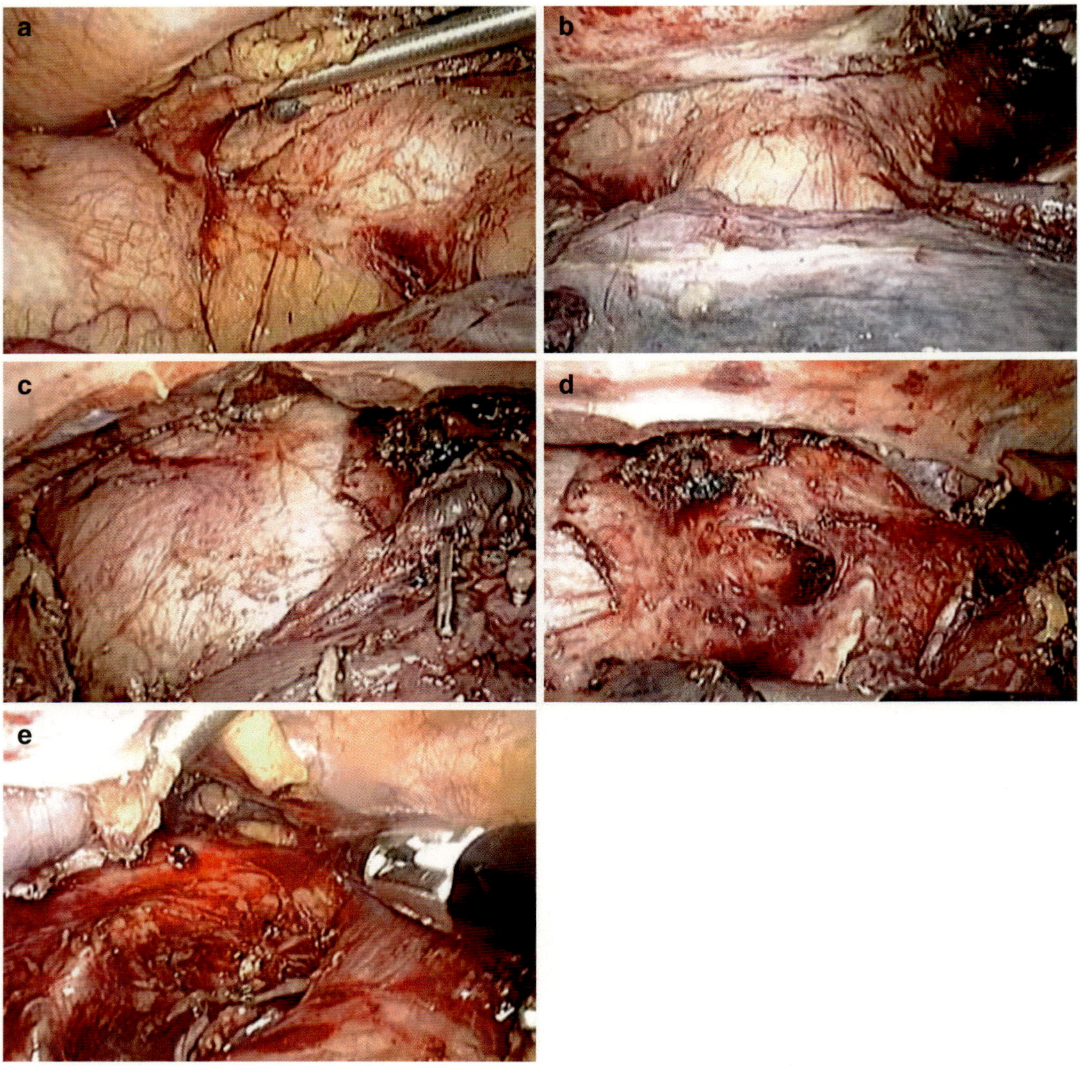

Fig. 12.4 (**a–e**) Inspection of mediastinum after esophageal resection: hiatus, pericard sac, carina and trachea

to the trachea, taking care not damage the right vagal nerve. The lymphadenectomy of the right recurrent laryngeal nerve is done after visualization of the nerve at the right subclavian artery (groups 2 and 4R). At the left side lymphadenectomy starts with careful dissection of the left recurrent nerve. Dissection should be done gently without tractions and not use of diathermia, only scissors.

11. After haemostasis and general inspection the thoracic cavity is drained and the ports closed.

12.1.2 Laparoscopy

1. Patient is placed for the laparoscopy and cervical phase of the operation. Five trocars are introduced in the upper abdomen (Fig. 12.5a).
2. Extensive lymphadenectomy of the celiac trunk and branches (D1+) is performed through the gastro-hepatic ligament after dividing the pars flaccida. After dissection and division of the left gastric artery and vein, dissection continues up to the hiatus.

Fig. 12.5 (a–e) Laparoscopy and positions of trocars. Lymphadenectomy of the celiac trunk and dissection of the stomach with preservation of gastroepiploic vessels

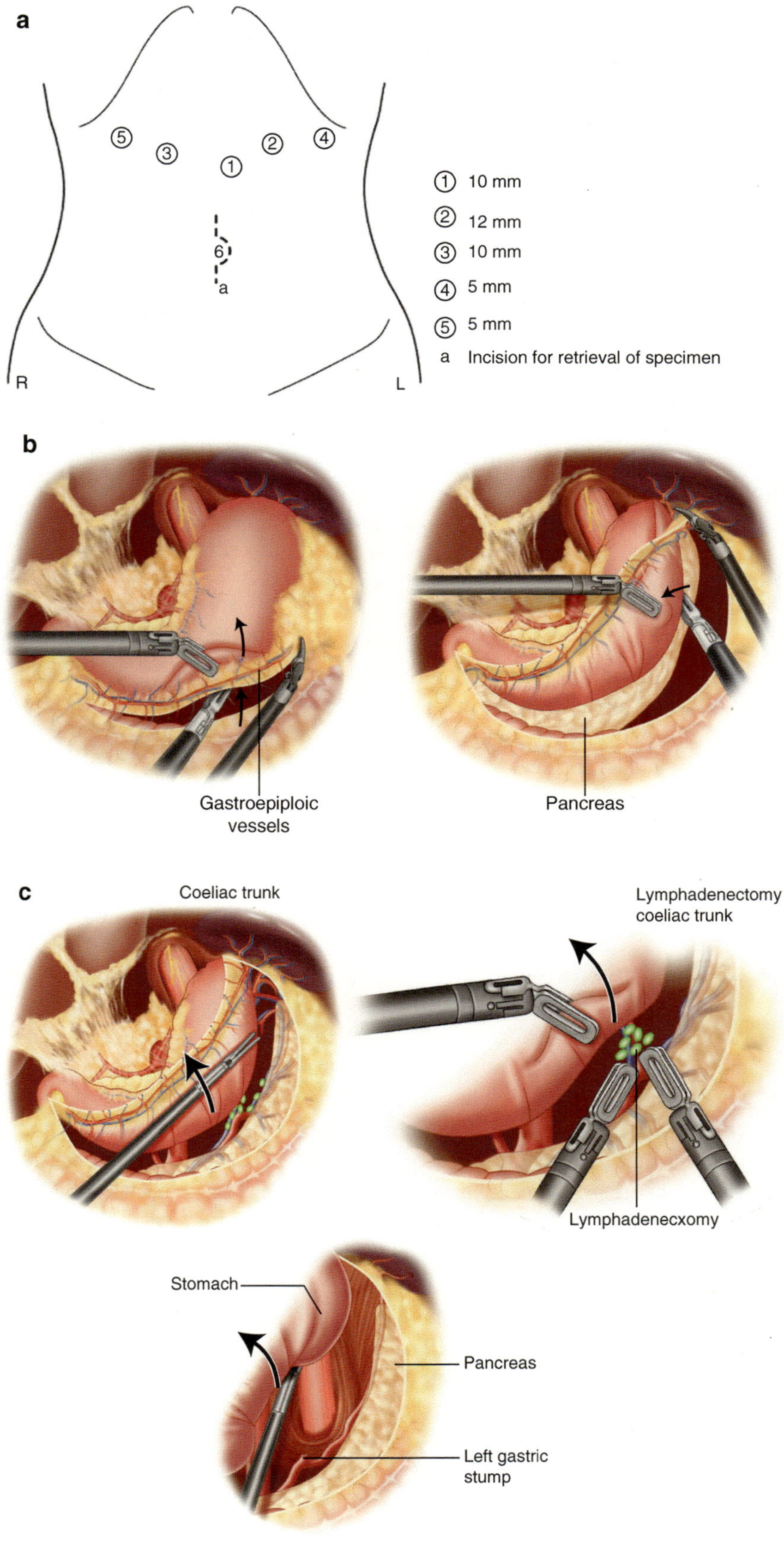

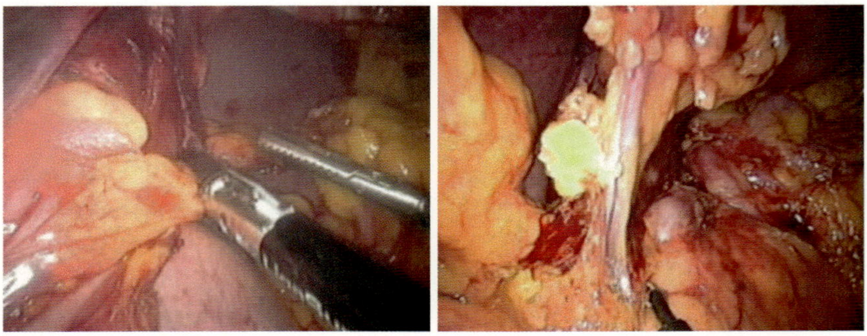

Fig. 12.5 (continued)

3. Gastrocolic ligament is opened and working first in direction to the hiatus and afterwards to the pylorus, the stomach is mobilized completely with preservation of the gastro-epiploic vessels (Fig. 12.6b–e). In this part of the intervention you can perform first the lymphadenectomy followed by the gastrolysis or first the gastrolysis followed by lymphadenectomy.
4. Last part of the laparoscopic approach is the dissection of the hiatal area in which the hiatus is enlarged anteriorly and carefully a communication is made with the thoracic dissection area (insufflation is lowered up to 8 mm Hg in order to avoid ventilation problems). Take care that all the specimen, esophagus and stomach are completely free!

12.1.3 Cervical Phase

1. At the same time a second team (if possible) approach the esophagus at the cervical area and after division the esophagus, the distal part is attached to a nasogastric tube in order to permit that the specimen can be retrieved by the abdominal surgeon through a well-protected supraumbilical incision of 7 cm. A 3–4 cm gastric tube is created by means of a linear stapler device. The gastric tube is fixed to the nasogastric tube, placed into the cervical area and anastomosed (Fig. 12.6a–d).

   Other option will be to create the gastric tube totally intracorporeally (intraabdominal). Once the gastric mobilization has been accomplished, the gastric tube of 3–4 cm is created by means of endostaplers leaving a bridge between the specimen and the gastric tube (other option is to divide the stomach completely and to attach the gastric tube to the specimen by means of two stitches) (Fig. 12.7). Through a well protected neck incision the specimen and the gastric tube can now be exteriorized. After resection, an esophago-gastric tube anastomosis will be performed.

12.2 Minimally Invasive Ivor-Lewis Esophagectomy (See the Video 12.2)

A two stage minimally invasive Ivor-Lewis approach with an intra-thoracic esophagus-gastric tube anastomosis is an increasingly performed intervention for many infracarinal located esophageal tumors (distal esophageal adenocarcinomas and Siewert 1 and 2).

1. The operation starts with the laparoscopic procedure with lymphadenectomy of the celiac trunk branches (D1+).
2. The stomach is mobilized with preservation of the gastro-epiploic vessels and a broad piece of proximal omentum.
3. The gastric tube (3–4 cm wide) is created by endostaplers.
4. The hiatus is dissected and distal esophagus dissected free along the oncological planes (aorta and pericard sac).
5. A jejunostomy is created
6. Patient is then placed in a prone decubitus position for right thoracoscopy.

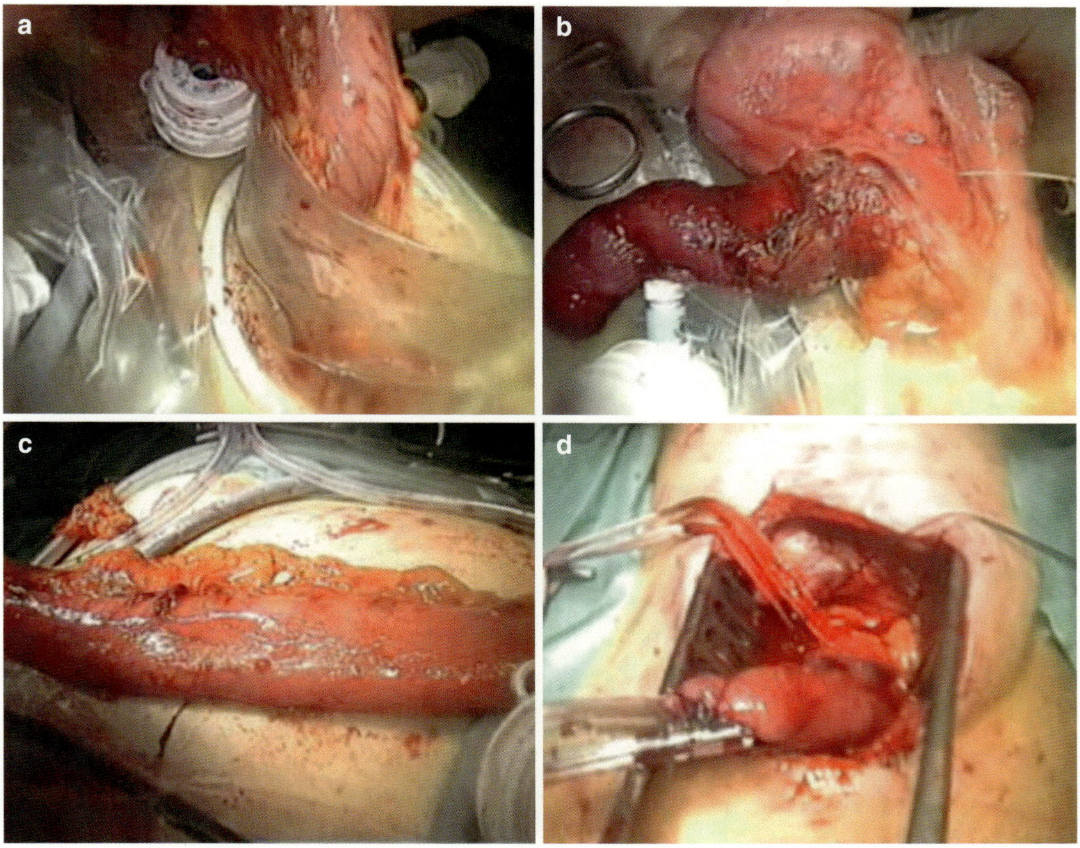

Fig. 12.6 (**a–d**) Exteriorization of the specimen, creation of gastric tube and neck anastomosis

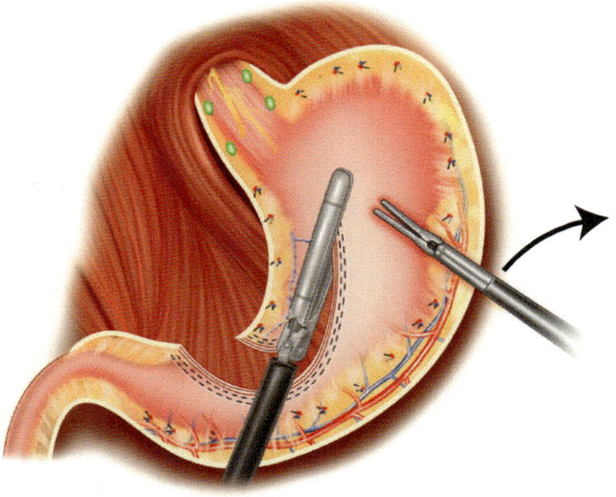

Fig. 12.7 Creation of gastric tube intracorporeally

7. After mobilization of the esophagus and lymphadenectomy up to the carina (if indicated a total lymphadenectomy should be performed), the esophagus is divided by staplers at the level of the azygos vein.
8. The gastric tube and the specimen are pulled into the thorax through a wide hiatus. There are different possibilities to perform the anastomosis.

Summary of intrathoracic anastomosis (Figs. 12.8, 12.9, 12.10, 12.11, and 12.12)

(a) Manual anastomosis (Fig. 12.8)
(b) Linear stapler anastomosis followed by closure of the opening (Fig. 12.9)
(c) Circular stapler anastomosis
   - Orvil device® anastomosis (21 or 25 mm) (Fig. 12.10a, b)

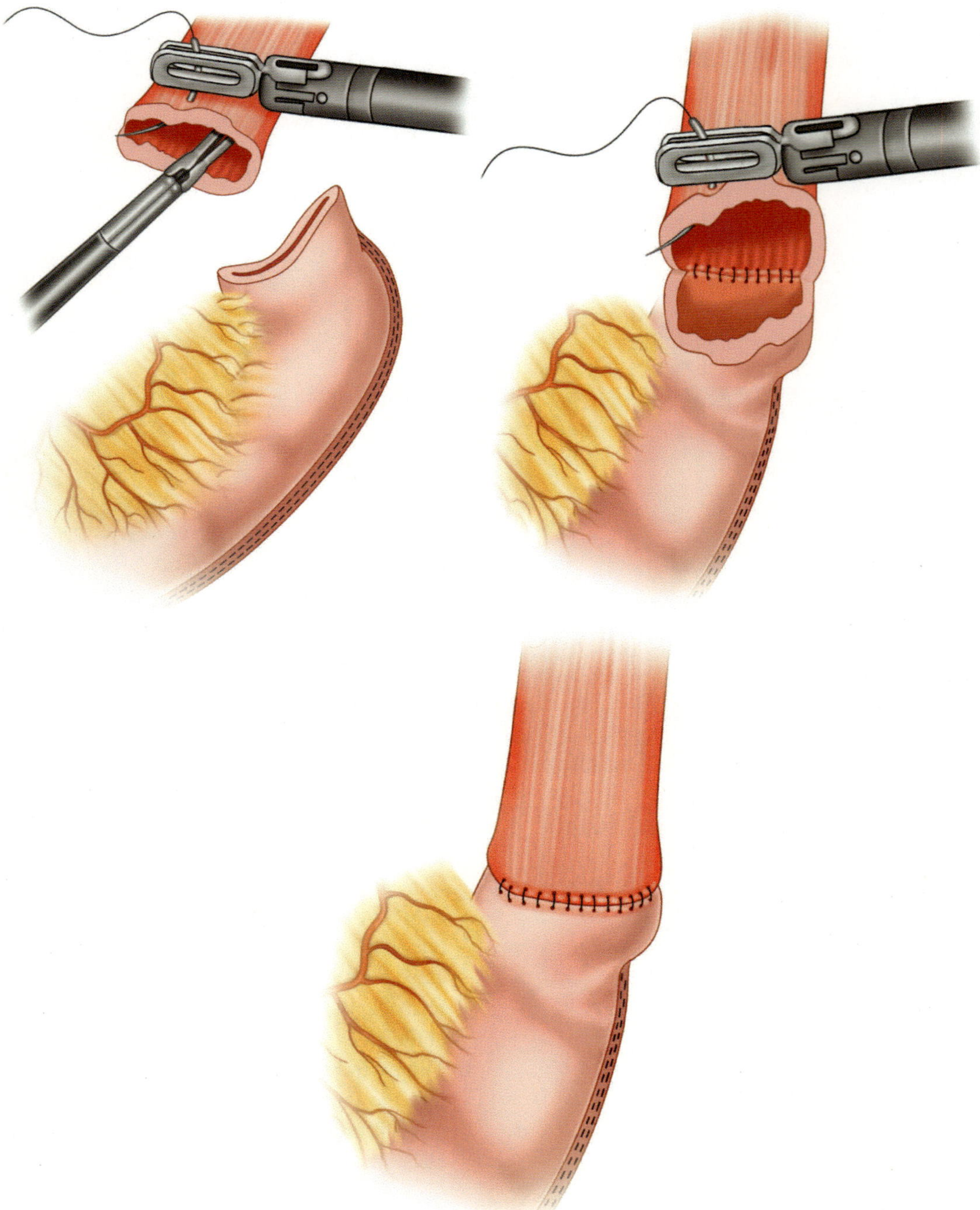

Fig. 12.8 Manual anastomosis

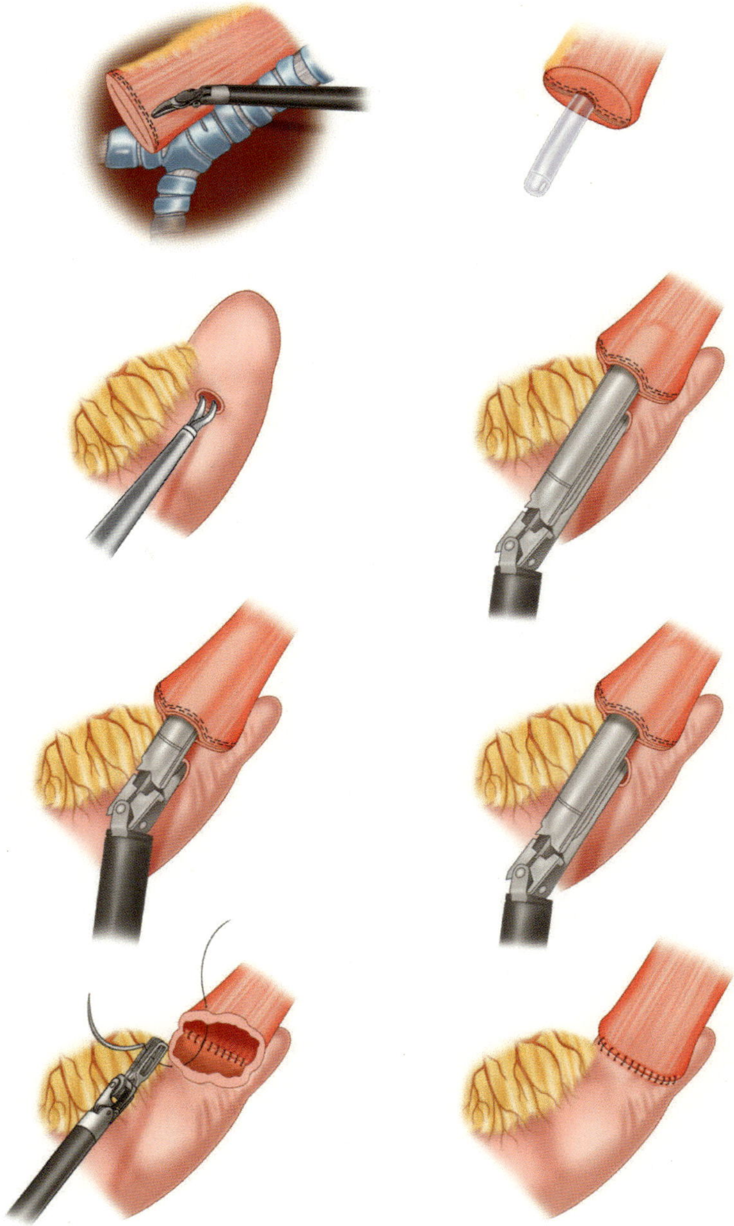

Fig. 12.9 Linear side to side anastomosis

- Conventional circular stapler around purse string (21, 25 or 28 mm) (Omental wrap anastomosis, Fig. 12.11)
- Robot assisted anastomosis (RAMIE) (Fig. 12.12).

9. A small protected thoracotomy is necessary for initiating the type of anastomosis in which a circular stapler will be positioned in the gastric tube and the anvil in the esophageal stump. For performing the manual, robot assisted and linear anastomosis, doing an initial small-assistance thoracotomy is not required. Only at the end of the procedure will the specimen need to be retrieved through the abdomen (patient must be repo-

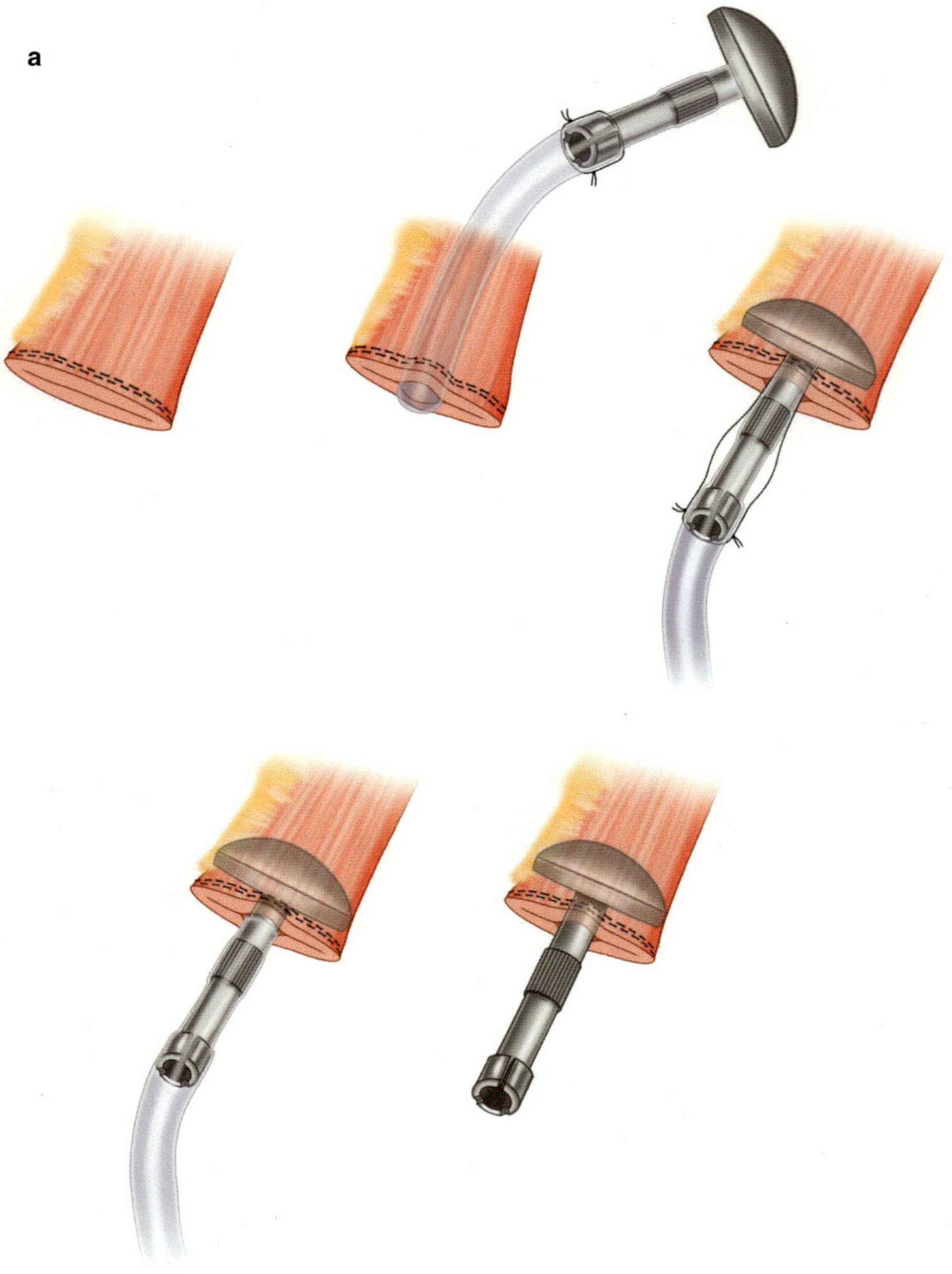

Fig. 12.10 (**a**) Circular anastomosis ORVIL. (**b**) Circular anastomosis ORVIL plus omental wrap, placement orvil in the esophagus stump

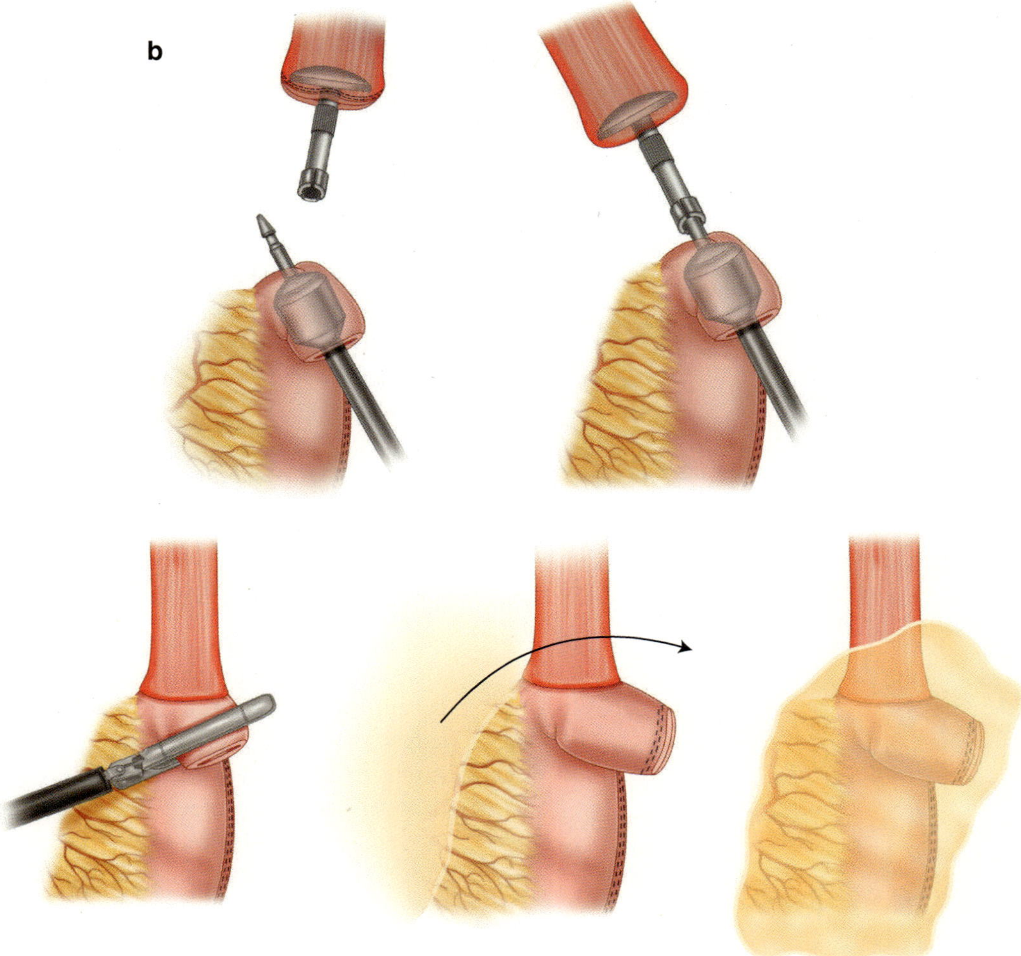

Fig. 12.10 (continued)

sitioned again) or retrieved at the end of the thoracoscopy by way of a small thoracotomy incision.

10. Concerning the type of intubation needed during the anastomosis phase, what is required for the manual, robot assisted, and the linear anastomosis is only a single intubation with two-lung ventilation (some anesthesiologists will use a selective intubation during the whole procedure). Whereas

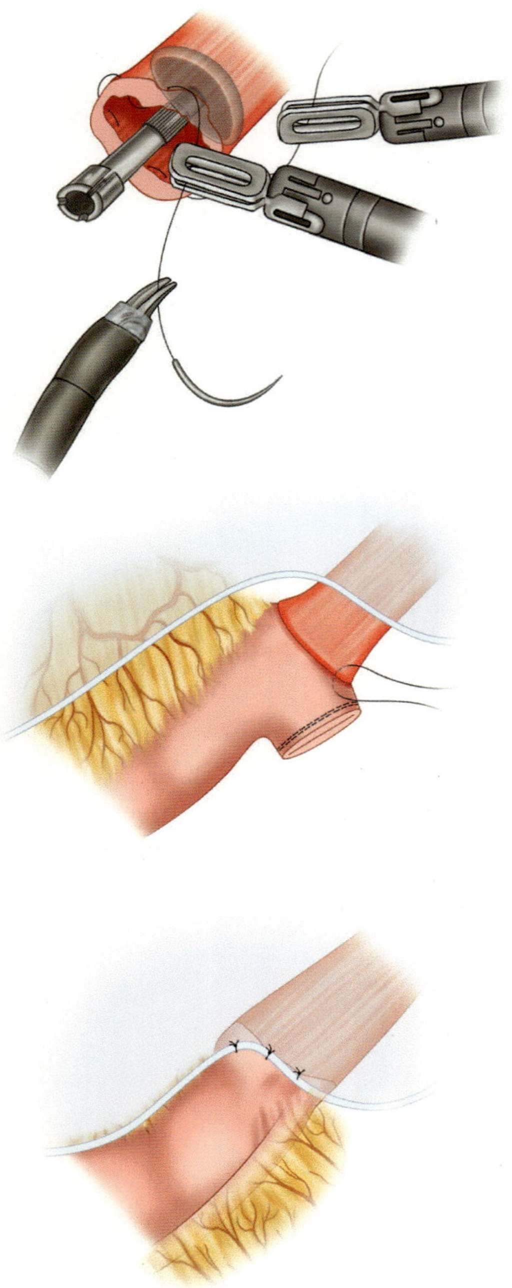

Fig. 12.11 Conventional circular stapler anastomosis and pleural flap

holding for the circular stapler anastomosis, a total collapse of the right lung during anastomosis is essential either by (a) selective intubation, or (b) placing a Fogarty catheter in the right bronchus to be inflated during the anastomosis phase or (3) applying to the wound a glove or some gel cap system along with maintaining a thoracic insufflation at 7–8 mmHg (Fig. 12.13).

12.3 Minimally Invasive Transhiatal Esophagectomy Operative Technique (see the Video 12.3)

The conventional operation technique described by Orringer and Sloan [1] is performed laparoscopically.

1. The patient is positioned in the supine position with the legs in the French position and the neck extended with exposure of the left side. The operating surgeon stands between the legs of the patient looking at two monitors placed at shoulder level of the patient. Two assistants stand on both sides of the patient, with the nurse on the right side of the surgeon.
2. A pneumoperitoneum is created by a 10-mm incision halfway between the xiphoid and the umbilicus on the left side of the middle line. The 30 degree camera is introduced through this trocar, and four other trocars are placed in the upper abdomen (Fig. 12.14).
3. Abdominal and local inspection at the hiatus takes place (Fig. 12.15). After displacement of the lateral segments of the left hepatic lobe and caudal traction of the stomach, a transhiatal dissection of the esophagus is laparoscopically performed in the plane between the pericardium, aorta, and both pleurae. For this part of the operation, a sealing device is used. After division of the hepatogastric ligament (pars flacida) and the most proximal short vessels, the space between the right crus and the esophagus is gentle opened in order to dissect the esophagus free and place a sling around it. In the case of junction tumors, a ring of the hiatus muscle is resected. The sling, placed around the esophagus, will permit traction of the esophagus in the caudal direction (Fig. 12.16).

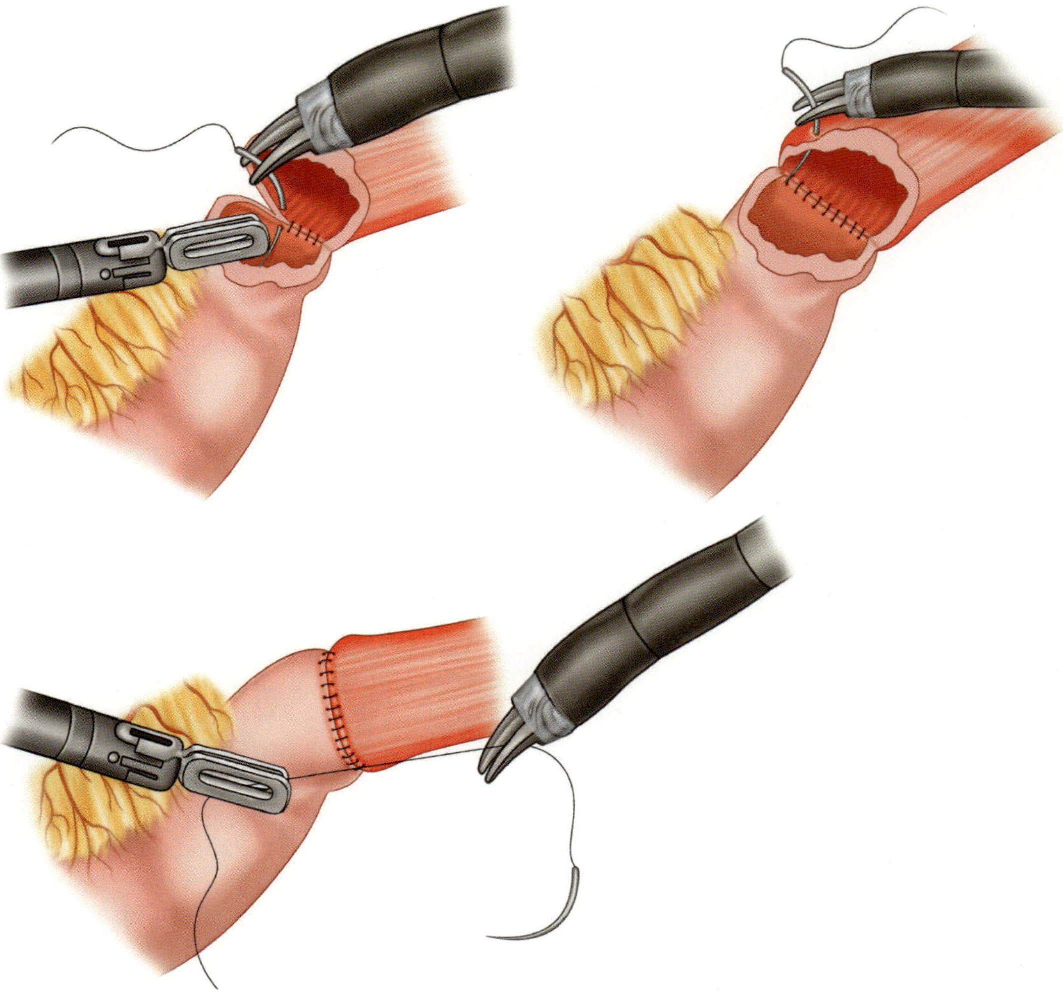

Fig. 12.12 Robot assisted anastomosis (RAMIE)

4. The hiatus is enlarged by dividing the anterior part with the division of the phrenic vein by means of the Ligasure device according to Pinotti [2] (Fig. 12.17). Anteriorly dissection is performed in an avascular plane in the anterior mediastinum with visualization of the pericardium and pulmonary vein (Fig. 12.18). Dissection continues anteriorly up to the level of the carina, in which the lymph nodes can be visualized but not resected.
5. On the right side of the esophagus, the aorta is approached at the level of the hiatus and in an avascular plane dissected free as high as possible in the posterior mediastinum.
6. Lateral dissection is performed on both sides at the level of the pleurae. The pleurae are always opened, on both sides in most cases, with resection of some part of it if necessary. The anaesthesiologist is warned of this situation because the mechanical ventilation must be adapted. Mechanical ventilation is corrected by means of increase of minute volume, use of positive end-expiratory pressure (PEEP) and decrease of the insufflation pressure to about 10 mmHg [3]. The esophagus is resected laparoscopically in this way, together with para-esophageal tissue and

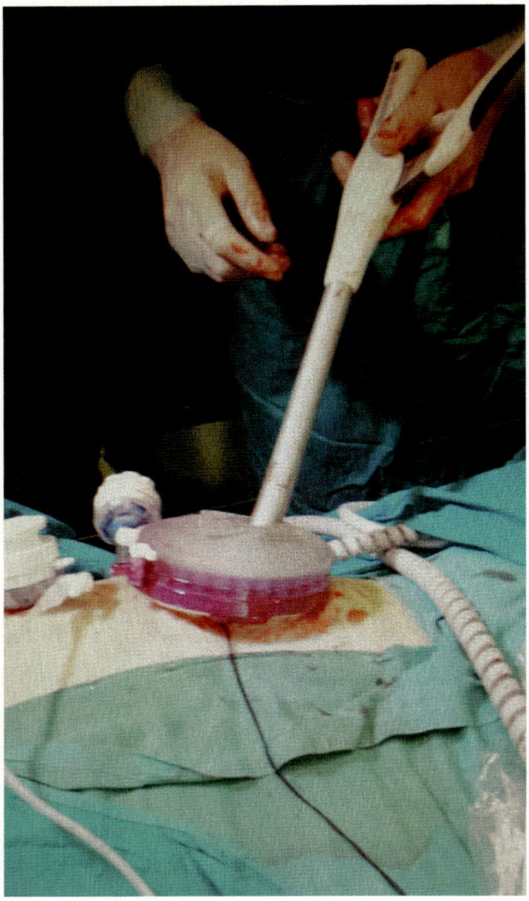

Fig. 12.13 Gel cap system used in the small thoracotomy wound in order to maintain the insufflation and permit introduction of staplers and work trocars

periesophageal lymph nodes, to the level of the carina (Fig. 12.19a–d).

7. By retracting the stomach to the left, a D1+ lymphadenectomy of the celiac trunk and their branches is performed, to be followed by division of the left gastric artery and vein by means of a sealing device or clips. From there, the dissection is completed up to the hiatus (Fig. 12.20a–c).
8. The sealing device is used to mobilize the greater curvature of the stomach by dividing the gastro-colic ligament from the antrum-body junction, with preservation of the gastroepiploic vessels. Afterwards, the short gastric vessels are approached and divided up to the left crus of the hiatus.

   (These two steps, 7 and 8, can be performed in different order, first lymphadenectomy followed by gastric dissection or first gastric dissection followed by lymphadenectomy).
9. The next step is dissection of the cervical esophagus by means of a left-side cervical incision.
10. At the same time (if possible), another surgeon performs a small assistance periumbilical incision (7 cm) with protection. Through the lateral left trocar, a venous stripper is introduced into the gastric lumen by a small incision in the lesser gastric curvature and then pushed up to the cervical dissected esophagus. If the stripper cannot be pushed because of the obstruction caused by the

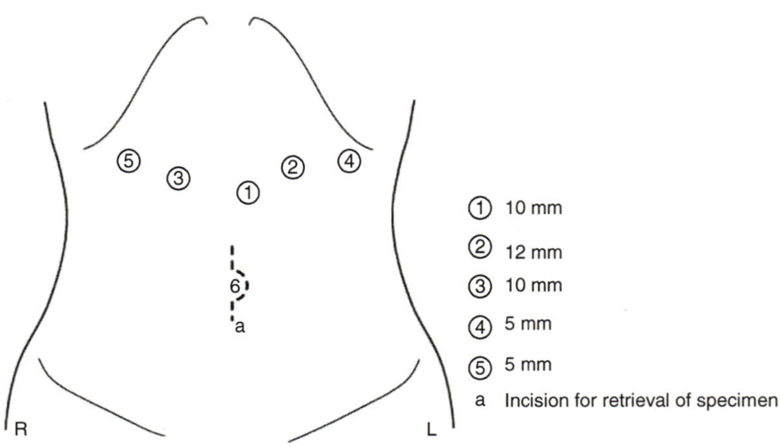

Fig. 12.14 Patient is placed for laparoscopic and cervical part of the procedure. Surgeon stands between the legs of the patient looking to the monitor at the level of the patient's shoulders (**a**). Position of the trocars along both subcostal margins (**b**)

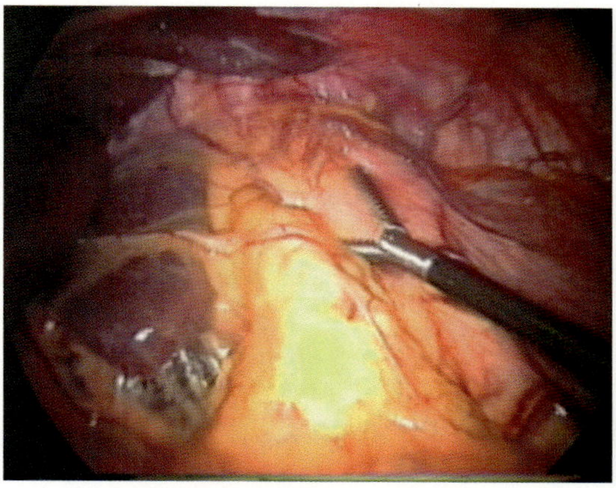

Fig. 12.15 Complete abdominal inspection is followed by local inspection of the hiatal area. Especially attention is paid, if tumor is located in the G-E junction, to its relation with the hiatal structures and lymph nodes

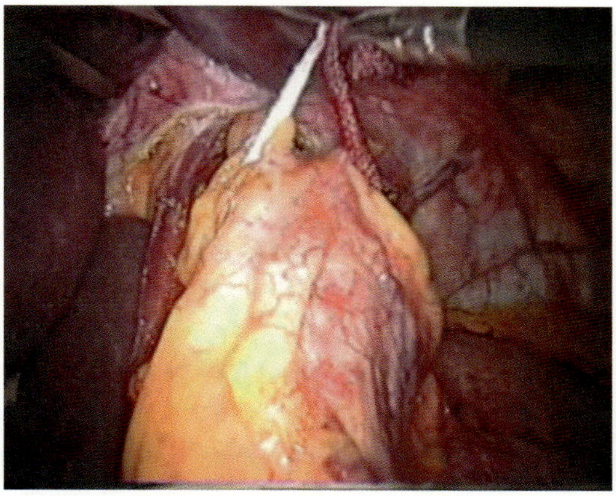

Fig. 12.16 In the case of a G-E junction tumor, a ring of the hiatus is excised in continuity with the tumor. Very gentle dissection permits to dissect the esophagus free and to put a sling around it for traction

tumour, the feeding tube can be withdrawn via the small opening in the stomach and then exteriorised. The cervical esophagus is divided, after which the most distal part is closed around the stripper. A nasogastric tube is attached to it. Through the abdominal incision and manual assisted stripping of the esophagus will take place. This nasogastric tube can be used afterwards to lead the gastric tube upside to the cervical incision.

11. In this way, with the hand of the surgeon in the abdomen, the controlled stripping can be safely

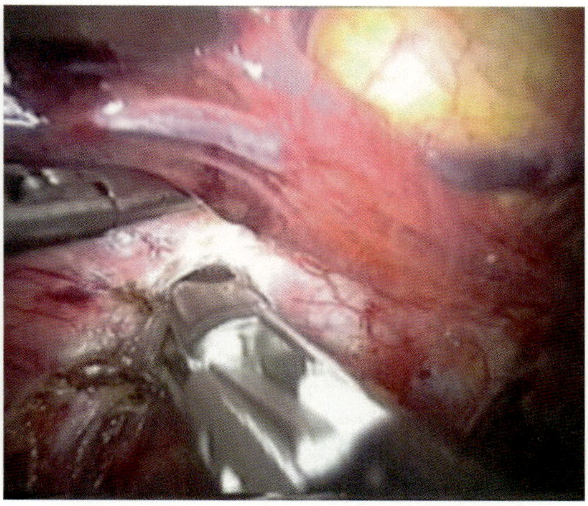

Fig. 12.17 Hiatus is open anteriorly according to Pinotti; the phrenic vein being divided by means of clips or sealing device

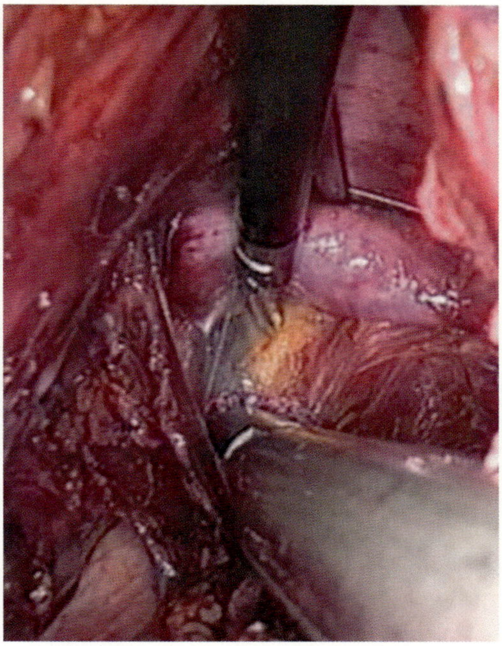

Fig. 12.18 Gentle blunt dissection is anteriorly performed along the plane of the pericard sac and inferior pulmonary vein

performed. In most patients, branches of the vagal nerves must be divided at this stage to retrieve the specimen through a fully protected periumbilical incision (Fig. 12.21a–c).

12. Once the specimen retrieved outside the abdomen, the mobilization of the stomach is completed, and the gastric tube is created,

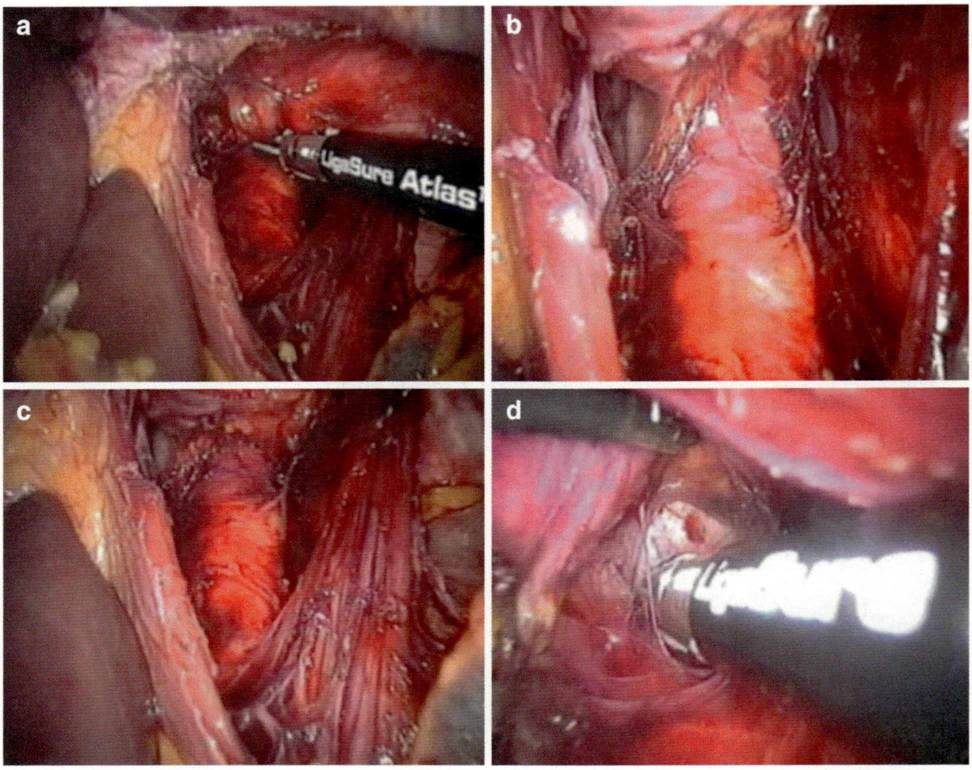

Fig. 12.19 (**a–d**) Posteriorly the aorta is dissected free at the level of the hiatus and dissected bluntly in proximal direction (**a–c**). Dissection proceeds at both lateral parts, taking down the lateral tissue (most of cases with a wedge of the pleura) by means of sealing device. (**d**): the carina is visualized

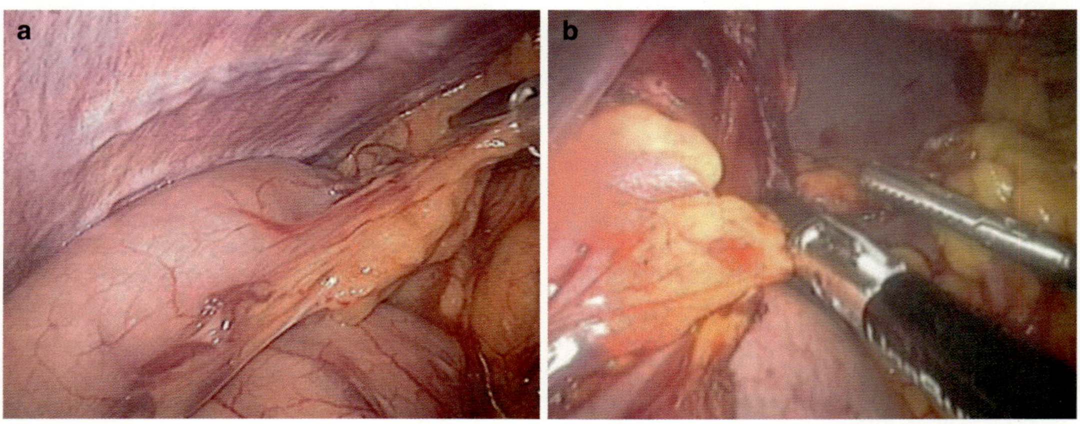

Fig. 12.20 (**a–c**) Procedure proceeds with gastrolysis along the greater curvature with preservation of the gastro-epiploic vessels (**a–b**). Lymphadenectomy of the celiac trunk should be now performed (**c**)

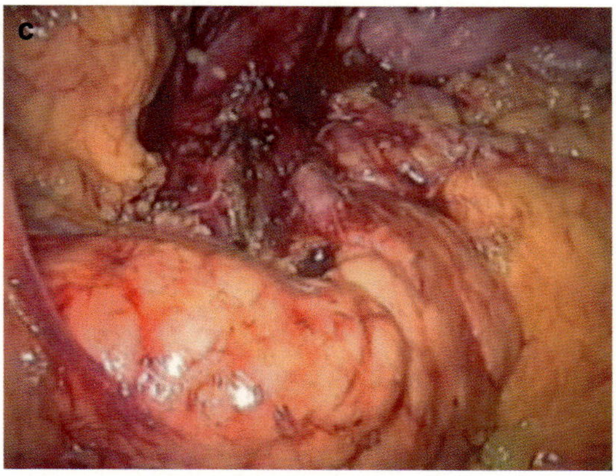

Fig. 12.20 (continued)

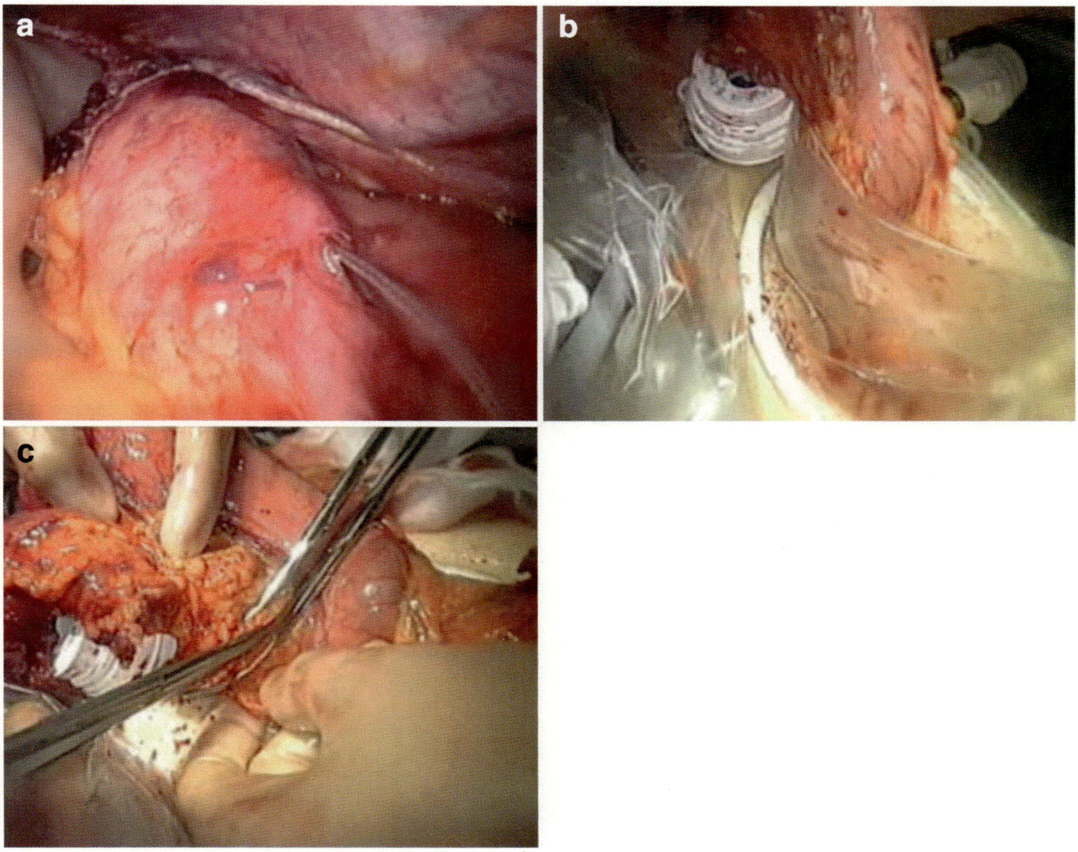

Fig. 12.21 (**a–c**) The cervical incision is done and after division of the esophagus, and by means of a stripper the specimen can be retrieved and exteriorized through the small and well protected abdominal wound

3–4 cm width, by using stapling device. The gastric tube then is oversewn and attached to the nasogastric tube and replaced in the abdomen. Next, the gastric tube is placed under vision into the cervical esophagus by traction of the nasogastric tube. A cervical anastomosis is created (Fig. 12.22a–c).

13. Through the transumbilical incision a jejunostomy feeding tube was placed for feeding and the two thoracic cavities were drained by two thoracic drains placed through the trocar openings. In none of the patients in this series was a Kocher manoeuvre, a pyloromyotomy, or a pyloroplasty performed.

Postoperatively patients were extubated after the operation when haemodinamically and respiratory stable.

Patients were fed through the jejunostomy feeding tube from the first day after their operation, until the oral feeding could be completely resumed.

Active mobilization and physiotherapy follows. On postoperative day 3 the nasogastric tube was removed and oral feeding was started.

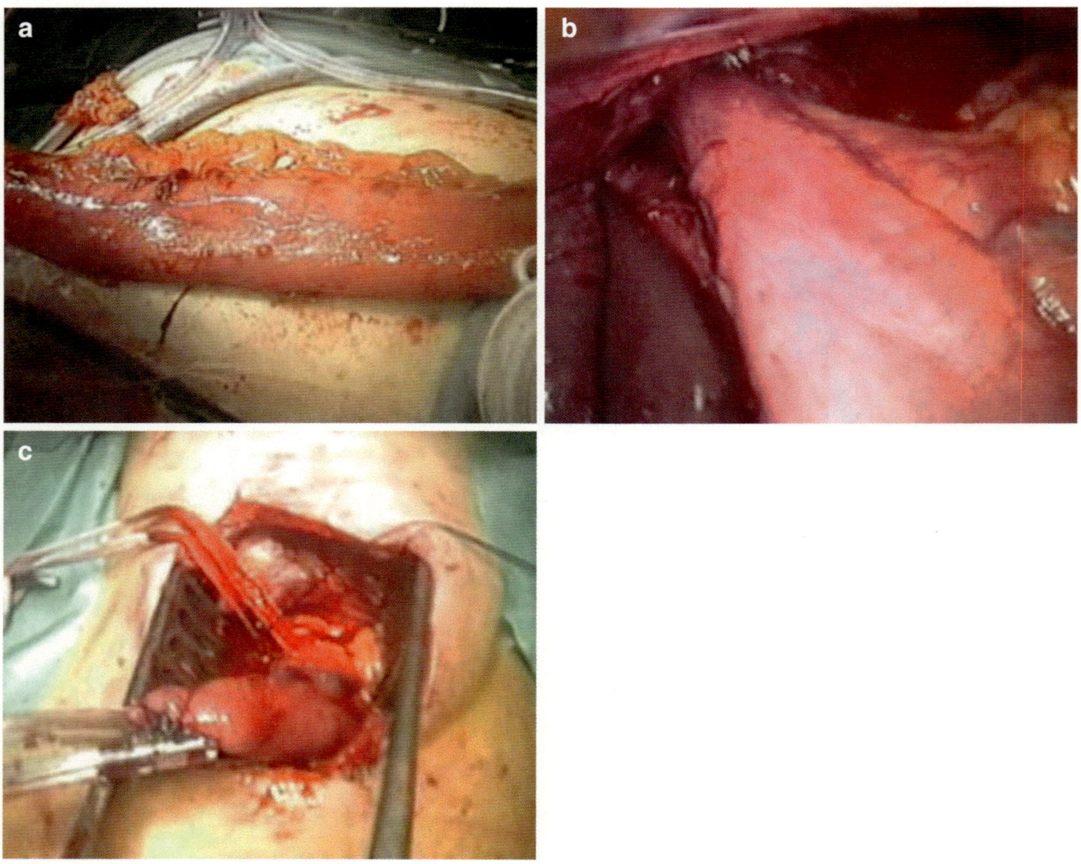

Fig. 12.22 (**a–c**) Once the specimen is exteriorized, gastric tube (3–4 cm) is created by means of staplers along the greater curvature. The good vascularized gastric tube is oversewn, attached to a nasogastric tube and pulled up into the cervical wound and anastomosed (**a–c**). Through the small laparotomy a jejunostomy catheter is introduced and both thoracic cavities are drained by means of drains introduced through the abdominal trocars ports

12.4 Comments

Current use of pyloroplasty remains controversial as well [4]. Even though many authors still include the drainage of the pylorus in the operative procedure. In our experience the avoidance of this pyloroplasty have not lead to any emptying problems of the gastric tube during the postoperative period but control of the pylorus passage at the third postoperative day is important. Therefore we do not recommend a routine pyloroplasty as part of the gastric tube formation.

References

1. Orringer MB, Sloan H. Esophagectomy without thoracotomy. J Thorac Cardiovasc Surg. 1978;76:643–54.
2. Pinotti HW, Zilberstein B, Pollara W, Raia A. Esophagectomy without thoracotomy. Surg Gynecol Obstet. 1981;152:345–7.
3. Makay O, van den Broek WT, Yuan JZ, et al. Anaesthesiological hazards during laparoscopic transhiatal esophageal resection: a case control study of the laparoscopic assisted versus the conventional approach. Surg Endosc. 2004;18:1263–7.
4. Mannell A, Mcknight A, Esser JD. Role of pyloroplasty in the retrosternal stomach – results of a prospective, randomized, controlled trial. Br J Surg. 1990;77:57–9.

Part III

Gastric Cancer

13 Surgical Anatomy of the Omental Bursa

Hylke J.F. Brenkman, Nicole I. van der Wielen, Ronald L.A. Bleys, Maarten S. van Leeuwen, Joris J. Scheepers, Donald L. van der Peet, Jelle P. Ruurda, Richard van Hillegersberg, and Miguel A. Cuesta

13.1 Introduction

During Minimally Invasive Surgery (MIS) of the Upper Gastrointestinal (GI) tract, such as esophagectomy, gastrectomy, pancreatectomy, and transverse colectomy, it is imperative to have a thorough knowledge of the omental bursa (or: lesser sac) in order to perform an adequate dissection of those organs and an appropriate lymphadenectomy. Yet the surgical anatomy of the omental bursa seems very complex as the rotational embryological development of the upper abdominal organs results in a crossroads of these organs with accompanying vessels and lymph nodes [1], hence making surgery around these organs quite difficult.

H.J.F. Brenkman (✉) • J.P. Ruurda
R. van Hillegersberg
Department of Surgical Oncology, University Medical Center Utrecht, Utrecht, The Netherlands
e-mail: H.J.F.Brenkman@umcutrecht.nl

N.I. van der Wielen • D.L. van der Peet • M.A. Cuesta
Department of Surgery, Vumc, Amsterdam, The Netherlands
e-mail: ma.cuesta@vumc.nl

R.L.A. Bleys
Department of Anatomy, University Medical Center Utrecht, Utrecht, The Netherlands

M.S. van Leeuwen
Department Radiology, University Medical Center Utrecht, Utrecht, The Netherlands

J.J. Scheepers
Department of Surgery, Reinier de Graaf Hospital, Delft, The Netherlands

Our observation and dissection of the omental bursa during MIS prompted a descriptive study of this area, based on laparoscopic observation, with the aim to devise an understandable surgical anatomical concept.

From our surgical-anatomic point of view we deemed the following two points important to know: (1) What are the boundaries of the omental bursa? (2) Which of the varying approaches to the omental bursa bring about the most complete lymphadenectomy?

13.1.1 Laparoscopic Gastrectomy

The surgical steps to perform a laparoscopic gastrectomy are

1. Omentectomy
2. Lymphadenectomy
3. Resection of the organ (distal or total gastrectomy)
4. Reconstruction by anastomosis

Cancer deposits and presence of cancer cells in lymph nodes in the greater omentum varies between 5 and 10% of the patients and it is associated with a relative worse prognosis. In laparoscopic gastrectomy, omentectomy is still a part of the procedure [1, 2].

M.A. Cuesta (ed.), *Minimally Invasive Surgery for Upper Abdominal Cancer*,
DOI 10.1007/978-3-319-54301-7_13

In order to perform the steps 2 and 3, surgical approach and knowledge of the omental bursa is essential.

13.2 Surgical Anatomy of the Omental Bursa

A schematic anterior view of the bursa is shown in Illustration 1. If the omental bursa is visualized as a square box, the anterior aspect of the omental bursa consists of the hepatogastric ligament (pars flaccida), the posterior wall of the stomach (main part), the gastrocolic ligament with the gastroepiploic vessels, and the gastrosplenic ligament with the short gastric vessels.

At the posterior wall, at the most cranial part, the gastropancreatic fold, from the aorta to the lesser gastric curvature, contains the celiac trunk and left gastric vessels and divides the cranial part of the omental bursa in two compartments (Fig. 13.1). The right space is commonly named the superior recess, whereas the left space is commonly known as the splenic recess. The connection between the superior recess and the splenic recess takes place at the level of the pancreas just caudal to the celiac trunk; this part of the omental bursa is called the vestibulum. During MIS, one enters the superior recess by opening the hepatogastric ligament (pars flaccida), and the splenic recess by opening the gastrocolic or gastrosplenic ligament.

From caudal to cranial, the posterior wall and floor of the splenic recess consists of the transverse mesocolon up to the inferior edge of the pancreas, the splenorenal ligament with the splenic artery and vein, and more cranially the retroperitoneum (covering the left adrenal gland and left kidney) up to the diaphragm. The left lateral wall is formed in the upper part by the gastrosplenic ligament, the short gastric vessels fold and the left gastroomental fold (Fig. 13.1). These two folds contain the short gastric vessels and the left gastroepiploic vessels, respectively originating from the distal splenic artery and running upward and downward to the greater gastric curvature. At the level of the head of the pancreas the right gastroomental fold, containing the right gastroepiploic vessels (originating from the gastroduodenal artery once this artery has passed under the duodenum) forms the right inferior side of the omental bursa (Fig. 13.2).

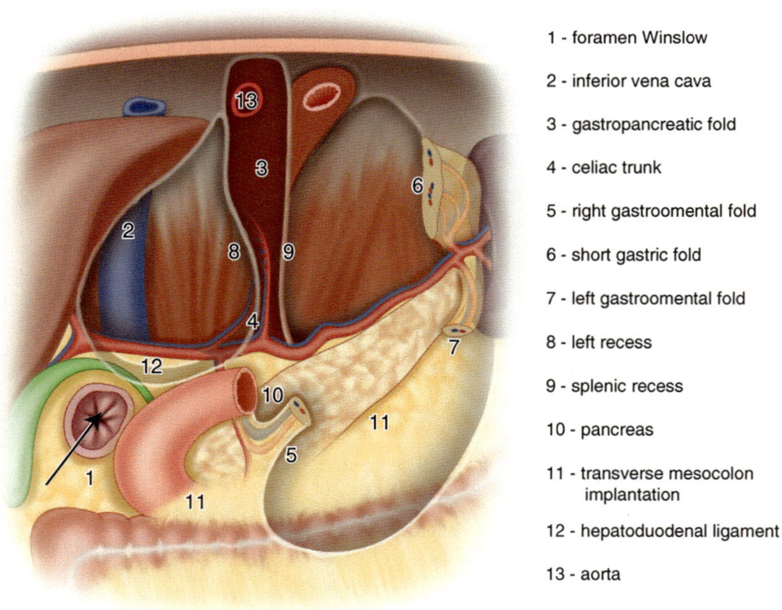

Fig. 13.1 Illustration of the bursa omentalis. (*1*) Foramen Winslow. (*2*) Inferior vena cava. (*3*) Gastropancreatic fold. (*4*) Celiac trunk. (*5*) Right gastroomental fold. (*6*) Short gastric fold. (*7*) Left gastroomental fold. (*8*) Left recess. (*9*) Splenic recess. (*10*) Pancreas. (*11*) Transverse mesocolon. (*12*) Hepatoduodenal ligament. (*13*) Aorta

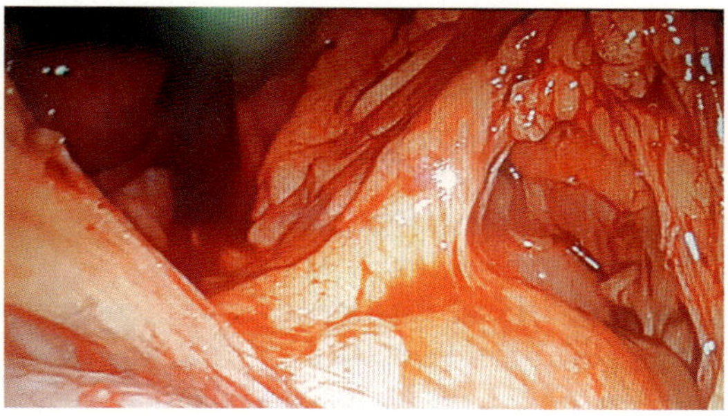

Fig. 13.2 Gastropancreatic plica (fold)

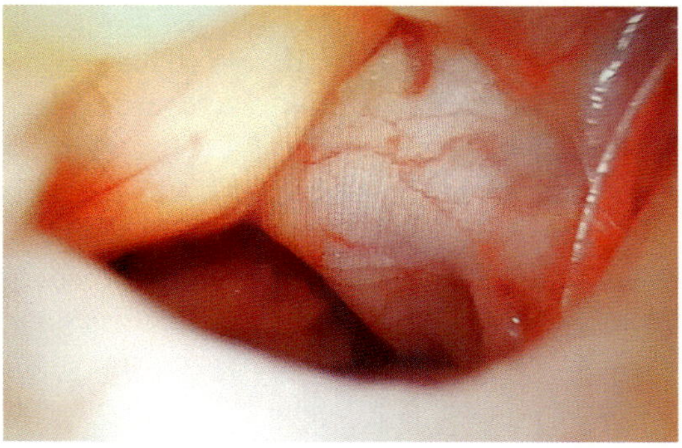

Fig. 13.3 Foramen of Winslow

This inferior part of the omental bursa is named the inferior recess. During MIS, one enters the inferior recess by opening the gastrocolic ligament or after omentectomy during laparoscopic gastrectomy.

At the superior recess and from caudal to cranial the posterior wall consists of the inferior vena cava and the caudate lobe (segment 1) of the liver up to the right crus of the diaphragm. The anterior side of the hepatoduodenal ligament is located inside the omental bursa and forms the most distal part of the superior recess (Fig 13.1). The greater sac of the peritoneal cavity and the omental bursa are connected through the omental foramen (foramen of Winslow). Boundaries of the foramen of Winslow are as follows: it is bounded cranially by the caudate lobe, caudally by the first part of the duodenum, ventrally by the hepatoduodenal ligament, and dorsally by the inferior vena cava (Illustration 1). In this way, both the anterior and posterior aspects of the hepatoduodenal ligament are covered by peritoneum of the omental bursa. After entering the omental foramen (Fig. 13.3), one enters the vestibulum of the omental bursa.

13.2.1 Lymphandenectomy for Gastric Cancer

The celiac trunk forms part of the posterior wall of the omental bursa (gastropancreatic fold, Fig. 13.2) and is covered by peritoneum, fat and lymph nodes. All D2 lymph nodes (LN) according to the Japanese classification are in relation with the celiac trunk or its branches (left gastric artery, splenic artery and the hepatic artery) whereas the D1 LN are located at the greater and lesser curvatures. D2 lymphadenectomy includes the groups number 8a–12a whereas in distal gastrectomy the groups number 8a–11p [3].

13.2.2 Surgical Approach of the Omental Bursa

During minimally invasive upper GI surgery, the omental bursa can be opened in three ways:

1. by incision of the hepatogastric ligament (pars flaccida of the lesser omentum).
2. through the gastrocolic and gastrosplenic ligament, and
3. by opening the transverse mesocolon at the level of the pancreas.

The first option starts by opening the lesser omentum and retraction of the stomach to the left, so that the superior edge of the pancreas can be visualized. Opening of the peritoneum above the pancreas permits dissection of the common hepatic artery and from there dissection proceeds up to the liver along the right gastric artery up to the level of proper hepatic artery.

At that point, lymphadenectomy is done starting with groups number 9, 8a and 12a up to the right crus of the hiatus along the portal vein and inferior vena cava. Proceeding from the common hepatic artery to the left, the celiac trunk is approached, the

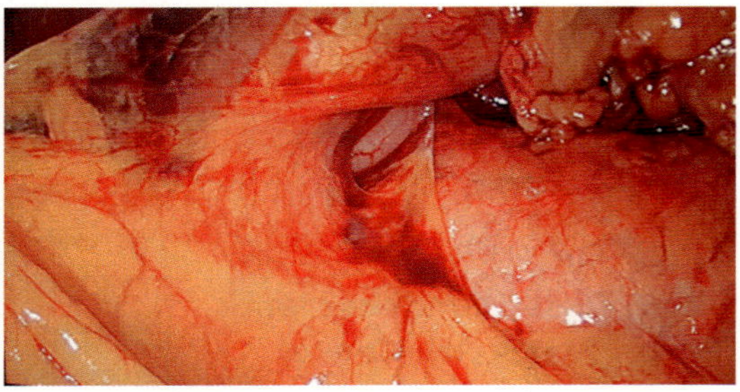

Fig. 13.4 Right gastroomental fold

left gastric vein and artery are dissected free and then divided (lymphadenectomy of group 7). The next step is to continue the lymphadenectomy along the splenic artery—as far as possible—on the superior edge of the body of the pancreas. In this way, all the D2 lymph nodes groups 11p, and 11d are excised "en bloc" with exception of station 10 located at the splenic hilum. Important to note is that LN groups, numbers 6 (D1), 10 (D2) and 12a (D2), considered as "extreme groups" and difficult to resect during gastrectomy are located at the edge of the omental bursa, as they lay inside the right gastroomental fold (Fig. 13.4b) and the hilum of the spleen and liver respectively. The gastroomental fold (with the right gastroepiploic vessels, number 6) have to be dissected free from the transverse mesocolon in order to be identified and the other two groups have to be approached at the hilum of both organs, liver (number 12a) and spleen (number 10) respectively.

The second option starts by entering the omental bursa through the gastrocolic and gastrosplenic ligament. This permits a good approach of the celiac trunk with its three arterial branches, but to a lesser extent visualization of the lymph nodes along the hepatic artery to the hilum of the liver. In many cases a combination of both approaches is necessary. The first two approaches are used in Upper GI surgery, being the approach through the gastrosplenic ligament used to create any type of fundoplication during surgery for Gastroesophageal Reflux disease. The last option, the opening of the transverse mesocolon at the level of the distal pancreas, is used in colorectal surgery for mobilization of the splenic flexure.

13.3 Discussion

A comprehensive concept of the live surgical anatomy is necessary for ensuring anatomical accuracy as well as reproducible radical surgery resections for cancer.

During MIS of the Upper GI tract, including esophageal, gastric and duodeno-pancreatic resections, the omental bursa may be a difficult area to visualize and to dissect when surgeons try to perform an adequate celiac trunk and branches lymphadenectomy and resection of the involved organ. It is a complex area in which during the ontogenesis the embryological anatomy developed into a crossroads of important vessels and digestive organs.

Particularly for the Upper GI surgeon—dedicated to MIS of the Upper GI tract—having a comprehensive knowledge of the omental bursa is imperative. MIS of the Upper GI organs is increasingly performed and certain interventions, such as the esophagectomy, gastrectomy and pancreatectomies are being evaluated through randomized controlled trials [4–6]. Our aim was to describe the surgical boundaries of the omental bursa, with surgical landmarks and folds that have to be visualized and dissected, and demonstrating how to perform an adequate lymphadenectomy followed by an oncological resection of the involved organ.

Moreover, the two ways for approaching the omental bursa, first through the lesser omentum and second through the gastrocolic ligament, are described. Both are not exclusive and in many events a combination of both approaches can help for gaining an adequate lymphadenectomy.

In conclusion, it appears that dissection of structures surrounding the bursa by MIS can be demanding because of the complex anatomy [7]. We have argued that having knowledge of the surgical anatomy and landmarks of the resection will enable a more adequate and reproducible surgical resection during Upper GI MIS. The conclusion can be that the advantages gained by MIS, such as visualization and magnification, contribute to a more complete knowledge of the omental bursa with its central location in the upper abdomen.

References

1. Haverkamp L, Brenkman HJ, Ruurda JP, et al. The oncological value of omentectomy in gastrectomy for cancer. J Gastroint Sur. 2016;20:885–90.
2. Jongerius EJ, Boerma D, Seldenrijk KA, et al. Role of omentectomy as a part of radical surgery for gastric cancer. Br J Surg. 2016;10:1497–503.
3. Japanese Gastric Cancer Association. Japanese gastric cancer treatment guidelines 2010 (ver. 3). Gastric Cancer. 2011;14(2):113–23.
4. Wang M, Cai H, Meng L, Cai Y, Wang X, Li Y, et al. Minimally invasive pancreaticoduodenectomy: a comprehensive review. Int J Surg. 2016;35:139–46.
5. Haverkamp L, Brenkman HJ, Seesing MF, Gisbertz SS, van Berge Henegouwen MI, Luyer MD, et al. Laparoscopic versus open gastrectomy for gastric cancer, a multicenter prospectively randomized controlled trial (LOGICA-trial). BMC Cancer. 2015;15(1):556-015-1551-z.
6. Straatman J, van der Wielen N, Cuesta MA, Gisbertz SS, Hartemink KJ, Alonso Poza A, et al. Surgical techniques, open versus minimally invasive gastrectomy after chemotherapy (STOMACH trial): study protocol for a randomized controlled trial. Trials. 2015;16:123-015-0638-9.
7. Larsen W. Development of the gastrointestinal tract. In: Sherman L, Potter S, Scott W, editors. Human embryology. 3rd ed. Churchill: Livingstone; 2001. p. 235–64.

14 Neoadjuvant Treatment of Gastric Cancer

Yvette H.M. Claassen, Henk H. Hartgrink, Wobbe O. De Steur, Marije Slingerland, and Cornelis J.H. Van de Velde

14.1 Introduction

Gastric cancer remains a significant health problem. Despite the fact that the incidence of gastric cancer over the last decades decreased considerably, it is still the fifth most common malignancy in the world with approximately one million new cases each year. With over 700,000 deaths yearly it is the third leading cause of cancer deaths in both sexes worldwide, with the highest mortality rates reported in Eastern Asia (14.0 per 100,000 males and 9.8 per 100,000 females) [1].

Surgery is still the cornerstone in treatment of curable gastric cancer. Nowadays, gastrectomies are increasingly minimally invasive performed. The results of gastrectomies have improved over the last years with respect to morbidity, postoperative mortality, and survival [2]. However, whether the extended lymph node dissection contributed to this improvement is still unclear as the last decades the role of extended lymph node dissection has been controversial. In Asian countries an extended lymph node dissection (D2) has been the standard procedure for the last two decades, whereas in Western countries only a limited lymph node dissection (D1) was common practice until recently [2]. Many studies have investigated the benefit of an extended lymph node dissection (D2) over the standard limited (D1) lymphadenectomy for Western patients, including three methodologically well performed randomized clinical trials, the UK Medical Research Council (MRC) surgical trial, the Dutch Gastric Cancer Trial (DGCT), and the Italian Gastric Cancer Trial [3–5]. Initially none of these trials showed a difference in overall survival, though a D2 lymphadenectomy was associated with a significant higher morbidity- and mortality rate [3–5]. Long term follow up in the Dutch trial, however, did show a benefit for the more extended lymph node dissection, especially if morbidity and mortality could be minimalized [4, 6]. Furthermore, the Italian trial showed that an extended lymph node dissection was beneficial for patients with node positive disease [5]. Nevertheless, survival after surgery alone with a D2 lymph node dissection remains poor with a 5-year survival rate around 50% in Western countries [2].

As no further great improvements were expected in the field of surgery, new treatment strategies were urgently needed to improve survival rates of gastric cancer. In order to achieve this, numerous studies were conducted with multimodal treatment strategies, such as (neo) adjuvant chemotherapy and/or radiotherapy, in addition to surgery. First, adjuvant chemotherapy was tested

Y.H.M. Claassen • H.H. Hartgrink • W.O. De Steur
C.J.H. Van de Velde (✉)
Department of Surgery, Leiden University Medical Center, Leiden, The Netherlands
e-mail: Y.H.M.Claassen@lumc.nl; C.J.H.van_de_Velde@lumc.nl

M. Slingerland
Department of Medical Oncology, Leiden University Medical Center, Leiden, The Netherlands

M.A. Cuesta (ed.), *Minimally Invasive Surgery for Upper Abdominal Cancer*, DOI 10.1007/978-3-319-54301-7_14

in several trials with limited patients, but with promising results [7]. Later on, the role of chemotherapy in neoadjuvant setting was evaluated, starting in the Dutch FAMTX trial, and developed to an essential part of the treatment of gastric cancer [8]. Application of radiotherapy in neoadjuvant setting has also gained space over time. The last years attention has risen increasingly for chemotherapy combined with targeted agents. Consequently, in the last 15 years, major advances in the field of multimodal treatment strategies have changed clinical management of gastric cancer.

This chapter comprises the current status of neoadjuvant therapy in treatment of gastric cancer in the Western world. Future directions in the treatment of gastric cancer are addressed.

14.2 Neo-Adjuvant/Perioperative Chemotherapy

The use of preoperative chemotherapy in gastric cancer was considered to achieve downstaging of the tumor, to improve resectability, and to increase the likelihood of completing multimodal treatment, as surgery is associated with substantial morbidity rates. An overview of studies investigating the impact of neo-adjuvant/perioperative chemotherapy in gastric cancer is shown in Table 14.1. One of the first randomized clinical trials investigating the added value of neoadjuvant chemotherapy in resectable gastric cancer was the Dutch FAMTX trial (also known as the POCOM (Preoperative Chemotherapy for Operable Gastric Cancer) trial) [8]. The aim of this trial was to investigate whether pre-operative chemotherapy led to a 15% higher curative resectability rate in patients with operable gastric cancer. After adequate staging, patients were randomized to receive either four courses of FAMTX (5-fluorouracil, doxorubicin, and methotrexate), followed by surgery or surgery alone. With a two-sided significance level of 5% and a power of 90%, 225 patients were required in each arm. Due to poor accrual an interim analysis was prematurely performed where no difference in resectability rates was observed between both arms. Based on these results and poor accrual, the trial was prematurely closed. Between 1993 and 1996, 59 patients were randomized of which 29 patients were allocated to the FAMTX regimen and 30 patients to surgery alone. A beneficial effect of the pre-operative FAMTX could not be shown as the results showed equal resectability rates in both groups. The response rate (complete or partial) in the FAMTX group was only 32%, which was comparable with lower results of previous reported data. The median survival was 18 months in the FAMTX group compared to 30 months in the surgery alone group ($P = 0.17$). At initiation of this trial in the early 90s, a FAMTX regimen was chosen because of its repeatedly demonstrated steady response rates, lower toxicity compared with EAP (etoposide, 5-fluorouracil (5-FU) and methotrexate), lower costs, and lower toxicity compared with FEMTX-P (5-FU, epidoxorubicin, methotrexate, and cisplatin). Moreover, at that time FAMTX

Table 14.1 Overview of studies investigating the impact of neoadjuvant/perioperative chemotherapy in resectable gastric cancer

Trial	Years	N	Treatment	Results	*P*
FAMTX trial [8]	1993–1996	29	FAMTX—S	Median survival: 18 months	0.17
		30	S	Median survival: 30 months	
MAGIC trial [9]	1994–2002	250	ECF—S—ECF	HR 0.75 (CI: 0.60–0.93)	0.009
		253	S		
FNLCC/FFDC trial [10]	1995–2003	113	CF—S—CF	HR 0.69 (CI: 0.50–0.95)	0.02
		111	S		
EORTC 40954 [11]	1999–2004	113	CF—S	HR 0.84 (CI: 0.52–1.35)	0.466
		111	S		

N number of patients, *P* *p*-value, *FAMTX* 5-fluorouracil, doxorubicin, and methotrexate, *S* surgery, *ECF* epirubicin, cisplatin, and 5-fluorouracil, *HR* hazard ratio, *CI* 95% confidence interval, *CF* cisplatin and 5-fluorouracil was considered the golden standard for future randomised trials. After prematurely closing the study investigators suggested that more active regimens than FAMTX are required for future randomised trials, such as epirubicin, cisplatin, and 5-fluorouracil (ECF).

A landmark study in the field of perioperative chemotherapy for gastric cancer is the United Kingdom Medical Research Council MAGIC study in which Dutch participants contributed significantly [9]. This trial was the first randomized clinical trial showing a survival benefit for perioperative chemotherapy in gastric cancer compared to surgery alone. Patients with resectable adenocarcinoma of the stomach, esophagogastric junction (GEJ), or lower esophagus were included. Between 1994 and 2002, 250 patients were randomly assigned to perioperative chemotherapy and 253 patients to surgery alone. Chemotherapy consisted of three preoperative and three postoperative cycles of intravenous epirubicin (50 mg/m^2 body surface) and cisplatin (60 mg/m^2) on day 1, and a continuous intravenous infusion of 5-fluorouracil (200 mg/m^2/day). The primary endpoint was overall survival. Postoperative complications rates were similar in the perioperative and the surgery alone group (46% vs. 45%), as were the numbers of death within 30 days (6% vs. 6%). In the perioperative chemotherapy group more patients were able to undergo surgery (79% vs. 70%) and tumors were significantly smaller (T1/T2 52% vs. 37%) with less involved lymph nodes (N0/N1 84% vs. 71%). The perioperative chemotherapy group improved both overall survival (HR 0.75; 95% CI: 0.60–0.93, P = 0.009; 5-year survival rate 36% vs. 23%) as disease-free survival (HR 0.66; 95% CI: 053–0.81, P < 0.001) compared to surgery alone. Despite these promising results, this trial was criticized for the fact that only 54% of the patients completed the entire treatment, suggesting that the benefit found was largely derived from neoadjuvant ECF.

Similar outcomes as the MAGIC trial were achieved in the French FNCLCC and FFCD multicentre phase III trial [10]. A total of 224 patients with resectable adenocarcinoma of the lower esophagus, GEJ, or stomach were randomized to receive either 2–3 cycles of preoperative and 3–4 cycles of perioperative chemotherapy (5-fluorouracil 800 mg/m^2 daily for 5 days plus cisplatin 100 mg/m^2 on day 1 or 2, every 4 weeks; n = 113) or surgery alone (n = 111). The perioperative chemotherapy group had a better overall survival (HR 0.69; 95% CI: 0.50–0.95, P = 0.02; 5-year survival rate 38% vs. 24%) and a better disease-free survival (HR 0.65; 95% CI: 0.48–0.89, P = 0.003; 5-year rate 34% vs. 19%).

The European Organisation for Research and Treatment of Cancer randomized trial (EORTC 40954) was closed due to poor accrual and was not able to demonstrate a survival benefit for neoadjuvant chemotherapy compared to surgery alone (HR 0.84; 95% CI: 0.52–1.35, P = 0.466) [11]. Possible explanations according the study investigators were a low statistical power, a high rate of proximal gastric cancer, and a better outcome than expected after surgery alone. This trial, however, did show a significantly increased R0 resection rate in favour of the neoadjuvant chemotherapy group (82% vs. 67%, P = 0.036).

A recent meta-analysis of *Yang et al.* investigated the effect of neoadjuvant chemotherapy on the survival outcomes of resectable gastric cancer [12]. Results showed that perioperative chemotherapy led to an increase in progression-free survival (HR = 0.66; 95% CI: 0.55–0.78, $P \leq 0.001$) and reduction in distant metastases (RR = 0.72, 95% CI: 0.59–0.87, P = 0.001) compared to surgery alone. A trend toward favouring neoadjuvant chemotherapy compared to no neo-adjuvant chemotherapy was observed in overall survival, but was not significant (HR = 0.68, 95% CI: 0.44–1.05, P = 0.08) [12].

14.3 Neoadjuvant Chemoradiotherapy

Application of radiotherapy in the neoadjuvant setting has gained ground over the years. In theory, the gastric tumor remains intact leading to a facile treatment planning by the conserved normal anatomy and there is limited toxicity to adjacent organs. An overview of studies investigating the impact of neoadjuvant chemoradiotherapy is

Table 14.2 Overview of trials investigating the impact of neoadjuvant chemoradiotherapy in resectable gastric cancer

Trial	Years	N	Treatment	Results	*P*
POET trial [13]	2000–2005	60	PLF—CRT[1]—S	HR 0.67 (CI: 0.41–1.07)	0.07
		59	PLF—S		
CROSS trial[a] [14]	2004–2008	178	CRT[2]—S	HR 0.66 (CI: 0.50–0.87)	0.003
		188	S		
TOPGEAR trial [15]	2009–2020[b]		ECF—CRT[3]—S	Ongoing	
			ECF—S		

N number of patients, *P* *p*-value, *PLF* cisplatin, 5-fluorouracil, and leucovorin, *CRT*[1] cisplatin, etoposide, and radiotherapy (30 Gy), *S* surgery, *HR* hazard ratio, *CI* 95% confidence interval, *CRT*[2] carboplatin, paclitaxel, and radiotherapy (41.4 Gy), *ECF* epirubicin, cisplatin, and 5-fluorouracil, *CRT*[3]5-fluorouracil and radiotherapy (45 Gy)
[a]Trial which included esophageal or esophagogastric-junction cancer
[b]Estimation

provided in Table 14.2. A German phase III randomized clinical trial (POET trial) aimed to address the question of whether adding chemoradiotherapy to neoadjuvant chemotherapy (cisplatin, 5-fluorouracil, and leucovorin) in tumors of the lower esophagus and gastric cardia would lead to survival benefit compared to chemotherapy alone [13]. The study was planned according a two-stage adaptive design. The alternative hypothesis was superiority of 10% in 3-year survival of the chemoradiotherapy arm compared with the chemotherapy arm. With one-sided significance level of 5% and power of 80% the required amount of 263 patients each arm was not achieved resulting in prematurely closing of the trial. From 2000 and 2006, 126 patients were randomly assigned. A significant higher probability of showing pathological complete response was found in favour of the chemoradiotherapy group (15.6% vs. 2.0%, $P = 0.03$). This study found a trend toward improved 3-year survival with the addition of chemoradiotherapy to chemotherapy alone (27.7% vs. 47.4%, $P = 0.07$). However, no statistical significance was seen, most likely due to prematurely closing of the study.

Later on, the Dutch CROSS trial was conducted to demonstrate the benefit of neoadjuvant chemoradiotherapy in esophageal or esophagogastric-junction cancer [14]. It should be notified that this study included primarily patients with esophageal cancer (76%) and a smaller part tumors of the GEJ (24%). Between 2004 and 2008, patients were randomly assigned to carboplatin (doses titrated to achieve an area under the curve of 2 mg/mL/min) and paclitaxel (50 mg/m^2/body surface) and concurrent radiotherapy (41.4 Gy in 23 fractions, 5 days per week), followed by surgery or surgery alone. Overall survival improved in the chemoradiation group (HR 0.66; 95% CI: 0.50–0.87, $P = 0.003$). Complete resection (R0) was achieved in 92% of the chemoradiation group vs. 69% in the surgery alone group ($P < 0.001$). Acceptable adverse event rates were observed.

Since 2009, the TOPGEAR trial is accruing. Patients with resectable adenocarcinoma of the stomach or GEJ are eligible for this trial. The hypothesis of this randomized phase III trial is that adding chemoradiation to standard perioperative chemotherapy (three cycles of ECF preoperative and postoperative) will have a positive effect on overall survival rates [15].

14.4 Adjuvant Therapy

Although the primary goal of this chapter is to focus on neoadjuvant treatment strategies in gastric cancer, a description of the present evidence for adjuvant therapy in gastric cancer is necessary to obtain a complete overview of the current multimodal treatment strategies of gastric cancer. Results of below mentioned studies are shown in Table 14.3.

Table 14.3 Overview of trials investigating the impact of adjuvant therapy in resectable gastric cancer

Trial	Years	N	Treatment	Results	*P*
Intergroup 0116 trial [16]	1991–1998	281	S—CRT[1]	HR 1.35 (CI: 1.09–1.66)	0.005
		275	S		
ARTIST trial [17]	2004–2008	211	S—XP—CRT[2]—XP	HR 1.130 (CI: 0.78–1.65)	0.527
		204	S—XP		
CRITICS trial [19]	2007–2015	395	ECC—S—CRT[3]	Median survival: 3.3 year	0.99
		393	ECC—S—ECC	Median survival: 3.5 year	

N number of patients, *P p*-value, *S* surgery, *CRT*[1] 5-fluorouracil, leucovorin, and radiotherapy (4500 cGy), *HR* hazard ratio, *CI* 95% confidence interval, *XP* capecitabine and cisplatin, *CRT*[2] capecitabine and radiotherapy (45 Gy), *ECC* epirubicin, cisplatin/oxaliplatin, and capecitabine, *CRT*[3] 5-fluorouracil, cisplatin, and radiotherapy (45 Gy)

In 2001, the SWOG/Intergroup 0116 trial showed an improvement in survival and locoregional control with the introduction of postoperative chemoradiotherapy [16]. In this trial, 556 patients were randomized to surgery and postoperative chemoradiotherapy (45 Gy in 25 fractions in 5 weeks and three cycles of 5-fluorouracil and leucovorin; n = 281) or surgery alone (n = 275). A survival benefit was seen in the chemoradiotherapy group with a median overall survival of 36 months compared to 27 months in the surgery group (HR 1.35; 95% CI: 1.09–1.66, $P = 0.005$). Relapse free survival was prolonged in the chemoradiotherapy group (19 months compared to 30 months in surgery alone group (HR 1.52; 95% CI: 1.23–1.86, $P < 0.001$)). This study was criticized for its poor adherence to the surgical protocol, as only 10% of the included patients underwent the intended D2-lymphadenectomy.

The South Korean ARTIST trial was the first study investigating the addition of radiotherapy to adjuvant chemotherapy for patients who underwent a curative gastric resection with a D2 lymph node dissection [17]. Between 2004 and 2008, 458 patients were randomized between either capecitabine plus cisplatin followed by chemoradiotherapy and two additional cycles capecitabine (n = 230) or only capecitabine plus cisplatin regime (n = 228). Overall, addition of chemoradiotherapy did not lead to a significant difference with regard to disease free survival (HR 0.740; 95% CI: 0.52–1.05, $P = 0.092$) nor overall survival (HR 1.130; 95% CI: 0.78–1.65, $P = 0.527$). Though, results showed a significant benefit in disease free survival benefit of chemoradiation in the subset of patients with node-positive disease. As a follow up of this trial the ARTIST 2 is ongoing and will evaluate the value of adjuvant chemotherapy and chemoradiation after a D2 lymph node dissection in patients with node positive gastric cancer. It should be notified that these trials are being performed in the Eastern world. Gastric cancer in the Eastern world differs compared to the Western world, regarding biology, epidemiology, stage, and prognosis. In the Eastern world, gastric cancer is characterised by a higher incidence, more distally located tumors, more often found in an early stage of the disease, more standardized surgery with a D2 lymph node dissection, and better prognosis [18].

In order to determine the most optimal adjuvant therapy for the Western gastric cancer patient with advanced disease, the CRITICS trial was conducted and recently completed. In this randomized clinical trial patients with resectable gastric cancer were treated with three cycles of preoperative epirubicin, cisplatin/oxaliplatin, and capecitabine (ECC/EOC) and surgery with adequate lymph node dissection, followed by either three cycles of ECC/EOC (CT) or concurrent chemoradiation (CRT; 45 Gy in 25 fractions with 5-fluorouracil and cisplatin) [19]. The first study results were presented during the ASCO convention in 2016 but are not published yet. The median follow up was 4.2 years. The 5-year overall survival was equal in both arms: 40.8% for CT and 40.9% for CRT, with a corresponding median survival of 3.5 years and 3.3 years. No differences were observed with regard to progression free survival across both arms (5-year 38.5% (CT) and 39.5% (CRT) with a median progression free survival of 2.3 years (CT) and 2.5 years (CRT)). Sixty-one percentage of the patients in the CT group and 63% in the CRT group started with postoperative treatment whereas 47% and 52% of the patients respectively were able to complete treatment. Further analyses of this trial are currently being performed.

In the near future, the CRITICS-II trial aims to establish the most optimal preoperative regimen in resectable gastric cancer by comparing chemotherapy, chemotherapy and subsequent chemoradiotherapy, and chemoradiotherapy.

In 2014, *Cao et al.* aimed to assess the value of adjuvant chemotherapy in patients with gastric cancer after radical surgical resection in a meta-analysis [20]. Results showed that adjuvant chemotherapy can improve overall survival rate (RR = 1.09, 95% CI: 1.06–1.23), as well as disease-free survival rate (RR = 1.11, 95% CI: 1.07–1.15), and can reduce the relapse rate after curative resection (RR = 0.79, 95% CI: 0.74–0.84) [20].

14.5 Targeted Therapy

Biomarker-targeted therapy has received increased attention in the recent years. Although high expectations, until this moment, targeted agents have no place in the standard care of curable Western gastric cancer patients after several trials obtained negative trial results. Currently, the INNOVATION trial is being conducted to investigate whether trastuzumab (a humanized monoclonal IgG antibody which inhibits the HER-2/neu receptor) or trastuzumab with pertuzumab shows more activity against standard chemotherapy after surgery in patients with HER-2 positive resectable gastric cancer and whether it can be safely administered (NCT02205047). The HER-2 positive rate in resectable gastric cancer is around 15%. Some studies suggested that HER-2 positive status is associated with a worse prognosis although the sample sizes of these studies were relatively small. Primary completion date for the INNOVATION trial is estimated for September 2020.

In contrast with the negative trial results of targeted therapy for curable gastric cancer, positive results are being achieved in trials with targeted therapy for incurable gastric cancer. The most important trials with targeted therapy in metastatic gastric cancer are discussed here and shown in Table 14.4.

In both neoadjuvant as adjuvant settings, trastuzumab has been shown to be effective regarding the treatment of HER-2 positive breast cancer. In 2010, the ToGA (Trastuzumab for Gastric Cancer) trial is conducted to evaluate the benefit of combining trastuzumab with chemotherapy vs. chemotherapy alone for treatment of HER-2 positive incurable gastric or GEJ cancer [21]. Chemotherapy regimen consisted of either capecitabine plus cisplatin or 5-fluorouracil plus cisplatin every 3 weeks for six cycles or this chemotherapy regimen in combination with intravenous trastuzumab.

Table 14.4 Overview of studies investigating the impact of neoadjuvant chemotherapy combined with targeted agents in incurable gastric cancer

Trial	Years	N	Regimen	Results	*P*
ToGa trial [21]	2005–2008	298	tra—CT	HR 0.74 (CI: 0.60–0.91)	0.005
		296	CT		
AVAGAST trial [22]	2007–2008	387	bev—CT	HR 0.87 (CI 0.73–1.03)	0.100
		387	CT		
REGARD trial [23]	2009–2012	238	ram	HR 0.776 (CI: 0.60–1.00)	0.047
		117	placebo		
RAINBOW trial [24]	2010–2012	330	ram—pac	HR 0.81 (CI: 0.68–0.96)	0.017
		335	placebo—pac		

N number of patients, *P* *p*-value, *tra* trastuzumab, *CT* chemotherapy, *HR* hazard ratio, *CI* 95% confidence interval, *bev* bevacizumab, *ram* ramucirumab, *pac* paclitaxel

Addition of trastuzumab significantly prolonged median overall survival compared to chemotherapy alone (HR 0.74; 95% CI: 0.60–0.91, $P = 0.005$). Rates of overall grade 3 or 4 adverse events did not differ between both groups. [21] Since the results of this trial were published, trastuzumab in combination with chemotherapy could be considered as a new standard option for patients with HER-2 positive incurable gastric of GEJ cancer.

Additional targeted therapies for metastatic diseases have been investigated the latest years with promising results. Bevacizumab, a vascular endothelial growth factor A (VEGF-A) inhibitor, has earlier been adding to chemotherapy in colon- and rectal cancer. In 2011, the results of the AVAGAST trial (Avastin in Gastric Cancer) have been published [22]. This randomized, double-blind, placebo-controlled phase III trial evaluated the addition of an antiangiogenic agent to chemotherapy with regard to survival in patients with incurable gastric cancer. Patients received bevacizumab (vascular endothelial growth factor A, VEGF-A, inhibitor) 7.5 mg/kg or placebo followed by cisplatin 80 mg/m^2 on day 1 plus capecitabine 1000 mg/m^2 twice daily for 14 days every 3 weeks. Cisplatin was given for six cycles; capecitabine and bevacizumab were administered until disease progression of unacceptable toxicity. In total, 774 patients were enrolled, both equally assigned to each treatment group. Overall survival improved in the bevacizumab plus fluoropyrimidine-cisplatin group compared to the placebo plus fluoropyrimidine-cisplatin (HR 0.87; 95% CI 0.73–1.03; $P = 0.100$). Although this trial did not reach its primary objective, it was shown that both median progression-free survival (6.7 vs. 5.3% months; HR 0.80; 95% CI: 0.68–0.93, $P = 0.004$) and overall response rate (46.0% vs. 37.4%; $P = 0.032$) significantly improved with bevacizumab vs. placebo [22].

Furthermore, increasing attention has been given to ramucirumab, a vascular endothelial growth factor (VEGF) receptor-2 antagonist. Recently the REGARD trial aimed to assess whether ramucirumab prolonged survival in patients with incurable gastric cancer [23]. Between 2009 and 2012, 355 patients were randomly assigned to receive either ramucirumab (8 mg/kg, n = 238) or best supportive care (n = 117). Ramucirumab improved overall survival (HR 0.78; 95% CI: 0.60–1.00, $P = 0.047$) and adverse events were mostly similar between groups [23]. This international trial showed that ramucirumab, as a single drug, is the first biological treatment prolonging survival in patients with advanced gastric or GEJ adenocarcinoma after first-line chemotherapy.

Between 2010 and 2012, 665 patients were randomized in the RAINBOW trial with previously treated advanced gastric cancer to receive either ramucirumab (n = 330) or placebo (n = 335), plus paclitaxel [24]. Overall survival was significantly higher in the ramucirumab plus paclitaxel group than in the placebo plus paclitaxel group (HR 0.81; 95% CI: 0.68–0.96, $P = 0.017$) [24]. From that moment, this combination of targeted therapy is regarded as a new standard second-line treatment for patients with advanced gastric cancer.

Conclusions

Gastric cancer is a common and highly lethal malignancy. The average age of patients has become higher in the past decades, leading to a higher rate of comorbidities to account for during treatment. This development gave rise to several new considerations to the approach of treatment of gastric cancer in the Western world.

Gastrectomy is considered as high-risk surgery in the Western world. Despite improved outcomes of gastric resections in centralized, high-volume centres, gastrectomies are still associated with surgical morbidity rates of 39% and mortality rates of approximately 4% [25, 26]. It is well known that morbidity rates in gastrectomies are greatly influenced by age. Previous studies showed that sarcopenia and frailty of patients, which are frequently seen in older gastric cancer patients, are strong risk factors to experience severe problems once a complication occurs [27]. This emphasizes the need for careful consideration to perform a gastrectomy (and to receive adjuvant therapy)

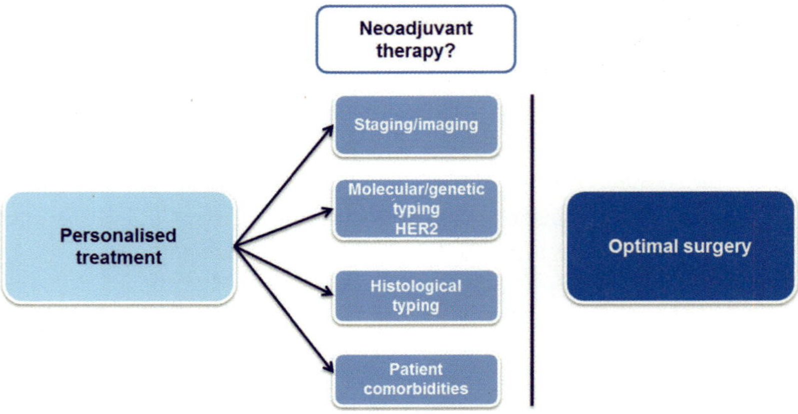

Fig. 14.1 Tailoring treatment for gastric cancer patients in the Western world

when patients are not able to complete neoadjuvant therapy.

Secondly, compliance of patients to therapy is an essential part in the multimodal treatment of gastric cancer. Several trials showed that protocol adherence to postoperative treatment is poor. For instance, treatment was completed as planned by 42% of patients in the MAGIC trial and in approximately 50% in the CRITICS trial [9]. Especially for the frail, older patient, the rate of postoperative therapy compliance is low, most likely due to the interplay between their pre-existing presence of comorbidity, diminished physical condition, and postoperative morbidity. Protocol adherence to *preoperative* treatment is evidently higher because these patients did not (yet) undergo gastric resection, which is considered high-impact surgery. For instance, more than 80% of the patients in the CRITICS trial were able to complete preoperative treatment. Considering the growing population of elderly patients, neo-adjuvant treatment is therefore the future in the multimodal treatment of gastric cancer in the Western world. Ongoing and future studies will determine the most optimal neoadjuvant therapy (chemotherapy and/ or radiation) combined with optimal dose and timing.

Lastly, due to the heterogeneity of older gastric cancer patients, tailored treatment for these patients is needed. Diagnostic tools like staging/imaging, molecular/genetic tools, and histological typing should be targeted, and should lead, together with the consideration of comorbidities, to a personalized treatment (Fig. 14.1). This approach requires a multidisciplinary collaboration between medical oncologists, radiologists, nuclear oncologists, radiation oncologists, pathologists, nutritionists, and surgeons.

In conclusion, neoadjuvant therapy is a key element in the multimodal way of treatment of gastric cancer in the Western world. This is an inevitable consequence of the ageing population, since neoadjuvant treatment is associated with a better compliance. For this future personalized treatment of gastric cancer, a multidisciplinary approach remains crucial.

References

1. Ferlay J, Soerjomataram I, Dikshit R, et al. Cancer incidence and mortality worldwide: sources, methods and major patterns in GLOBOCAN 2012. Int J Cancer. 2015;136(5):E359–86.
2. Papenfuss WA, Kukar M, Oxenberg J, et al. Morbidity and mortality associated with gastrectomy for gastric cancer. Ann Surg Oncol. 2014;21(9):3008–14.
3. Cuschieri A, Weeden S, Fielding J, et al. Patient survival after D1 and D2 resections for gastric cancer: long-term results of the MRC randomized surgical trial. Surgical Co-operative Group. Br J Cancer. 1999;79(9–10):1522–30.
4. Songun I, Putter H, Kranenbarg EM, et al. Surgical treatment of gastric cancer: 15-year follow-up results of the randomised nationwide Dutch D1D2 trial. Lancet Oncol. 2010;11(5):439–49.
5. Degiuli M, Sasako M, Ponti A, et al. Randomized clinical trial comparing survival after D1 or D2

gastrectomy for gastric cancer. Br J Surg. 2014; 101(2):23–31.
6. Hartgrink HH, van de Velde CJ, Putter H, et al. Extended lymph node dissection for gastric cancer: who may benefit? Final results of the randomized Dutch gastric cancer group trial. J Clin Oncol. 2004;22(11):2069–77.
7. Hermans J, Bonenkamp JJ, Boon MC, et al. Adjuvant therapy after curative resection for gastric cancer: meta-analysis of randomized trials. J Clin Oncol. 1993;11(8):1441–7.
8. Hartgrink HH, van de Velde CJ, Putter H, et al. Neo-adjuvant chemotherapy for operable gastric cancer: long term results of the Dutch randomised FAMTX trial. Eur J Surg Oncol. 2004;30(6):643–9.
9. Cunningham D, Allum WH, Stenning SP, et al. Perioperative chemotherapy versus surgery alone for resectable gastroesophageal cancer. N Engl J Med. 2006;355(1):11–20.
10. Ychou M, Boige V, Pignon JP, et al. Perioperative chemotherapy compared with surgery alone for resectable gastroesophageal adenocarcinoma: an FNCLCC and FFCD multicenter phase III trial. J Clin Oncol. 2011;29(13):1715–21.
11. Schuhmacher C, Gretschel S, Lordick F, et al. Neoadjuvant chemotherapy compared with surgery alone for locally advanced cancer of the stomach and cardia: European Organisation for Research and Treatment of Cancer randomized trial 40954. J Clin Oncol. 2010;28(35):5210–8.
12. Yang Y, Yin X, Sheng L, et al. Perioperative chemotherapy more of a benefit for overall survival than adjuvant chemotherapy for operable gastric cancer: an updated meta-analysis. Sci Rep. 2015;5:12850.
13. Stahl M, Walz MK, Stuschke M, et al. Phase III comparison of preoperative chemotherapy compared with chemoradiotherapy in patients with locally advanced adenocarcinoma of the esophagogastric junction. J Clin Oncol. 2009;27(6):851–6.
14. van Hagen P, Hulshof MC, van Lanschot JJ, et al. Preoperative chemoradiotherapy for esophageal or junctional cancer. N Engl J Med. 2012;366(22):2074–84.
15. Leong T, Smithers BM, Michael M, et al. TOPGEAR: a randomised phase III trial of perioperative ECF chemotherapy versus preoperative chemoradiation plus perioperative ECF chemotherapy for resectable gastric cancer (an international, intergroup trial of the AGITG/TROG/EORTC/NCIC CTG). BMC Cancer. 2015;15:532.
16. Macdonald JS, Smalley SR, Benedetti J, et al. Chemoradiotherapy after surgery compared with surgery alone for adenocarcinoma of the stomach or gasroesophageal junction. N Engl J Med. 2001;345(10): 725–30.
17. Park SH, Sohn TS, Lee J, et al. Phase III trial to compare adjuvant chemotherapy with capecitabine and cisplatin versus concurrent chemoradiotherapy in gastric cancer: final report of the adjuvant chemoradiotherapy in stomach tumors trial, including survival and subset analyses. J Clin Oncol. 2015;33(28): 3130–6.
18. Bickenbach K, Strong VE. Comparisons of gastric cancer treatments: east vs. west. J Gastric Cancer. 2012;12(2):55–62.
19. Dikken JL, van Sandick JW, Swellengrebel HA, et al. Neo-adjuvant chemotherapy followed by surgery and chemotherapy or by surgery and chemoradiotherapy for patients with resectable gastric cancer (CRITICS). BMC Cancer. 2011;11:329.
20. Cao J, Qi F, Liu T. Adjuvant chemotherapy after curative resection for gastric cancer: a meta-analysis. Scand J Gastroenterol. 2014;49(6):690–704.
21. Bang YJ, Van Cutsem E, Feyereislova A, et al. Trastuzumab in combination with chemotherapy versus chemotherapy alone for treatment of HER2-positive advanced gastric or gastro-oesophageal junction cancer (ToGA): a phase 3, open-label, randomised controlled trial. Lancet. 2010;376(9742):687–97.
22. Ohtsu A, Shah MA, Van Cutsem E, et al. Bevacizumab in combination with chemotherapy as first-line therapy in advanced gastric cancer: a randomized, double-blind, placebo-controlled phase III study. J Clin Oncol. 2011;29(30):3968–76.
23. Fuchs CS, Tomasek J, Yong CJ, et al. Ramucirumab monotherapy for previously treated advanced gastric or gastro-oesophageal junction adenocarcinoma (REGARD): an international, randomised, multicentre, placebo-controlled, phase 3 trial. Lancet. 2014; 383(9911):31–9.
24. Wilke H, Muro K, Van Cutsem E, et al. Ramucirumab plus paclitaxel versus placebo plus paclitaxel in patients with previously treated advanced gastric or gastro-oesophageal junction adenocarcinoma (RAINBOW): a double-blind, randomised phase 3 trial. Lancet Oncol. 2014;15(11):1224–35.
25. Bartlett EK, Roses RE, Kelz RR, et al. Morbidity and mortality after total gastrectomy for gastric malignancy using the American College of Surgeons National Surgical Quality Improvement Program database. Surgery. 2014;156(2):298–304.
26. Pasquer A, Renaud F, Hec F, et al. Is centralization needed for esophageal and gastric cancer patients with low operative risk?: A nationwide study. Ann Surg. 2016;264(5):823–30.
27. Wagner D, DeMarco MM, Amini N, et al. Role of frailty and sarcopenia in predicting outcomes among patients undergoing gastrointestinal surgery. World J Gastrointest Surg. 2016;8(1):27–40.

15 Open or Minimally Invasive Gastrectomy

Nicole I. van der Wielen, Jennifer Straatman, Freek Daams, Miguel A. Cuesta, and Donald L. van der Peet

15.1 Introduction

Gastric cancer has been amongst the most commonly diagnosed malignancies worldwide since 1975 with the highest incidence in Eastern Asia (13.3%) followed by Central and Eastern Europe (6.7%) [1]. Japan was the first country to start with the implementation of a screening program for gastric cancer in 1983 to facilitate early detection of the disease [2]. Consequently, other countries with a high prevalence of gastric cancer also implemented a screening program, such as Korea and China [3]. This resulted in a high incidence of early gastric cancer. Despite the early detection of this disease, the overall mortality is still amongst the highest in the world [1].

15.2 Gastrectomy

To this day the only curative treatment for gastric cancer is a surgical resection with an adequate lymph node dissection. According to the Japanese Gastric Cancer Association, a radical resection of the stomach with a proximal margin of at least 3 cm is recommended for T2 or deeper tumors with an expansive growth pattern and 5 cm for those with an infiltrative growth pattern. For tumors invading the esophagus, a margin of 5 cm is not required, but frozen section examination is desirable to ensure a R0 resection. The number of dissected lymph nodes and the correlating lymph node stations are a marker for the quality of the resection. According to the Japanese Gastric Cancer treatment guidelines, extent of the lymph node dissection has to be in accordance with tumor-stage and the type of gastrectomy conducted. Lymph node stations are depicted in Fig. 15.1. Type of gastrectomy consists of a total, distal or proximal gastrectomy. For cT1N0 tumors a D1 or D1+ lymphadenectomy is recommended, whereas for cN+ or cT2–T4 tumors a D2 lymphadenectomy is recommended. In distal gastrectomy D1 lymphadenectomy consists of lymph node stations 1, 3, 4sb, 4d, 5, 6 and 7. D1+ lymphadenectomy consists of lymph node stations D1 plus station 8a and 9. D2 lymphadenectomy consists of D1 plus station 8a, 9, 11p and 12a. In total gastrectomy D1 lymphadenectomy consists of a dissection of lymph node stations 1 to 7. D1+ consists of D1 plus station 8a, 9 and 11p. D2 lymphadenectomy consists of D1 plus station 8a, 9, 10, 11d, 11p and 12a. However, if there is a suspicion of nodal involvement, a D2 lymphadenectomy should always be performed. A minimum of 15 regional lymph nodes should be assessed by the pathologist [4].

N.I. van der Wielen (✉) • J. Straatman • F. Daams
M.A. Cuesta • D.L. van der Peet
Department of Surgery, VU University Medical Center, Amsterdam, The Netherlands
e-mail: ni.vanderwielen@vumc.nl; ma.cuesta@vumc.nl

M.A. Cuesta (ed.), *Minimally Invasive Surgery for Upper Abdominal Cancer*,
DOI 10.1007/978-3-319-54301-7_15

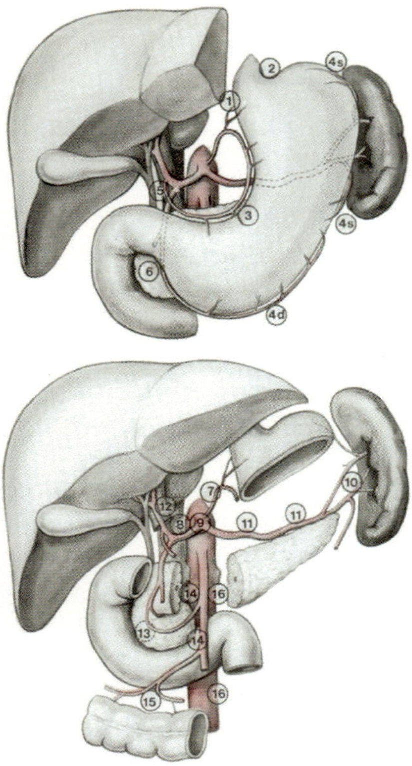

Fig. 15.1 Lymph node stations [6]

As regards to omentectomy, the Japanese Gastric Cancer Association recommends the removal of the greater omentum for T3 or deeper tumors. For T1 or T2 tumors, the part of the omentum that is more than 3 cm away from the gastroepiploic arcade may be preserved [5].

15.3 Sentinel Lymph Node

The screening program has led to a high incidence of early gastric cancer in Eastern Asian countries, subsequent early diagnosis and treatment is associated with better survival rates. Hence, postoperative quality of life has gained more importance in the overall treatment. The extent of gastrectomy and the extent of lymphadenectomy is of influence on postoperative morbidity and survival. In early gastric cancer, the incidence of lymph node metastasis is reported to be 14.1% overall and 4.8–23.6% depending on cancer depth [7]. Therefore, the concept of sentinel lymph node navigation surgery is obtaining more interest. If only a small group of patients with early gastric cancer have lymph node metastases, the majority may not benefit from such an extensive lymphadenectomy. The optimal method to perform sentinel lymph node navigation surgery is still under debate. Current research is assessing the use of a radioactive tracer, dye fluorescence imaging or a combination of both [8].

15.4 Neoadjuvant Therapy

The feasibility of perioperative chemotherapy as part of the treatment of gastric cancer is still under debate. The MAGIC trial compared perioperative chemotherapy plus surgery vs. surgery alone in patients with resectable gastroesophageal cancer. This study showed a significant better disease free and overall survival in the chemotherapy group. As a result, the use of perioperative chemotherapy has become a part of the standard treatment in several European countries [9]. The CRITICS trial compared survival between patients receiving chemotherapy or chemoradiotherapy after surgery with curative intent. This trial showed no difference in survival between both groups [10].

15.5 Minimally Invasive Gastrectomy

Studies have shown that minimally invasive techniques for malignancies are safe and have several important advantages in comparison to the conventional open surgical techniques. Several randomized controlled trials compared minimally invasive with open surgery, such as the LAFA, COLOR I, COLOR II for colorectal cancer and the TIME trial for esophageal cancer. These studies showed favorable short-time outcomes for the minimally invasive technique, such as less perioperative blood loss, faster patient recovery and fewer complications with similar oncological outcomes [11–14]. The first minimally invasive distal gastrectomy was described by Kitano et al. in 1994 [15]. This was followed in 1996 by the first minimally invasive total gastrectomy for cancer, described by Azagra et al. [16]. Since then, minimally invasive techniques for gastric cancer have gained an increasing interest worldwide. The first randomized controlled trial comparing open vs. minimally invasive distal gastrectomy was performed by Huscher et al. between 1992 and 1996. The study showed less perioperative blood loss and a better postoperative recovery in the minimally invasive group. No significant differences were found regarding the number of resected lymph nodes, postoperative morbidity and mortality and 5-year survival [17]. Since then, several meta-analysis and randomized controlled trials have been performed, all in Asian countries.

Twenty-eight systematic reviews and meta-analysis have been published since 2009, being the majority from Asian countries were the incidence of gastric cancer is many times higher than in Western countries. They compared early and advanced gastric cancer being dedicated the majority to distal gastrectomy. Moreover there are meta-analysis about robot-assisted gastrectomy. A minority is dedicated to the study of total gastrectomy. Best et al. have performed a Cochrane Database Systematic Review on this subject in 2016 [18]. They found that based on low quality evidence, no difference in short term mortality between laparoscopy and open gastrectomy. Moreover, there is no evidence for any differences in short-term or long-term outcomes between laparoscopic and open gastrectomy. However, the data was found sparse and the confidence intervals wide suggesting that significant benefits or harms of laparoscopic gastrectomy cannot be ruled out. Trials are currently being performed and will clarify the role of MIG.

Large cohort studies have been performed by the Korean Laparoscopic Gastrointestinal Surgery Study (KLASS) Group. The KLASS-01 trial is a randomized controlled trial, comparing minimally invasive distal gastrectomy with open distal gastrectomy for stage I gastric cancer. This trial showed a significantly lower overall complication rate in the minimally invasive group in comparison to the open group, with a significant difference in wound infections [19].

Additionally, several studies are still examining the differences between minimally invasive and open techniques. The KLASS-02 trial has been set up to compare minimally invasive D2 lymphadenectomy with open D2 lymphadenectomy for patients with locally advanced gastric cancer. The KLASS-02-QC trial investigates the quality control of a D2 lymphadenectomy. The KLASS-03 trial compares minimally invasive total gastrectomy to open total gastrectomy for clinical stage I gastric cancer. KLASS-04 is a trial comparing laparoscopic pylorus preserving gastrectomy with laparoscopic distal gastrectomy for the middle third early gastric cancer. And the KLASS-05 trial will be comparing laparoscopic proximal gastrectomy with laparoscopic total gastrectomy for upper third early gastric cancer. Results from these trials are expected to be published soon [20].

Our research group has performed two meta-analysis comparing minimally invasive distal with open distal gastrectomy (Table 15.1) and

Table 15.1 Study characteristics of studies comparing open with minimally invasive distal gastrectomies

Author	Publication year	Study period	Design	Country	Sample size MIDG	ODG	Tumor stage (%) I	II	III	IV	Lymph node dissection
Adachi	2000	01/1993–07/1999	Retrospective	Japan	49	53	100	0	0	0	
Du	2009	06/2004–12/2008	Retrospective	China	78	90	10.1	33.9	45.8	9.5	D2
Fang	2013	08/2009–12/2010	Retrospective	China	50	62					D2
Huang	2010	01/2007–06/2008	Retrospective	China	66	69	25.2	31.1	41.5	2.2	D2
Jung	2008	11/2004–02/2005	Retrospective	Korea	10	10	100	0	0	0	D1+
Kawamura	2010	01/2003–12/2008	Retrospective	Japan	192	190	100	0	0	0	
Naka	2005	1998–2001	Retrospective	Japan	20	22	100	0	0	0	D1+/D2
Noshiro	2005	01/1996–04/2004	Matched cohort	Japan	37	31					D2
Shimizu	2000	01/1996–08/1998	Retrospective	Japan	21	31	100	0	0	0	D1/D1+/D2
Zhao	2011	01/2004–06/2009	Retrospective	China	346	313	12	28.2	57.7	2.1	D1/D1+/D2
Zheng	2015	02/2013–01/2014	Matched cohort	China	23	27	16	14	70	0	D2
Ziqiang	2006	03/2004–05/2005	Retrospective	China	44	58	26.5	20.6	46	6.9	D1+/D2
Fujii	2003	04/1999–01/2002	RCT	Japan	10	10	95	5	0	0	
Hayashi	2005	12/1999–11/2001	RCT	Japan	14	14	100	0	0	0	D1
Hu	2016	09/2012–12/2014	RCT	China	508	507	29.2	26.5	42.4	1.8	D2
Huscher	2005	11/1992–02/1996	RCT	Italy	30	29	37.3	15.2	32.2	15.3	D1/D2
Kim	2008	07/2003–11/2005	RCT	Korea	82	82	96.3	3.7	0	0	D1+/D2
Kim	2016	02/2006–08/2010	RCT	Korea	644	612	90.3	6.2	2.9	0.6	D1+/D2
Kitano	2002	10/1998–13/2001	RCT	Japan	14	14	96.4	3.6	0	0	
Lee	2005	11/2001–08/2003	RCT	Korea	24	23	97.9	2.1	0	0	D2
Sakuramoto	2013	10/2005–02/2008	RCT	Japan	31	32	96.8	1.6	1.6	0	D1+

minimally invasive total with open total gastrectomy (Table 15.2). These meta-analyses showed a significantly longer operation time in the minimally invasive group with significantly less blood loss. Postoperative recovery was significantly in favor of the minimally invasive group. It showed a shorter hospital stay and an earlier time to first bowel movement. There were also significant differences in postoperative complications in favor of the minimally invasive group with equal mortality rates. Additionally, there was no difference in the number of resected lymph nodes between both groups. Furthermore, a meta-analysis regarding minimally invasive gastrectomy in

Table 15.2 Study characteristics of studies comparing open with minimally invasive total gastrectomies

Author	Year	Study period	Design	Country	Sample size		Tumor stage (%)				Lymph node dissection
					MITG	OTG	I	II	III	IV	
Bo	2013	01/2004–12/2010	Retrospective	China	117	117	4.3	33.3	45.7	16.7	D2
Du	2010	11/2005–05/2009	Retrospective	China	82	94	5.1	38.1	56.8	0	D2
Dulucq	2005	04/1995–03/2004	Retrospective	France	8	11					D1 + β
Kawamura	2010	01/2003–12/2008	Retrospective	Japan	42	30					D2
Kim	2008	01/2004–07/2006	Retrospective	Korea	27	33					D1 + α/β/D2
Kim	2011	01/2009–04/2010	Retrospective	Korea	63	127					D2
Lee	2013	06/2003–05/2010	Matched cohort	Korea	120	228	40.8	18.7	23.8	16.7	D2
Mochiki	2008	04/1998–12/2007	Retrospective	Japan	20	18					D1 + β
Sakuramoto	2009	07/2003–07/2007	Retrospective	Japan	30	44	54	25.7	20.3	0	D1 + β/D2
Siani	2012	01/2003–10/2009	Matched cohort	Italy	25	25	20	20	60	0	D1 + α/β/D2
Topal	2008	01/2003–12/2006	Retrospective	Belgium	38	22	40	23.3	26.7	10	D2
Usui	2005	05/2001–08/2004	Retrospective	Japan	20	19	46.2	7.7	0	0	

advanced gastric cancer has been performed. This study showed similar outcomes between both approached in terms of lymph node yield and survival. With similar mortality rates in minimally invasive techniques, more consideration regarding quality of life has arisen. A large number of studies regarding distal gastrectomies have been performed. The evidence for total gastrectomies however is less validated due to fewer studies regarding this subject that have been performed [21, 22].

15.6 Robotic Gastrectomy

Several studies have examined the safety and feasibility of robotic surgery in the treatment of gastric cancer. These showed a longer operation duration in comparison to open surgery, with less blood loss and a comparable oncological resection. Additionally, postoperative recovery was better in the robotic group, with a shorter hospital stay and earlier recovery of bowel function. Robotic gastrectomy could help overcome some intrinsic limitations of laparoscopic surgery. Three dimensional, high-definition imaging is provided, tremors can be filtered and a steady surgical field is accommodated. The ability to move in restricted fields and around important structures could help with the complexity of a well performed extended lymph node dissection. Outcomes regarding long-term oncological safety in robotic surgery has yet to be examined [23, 24].

15.7 East Vs. West

Considering a high incidence of gastric cancer in Eastern Asia, most of these results are based on Asian studies. With the implementation of a screening program for gastric cancer, the incidence of stage I gastric cancer is well over 50% of all diagnosed gastric cancers in Japan and

Korea [25]. The treatment for early gastric cancer is different than the treatment for advanced gastric cancer, where in early gastric cancer a more limited resection could be sufficient. Additionally, with the developing endoscopic techniques, some superficial gastrointestinal lesions cannot only be diagnosed but can also be treated through an endoscopic mucosal resection.

However, the incidence and treatment for gastric cancer in Asia is in stark contrast to other countries in the world. In Western countries a screening program for gastric cancer is not feasible due to the low incidence of gastric cancer in comparison with the high incidence of other malignancies. In some countries in North-West Europe like the Netherlands, the incidence of gastric cancer is decreasing notably and the incidence of esophageal and gastroesophageal junction cancers is higher than the incidence of gastric cancer [26]. Thus diagnosis of gastric cancer is usually made when patients get clinical symptoms of a tumor, such as anemia or obstructive problems, resulting in a much more advanced stage of disease. Moreover, the patient characteristics are different between East and West. In the more developed countries in Europe a higher proportion of obese and morbid patients exists, influencing the outcome of the surgical techniques [25].

The implementation of a minimally invasive technique has shifted from the application in early gastric cancer to the application in more advanced stages of disease. Surgeons in the Eastern part of the world have gained a lot of experience with minimally invasive gastrectomies. Therefore the outcomes of this technique proved to have more advantages for the patient in comparison to the open technique. However, surgeons in Central Europe and the United States are less exposed to this technique due to a lower incidence. Additionally, the disease is usually in a more advanced stage, resulting in a gradual implementation of this minimally invasive technique in the West.

There have been several Western studies examining the safety and feasibility of minimally invasive techniques for gastric cancer. These studies show similar outcomes in comparison to Asian studies, thus the advantages of a minimally invasive technique with a similar oncological safety. However, due to small study populations and all studies being retrospective of nature, more evidence has to be provided to make it as acceptable in the West as it is in the East.

Conclusion

In search of evidence regarding the safety of a minimally invasive gastrectomy in comparison to an open approach several meta-analysis have been published. However, most studies are conducted in Asian countries and consist of a partial gastrectomy. These studies show better short term outcomes for the minimally invasive approach. For total gastrectomy, hard evidence is lacking and outcomes are based on retrospective databases. Furthermore, these outcomes are all based on Asian studies.

To provide evidence for implementation in the rest of the World, randomized controlled trials outside Asia are necessary. In the Netherlands there are two randomized controlled trials comparing minimally invasive with open gastrectomies. The STOMACH trial is a European, multicenter trial comparing only total gastrectomies. Primary outcome will be the quality of the resected specimen and lymphadenectomy. The LOGICA trial is a Dutch multicenter trial comparing distal and total gastrectomies. Primary outcome will be hospital stay and postoperative recovery [27, 28]. The results of these trials will give more insight in the evidence whether minimally invasive gastrectomy is as feasible and safe in the West as it is in the East in the treatment of gastric cancer patients.

References

1. Ferlay J, Soerjomataram I, Dikshit R, Eser S, Mathers C, Rebelo M, et al. Cancer incidence and mortality worldwide: sources, methods and major patterns in GLOBOCAN 2012. Int J Cancer. 2015;136(5):E359–86.
2. Hamashima C, Shibuya D, Yamazaki H, Inoue K, Fukao A, Saito H, et al. The Japanese guidelines for gastric cancer screening. Jpn J Clin Oncol. 2008;38(4):259–67.

3. Lee S, Jun JK, Suh M, Park B, Noh DK, Jung KW, et al. Gastric cancer screening uptake trends in Korea: results for the National Cancer Screening Program from 2002 to 2011: a prospective cross-sectional study. Medicine (Baltimore). 2015;94(8):e533.
4. Cancer AJCo. In: Greene FD, Page DL, Fleming ID, Fritz AG, Balch CM, Haller DG, Morrow M, editors. AJCC cancer staging manual. 6th ed. Chicago: Springer; 2002.
5. Association JGC. Japanese gastric cancer treatment guidelines 2014 (version 4). Gastric Cancer. 2016; 20:1–19.
6. Nederland IIK. Maagcarcinoom versie 2.1. www.oncoline.nl/maagcarcinoom. Accessed 08 Nov 2016.
7. Akagi T, Shiraishi N, Kitano S. Lymph node metastasis of gastric cancer. Cancers (Basel). 2011;3:2141–59.
8. Wang Z, Dong ZY, Chen JQ, Liu JL. Diagnostic value of sentinel lymph node biopsy in gastric cancer: a meta-analysis. Ann Surg Oncol. 2012;19:1541–50.
9. Cunningham D, Allum WH, Stenning SP, Thompson JN, Van de Velde CJ, Nicolson M, et al. Perioperative chemotherapy versus surgery alone for resectable gastroesophageal cancer. N Engl J Med. 2006;355(1):11–20.
10. Verheij M. A multicenter randomized phase III trial of neo-adjuvant chemotherapy followed by surgery and chemotherapy or by surgery and chemoradiotherapy in resectable gastric cancer: first results from the CTITICS study. Chicago: American Society of Clinical Oncology; 2016.
11. Vlug MSWJ, Hollmann MW, Ubbink DT, Cense HA, Engel AF, Gerhards MF, van Wagensveld BA, van der Zaag ES, van Geloven AAW, Sprangers MAG, Cuesta MA, Bemelman WA. Laparoscopy in combination with fast track multimodal management is the best perioperative strategy in patients undergoing colonic surgery (LAFA-study). Ann Surg. 2011;254(6): 868–75.
12. Buunen MVR, Hop WCJ, Kuhry E, Jeekel J, Haglind E, Pahlman L, Cuesta MA, Msika S, Morino M, Lacy A, Bonjer HJ. Survival after laparoscopic surgery versus open surgery for colon cancer: long-term outcome of a randomised clinical trial. Lancet Oncol. 2009;10:44–52.
13. van der Pas MH, Haglind E, Cuesta MA, Furst A, Lacy AM, Hop WC, et al. Laparoscopic versus open surgery for rectal cancer (COLOR II): short-term outcomes of a randomised, phase 3 trial. Lancet Oncol. 2013;14(3):210–8.
14. Biere SS, van Berge Henegouwen MI, Maas KW, Bonavina L, Rosman C, Garcia JR, et al. Minimally invasive versus open oesophagectomy for patients with oesophageal cancer: a multicentre, open-label, randomised controlled trial. Lancet. 2012;379(9829): 1887–92.
15. Kitano S, Iso Y, Moriyama M, Sugimachi K. Laparoscopy-assisted Billroth I gastrectomy. Surg Laparosc Endosc. 1994;4(2):146–8.
16. Azagra JS, Goergen M, De Simone P, Ibanez-Aguirre J. Minimally invasive surgery for gastric cancer. Surg Endosc. 1999;13(4):351–7.
17. Huscher CGS, Mingoli A, Sgarzini G, Sansonetti A, Di Paola M, Recher A, Ponzano C. Laparosocpic versus open subtotal gastrectomy for distal gastric cancer. Five year results of a randomized prospective trial. Ann Surg. 2005;241(1):232–7.
18. Best LM, Mughal M, Gurusamy KS, et al. Laparoscopic versus open gastrectomy for gastric cancer. Cochrane Database Syst Rev. 2016;31;3: CD011389. doi:10.1002/14651858.
19. Kim W, Kim HH, Han SU, Kim MC, Hyung WJ, Ryu SW, et al. Decreased morbidity of laparoscopic distal gastrectomy compared with open distal gastrectomy for Stage I gastric cancer: short-term outcomes from a multicenter randomized controlled trial (KLASS-01). Ann Surg. 2016;263(1):28–35.
20. https://clinicaltrials.gov/ct2/results?term=KLASS+trial&Search=Search
21. Straatman J, van der Wielen N, Cuesta MA, de Lange-de Klerk ES, Jansma EP, van der Peet DL. Minimally invasive versus open total gastrectomy for gastric cancer: a systematic review and meta-analysis of short-term outcomes and completeness of resection: surgical techniques in gastric cancer. World J Surg. 2016;40(1):148–57.
22. Martínez-Ramos D, Miralles-Tena JM, Cuesta MA, Escrig-Sos J, van der Peet DL, Hoashi JS, Salvador-Sanchis JL. Laparoscopy versus open surgery for advances and resectable gastric cancer: a meta-analysis. Rev Esp Enferm Dig. 2011;103(3):133–41.
23. Wang G, Jiang Z, Zhao J, Liu J, Zhang S, Zhao K, Feng X, Li J. Assessing the safety and efficacy of full robotic gastrectomy with intracorporeal robot-sewn anastomosis for gastric cancer: a randomized clinical trial. J Surg Oncol. 2016;113:387–404.
24. Amore Bonapasta S, Guerra F, Linari C, Annecchiarico M, Boffi B, Calistri M, Coratti A. Robot-assisted gastrectomy for cancer. Der Chirurg. 2016;88(1):12–8.
25. Kodera Y. The current state of stomach cancer surgery in the world. Jpn J Clin Oncol. 2016;46(11):1062–71.
26. Jaarraportage. Dutch institute for clinical auditing. 2015. www.dica.nl/jaarraportage-2015. Accessed 08 Nov 2016.
27. Straatman J, van der Wielen N, Cuesta MA, Gisbertz SS, Hartemink KJ, Alonso Poza A, Weitz J, Mateo Vallejo F, Akhtar K, Diez del Val I, Roig Garcia J, van der Peet DL. Surgical techniques, open versus minimally invasive gastrectomy after chemotherapy (STOMACH trial): study protocol for a randomized controlled trial. Trials. 2015;16:123.
28. Haverkamp L, Brenkman HJF, Seesing MFJ, Gisbert SS, van Berge Henegouwen MI, Luyer MDP, Nieuwenhuijzen GAP, Wijnhoven BPL, van Lanschot JJB, de Steur WO, Hartgrink HH, JHMB S, Hulsewé KWE, Spillenaar Bilgen EJ, Rütter JE, Kouwenhoven EA, van Det MJ, van der Peet DL, Daams F, Draaisma WA, Broeders IAMJ, van Stel HF, Lacle MM, Ruurda JP, van Hillegersberg R. Laparoscopic versus open gastrectomy for gastric cancer, a multicenter prospectively randomized controlled trial (LOGICA trial). BMC Cancer. 2015;15:556.

16 Minimally Invasive Surgery of Gastric Cancer

Ali Guner and Woo Jin Hyung

Medicine including surgical techniques has been flourishing since ancient societies. All efforts have aimed to increase patient's survival in addition to quality of life. Lately, along with the increased popularity of laparoscopic surgery, minimally invasive surgical techniques have taken its place in surgical practice for various type of procedures, owing to several advantages such as rapid recovery, less pain as well as improved cosmetic outcomes [1]. However, for treatment of malignant diseases, safety and feasibility of minimally invasive surgery (MIS) has remained under debate for years until recently. With the increasing amount of evidence and surgical experience, MIS is now commonly favored practice for oncological surgery that made of more sophisticated processes compared to those of surgery for benign diseases [2]. Whereas MIS represents a developing trend, some limitations faced by surgeon during conventional laparoscopy led surgeons for innovative solutions and robotic technology has been introduced with many advantages including articulated instruments, three-dimensional images, and tremor filtering. Although several robotic systems have been developed, its popularity has increased just after the approval of Da Vinci robotic system (Intuitive Surgical, California, USA), many robotic systems have been started being used worldwide [3].

Despite the decreasing trend for overall incidence, gastric cancer is still one of the most common cancer type and one of the most common cause of cancer-related mortality worldwide. Radical gastrectomy with en-bloc lymphadenectomy is fundamental cornerstone for curative treatment in resectable gastric cancer patients. With the mass-screening programs and advances in diagnostic tools, the incidence of early gastric cancer (EGC) has increased particularly in eastern countries. Subsequent studies using conventional open surgery reported over 90% survival rate for EGC and surgeons' interest have increased for function preservation and quality of life in addition to the oncological curability for patients with gastric cancer particularly for EGC [4].

Laparoscopic surgery for gastric cancer have been used for limited resections in the early

A. Guner
Department of Surgery, Yonsei University College of Medicine, 50-1 Yonsei-ro, Seodaemun-gu, Seoul 120-752, Republic of Korea

Department of General Surgery, Karadeniz Technical University College of Medicine, Farabi Hospital, Trabzon, Turkey

W.J. Hyung, M.D., Ph.D. (✉)
Department of Surgery, Yonsei University College of Medicine, 50-1 Yonsei-ro, Seodaemun-gu, Seoul 120-752, Republic of Korea
e-mail: wjhyung@yuhs.ac

Gastric Cancer Center, Yonsei Cancer Center, Yonsei University Health System, Seoul, South Korea

M.A. Cuesta (ed.), *Minimally Invasive Surgery for Upper Abdominal Cancer*,
DOI 10.1007/978-3-319-54301-7_16

1990s. Laparoscopic intragastric mucosal resections and laparoscopic wedge resection were two methods that historically used for lesions without the risk of lymph node metastasis. However, with the advance of endoscopic resection techniques such as mucosal resection and submucosal dissection, their usage has declined recently. Currently, only laparoscopic wedge resection is being investigated within sentinel lymph node mapping concept. Following the Kitano's report presenting first laparoscopic-assisted gastrectomy for gastric cancer in 1994, laparoscopic gastrectomy (LG) has been introduced as an alternative to conventional open surgery [5]. LG that is initially used for EGC located in distal stomach has been started being used for tumors located in proximal stomach and for advanced gastric cancers (AGC) including extended lymphadenectomy. Number of cases that LG was used has increased tenfold between 1991 and 2009 in Japan mainly for Stage I disease, and from 6.6 to 25.8% between 2004 and 2009 in South Korea, even for the Western countries but with slower trend [6]. During this development period, improvements in robotic surgery has also followed the those of LG, and robotic gastrectomy (RG) for gastric cancer now became a frequently performed procedure especially in Korea, Japan and Italy.

16.1 Indications for Minimally Invasive Gastrectomy

Although endoscopic treatment modalities are the ideal approaches to preserve patient's functions and quality of life, these techniques can be used only for a limited number of patient that meet rigorous criteria. Regarding LG, while previous Japanese Gastric Cancer Treatment guideline recommends LG as an investigational treatment, in the fourth edition that was published in 2016, laparoscopic surgery is recognized as an option in general clinical practice for clinical Stage I gastric cancer that is indicated only for distal gastrectomy but patients require total gastrectomy [7]. Correspondingly, in South Korea, patients that does not required extended lymphadenectomy such as cN-, patients that does not required total gastrectomy and tumors that limited to the submucosa can be considered as initial indication for laparoscopic surgery with the exception of the patients that are suitable for endoscopic treatment.

In experienced centers from East Asia, the current indication for LG has been extended beyond EGC to AGC irrespective of perigastric node involvement. However, outcomes of ongoing studies are needed to utilize LG with extended indications. The indications for RG does not differ from those of LG.

16.2 Operative Strategy

Terminology: Gastrectomy procedures have various definitions based on the extent of resection such as distal, total, proximal or pylorus-preserving. Besides, when MIS techniques are used, it can be defined as laparoscopic assisted or totally laparoscopic. For cases which anastomosis are made extracorporeally, it is defined as laparoscopic assisted and when intracorporeal anastomosis is used, as totally laparoscopic. Despite the variations in the literature, usual definitions include laparoscopic assisted distal gastrectomy (LADG), laparoscopic assisted total gastrectomy (LATG), totally laparoscopic distal gastrectomy (TLDG), totally laparoscopic total gastrectomy (TLTG). When robotic systems are used, they can be called as robotic-assisted distal gastrectomy (RADG or RDG) or robotic-assisted total gastrectomy (RATG or RTG). In addition to LADG and LATG, proximal gastrectomy and pylorus preserving distal gastrectomy are the other procedures can be performed by either laparoscopic and robotic.

Port placement. While some surgeons prefer using six port including one for liver retraction, most surgeons prefer a total of five ports (Fig. 16.1a, b) [8]. For LG, the first 10-mm camera port is placed using open method at the infra-umbilical area, and pneumoperitoneum is achieved at 12 mmHg. Four other trocars are inserted, one in the right upper quadrant, one in the upper left quadrant, one in the right lateral

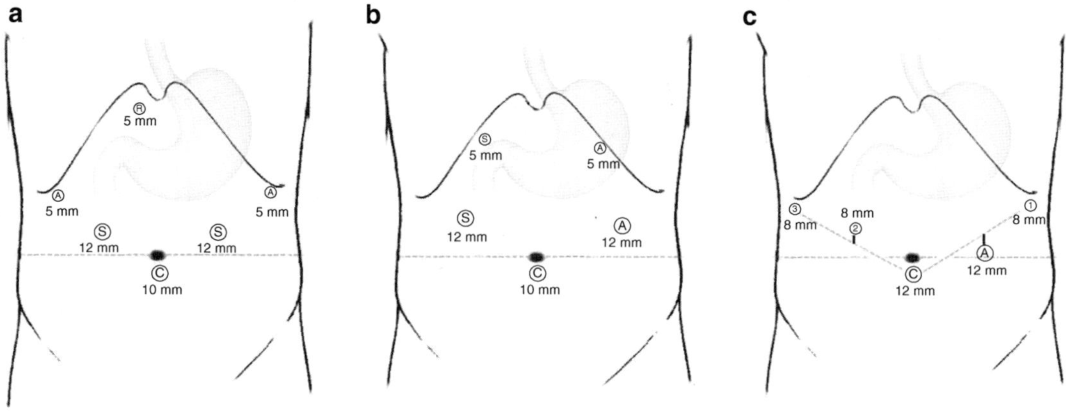

Fig. 16.1 Port placement for minimally invasive gastrectomy. 6-port (**a**) or 5-port (**b**) surgery can be used for laparoscopic gastrectomy. (**c**) Shows the place for ports in robotic gastrectomy (*C* camera, *S* surgeon, *A* assistant, *R* retractor)

side, and one to the left lateral side of the abdomen. The surgeon and scope operator are located on the right side of the patient and an assistant is on patient's left side. The RG procedure follows the identical steps as those of LG with some modifications in port placements (Fig. 16.1c). A 12-mm camera port placed below the umbilicus, and four other trocars including three 8-mm port for the robotic arms and one 12-mm assistant's port are placed. Assistant port is usually placed between the camera port and first arm that placed patient's left side below the costal margin. Then, robotic arms are docked to initiate the procedure.

Liver retraction. Various techniques have been defined thus far to retract the liver and to have clear visualization for hepatogastric/hepatoduodenal ligaments. Although using liver retractor requires one extra port, using suture-gauze technique maintains ideal liver retraction and allows surgeon to use one less port [9].

Intraoperative tumor localization. Particularly for EGC, it is challenging to locate tumor by using laparoscopic or robotic instruments, therefore surgeon needs to use some techniques to determine safe surgical margin. Various methods such as intraoperative ultrasound, intraoperative endoscopy, and abdominal plain radiograph following preoperative endoscopic clipping have been defined for this key step [10].

Extent of omentectomy. Although total omentectomy is recommended for T3–T4 tumors, partial omentectomy which removes the 3 cm away from gastroepiploic vessels can be used for T1 and T2 tumors.

Extent of lymphadenectomy. Clinical stage of the tumor and type of gastrectomy are the markers to decide the extent of lymphadenectomy. For distal gastrectomy, D1+ lymphadenectomy includes the lymph nodes numbered as #1, #3, #4sb, #4d, #5, #6, #7, #8a and #9. D2 lymphadenectomy includes #11p and #12a in addition to D1+ lymphadenectomy. For total gastrectomy, D1+ lymphadenectomy includes #1–7, #8a, #9, #11p and D2 lymphadenectomy includes #10, #11d, #12a in addition to D1+ lymphadenectomy. D1+ lymphadenectomy for proximal gastrectomy requires the dissection of #1, #2, #3a, #4sa, #4sb, #7, #8a, #9, #11p.

Left side dissection. Despite minor differences among surgeons, each individual surgeon uses standardized steps for minimally invasive gastrectomy. It is usually preferred to start from the left side. Following the division of gastrocolic ligament, the left gastroepiploic vessels are divided at their root on the left side, #4sb and #4d are removed for distal gastrectomy and then greater curvature is cleared for transection and anastomosis (Fig. 16.2a). If total gastrectomy is intended, short gastric vessels are divided up to left diaphragmatic crus and #2 and #4a are

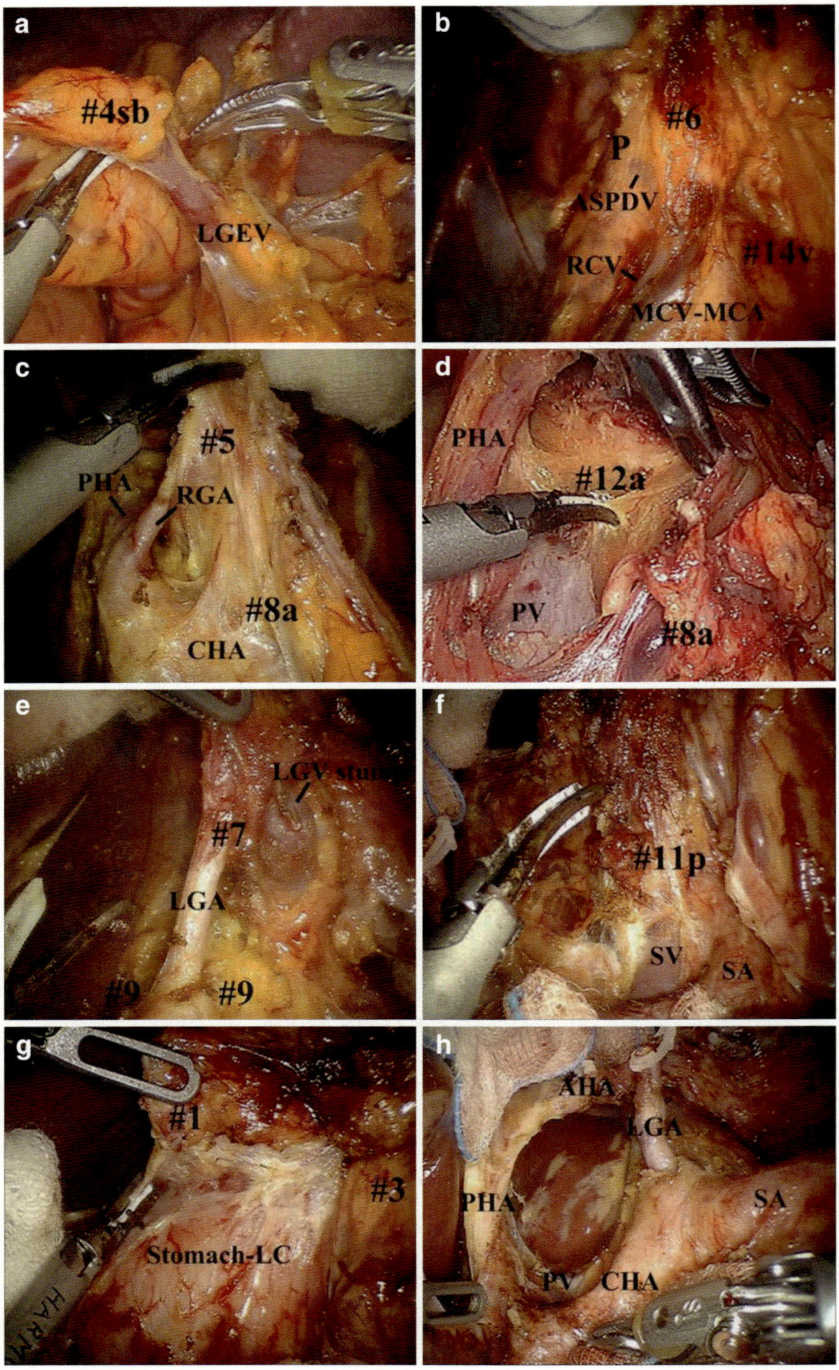

Fig. 16.2 Steps for lymphadenectomy during minimally invasive gastrectomy. (**a**): left side dissection for #4sb around LGEV. (**b**): right side dissection for #6 lymph nodes above the pancreas. (**c**): for #5 and #8a, RGA is exposed and soft tissues around the CHA are dissected. (**d**): soft tissues medial to the PV and PHA are dissected for proper #12a dissection in D2 lymphadenectomy. (**e**): LGA is exposed above the celiac trunk. (**f**): for #11p dissection, SV and SA are exposed and all soft tissues are cleaned along these vessels. (**g**): lesser curvature is cleaned to remove #1 lymph nodes. (**h**): final view of lymph node dissection. (*LGEV* left gastroepiploic vessels, *ASPDV* anterior superior pancreaticoduodenal vein, *RCV* right colic vein, *MCV* middle colic vein, *MCA* middle colic artery, *RGA* right gastric artery, *PHA* proper hepatic artery, *CHA* common hepatic artery, *PV* portal vein, *LGA* left gastric artery, *LGV* left gastric vein, *SV* splenic vein, *SA* splenic artery, *LC* lesser curvature, *AHA* accessory hepatic artery arising from LGA)

removed. To maintain D2 dissection when necessary, #10 and #11d should be removed with or without splenectomy.

Right side dissection and duodenal division. After completion of left side, procedure move to right side and tissues around the gastrocolic trunk are cleared (Fig. 16.2b). right gastroepiploic vein is divided and the soft tissues above the pancreas are retrieved (#6). Right gastroepiploic artery is divided and dissection continues up to the root of gastroduodenal artery to mobilize the duodenum from the pancreas. In supraduodenal area, minor periduodenal vessels are divided and duodenum is transected by using linear endoscopic stapler.

Suprapancreatic dissection. Right gastric vessels are divided and soft tissues around the common hepatic artery are dissected (#5–8a) (Fig. 16.2c). For D2 dissection, soft tissues medial to the portal vein and proper hepatic artery are included in the specimen (#12a) (Fig. 16.2d). After left gastric vein division, soft tissues around left gastric artery are dissected on the right side (#7, #9), and splenic artery on the left side (#11p) (Fig. 16.2e, f). Retroperitoneal attachments of stomach including posterior gastric vessels if present are detached. Right diaphragmatic crus is reached and lesser curvature of the stomach is cleaned to remove #1 and some parts of #3 for distal gastrectomy (Fig. 16.2g, h).

Reconstruction. It is possible to perform anastomosis by either intra- or extracorporeally after gastrectomy. After distal gastrectomy, Billroth-I gastroduodenostomy, Billroth-II gastrojejunostomy, or Roux-en-Y gastrojejunostomy are the options to maintain intestinal continuity. For Billroth-I gastroduodenostomy, small full-layer incisions are created on the edge of greater curvature side of the stomach and on the edge of the posterior side of the duodenum. The 45-mm endoscopic linear stapler is inserted towards both intestinal lumens and the posterior walls of the stomach and duodenum are anastomosed (Fig. 16.3a). The entry hole is closed with another endoscopic linear stapler and Delta-Shaped Anastomosis is achieved (Fig. 16.3b) [11]. For Billroth-II gastrojejunostomy roughly 20 cm distal to the treitz ligament is brought up and anastomosis is performed by using two linear staplers (Fig. 16.3c, d). When jejenum is divided from same distance, it is possible to perform roux-en-Y gastrojejunostomy by using linear staplers and then jejunojejunostomy is added 25–30 cm distal to the gastrojejunostomy with similar stapling technique. After total gastrectomy, most common anastomosis type is Roux-en-Y esophagojejunostomy. For years, it has been performed by circular stapling technique which require mini-laparotomy, however, it is now possible to perform safely with side-to-side linear stapling technique (Fig. 16.3e, f). Linear staplers can also be used for esophagogastrostomy after proximal gastrectomy and for gastro-gastrostomy after pylorus-preserving gastrectomy to achieve all reconstructive process intracorporeally. For reconstruction, in addition to the techniques mentioned above, jejunal interposition and double-tract method are alternative options.

16.3 Current Evidences for Minimally Invasive Gastrectomy

After first report of LG, many studies including randomized controlled trials (RCT) are conducted in various centers. However, because the stage of tumor (EGC vs. AGC) and type of gastrectomy (distal vs. total) determine the extent and invasiveness of surgery, it is not possible to gather all studies in one pool, and short-term and long-term outcomes should be evaluated with distinct subgroups.

16.3.1 Laparoscopic Gastrectomy Versus Open Gastrectomy

Up to now, there are several published retrospective series, RCTs and meta-analysis comparing LADG vs. open distal gastrectomy (ODG) for EGC located in the mid-to-lower part of the stomach. The most recent meta-analysis including seven RCTs (five from Japan and two from South Korea) published in 2015 demonstrated that LADG provides less blood loss (WMD: −108.11; 95% CI: −145.97 to −70.26), less

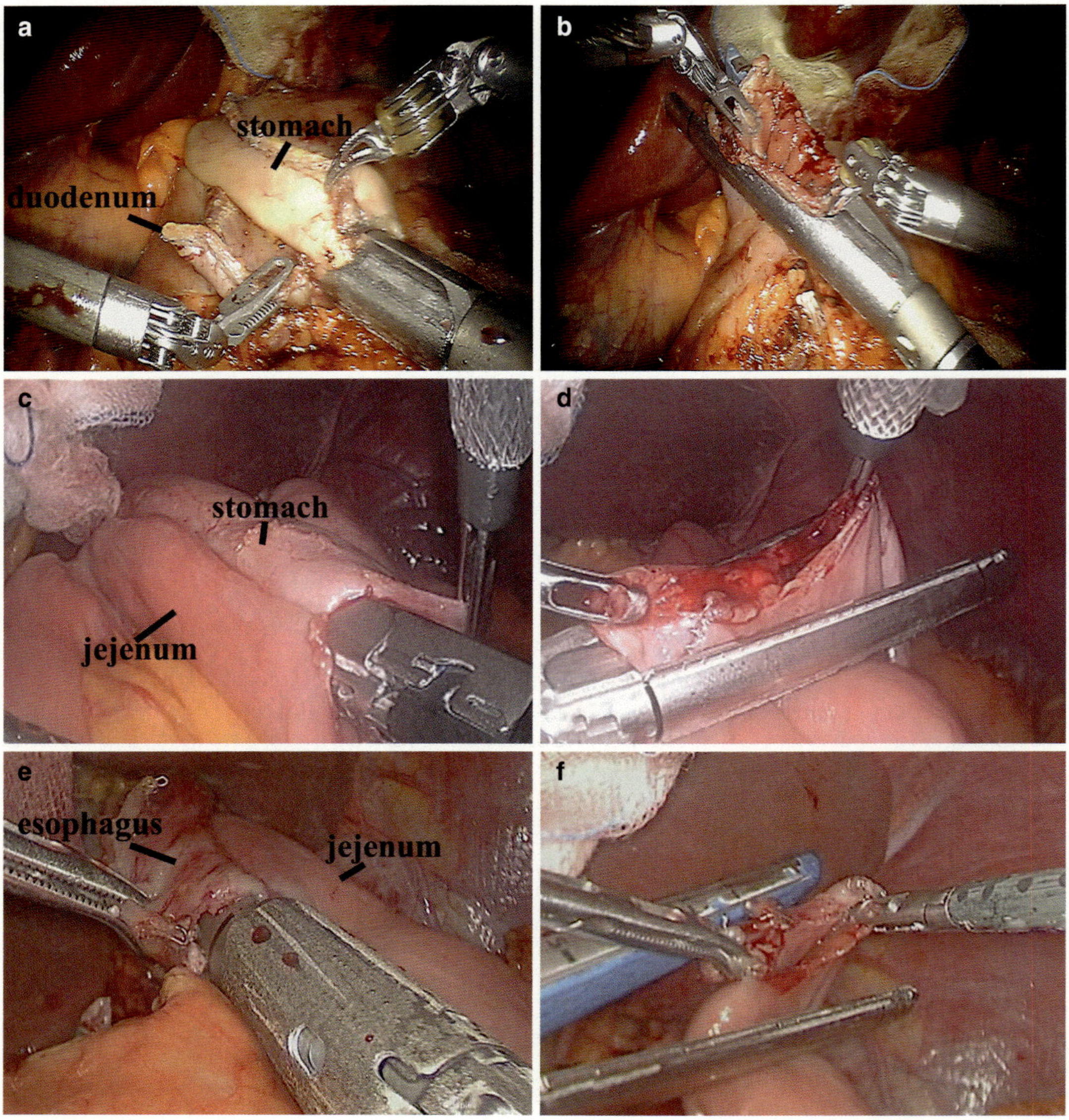

Fig. 16.3 Intracorporeal anastomosis for Billroth-I gastroduodenostomy (**a**, **b**), Billroth-II gastrojejunostomy (**c**, **d**) after distal gastrectomy, and intracorporeal Roux-en-Y esophagojejunostomy (**e**, **f**) after total gastrectomy

analgesic requirement (WMD: −1.70; 95% CI: −2.19 to −1.22), lower incidence of complications (OR: 0.26; 95% CI: 0.13–0.54), shorter hospital stay (WMD: −1.0; 95% CI: −1.83 to −0.16), and earlier passage of flatus (WMD: −0.62; 95% CI: −0.96 to −0.27), though at the price of longer operative times (WMD: 79.60; 95% CI: 59.86–99.35) and the number of harvested lymph nodes (WMD: −2.77; 95% CI: −4.38 to −1.16) lesser as compared to ODG [12]. Despite the combination of several RCTs, total number of patients was 390 (195 LADG and 195 ODG) in this meta-analysis and might be considered as a limitation for proper conclusion. To overcome this limitation, we need to look into the outcomes of phase III studies. Multi-institutional randomized KLASS-01 study conducted by the Korea Laparoscopic

Gastrointestinal Surgery Study Group (KLASS), that started in 2006, is a study that compares LDG and ODG and short-term outcomes were published recently [13]. While the major intraabdominal complication (LADG vs. ODG; 7.6% vs. 10.3%) and mortality rates (0.6% vs. 0.3%) were comparable between two groups, overall complication rate (13.0% vs. 19.9%) including wound complication rate (3.1% vs. 7.7%) were lower in LADG group. In addition to these findings, LADG was associated with significantly longer operation time (184.1 ± 53.3 vs. 139.4 ± 42.7), less blood loss (110.8 ± 135.7 vs. 190.6 ± 156.3), shorter hospital stay (7.1 ± 3.1 vs. 7.9 ± 4.1), and less number of harvested lymph nodes (40.5 ± 15.3 vs. 43.7 ± 15.7). The other randomized study JCOG0912, which was carried out by the Japan Clinical Oncology Group (JCOG), demonstrated similar outcomes and concluded that LADG can be considered as a safe alternative to open surgery in terms of adverse events and short-term outcomes [14]. The study showed longer operation time (LADG vs. ODG, median 278 min vs. 194 min) with less blood loss (median 38 mL vs. 115 mL) in LADG group, and no difference was found in terms of major complications (3.3% vs. 3.7%), only liver enzymes elevation was observed more (16.4% vs. 5.3%) in LADG group possibly due to long duration of liver retraction. As for oncologic safety of LADG for EGC, while a recent meta-analysis demonstrated comparable oncological outcomes in terms of long-term mortality and relapse rate, we need to wait little bit more to obtain the long-term outcomes of large-scale RCTs.

Apart from the increasing number of evidence on LADG for EGC, high-level evidences neither for LATG and nor for advanced stage disease are available, because of the technical difficulties and the technical heterogeneity among the surgeons during LATG or lymphadenectomy for AGC. Because AGC requires extensive lymphadenectomy for patients with gastric cancer, it is difficult to standardize the surgery and to have high-quality evidence. Recently published Chinese study includes total 1056 patients (The Chinese Laparoscopic Gastrointestinal Surgery Study, CLASS-01) showed no difference in terms of morbidity and mortality in patients with AGC require distal gastrectomy [15]. Postoperative morbidity was 15.2% for LDG and 12.9% in ODG group, while 0.4% mortality rate in LDG and no mortality was observed in ODG group. As for oncological safety, the only RCT showing long-term outcomes demonstrated 67.1 and 53.8% survival rates respectively for LG and open gastrectomy with no statistical difference. There are two ongoing large-scale study in South Korea and Japan, KLASS-02 and JLSSG0901 (Japanese Laparoscopic Surgery Study Group). The oncological outcomes of these two as well as the CLASS-01 study will answer the questions on the safety and efficacy of LG for AGC [3].

Because the incidence of proximal gastric cancer is low in Asian countries, and owing to difficulties in the reconstruction phase after total gastrectomy, LTG could not have been generalized in surgical practice. Although recent meta-analysis that includes EGC or AGC regardless of stage and compare LTG vs. open total gastrectomy demonstrated the benefits of LTG in terms of blood loss, pain, hospital stay and morbidity with the comparable long-term outcomes, relatively small sample size of studies and the lack of RCTs are the obstacles to have exact conclusion. Although the outcomes of prospective phase-II KLASS-03 study aiming to evaluate the feasibility of LTG for patients with EGC will shed light on the future of LTG, randomized trials are still required [16].

16.3.2 Robotic Gastrectomy Versus Open Gastrectomy

Following the first report of large case series evaluating RG that was published in 2009, and that demonstrated RG as a safe and effective alternative, surgeons have conducted some comparative studies [17]. Meta-analysis of seven retrospective case-matched series argued that RG is safe and efficient method and may be a more practical and feasible alternative to open gastrectomy [18]. Similarly, recent RCT comparing RG with intra-corporeal robot-sewn anastomosis and open gastrectomy demonstrated that RG ensures less blood loss (94.2 ± 51.5 vs. 152.8 ± 76.9 mL), shorter hospital stay (5.6 ± 1.9 vs. 6.7 ± 1.9 days) and earlier restoration of bowel function (2.6 ± 1.1 vs. 3.1 ± 1.2 days), however surgical duration was longer (242.7 ± 43.8 vs. 192.4 ± 31.5 min) in RG group [19]. Neither complication rates (10.3 vs. 9.3%) nor number of harvested lymph node (30.9 ± 10.4 vs. 29.3 ± 9.7 days) were different. As was shown in this RCT and previous large series, besides the benefits of minimal invasiveness of RG compared to open surgery, some issues such as cost and surgical duration are the shortcomings to be solved in the future. For oncological safety, a matched-case control study showed comparable outcomes between RG and open gastrectomy, however, further studies are needed [20].

16.3.3 Robotic Gastrectomy Versus Laparoscopic Gastrectomy

Even though both are minimally invasive techniques, some studies try to find out whether there is a difference between RG and LG. Recent multicenter prospective study from South Korea, both groups showed comparable overall complication rates (robotic: 11.9% vs. laparoscopic: 10.3%) and major complication rates (robotic: 1.1% vs. laparoscopic: 1.1%) [21]. Owing to the higher cost of robotic surgery and longer operative time in RG group, any superiority of RG over LG could not have been demonstrated in this study. Furthermore, in subgroup analysis of that study showed that RG compared to LG is more beneficial in terms of blood loss for the patients underwent D2 lymph node dissection [22]. However, robotic assistance was not helpful to overcome the obstacles of LG for obese patients or for patients underwent total gastrectomy. Given that use of robot for gastrectomy has a short history, long-term oncologic outcomes of RG still remains controversial. Even so, retrospective series comparing survival between RG and LG revealed that survival was comparable between the two approaches [23].

16.3.4 Robotic Gastrectomy Versus Laparoscopic Gastrectomy Versus Open Gastrectomy

In a study comparing three approaches in terms of major early complications in a total of 5839 patients (4542 open gastrectomy, 861 LG and 436 RG), while no significant difference was found between the three groups, intestinal obstruction and intra-abdominal fluid collection was observed more after open gastrectomy and MIS led to more anastomotic leakage [24].

16.3.5 Overview to Evidences

Because gastric cancer treatment depends on various factors such as tumor location, tumor stage, and patient characteristics, it is not rational to place all gastric cancer patients in one pool to evaluate the efficacy of MIS. Indeed, MIS for gastric cancer does not have a long history, thus we have recently started having some evidence as regard to its safety and feasibility. The evidences we have had thus far may demonstrate that MIS is safe, technically feasible and oncological effective approach for early gastric cancer patients requiring distal gastrectomy. Although we have some evidence concerning the safety for advanced gastric cancer and for patients requiring total gastrectomy, we need to wait the outcomes of ongoing Korean and Japanese studies to have exact conclusion.

Less blood loss, improved recovery, and shorter hospital stay are the main advantages of the laparoscopic surgery as was observed in other gastrointestinal malignancies. Given that gastric cancer surgery including lymphadenectomy is a complex procedure, it is conceivable to suppose that robotic instruments will assist surgeons overcome the difficulties during laparoscopic gastrectomy. Surgical duration is one of the disadvantage of MIS, however, it should be kept in mind that learning curve effect is a key point for complex procedures. And, as recent studies revealed, with the increasing surgeon experience, time having spent in operation room is getting shorter not only for LG and also for RG. The cost is another obstacle for MIS and this should be investigated and solved in future studies.

In the lights of current evidences, although LG and RG are complex procedures for surgeon, can be performed safely with the expected advantages of minimally invasive surgery. Given the difficulties during laparoscopic surgery, robotic surgery may offer a promising alternative to traditional open or conventional laparoscopic gastrectomy.

References

1. Arezzo A. The past, the present, and the future of minimally invasive therapy in laparoscopic surgery: a review and speculative outlook. Minim Invasive Ther Allied Technol. 2014;23(5):253–60. doi:10.3109/13645706.2014.900084.
2. Son T, Hyung WJ. Laparoscopic gastric cancer surgery: current evidence and future perspectives. World J Gastroenterol. 2016;22(2):727–35. doi:10.3748/wjg.v22.i2.727.
3. Son T, Kwon IG, Hyung WJ. Minimally invasive surgery for gastric cancer treatment: current status and future perspectives. Gut Liver. 2014;8(3):229–36. doi:10.5009/gnl.2014.8.3.229.
4. Jeong O, Park YK. Clinicopathological features and surgical treatment of gastric cancer in South Korea: the results of 2009 nationwide survey on surgically treated gastric cancer patients. J Gastric Cancer. 2011;11(2):69–77. doi:10.5230/jgc.2011.11.2.69.
5. Kitano S, Iso Y, Moriyama M, Sugimachi K. Laparoscopy-assisted Billroth I gastrectomy. Surg Laparosc Endosc. 1994;4(2):146–8.
6. Antonakis PT, Ashrafian H, Isla AM. Laparoscopic gastric surgery for cancer: where do we stand? World J Gastroenterol. 2014;20(39):14280–91. doi:10.3748/wjg.v20.i39.14280.
7. Japanese Gastric Cancer Association. Japanese gastric cancer treatment guidelines 2014 (ver. 4). Gastric Cancer. 2016;20(1):1–19. doi:10.1007/s10120-016-0622-4.
8. Guner A, Hyung WJ. Minimally invasive surgery for gastric cancer. Ulus Cerrahi Derg. 2014;30(1):1–9. doi:10.5152/ucd.2014.2607.
9. Woo Y, Hyung WJ, Kim HI, Obama K, Son T, Noh SH. Minimizing hepatic trauma with a novel liver retraction method: a simple liver suspension using gauze suture. Surg Endosc. 2011;25(12):3939–45. doi:10.1007/s00464-011-1788-9.
10. Kim HI, Hyung WJ, Lee CR, Lim JS, An JY, Cheong JH, Choi SH, Noh SH. Intraoperative portable abdominal radiograph for tumor localization: a simple and accurate method for laparoscopic gastrectomy. Surg Endosc. 2011;25(3):958–63. doi:10.1007/s00464-010-1288-3.
11. Kanaya S, Kawamura Y, Kawada H, Iwasaki H, Gomi T, Satoh S, Uyama I. The delta-shaped anastomosis in laparoscopic distal gastrectomy: analysis of the initial 100 consecutive procedures of intracorporeal gastroduodenostomy. Gastric Cancer. 2011;14(4):365–71. doi:10.1007/s10120-011-0054-0.
12. Deng Y, Zhang Y, Guo TK. Laparoscopy-assisted versus open distal gastrectomy for early gastric cancer: a meta-analysis based on seven randomized controlled trials. Surg Oncol. 2015;24(2):71–7. doi:10.1016/j.suronc.2015.02.003.
13. Kim W, Kim HH, Han SU, Kim MC, Hyung WJ, Ryu SW, Cho GS, Kim CY, Yang HK, Park DJ, Song KY, Lee SI, Ryu SY, Lee JH, Lee HJ. Decreased morbidity of laparoscopic distal gastrectomy compared with open distal gastrectomy for stage I gastric cancer: short-term outcomes from a multicenter randomized controlled trial (KLASS-01). Ann Surg. 2016;263(1):28–35. doi:10.1097/sla.0000000000001346.
14. Katai H, Mizusawa J, Katayama H, Takagi M, Yoshikawa T, Fukagawa T, Terashima M, Misawa K, Teshima S, Koeda K, Nunobe S, Fukushima N, Yasuda T, Asao Y, Fujiwara Y, Sasako M. Short-term surgical outcomes from a phase III study of laparoscopy-assisted versus open distal gastrectomy with nodal dissection for clinical stage IA/IB gastric cancer: Japan Clinical Oncology Group Study JCOG0912. Gastric Cancer. 2016. [Epub ahead of print]. doi:10.1007/s10120-016-0646-9
15. Hu Y, Huang C, Sun Y, Su X, Cao H, Hu J, Xue Y, Suo J, Tao K, He X, Wei H, Ying M, Hu W, Du X, Chen P, Liu H, Zheng C, Liu F, Yu J, Li Z, Zhao G, Chen X, Wang K, Li P, Xing J, Li G. Morbidity and mortality of laparoscopic versus open D2 distal gastrectomy for advanced gastric cancer: a randomized controlled trial. J Clin Oncol. 2016;34(12):1350–7. doi:10.1200/jco.2015.63.7215.
16. Kim KH, Kim SH, Kim MC. How much progress has been made in minimally invasive surgery for gastric cancer in Korea?: a viewpoint from Korean prospective clinical trials. Medicine (Baltimore). 2014;93(28):e233. doi:10.1097/MD.0000000000000233.
17. Song J, Oh SJ, Kang WH, Hyung WJ, Choi SH, Noh SH. Robot-assisted gastrectomy with lymph node dissection for gastric cancer: lessons learned from an initial 100 consecutive procedures. Ann Surg. 2009;249(6):927–32. doi:10.1097/01.sla.0000351688.64999.73.
18. Yang Y, Wang G, He J, Wu F, Ren S. Robotic gastrectomy versus open gastrectomy in the treatment of gastric cancer. J Cancer Res Clin Oncol. 2016;143(1):105–14. doi:10.1007/s00432-016-2240-2.
19. Wang G, Jiang Z, Zhao J, Liu J, Zhang S, Zhao K, Feng X, Li J. Assessing the safety and efficacy of full robotic gastrectomy with intracorporeal robot-sewn anastomosis for gastric cancer: a randomized clinical trial. J Surg Oncol. 2016;113(4):397–404. doi:10.1002/jso.24146.
20. Caruso S, Patriti A, Marrelli D, Ceccarelli G, Ceribelli C, Roviello F, Casciola L. Open vs robot-assisted laparoscopic gastric resection with D2 lymph node dissection for adenocarcinoma: a case-control study.

Int J Med Rob Comput Assisted Surg. 2011;7(4):452–8. doi:10.1002/rcs.416.
21. Kim HI, Han SU, Yang HK, Kim YW, Lee HJ, Ryu KW, Park JM, An JY, Kim MC, Park S, Song KY, Oh SJ, Kong SH, Suh BJ, Yang DH, Ha TK, Kim YN, Hyung WJ. Multicenter prospective comparative study of robotic versus laparoscopic gastrectomy for gastric adenocarcinoma. Ann Surg. 2016;263(1):103–9. doi:10.1097/SLA.0000000000001249.
22. Park JM, Kim HI, Han SU, Yang HK, Kim YW, Lee HJ, An JY, Kim MC, Park S, Song KY, Oh SJ, Kong SH, Suh BJ, Yang DH, Ha TK, Hyung WJ, Ryu KW. Who may benefit from robotic gastrectomy?: a subgroup analysis of multicenter prospective comparative study data on robotic versus laparoscopic gastrectomy. Eur J Surg Oncol. 2016;42(12):1944–9. doi:10.1016/j.ejso.2016.07.012.
23. Son T, Lee JH, Kim YM, Kim HI, Noh SH, Hyung WJ. Robotic spleen-preserving total gastrectomy for gastric cancer: comparison with conventional laparoscopic procedure. Surg Endosc. 2014;28(9):2606–15. doi:10.1007/s00464-014-3511-0.
24. Kim KM, An JY, Kim HI, Cheong JH, Hyung WJ, Noh SH. Major early complications following open, laparoscopic and robotic gastrectomy. Br J Surg. 2012;99(12):1681–7. doi:10.1002/bjs.8924.

17 Laparoscopic and Robot Assisted Gastrectomy

Seong-Ho Kong, Hyuk-Joon Lee, and Han-Kwang Yang

The advantages of minimally invasive approaches would be less postoperative pain, better cosmesis, less inflammatory reaction, rapid recovery of bowel function, well-preserved immune function, short hospital stay, and a rapid return to normal social activity. After the initial introduction of laparoscopic gastrectomy for gastric cancer by Kitano and colleagues in 1993 [1], it has rapidly spread out, and now it is considered as one of the standard minimally invasive procedures for the treatment of gastric cancer especially for early stage. For example, in Korea, the number of laparoscopic surgery for gastric cancer increased from 740 in 2004 to 3783 in 2009 respectively, which accounts for 6.6 and 25.8% of all gastric cancer surgeries in each year [2]. Now most of early gastric cancer is done by laparoscopic procedure. Over the last two decades, important clinical evidences for laparoscopic gastrectomy came mainly from Korea to Japan.

Electronic Supplementary Material The online version of this chapter (doi:10.1007/978-3-319-54301-7_17) contains supplementary material, which is available to authorized users. On http://springerlink.com enter the DOI number given above.

S.-H. Kong, M.D., Ph.D. • H.-J. Lee, M.D., Ph.D.
H.-K. Yang, MD, PhD, FACS, Hon ASA, ESA (✉)
Department of Surgery, Seoul National University Hospital, Seoul National University College of Medicine, Seoul, South Korea
e-mail: yangh@me.com

17.1 Laparoscopic Distal Gastrectomy

Laparoscopic distal gastrectomy (LDG) is the most commonly performed laparoscopic gastrectomy for gastric cancer. Operator is usually on the right side of the patient because dissection along the major vessels such as gastro-duodenal artery, common hepatic artery, and splenic artery is favored by this operator's position (Fig. 17.1). In this position, ultrasonic instrument can be applied for dissection of lymph nodes along these vessels more safely. Three types of reconstruction are usually performed; gastroduodenostomy (Billroth I), loop gastrojejunostomy (Billroth II), and roux-en-Y gastrojejunostomy. The range of LN dissection covered no. 1, 3, 4sb, 4d, 5, 6, 7, 8a, 9, with or without no. 11p and 12a according to Japanese gastric cancer classification [3]. For the anastomosis, circular or linear stapler was commonly used through 4–5 cm vertical or transverse mini-laparotomy on the upper abdomen in case of extracorporeal gastroduodenostomy or gastrojejunostomy [4]. In case of intracorporeal anastomosis, Delta-shaped anastomosis is commonly applied for the gastroduodenostomy [5]. Although intracorporeal anastomosis has some advantages providing a better operative view and a wider range for movement during the reconstruction, especially in obese patients, it is still controversial to be routinely used because of its higher cost for more staplers and similar clinical

M.A. Cuesta (ed.), *Minimally Invasive Surgery for Upper Abdominal Cancer*,
DOI 10.1007/978-3-319-54301-7_17

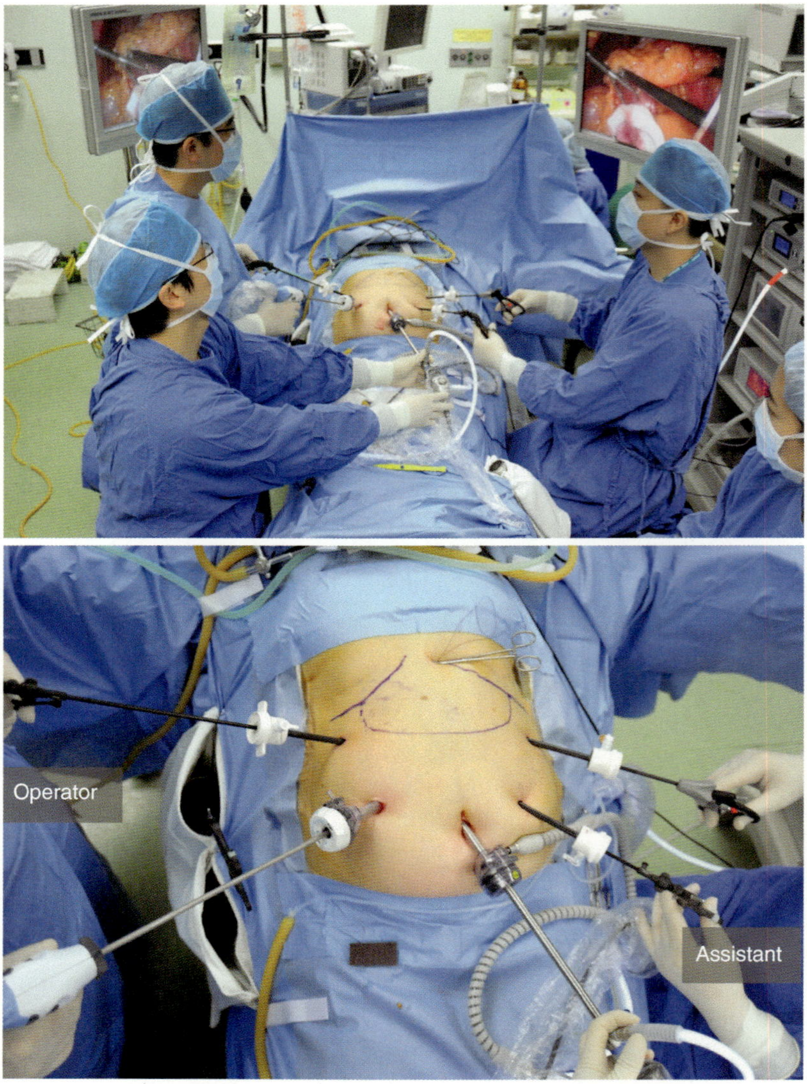

Fig. 17.1 Location of ports and operator for distal gastrectomy

outcomes, compared with extracorporeal anastomosis. Another concern is that intraluminal content has cytology positive even in early stage, which can possibly result in peritoneal recurrence [6].

Several randomized controlled trials comparing LDG versus ODG were published [2]. Among several RCTs, the largest and most noticeable one is the Korean multicenter trial, named KLASS (Korean Laparoendoscopic gAstrointestinal Surgery Study Group) trial (NCT00452751). The indication was clinical stage I (cT1N0M0, cT1N1M0, and cT2N0M0) gastric adenocarcinoma. The primary endpoint was overall survival, and the secondary endpoints were disease-free survival, morbidity, mortality, quality of life, inflammatory and immune responses, and cost-effectiveness. A distal gastrectomy with D1+ or D2 LN dissection was performed in both groups. Reconstruction was performed by Billroth I or Billroth II or roux-en-Y fashion, depending on the surgeons' preference. Surgery was performed by 15 surgeons at 13 institutes, who had performed at least 50 cases each of LDG and ODG and their institutions performed more than 80 cases of distal gastrectomy per year, to assure high surgical quality. The initial sample size was 1400. From February 2006 to August 2010, 1416 patients (705 LDG and 711 ODG) were enrolled. According to the short term outcomes, the overall complication rate was significantly lower in the LDG group (LDG vs. ODG; 13.0% vs. 19.9%, P = 0.001). In detail, the wound complication rate of the LDG group was significantly lower than that of the ODG group (3.1% vs. 7.7%, P < 0.001). The major intra-abdominal complication (7.6% vs. 10.3%, P = 0.095) and mortality rates (0.6% vs. 0.3%, P = 0.687) were similar between two groups [7].

For the long term outcome of LDG, several case-control study or case series are available at this time. Japanese Laparoscopic Surgery Study Group (JLSSG) reported a retrospective multi-center study of laparoscopic gastrecomy for EGC in 2007. Analyzing 1294 patients from 16 hospitals from 1994 to 2003, they showed that only 6 (0.6%) patients recurred during 36 month of median follow-up (range: 13–113 months), and the 5-year disease free survival rate was 99.8% for stage Ia, 98.7% for stage Ib, and 85.7% for stage II disease. In this cohort, LDG was performed in 1185 patients (91.5%), and the 5-year disease free survival after LDG was 99.4% [8].

KLASS group also reported a similar retrospective multicenter long-term outcome of 2976 patients who underwent laparoscopic (n = 1477) or open gastrectomy (n = 1499) from 10 hospitals from 1998 to 2005. The overall survival and recurrence-free survival were not statistically different at each cancer stage with the exception of an increased overall survival rate for patients with stage IA cancer treated via laparoscopy. After matching using a propensity scoring system, the overall survival, disease-specific survival, and recurrence-free survival rates were not statistically different at each stage [9].

17.2 Laparoscopic Total Gastrectomy

Unlike LDG, laparoscopic total gastrectomy (LTG) remains challenging procedure and the technique has not yet been standardized. The general indication is EGC located in the upper third of the stomach. However, compared to LDG, LTG seems to be selectively performed, even in Korea and Japan.

Esophagojejunostomy is usually made by roux-en-Y fashion, either by extracorporeal or intracorporeal approach using either circular stapler or linear stapler. Transoral introduction of the anvil head of the circular stapler (Orvil) is one available method. Sakuramoto and colleagues reported that intracorporeal esophagojejunostomy with this technique was achieved successfully in 26 out of 27 patients. No other complications, such as hypopharyngeal or esophageal injury, occurred during passage, and no postoperative complications occurred except one anastomotic stenosis [10]. On the other hands, Nagai and colleagues reported a case series of 94 patients who underwent intracorporeal esophagojejunostomy with linear stapler. Only two cases of anastomotic leakage were developed after surgery, but there was no open conversion or mortality in this cohort [11].

Recently, a meta-analysis was reported including eight non-RTCs with 314 LTG and 384 open total gastrectomy (OTG) in patients with gastric cancer. LTG showed less intraoperative blood loss, less postoperative complications, and shorter hospital stay compared with OTG, although operation time was longer in LTG group. In-hospital mortality rates were comparable for LTG (0.9%) and OTG (1.8%). Authors concluded that LTG shows better short-term outcomes compared with OTG in patients with gastric cancer [12].

KLASS group also reported a retrospective multicenter cohort study with 131 patients who underwent LTG. Only one patient required conversion to open procedure. The mean number of retrieved lymph nodes was 34.7. The mean duration of postoperative hospital stay was 11.3 days, and postoperative morbidity rate was 19% without operative mortality. The most common postoperative morbidity was wound complications at the mini-laparotomy site, and there were three cases of anastomotic leakage. Six patients (5%) had recurrence of cancer, and nine patients (7%) died during the follow-up period [13].

17.3 Laparoscopic Pylorus Preserving Gastrectomy

Early gastric cancer located in the middle portion of stomach with the distal tumor border at least 4 cm proximal to the pylorus can be managed by pylorus preserving gastrectomy (PPG) [14, 15]. Compared to distal gastrectomy, PPG has several advantages such as nutritional benefit, lower incidence of dumping syndrome, bile reflux or gallstone formation [16]. Recently, several clinical data were reported to validate the role of PPG performed by laparoscopy. PPG is different from DG, in terms of the preservation of distal antrum (about 3 cm), hepatic branch of vagus nerve, right gastric vessel and infrapyloric vessel. For the LN dissection, No. 5 and No. 12a stations are not dissected to preserve pyloric branch of vagus nerve but No. 6 station is well dissected even with preserving infra-pyloric vessels. Gastrogastrostomy is mostly done by end-to-end manner. In laparoscopic procedure, it is usually performed by extracorporeal hand-sewn method, since antrum is too thick to be cut and anastomosed by linear stapler. Hiki and colleagues reported the short-term outcome of 307 patients who underwent laparoscopic pylorus preserving gastrectomy (LPPG) from 2005 to 2009. The mean operation time for LPPG was 229.4 min and estimated blood loss was 49.1 mL. The mean number of dissected lymph nodes was 31.6. Complications developed in 53 patients (17.3%), and major complications were observed in only four patients (1.3%). The most frequent complication was gastric stasis, occurring in 19 patients (6.2%) [17].

Our group performed a retrospective analysis comparing those who underwent LPPG (n = 116) and LDG (n = 176) for middle third EGC. The overall postoperative morbidity rate was similar between two groups, although delayed gastric emptying was more frequent in LPPG than in LDG (7.8% vs. 1.7%). The number of retrieved lymph nodes was not significantly different (35.9 in LPPG vs. 35.2 in LDG), and 3-year recurrence free survival rates were also similar between LPPG and LDG (98.2% vs. 98.8%). Serum protein and albumin at postoperative 1 and 6 months, and abdominal fat area at postoperative 1 year were significantly less decreased in LPPG. The 3-year cumulative incidence of gallstone was also significantly lower in LPPG than in LDG (0% vs. 6.5%) [18]. Therefore, LPPG can be considered as a better treatment option than LDG in terms of nutritional advantage and lower incidence of gallstone for middle-third EGC.

In order to determine whether the postoperative quality of life and nutritional status are better, and if survival is comparable after LPPG, the KLASS group has started a multicenter RCT (KLASS-04 study) to compare LPPG and LDG for middle-third EGC (NCT No.02595086). A total of 256 patients, diagnosed with a cT1N0M0 primary gastric adenocarcinoma located at the middle-third of the stomach by endoscopic ultrasonography or CT, will be enrolled (128 patients in each group). The primary endpoint is the incidence of dumping syndrome, assessed using the Sigstad score (≥7) at 1 year after surgery. The secondary endpoints are: the 3-year relapse-free survival and overall survival; the 30-day operative morbidity and mortality; changes in body weight and fat volume on abdominal CT; changes in hemoglobin, protein, albumin, and pre-albumin levels; symptoms and quality of life measurement using the JSGIS-Q, EORTC C30, and STO22; the incidence of gallstones; and the gross and microscopic findings on gastroscopy.

17.4 Laparoscopic Gastrectomy for Advanced Cancer

As surgical experience increased, some surgeons are now applying laparoscopic gastrectomy with D2 LN dissection for the patients with AGC. The short term outcomes were reported as 11–16% of morbidity and 1–2% of mortality which were comparable to those of open surgery [2]. Recent meta-analysis, including seven case-control studies with 1271 AGC patients (626 LDG and 645 ODG), showed that LDG patients had a longer operative time but a less estimated blood loss, a few analgesic requirements, and a shorter hospital stay, compared with patients undergoing ODG. There were no significant differences between the two groups in number of LN dissections, postoperative mortality, overall complications, and 3-year overall survival rate. Therefore, authors concluded that the oncologic outcomes of LDG for AGC patients were comparable with open approach [19].

KLASS group also studied the efficacy of LDG with D2 LN dissection for cT2-T4a/cN0-N1 gastric cancer (KLASS-02, NCT01456598). The estimated sample size is 1050 and the primary endpoint is 3-year disease free survival rate. As the surgical quality may become one of the most important issues in this clinical trial, surgeons are required to be standardized and qualified by participating a surgical quality control trial. Each applicant should submit three unedited videos each for LDG and ODG, respectively, which were evaluated by independent reviewers. As a result, 18 certified surgeons from 11 institutes were entered in KLASS-02, and enrolment of 1050 was completed at April 2105 [20]. Short and long term outcomes have been presented at ASCO and will be reported in the near future.

Chinese surgeons also started a similar multicentre RCT, named CLASS-01, comparing LDG versus ODG for advanced gastric cancer and short term result has been reported. Patients with cT2-4aN0-3M0 gastric cancer were eligible for inclusion. They were randomly assigned to either the LG with D2 lymphadenectomy group ($n = 528$) or the open gastrectomy (OG) with D2 lymphadenectomy group ($n = 528$). The postoperative morbidity was 15.2% in the LG group and 12.9% in OG group with no significant difference ($P = 0.285$). The mortality rate was 0.4% for the LG group and zero for the OG group ($P = 0.249$) [21].

Japanese group also started another multicentre phase II/III trial evaluating LDG with D2 LN dissection for cT2-T4a gastric cancer. After accrual of 180 patients, of which 90 are to be treated with the laparoscopic approach, the incidence of major surgical complications will be assessed. If an early-stopping rule because of high incidence of complications does not apply, the trial will continue accrual for a total of 500 patients to show non-inferiority of the laparoscopic approach [22].

These three prospective clinical trials are expected to confirm the role of laparoscopic surgery for AGC [23].

17.5 Robotic Gastrectomy

Robot assisted gastrectomy is laparoscopic surgery using robot as an instrument. Robotic surgery, currently referring the surgery using the da Vinci® surgical system (Intuitive Surgical, Sunnyvale, California, USA), has been increasingly applied in a variety of surgical procedures in urology, gynecology, thoracic surgery, and general surgery. While the "robotic" platform contains intention of the automatized procedure, for example industrial robots, the da Vinci surgical system lacks of autonomy and it is rather a remote controlling master-slave system to manipulate the surgical instrument, initially designed to be used for extreme situation such as in spacecrafts or battlefields [24]. Considering this aspect, better terms to understand the current surgeries using the da Vinci system can be "remote access surgery" or "remote control surgery" using the robotic tele-manipulating system (Video 17.1).

Nevertheless, the da Vinci system is a concentrate of diverse cutting edge technologies, such as high quality 3D camera system with a stable vision, tenfold magnified view, scaled maneuver to enable fine movement of the instruments, tremor compensating mechanism, and near-infrared fluorescent camera adds-on, etc. The most discriminating feature of the system is articulating instruments with seven degrees of freedom, which is hard to be replaced by simple bendable instruments for conventional laparoscopic surgery. These features of the da Vinci system well met the need of minimally invasive surgery in urology, where fine spatial movement is required in limited space, and rapidly replaced open surgery in tertiary centers worldwide [25]. The situation in gastric surgery was not the same as urologic surgery. Unlike the urologic surgery shifted from the open surgery to the robotic surgery directly, the techniques and skills of conventional laparoscopic gastrectomy has been already developed to very high level in Korea and Japan before application of the da Vinci system to gastrectomy, and the operative field is too broad to maximize the features of the da Vinci system compared to prostatectomy. In spite of the beneficial features of the system, debates are continued on the cost-effectiveness in gastrectomy.

17.6 Set-Up of Robotic Gastrectomy

The procedure of robotic gastrectomy has been developed based on conventional laparoscopic surgery. The port placement and goals of each step of the procedures are similar with minor differences among the operators. Our preference of the port placement is as Fig. 17.2 [26]. It is recommended to separate each port at least 8 cm to minimize the collision between robotic arms, especially for the old version of the da Vinci system (S or Si). We set the Harmonic scalpel, the PK bipolar forceps, and the Cardiere forceps at the 1st, 2nd, and 3rd robotic arm, respectively Fig. 17.3. The Harmonic scalpel is the main dissecting device, and is installed in the 1st arm to be manipulated by the right hand, which is the dominant hand of most of our surgeons. This place is opposite to that in conventional laparoscopic gastrectomy, in which most of Korean surgeons and many Japanese surgeons stand at the right side of the patient and use the harmonic scalpel with their right hand. The direction provides good direction of dissection in infrapyloric area and around the hepatic artery, however, sometimes the 1st arm and the 2nd arm instruments can be exchanged for better dissection plane along the gastroduodenal artery and splenic artery. The time for changing instruments takes only a minute. It is suggested that the manipulation of the harmonic scalpel with the left hand of the right-handed surgeon is much easier that in conventional laparoscopy. However, there is a still correlation between the proficiency of the robotic procedure and the manual ambidexterity, and most right-hand dominant operators prefer to manipulate the main surgical instruments with their dominant hand [27]. The PK forceps have a fine tip and the adequate grip power optimized for the fine grasping of the tissues for the dissection. The bipolar coagulation provides effective hemostasis of minute bleeding where the jaw of the harmonic scalpel is difficult to be applied. The Cardiere forceps are one of the powerful grasper enough to hold and retract the stomach and major vessels. The articulating wrist of the Cardiere forcep is useful when it holds up the left gastric artery, because it can effectively lift up the left liver in the same time (Fig. 17.4). Compared to the human assistant, Cardiere forceps cannot be used reactively to the movement of the other forceps because both the 1st arm and the 3rd arm are manipulated by the right hand alternatively, however, it provides more consistent and

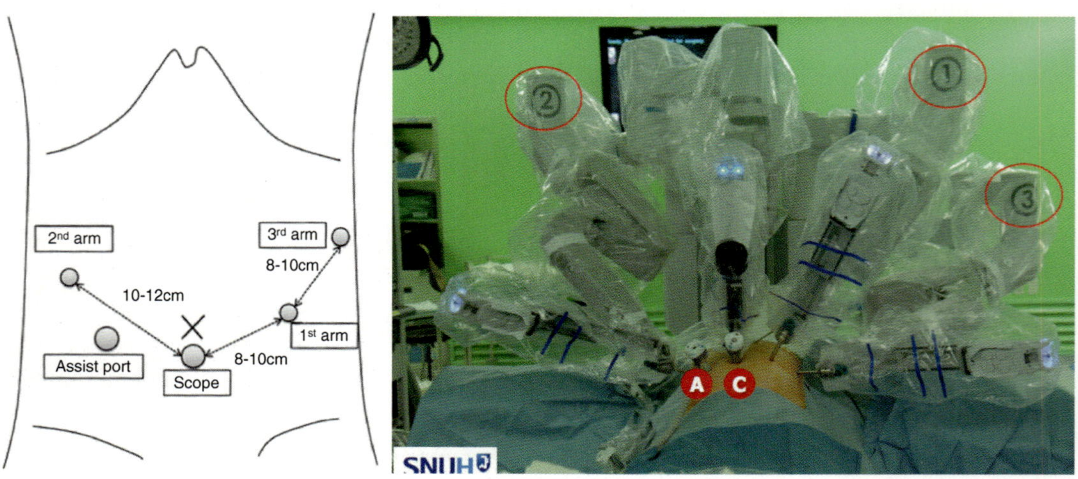

Fig. 17.2 Poor placement. Ⓐ: assistant port, Ⓒ: camera port

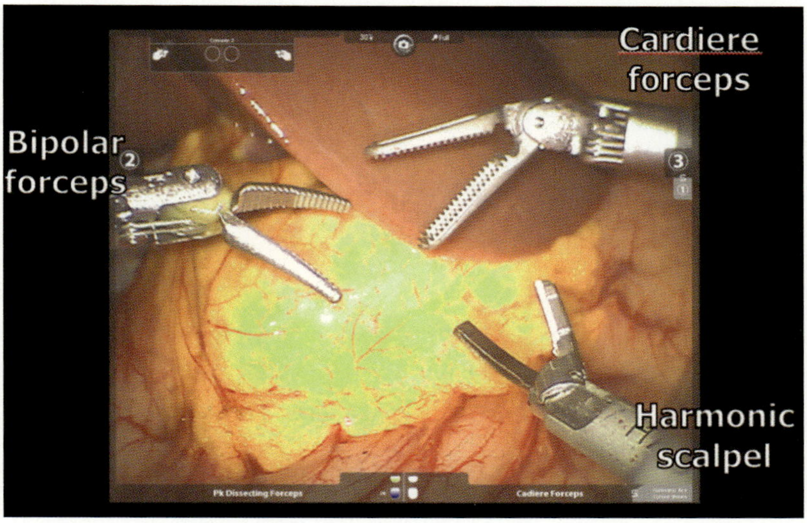

Fig. 17.3 Instrument setting

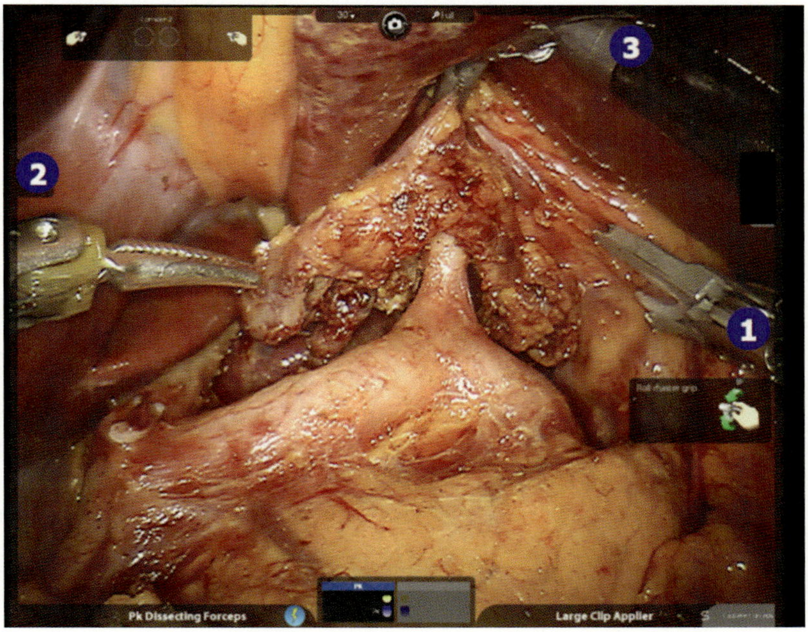

Fig. 17.4 Retraction of the tissue by the 2nd and 3rd arm. The Cadiere forceps at the 3rd hold up the pedicle of the left gastric artery, and lift up the left liver by articulating wrist at the same time

stable retraction. Finally, the assistant port is also play important role of counter-traction and application of additional devices such as suction device, clips, and surgical staplers (Fig. 17.5). Although the articulating function of the devices provides better direction of the retraction of the tissues, there has been still limitation of the spatial dissection due to lack of articulating energy-based dissection devices. Some surgeons used articulating monopolar or bipolar electrocautery devices instead of the energy-based devices for gastrectomy [28, 29]. However, there is a theoretically higher risk of free cancer cell spillage from the lymphatic channels with mono-polar electrocautery compared to that with energy-based devices, because the lymphatic channel is easily open when cut by the electrocautery and can spill out the free cancer cell that may exist in the lymphatic fluid [6]. Recently launched articulating advanced bipolar device EndoWrist® One™ Vessel Sealer

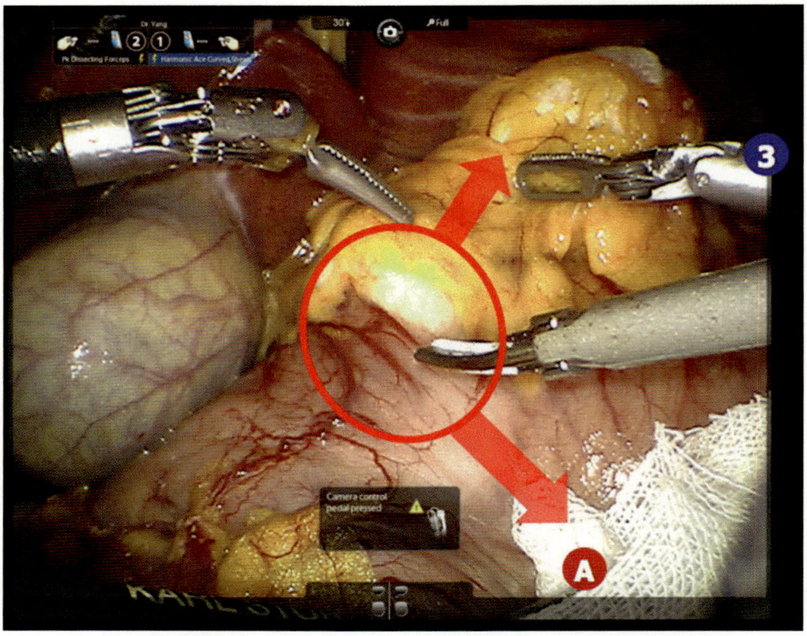

Fig. 17.5 Triangulation for retraction of the tissue. Assistant's instrument (Ⓐ) counter-tracts against the main retracting device Cardiere forcep at the 3rd robot arm

might be an option, and it requires to be tested in gastrectomy [30].

As in other robotic surgery, caution is needed to prevent machine-related injury. The da Vinci surgical system consists of very powerful robotic arms and lacks of haptic feedback to the hand of the surgeon. Careless misuse of the system can cause significant organ injury or even death of the patients. It is generally recommended deeper anesthesia, because the movement of the patient with heavy robotic instruments can cause serious organ injuries. It is also emphasized that the robotic arm outside the abdominal cavity should not press any part of the patient body. The power of traction should be well managed by visual haptic sense, and the movement of the robotic arm should be done under vision not outside of the visual field, which can cause serious injury to other organs.

17.7 Outcomes

Most of reports on the robotic gastrectomy were based on the results of the operations performed surgeons who are highly experienced in conventional laparoscopic surgery. At least for the experienced laparoscopic surgeon, the adaption of the robotic gastrectomy was rapid [31, 32]. It is not surprising considering the robot surgery is a kind of laparoscopic surgery. Simply it is a matter of whether the operator be familiar how to drive the robot.

While there have been scores of case series to show the feasibility and safety of the robotic gastrectomy, and several comparative studies comparing robotic versus open gastrectomy, the main issue of the debate on the robot gastrectomy has been whether it is superior to conventional laparoscopic surgery enough to justify higher cost. So far, there has been no large scaled randomized controlled trials to compare robotic versus laparoscopic surgery. It might have been very difficult to randomly assign the patients into different groups which costs are different by a few folds, without any financial support of the medical industry. Several not-randomized comparative studies showed no benefit or benefit in soft parameters, such as less intraopeartive blood loss and shorter hospital stay. However, benefit in relatively small amount of blood loss (<100 mL) and a flexible paramenter like hospital stay are not sufficient for justifying the "financially invasiveness" of the da Vinci surgery [33–36].

One of the largest comparative study with comparative control group is a Korean multicenter study to compare the result of the robotic gastrectomy for with those of the very next case fit the matching condition including the surgeon, extent of the gastric resection, and sex [37]. There was no difference in the complication rate (11.9% vs. 10.3%, $p = 0.619$), major complication rate (Clavien-Dindo classification 3 or more) (1.1% vs. 1.1%, $p = 0.999$), blood loss (50 mL vs. 55 mL, $p = 0.318$), number of retrieved lymph nodes (34 vs. 32, $p = 0.587$), length of hospital stay (6 days vs. 6 days, $p = 0.889$) between robot gastrectomy group and conventional laparoscopic group. On the other hand, robot gastrectomy group showed longer operative time (221 min vs. 178 min, $p < 0.001$) and higher total cost (13,748,422 KRW vs. 9,165,862 KRW, $p < 0.001$).

There could be arguments that the robotic gastrectomy may have benefit in more experienced hand or more sophisticated procedures. Pylorus-preserving gastrectomy may be one of the procedure requiring fine dissection of the infrapyloric area to obtain both sufficient lymph node dissection and preservation of the infrapyloric vessels. Our institution compared 68 cases of robotic pylorus-preserving gastrectomy and 68 cases laparoscopic pylorus-preserving gastrectomy by a propensity score matching analysis. There was no difference in the number of total examined lymph nodes (33.4 ± 11.9 vs. 36.5 ± 12.3, $p = 0.153$), number of infrapyloric area (station #6) (5.1 ± 3.2 vs. 4.9 ± 2.8, $p = 0.696$), complication rate (19.1% vs. 22.1% $p = 0.671$), and delayed gastric emptying (two cases vs. one case) [26]. There was report to suggest potential advantage of robotic gastrectomy to reduce the postoperative complication by robot-experienced surgeon's group, however, it is not reproduced by other surgeons [38]. Results in the high BMI patients are compelling each other, too [39–41]. Some surgeons expect the potential benefits of the robotic surgery over laparoscopic surgery in D2 dissection for advanced gastric cancer. One Japanese retrospective cohort study showed 3-year survival after robot gastrectomy, and the result of the stage II ($n = 19$) and III ($n = 16$) were comparable to those of laparoscopic gastrectomy [42]. In spite of potential benefit of the da Vinci surgical system, it is questionable whether it can show oncologic superiority over conventional laparoscopy. If robotic D2 dissection for advanced gastric cancer is not proven to be superior to the laparoscopic surgery in terms of long-term survival, alternative benefit such as less complication rate should be as powerful as to justify higher cost and longer operation time. To test feasibility, safety, effectiveness, and economical efficiency of robotic gastrectomy for resectable gastric cancer, a multi-institutional historically controlled prospective cohort study is undergoing now in Japan (personal communication with Professor Uyama and Terashima).

Conclusion

Laparoscopic gastrectomy is promising minimally invasive surgery for gastric cancer. As surgical experiences accumulated, laparoscopic surgery for gastric cancer is now popularized and standardized. LDG shows better or comparable outcomes compared to ODG in terms of short-term results. The long-term outcome after LDG has been shown comparable to ODG in EGC. Clinical evidence of LDG for AGC are accumulating, and ongoing Korean Chinese and Japanese multicenter RCT will reveal more clinical evidences. Evidences of LTG are still limited. LPPG seems to have benefit over conventional DG and will be confirmed by an ongoing trial.

The da Vinci surgical system has several technically beneficial features for the complexed oncologic surgery. Its use in gastric surgery has been shown to be safe and feasible, and at least not-inferior to the conventional laparoscopic gastrectomy, however, objective benefit has not been proven by high-level evidences. Some of soft parameters shown to be superior in robotic gastrectomy is not sufficient to justify the financially invasiveness of the da Vinci system. More possibilities including those in D2 dissection of advanced gastric cancer are waiting for investigation, and the medical industry's responsibility to support the clinical trials should be considered. On the other hand, this integrated tele-manipulating system has opened many opportunities and direction of development in future. We can expect a variety of robotic platforms with reasonable prices in competing market, which can facilitate the development of future surgery such as telementoring, image-guided surgery, and artificial intelligence-assistant surgery.

References

1. Kitano S, Iso Y, Moriyama M, Sugimachi K. Laparoscopy-assisted Billroth I gastrectomy. Surg Laparosc Endosc. 1994;4:146–8.
2. Lee HJ, Yang HK. Laparoscopic gastrectomy for gastric cancer. Dig Surg. 2013;30(2):132–41.
3. Japanese Gastric Cancer Association. Japanese classification of gastric carcinoma: 3rd English edition. Gastric Cancer. 2011;14:101–12.
4. Lee HJ, Shiraishi N, Kim HH, Hiki N, Uyama I, Choi SH, Yang HK, Kitano S. Standard of practice on laparoscopic gastric cancer surgery in Korea and Japan: experts' survey. Asian J Endosc Surg. 2012;5:5–11.
5. Kanaya S, Kawamura Y, Kawada H, Iwasaki H, Gomi T, Satoh S, Uyama I. The delta-shaped anastomosis in laparoscopic distal gastrectomy: analysis of the initial 100 consecutive procedures of intracorporeal gastroduodenostomy. Gastric Cancer. 2011;14:365–71.
6. Han TS, Kong SH, Lee HJ, Ahn HS, Hur K, Yu J, Kim WH, Yang HK. Dissemination of free cancer cells from the gastric lumen and from perigastric lymphovascular pedicles during radical gastric cancer surgery. Ann Surg Oncol. 2011;18(10):2818–25. doi:10.1245/s10434-011-1620-8.
7. Kim W, Kim HH, Han SU, Kim MC, Hyung WJ, Ryu SW, Cho GS, Kim CY, Yang HK, Park DJ, Song KY, Lee SI, Ryu SY, Lee JH, Lee HJ. Korean Laparoendoscopic Gastrointestinal Surgery Study (KLASS) Group: decreased morbidity of laparoscopic distal gastrectomy compared with open distal gastrectomy for stage I gastric cancer: short-term outcomes from a multicenter randomized controlled trial (KLASS-01). Ann Surg. 2016;263(1):28–35.
8. Kitano S, Shiraishi N, Uyama I, Sugihara K, Tanigawa N. Japanese Laparoscopic Surgery Study Group: a multicenter study on oncologic outcome of laparoscopic gastrectomy for early cancer in Japan. Ann Surg. 2007;245:68–72.
9. Kim HH, Han SU, Kim MC, Hyung WJ, Kim W, Lee HJ, Ryu SW, Cho GS, Song KY, Ryu SY. Long-term results of laparoscopic gastrectomy for gastric cancer: a large-scale case-control and case-matched Korean multicenter study. J Clin Oncol. 2014; 32(7):627–33.
10. Sakuramoto S, Kikuchi S, Futawatari N, Moriya H, Katada N, Yamashita K, Watanabe M. Technique of esophagojejunostomy using transoral placement of the pretilted anvil head after laparoscopic gastrectomy for gastric cancer. Surgery. 2010;147:742–7.
11. Nagai E, Ohuchida K, Nakata K, Miyasaka Y, Maeyama R, Toma H, Shimizu S, Tanaka M. Feasibility and safety of intracorporeal esophagojejunostomy after laparoscopic total gastrectomy: inverted T-shaped anastomosis using linear staplers. Surgery. 2013; 153(5):732–8.
12. Haverkamp L, Weijs TJ, van der Sluis PC, van der Tweel I, Ruurda JP, van Hillegersberg R. Laparoscopic total gastrectomy versus open total gastrectomy for cancer: a systematic review and meta-analysis. Surg Endosc. 2013;27(5):1509–20. doi:10.1007/s00464-012-2661-1.
13. Jeong GA, Cho GS, Kim HH, Lee HJ, Ryu SW, Song KY. Laparoscopy-assisted total gastrectomy for gastric cancer: a multicenter retrospective analysis. Surgery. 2009;146:469–74.
14. Japanese Gastric Cancer Association. Japanese gastric cancer treatment guidelines 2010 (ver. 3). Gastric Cancer. 2011;14:113–23.
15. Kong SH, Kim JW, Lee HJ, Kim WH, Lee KU, Yang HK. The safety of the dissection of lymph node stations 5 and 6 in pylorus-preserving gastrectomy. Ann Surg Oncol. 2009;16(12):3252–8.
16. Park DJ, Lee HJ, Jung HC, Kim WH, Lee KU, Yang HK. Clinical outcome of pylorus-preserving gastrectomy in gastric cancer in comparison with conventional distal gastrectomy with Billroth I anastomosis. World J Surg. 2008;32:1029–36.
17. Jiang X, Hiki N, Nunobe S, Fukunaga T, Kumagai K, Nohara K, Sano T, Yamaguchi T. Postoperative outcomes and complications after laparoscopy-assisted pylorus-preserving gastrectomy for early gastric cancer. Ann Surg. 2011;253:928–33.
18. Suh YS, Han DS, Kong SH, Kwon S, Shin CI, Kim WH, Kim HH, Lee HJ, Yang HK. Laparoscopy-assisted pylorus-preserving gastrectomy is better than laparoscopy-assisted distal gastrectomy for middle-third early gastric cancer. Ann Surg. 2014; 259(3):485–93.
19. Qiu J, Pankaj P, Jiang H, Zeng Y, Wu H. Laparoscopy versus open distal gastrectomy for advanced gastric cancer: a systematic review and meta-analysis. Surg Laparosc Endosc Percutan Tech. 2013;23:1–7.
20. Hur H, Lee HY, Lee HJ, Kim MC, Hyung WJ, Park YK, Kim W, Han SU. Efficacy of laparoscopic subtotal gastrectomy with D2 lymphadenectomy for locally advanced gastric cancer: the protocol of the KLASS-02 multicenter randomized controlled clinical trial. BMC Cancer. 2015;15:355.
21. Hu Y, Huang C, Sun Y, Su X, Cao H, Hu J, Xue Y, Suo J, Tao K, He X, Wei H, Ying M, Hu W, Du X, Chen P, Liu H, Zheng C, Liu F, Yu J, Li Z, Zhao G, Chen X, Wang K, Li P, Xing J, Li G. Morbidity and mortality of laparoscopic versus open D2 distal gastrectomy for advanced gastric cancer: a randomized controlled trial. J Clin Oncol. 2016;34(12):1350–7.

22. Kodera Y, Fujiwara M, Ohashi N, Nakayama G, Koike M, Morita S, Nakao A. Laparoscopic surgery for gastric cancer: a collective review with meta-analysis of randomized trials. J Am Coll Surg. 2010;211:677–86.
23. Kitano S, Yang HK, editors. Textbook: Laparoscopic gastrectomy for cancer. Tokyo: Springer; 2012.
24. Diana M, Marescaux J. Robotic surgery. Br J Surg. 2015;102(2):e15–28. doi:10.1002/bjs.9711.
25. Alemozaffar M, Sanda M, Yecies D, Mucci LA, Stampfer MJ, Kenfield SA. Benchmarks for operative outcomes of robotic and open radical prostatectomy: results from the Health Professionals Follow-up Study. Eur Urol. 2015;67(3):432–8. doi:10.1016/j.eururo.2014.01.039.
26. Han DS, Suh YS, Ahn HS, Kong SH, Lee HJ, Kim WH, Yang HK. Comparison of surgical outcomes of robot-assisted and laparoscopy-assisted pylorus-preserving gastrectomy for gastric cancer: a propensity score matching analysis. Ann Surg Oncol. 2015;22(7):2323–8. doi:10.1245/s10434-014-4204-6.
27. Yang JY, Son YG, Kim TH, Park JH, Huh YJ, Suh YS, Kong SH, Lee HJ, Kim S, Yang HK. Manual ambidexterity predicts robotic surgical proficiency. J Laparoendosc Adv Surg Tech A. 2015;25(12):1009–18. doi:10.1089/lap.2015.0288.
28. Uyama I, Kanaya S, Ishida Y, Inaba K, Suda K, Satoh S. Novel integrated robotic approach for suprapancreatic D2 nodal dissection for treating gastric cancer: technique and initial experience. World J Surg. 2012; 36(2):331–7. doi:10.1007/s00268-011-1352-8.
29. Park JY, Kim YW, Ryu KW, Eom BW, Yoon HM, Reim D. Emerging role of robot-assisted gastrectomy: analysis of consecutive 200 cases. J Gastric Cancer. 2013;13(4):255–62. doi:10.5230/jgc.2013.13.4.255.
30. Hoste G, Van Trappen P. Robotic hysterectomy using the Vessel Sealer for myomatous uteri: technique and clinical outcome. Eur J Obstet Gynecol Reprod Biol. 2015;194:241–4. doi:10.1016/j.ejogrb.2015.09.030.
31. Zhou J, Shi Y, Qian F, Tang B, Hao Y, Zhao Y, Yu P. Cumulative summation analysis of learning curve for robot-assisted gastrectomy in gastric cancer. J Surg Oncol. 2015;111(6):760–7. doi:10.1002/jso.23876.
32. Kim HI, Park MS, Song KJ, Woo Y, Hyung WJ. Rapid and safe learning of robotic gastrectomy for gastric cancer: multidimensional analysis in a comparison with laparoscopic gastrectomy. Eur J Surg Oncol. 2014;40(10):1346–54. doi:10.1016/j.ejso.2013.09.011.
33. Hyun MH, Lee CH, Kwon YJ, Cho SI, Jang YJ, Kim DH, Kim JH, Park SH, Mok YJ, Park SS. Robot versus laparoscopic gastrectomy for cancer by an experienced surgeon: comparisons of surgery, complications, and surgical stress. Ann Surg Oncol. 2013;20(4):1258–65. doi:10.1245/s10434-012-2679-6.
34. Woo Y, Hyung WJ, Pak KH, Inaba K, Obama K, Choi SH, Noh SH. Robotic gastrectomy as an oncologically sound alternative to laparoscopic resections for the treatment of early-stage gastric cancers. Arch Surg. 2011;146(9):1086–92. doi:10.1001/archsurg.2011.114.
35. Chuan L, Yan S, Pei-Wu Y. Meta-analysis of the short-term outcomes of robotic-assisted compared to laparoscopic gastrectomy. Minim Invasive Ther Allied Technol. 2015;24(3):127–34. doi:10.3109/13645706.2014.985685.
36. Wall J, Marescaux J. Robotic gastrectomy is safe and feasible, but real benefits remain elusive. Arch Surg. 2011;146(9):1092.
37. Kim HI, Han SU, Yang HK, Kim YW, Lee HJ, Ryu KW, Park JM, An JY, Kim MC, Park S, Song KY, Oh SJ, Kong SH, Suh BJ, Yang DH, Ha TK, Kim YN, Hyung WJ. Multicenter prospective comparative study of robotic versus laparoscopic gastrectomy for gastric adenocarcinoma. Ann Surg. 2016;263(1):103–9. doi:10.1097/sla.0000000000001249.
38. Suda K, Man IM, Ishida Y, Kawamura Y, Satoh S, Uyama I. Potential advantages of robotic radical gastrectomy for gastric adenocarcinoma in comparison with conventional laparoscopic approach: a single institutional retrospective comparative cohort study. Surg Endosc. 2015;29(3):673–85. doi:10.1007/s00464-014-3718-0.
39. Park JY, Ryu KW, Reim D, Eom BW, Yoon HM, Rho JY, Choi IJ, Kim YW. Robot-assisted gastrectomy for early gastric cancer: is it beneficial in viscerally obese patients compared to laparoscopic gastrectomy? World J Surg. 2015;39(7):1789–97. doi:10.1007/s00268-015-2998-4.
40. Park JM, Kim HI, Han SU, Yang HK, Kim YW, Lee HJ, An JY, Kim MC, Park S, Song KY, Oh SJ, Kong SH, Suh BJ, Yang DH, Ha TK, Hyung WJ, Ryu KW. Who may benefit from robotic gastrectomy?: a subgroup analysis of multicenter prospective comparative study data on robotic versus laparoscopic gastrectomy. Eur J Surg Oncol. 2016;42(12):1944–9. doi:10.1016/j.ejso.2016.07.012.
41. Lee J, Kim YM, Woo Y, Obama K, Noh SH, Hyung WJ. Robotic distal subtotal gastrectomy with D2 lymphadenectomy for gastric cancer patients with high body mass index: comparison with conventional laparoscopic distal subtotal gastrectomy with D2 lymphadenectomy. Surg Endosc. 2015;29(11):3251–60. doi:10.1007/s00464-015-4069-1.
42. Nakauchi M, Suda K, Susumu S, Kadoya S, Inaba K, Ishida Y, Uyama I. Comparison of the long-term outcomes of robotic radical gastrectomy for gastric cancer and conventional laparoscopic approach: a single institutional retrospective cohort study. Surg Endosc. 2016;30(12):5444–52. doi:10.1007/s00464-016-4904-z.

18 Minimally Invasive Treatment of Gastric GIST

Carlos Moreno-Sanz and Miguel A. Cuesta

18.1 Introduction

Gastrointestinal stromal tumours (GIST) form 5% of all gastrointestinal tumours and 40–60% of these are located in the stomach. GIST derive from the interstitial cells of Cajal [1] and constitute a separate entity from leiomyoma and leiomyosarcoma, which were previously thought to be the most common soft-tissue neoplasms in the gastrointestinal tract. Gastrointestinal stromal tumours are classified by molecular and immunohistological features and are characterized by overexpression of the tyrosine kinase receptor KIT. The criteria for differentiating benign from malignant gastric GISTs have been debated for several years. Tumour size and mitotic index, but not microscopic margins of resection, have been shown to be significant factors for predicting survival. Gastric GISTs that are smaller than 5 cm and have fewer than 5 mitoses per high-power field are considered to have low malignant potential. Tumours measuring 5–10 cm or having 5–10 mitoses per high-power field are considered intermediate risk, and those measuring greater than 10 cm or having more than 10 mitoses per high-power field are considering high risk [2]. Location and staging have been performed by a combination of endoscopy with detailed information about the exact location and size of the tumour, endoscopic ultrasonography and CT-scan.

The treatment of choice for primary non-metastatic gastric GIST is complete surgical resection; performing a complete bloc resection (R0) of the tumour and surrounding tissue.

The advent and improvement of endoscopic linear stapling devices have facilitated the laparoscopic approach to the point where laparoscopic partial resection by means of wedge resection or segmental resection of the stomach without lymphadenectomy forms the recommended standard treatment for gastric GIST. An important review of 50 laparoscopically treated patients has demonstrated a 92% disease-free long-term survival—despite an average tumour size of 4.4 cm (range, 1.0–8.5 cm); thereby supporting not only the technical feasibility of laparoscopic resection, but also its efficacy [3].

Moreover, in our experience, the laparoscopic approach has not been necessarily limited by

Electronic Supplementary Material The online version of this chapter (doi:10.1007/978-3-319-54301-7_18) contains supplementary material, which is available to authorized users. On http://springerlink.com enter the DOI number given above.

C. Moreno-Sanz (✉)
Department of General and Digestive Surgery, Hospital General La Mancha Centro, Alcazar de San Juan, Ciudad Real, Spain
e-mail: cmsurgery@hotmail.com

M.A. Cuesta
VUmc, Amsterdam, The Netherlands
e-mail: ma.cuesta@vumc.nl

M.A. Cuesta (ed.), *Minimally Invasive Surgery for Upper Abdominal Cancer*,
DOI 10.1007/978-3-319-54301-7_18

tumour size, as previously suggested by the GIST Consensus Conference [4]. Although previous authors have recommended limiting the application of their approach to tumours smaller than 2.5–4 cm, we were able to perform the procedure successfully with larger tumours (up to 10 cm) while still achieving negative margins in all cases with low morbidity and no compromise of oncologic principles [5].

Various Minimally Invasive Techniques can be used to approach GIST, such as endoscopic resection, atypical gastric resections (wedge), standard gastric resections and combination techniques involving endoscopic guided laparoscopic resection or laparoscopic guided endoscopic resection. When there is suspicion of a gastric GIST, the first rule is to consider the size of the tumour. For very small tumours (<1 cm) it is possible—regardless of the location of the tumour—to combine the endoscopic approach with laparoscopic support. Whereas for tumours with a size >1 cm, we can combine the laparoscopic approach with endoscopic support.

Potential combinations of procedures for resecting gastric GIST tumours:

1. EAWR (endoscopically assisted wedge resection). The endoscopist controls whether the surgeon has placed the stapler at the proper place and done so without tumour manipulation. The surgeon can simultaneously see the endoscopy [6].
2. The non-touch lifting method: the tumour can be lifted by sutures before applying the stapler [7].
3. Laparoscopically assisted endoscopic resection (LAER) being useful for small intragastric lesions. The endoscopist performs the submucosal resection while the surgeon assists in manipulating the tumour and if necessary in suturing the caused perforation [8].
4. Laparoscopic and Endoscopic Cooperative Surgery (LECS) by Hiki et al. The procedure starts with an endoscopic submucosal dissection around the tumour followed by a laparoscopic resection at the proper place. Defect is closed by suturing or by linear stapler [9].
5. The CLEAN-NET technique as modification of the LECS in which the submucosal dissection is avoided [10].
6. EATR (endoscopically assisted transgastric resection). The laparoscopic trocars are inserted directly in an insufflated stomach under endoscopic guidance. Lesion can be directly dissected, resected and the gastric opening sutured [11].

Using all necessary information, a proper surgical strategy can be devised. The goal is knowing how to resect the GIST in a specific location with a determined size. Although the technical effectiveness of laparoscopic resection has been demonstrated, an attempt to standardize the approach of laparoscopic resection of gastric GIST based on the location of the tumour is meaningful, as demonstrated here.

Regarding the gastric location of the GIST, we need to take into account the anterior and posterior walls of the stomach and the two curvatures, thereby allowing us to differentiate and classify these in three zones:

Zone A: Tumour localized from yuxtacardial area along the lesser curvature (1/3 medial anterior and 2/3 posterior wall of gastric body) (Fig. 18.1).

In all locations of this zone, and when the size of the tumour is limited, we prefer applying the trans-gastric laparoscopic approach (with endoscopic guidance) so that the tumour can be identified by an anterior gastrostomy, lifted with a suture and resected. In tumours located in this area in the anterior wall of the stomach, a EAWR technique should be proposed. This procedure allows complete resection of the tumour without compromise to the gastric inlet. In special cases in which the size and extension of the tumour require such, a proximal gastrectomy or an transhiatal esophagogastrectomy will be performed. Moreover, this procedure is a much more technically demanding procedure, requiring advanced laparoscopic skills. Finally, it is technically possible to place intragastric trocar-ports to perform laparoscopic transgastric resection in order to avoid the gastrostomy (EATR technique).

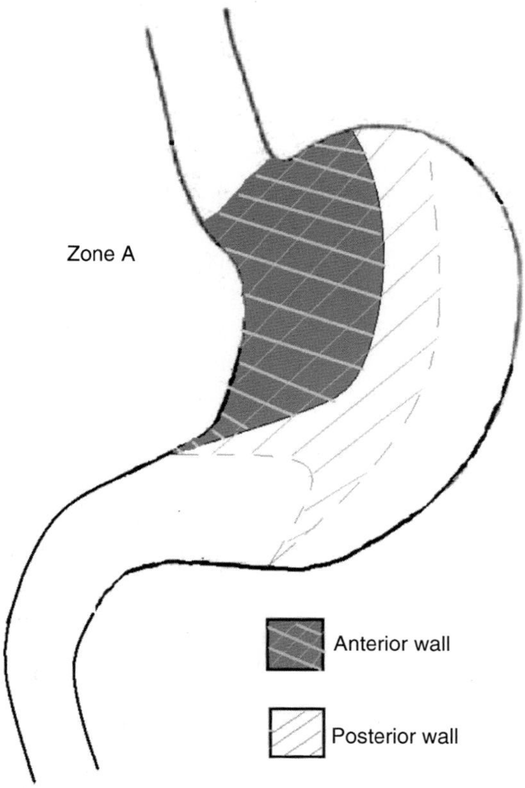

Fig. 18.1 Zone A, tumor localized from yuxtacardial area along the lesser curvature (1/3 medial anterior and 2/3 posterior wall of gastric body)

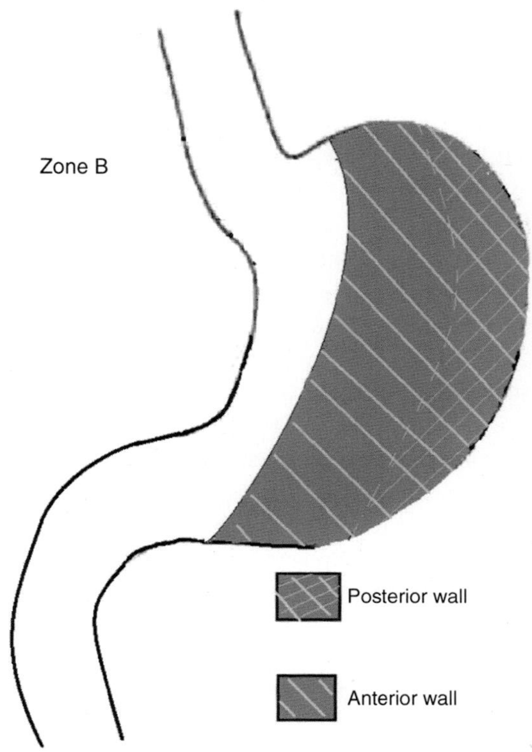

Fig. 18.2 Zone B. Tumor localized in the 2/3 anterior and 1/3 posterior wall of fundus and corpus along greater curvature

Zone B: Tumour localized in the 2/3 anterior and 1/3 posterior wall of fundus and corpus along greater curvature (Fig. 18.2).

After endoscopic localization and an adequate mobilization of the greater curvature, doing a stapled transection under simultaneous endoscopic guidance (EAWR technique) is a safe and effective technique—thanks to the extreme mobility of the stomach in this zone.

Zone C: Tumour localized in the anterior and posterior wall of antrum and prepyloric region (Fig. 18.3).

Stapled wedge resection is often difficult to realize due to the risk of gastric outlet-narrowing. When treating small tumours (and early gastric cancer) in this area, some authors propose using the transgastric approach with a submucosal resection (LECS or CLEAN-NET techniques) or even a wedge resection if located along the greater curvature. For larger tumours we prefer a distal gastrectomy, which precludes the possibility of

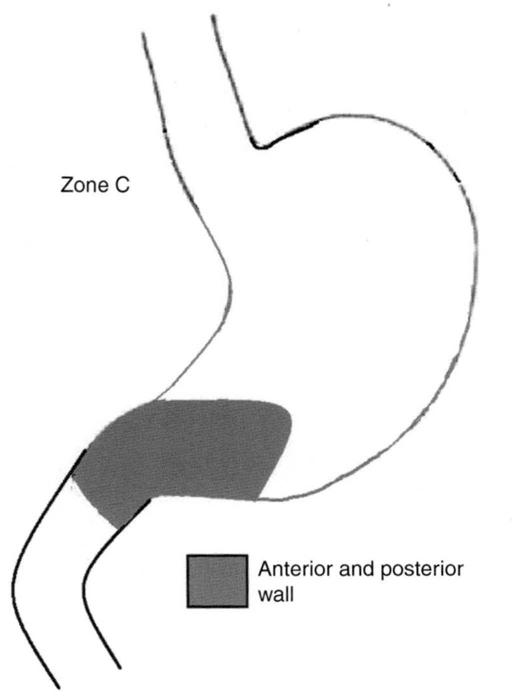

Fig. 18.3 Tumor localized in the anterior and posterior wall of antrum and prepyloric area

outlet obstruction and that can be performed laparoscopically with relative ease.

18.2 Own Series

From November 2002 to November 2016, 43 patients underwent laparoscopic treatment for gastric GIST. There were 21 men and 22 women with a mean age of 56.2 ± 6.2 years (range: 22–76 years). Main presenting symptoms are summarized in Table 18.1.

No patient received preoperative treatment with imatinib. Surgical procedures are summarized in Table 18.2. The mean operative times was 147 min (range 60–290 min). There were no postoperative complications III–V according to Clavien-Dindo.

In all patients GIST was confirmed by pathological examination, showing all of them low grade malignant potential except five with intermediate risk and six with high risk of recurrence according to Fletcher's classification. Pathologic margins were microscopically negative for all the patients. Six patients underwent treatment with imatinib due to high risk of recurrence. Patients have planned follow-up assessment with surveillance imaging every 6 months for a 2 year period, then yearly thereafter. The follow-up period for all the patients ranged from 6 month to 14 years.

To date, there has been one distant recurrence on the liver in one patient with a high risk tumor that did not complete the adjuvant treatment due to imatinib toxicity. This patient underwent a metastectomy of the liver.

Conclusion

The exact location and size of resectable non-metastasized gastric GIST are important factors when devising a laparoscopic strategy. Also by taking into account that the stomach can be divided into three zones in which a resection strategy should be accordingly performed. Special difficult zones are at locations A and C where an adequate strategy should be establish, according to size and location, to avoid narrowing of the esophago-gastric or gastric outlet. In small tumors combined treatments with the gastroenterologist is indicated.

It is our experience with more than 43 patients operated in this way, the standardized laparoscopic approach for gastric GIST tumours can be deemed as safe (Videos 18.1 and 18.2).

Table 18.1 Main presenting symptoms

Symptoms	
Anemia	30%
Abdominal pain	30%
Dysphagia	20%
Gastroesophageal reflux	20%
Active gastrointestinal bleeding	10%
Dyspepsia	10%

Table 18.2 Surgical procedures

Zone	Patients	Size (cm)	Wedge resection	Transgastric resection	Gastrectomy	Length of stay (days)
A	13	5 (2–10)	–	10	3	4.6 (3–9)
B	18	5.2 (2.5–14)	16	–	2	3.5 (3–6)
C	12	5 (1–10)	3	–	9	6.5 (3–8)

References

1. Min KW. Gastrointestinal stromal tumour: an ultrastructural investigation on regional differences with considerations on their histogenesis. Ultrastruct Pathol. 2010;34:174–88.
2. Fletcher CD, Berman JJ, Corless C, et al. Diagnosis of gastrointestinal stromal tumors: a consensus approach. Hum Pathol. 2002;33(5):459–65.
3. Bedard EL, Mamazza J, Schlachta CM, Poulin EC. Laparoscopic resection of gastrointestinal stromal tumors: not all tumors are created equal. Surg Endosc. 2006;20:500–3.
4. Blay JY, Bonvalot S, Casali P, Choi H, Debiec-Richter M, Dei Tos AP, Emile JF, Gronchi A, Hogendoorn PC, Joensuu H, Le Cesne A, McClure J, Maurel J, Nupponen N, Ray-Coquard I, Reichardt P, Sciot R, Stroobants S, van Glabbeke M, van Oosterom A, Demetri GD. GIST consensus meeting panelists. Consensus meeting for the management of gastrointestinal stromal tumors. Report of the GIST Consensus Conference of 20–21 March 2004, under the auspices of ESMO. Ann Oncol. 2005;16:566–78.
5. Takahasi T, Nakajima K, Miyazaki Y. Surgical strategy for the gastric gastrointestinal stromal tumors (GISTs) larger than 5 cm: laparoscopic surgery is feasible, safe and oncologically acceptable. Surg Laparosc Endosc Percutan Tech. 2015;25:114–8.
6. Ismael H, Ragoza Y, Caccitolo J, Cox S. Optimal management of GIST tumors located near the gastroesophageal junction: case report and review of the literature. Int J Surg Case Rep. 2016;25:91–6.
7. Kiyozaki H, Saito M, Chiba H. Laparoscopioc wedge resection of the stomach for gastrointestinal stromal tumor (GIST): non touch lesion lifting method. Gastric Cancer. 2014;17:337–40.
8. Wilhelm D, Delius V, Burian M. Simultaneous use of laparoscopy and endoscopy for minimally invasive resection of gastric subepithelial masses-analysis of 93 interventions. World J Surg. 2008;32:1021–8.
9. Hiki N, Yamamoto Y, Fukunaga T. Laparoscopic and endoscopic cooperative surgery for gastrointestinal tumour dissection. Surg Endosc. 2007;22:1729–35.
10. Kato M, Uraoka T, Isobe Y. A case of gastric adenocarcinoma of fundic gland type resected by combination of laparoscopic and endoscopic approaches to neoplasia with non-exposure technique (CLEAN-NET). Clin J Gastroenterol. 2015;8:393–9.
11. Gayer C, Edelman D, Curtis B. Combined endoscopic and laparoscopic approach to Gastroesophageal tumour. JSLS. 2011;15:228–31.

19 Minimally Invasive Gastrectomy Step by Step: How I Do It

Antonio Talvane Torres de Oliveira, Croider Franco Lacerda, Paulo A. Bertulucci, and Miguel A. Cuesta

19.1 Step by Step: Laparoscopic Total Gastrectomy (Video 19.1)

1. Positioning of patient and placement of trocars (Fig. 19.1)
2. Dissection of greater omentum from transverse colon from the middle to the left. Division of the left gastroepiploic vessels and short vessels up to the right crus of the hiatus (Figs. 19.2, 19.3, 19.4, and 19.5)
3. Dissection of the greater omentum to the right up to hepatic flexure
4. Dissection of the right gastroepiploic vessels, lymphadenectomy (station 6) and division of the vessels at the level of the pancreas (Figs. 19.6, 19.7, and 19.8)
5. Opening of the hepatoduodenal ligament (in the length). Lymphadenectomy of the common and proper hepatic artery (stations 8a and 12a), and division of the right gastric artery (Figs. 19.9, 19.10, 19.11, 19.12, and 19.13)
6. Dissection of proximal duodenum and division by stapler (Figs. 19.14 and 19.15)
7. Retraction of the stomach to the left

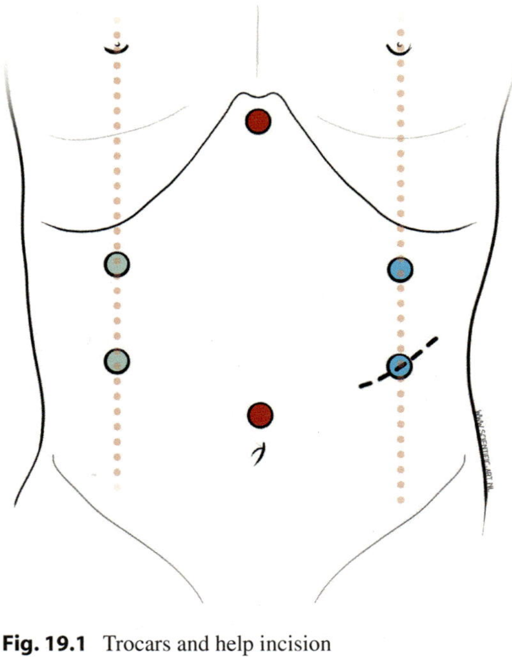

Fig. 19.1 Trocars and help incision

Electronic Supplementary Material The online version of this chapter (doi:10.1007/978-3-319-54301-7_19) contains supplementary material, which is available to authorized users. On http://springerlink.com enter the DOI number given above.

A.T.T. de Oliveira • C.F. Lacerda • P.A. Bertulucci
Department of Upper GI Surgery, Americas Medical City Hospital, Rio de Janeiro, Brazil

M.A. Cuesta (✉)
Emeritus professor, VUmc, Amsterdam, The Netherlands
e-mail: ma.cuesta@vumc.nl

M.A. Cuesta (ed.), *Minimally Invasive Surgery for Upper Abdominal Cancer*, DOI 10.1007/978-3-319-54301-7_19

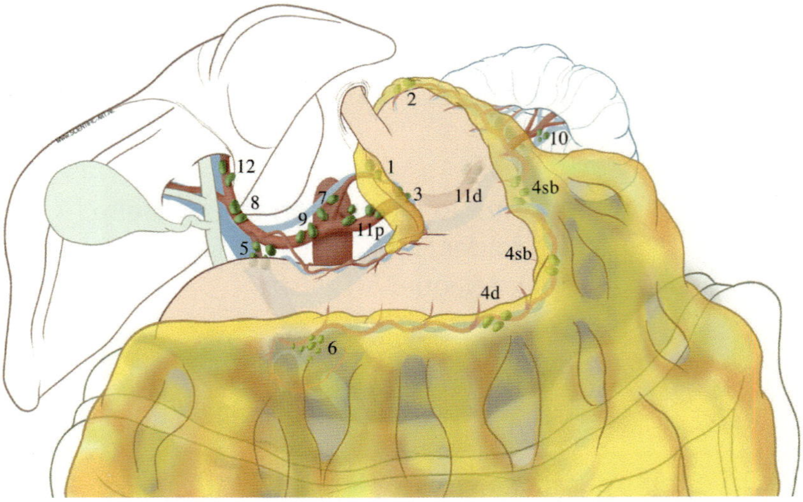

Fig. 19.2 Operative field with lymph node stations

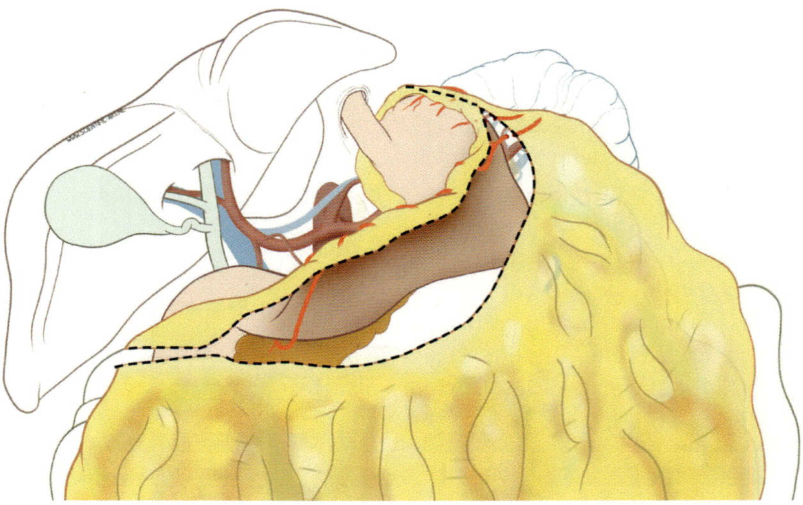

Fig. 19.3 Omentectomy in total gastrectomy

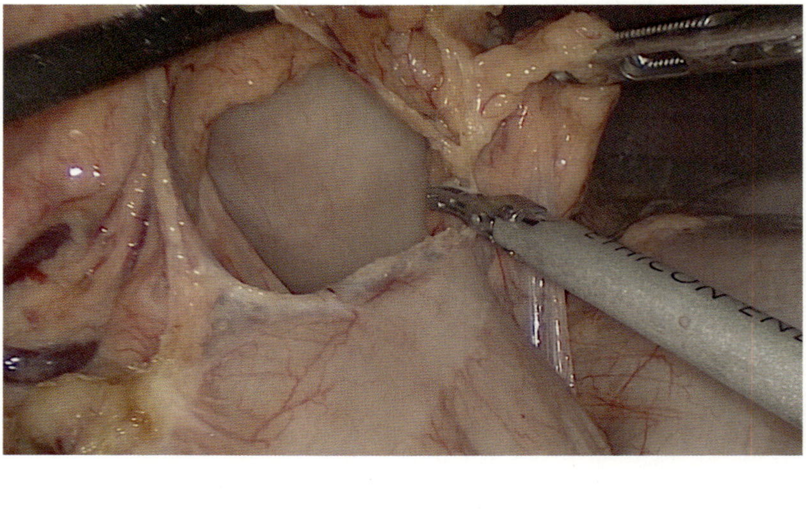

Fig. 19.4 Omentectomy

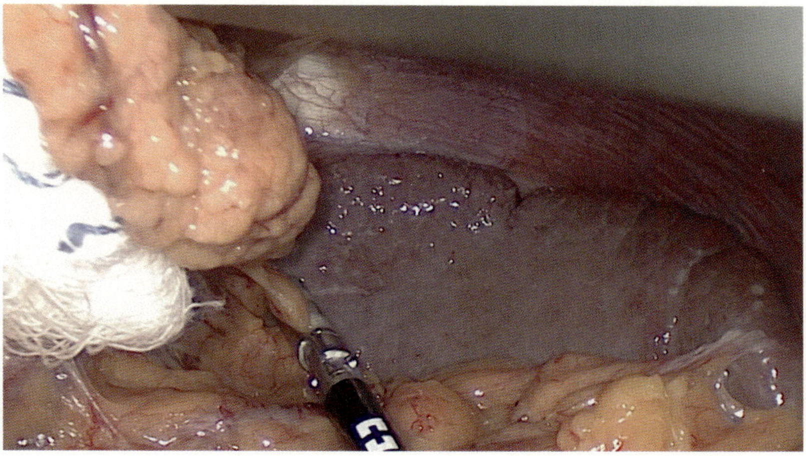

Fig. 19.5 Section of the short vessels

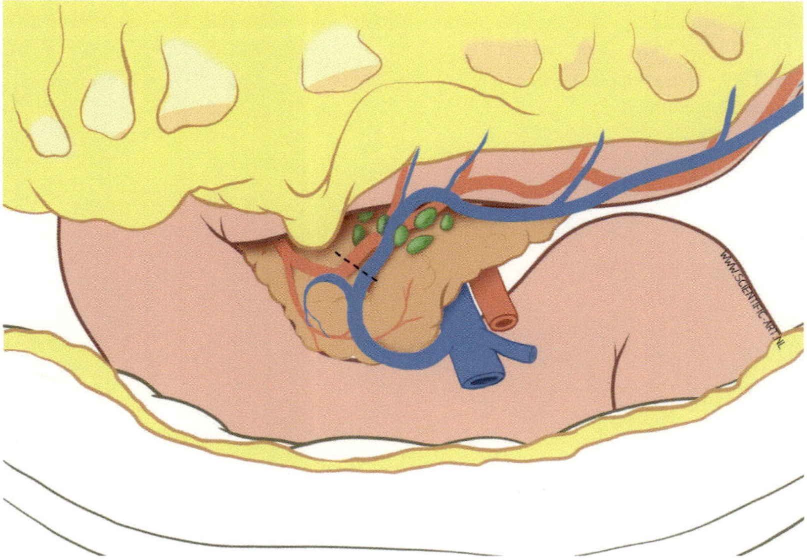

Fig. 19.6 Right gastroepiploic vessels dissection

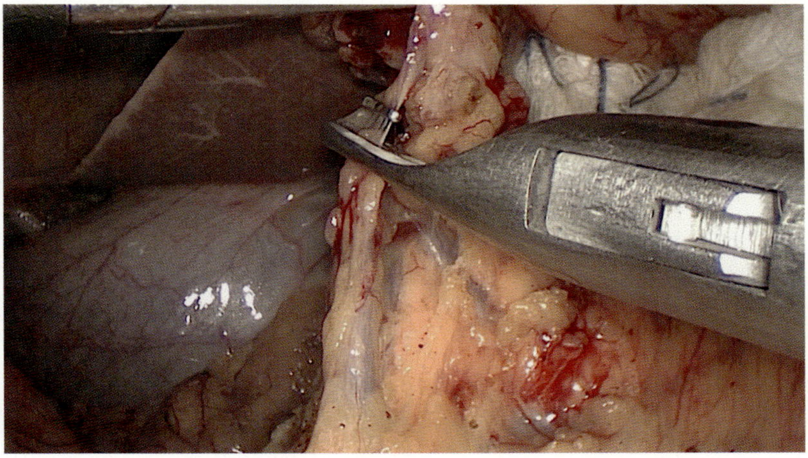

Fig. 19.7 Dissection of the right gastroepiploic vein

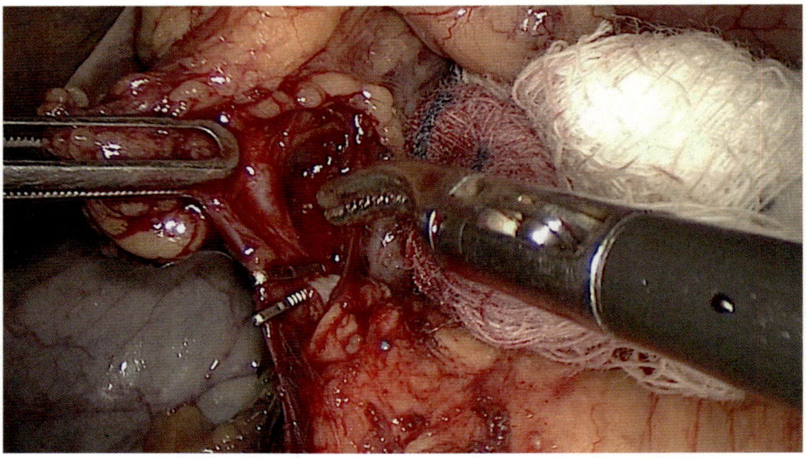

Fig. 19.8 Lymphadenectomy station 6

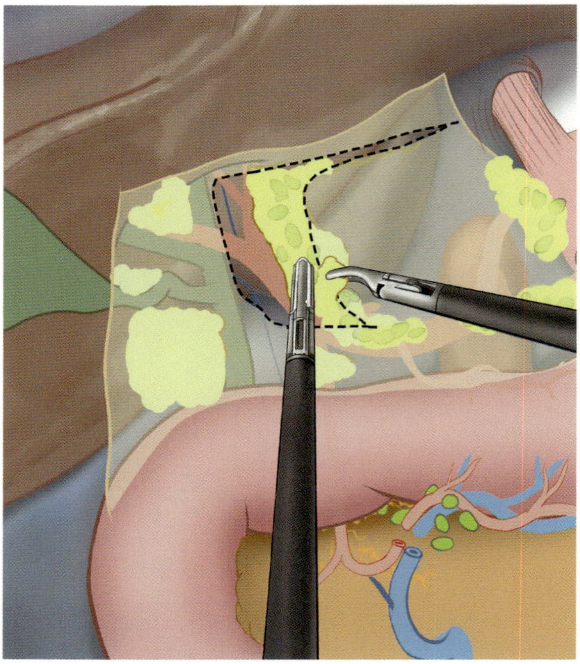

Fig. 19.9 Hepatoduodenal ligament lymphadenectomy

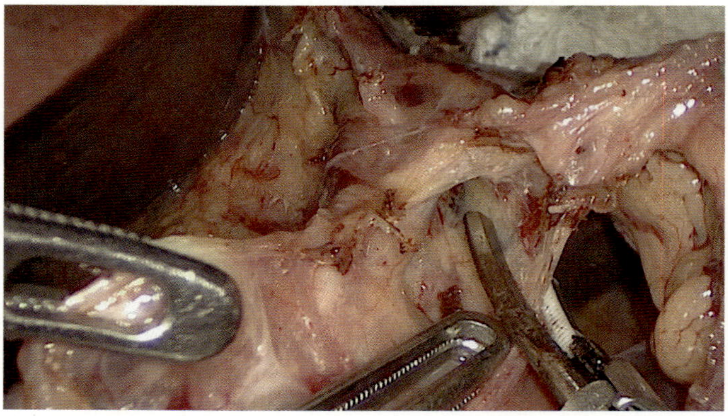

Fig. 19.10 Hepatoduodenal ligament dissection

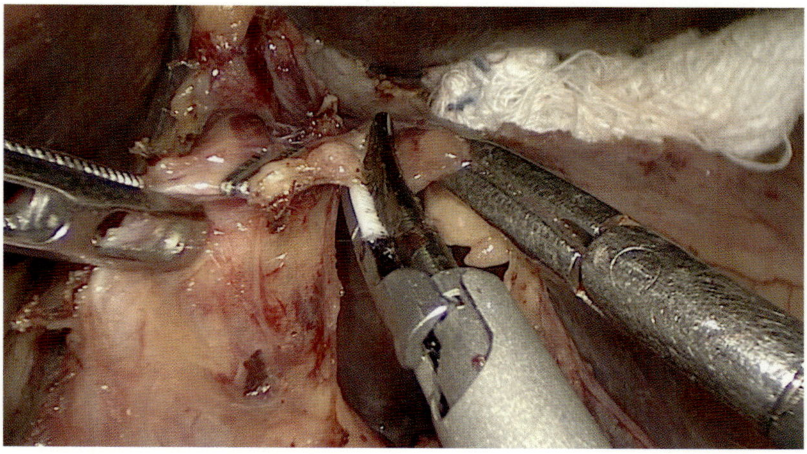

Fig. 19.11 Division right gastric artery

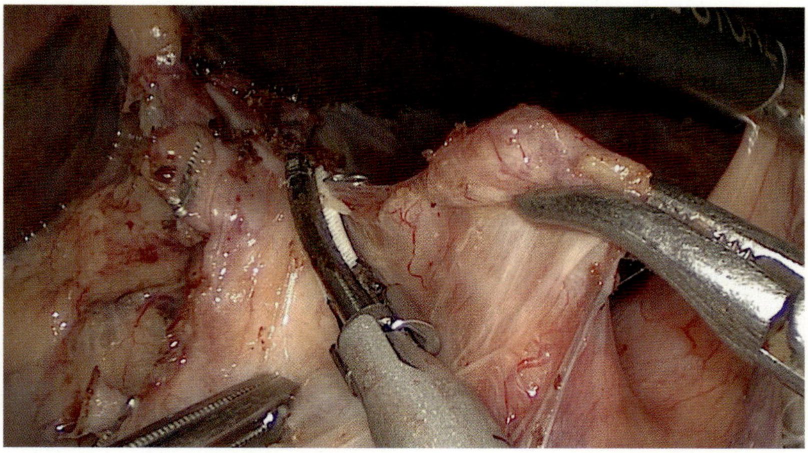

Fig. 19.12 Lymphadenectomy station 8a

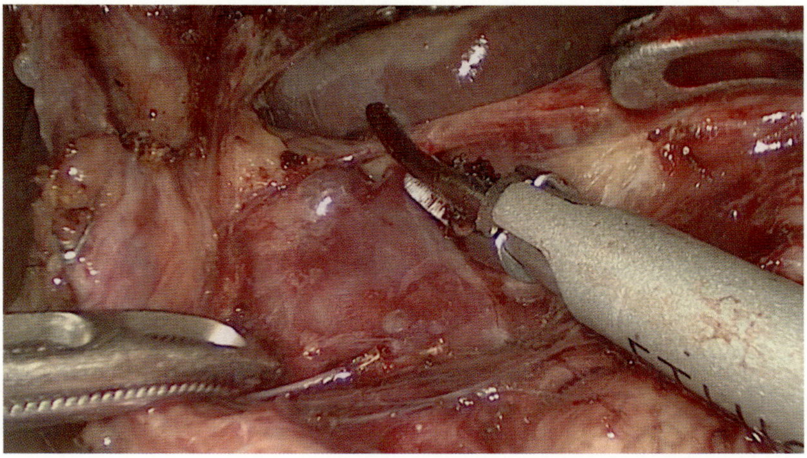

Fig. 19.13 Lymphadenectomy station 12a along portal vein

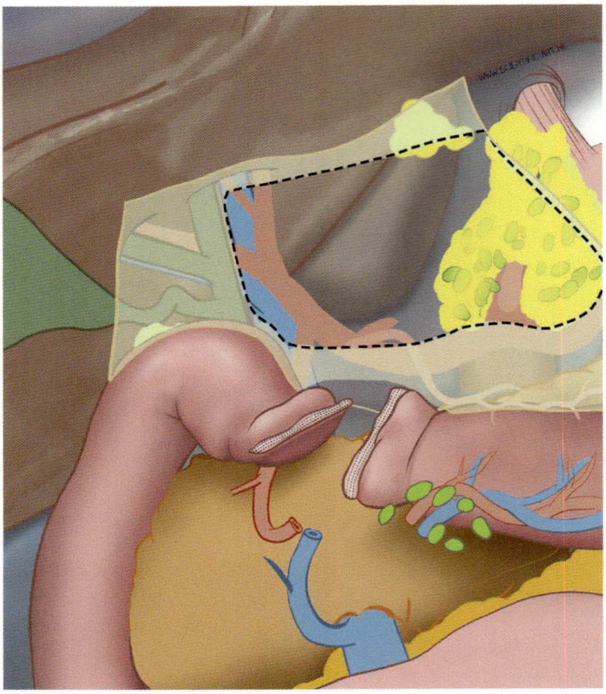

Fig. 19.14 Division duodenum by staplers

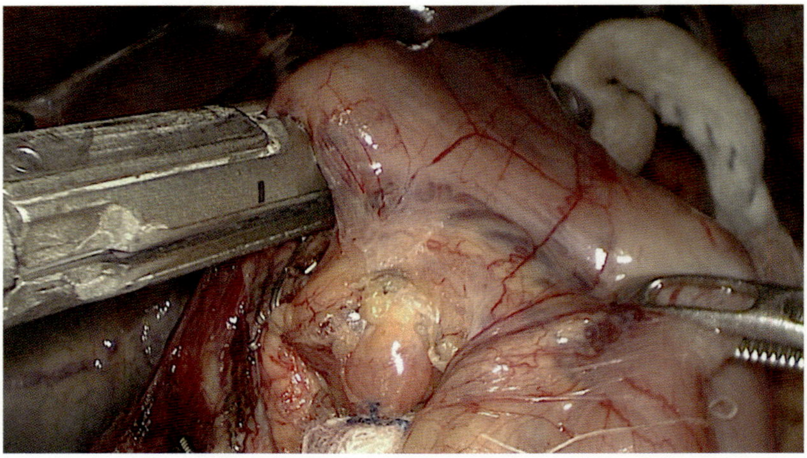

Fig. 19.15 Division of duodenum

8. Continuing the lymphadenectomy of the celiac trunk, left gastric vein and artery and along the proximal splenic artery (groups 9, 7 and 11p). Division of the left gastric vein and artery (Figs. 19.16, 19.17, and 19.18)
9. Continuing the dissection from here to the hiatus where the esophagus is dissected free and divided at the proper level by stapler and prepared for any type of anastomosis (Figs. 19.19, 19.20, 19.21, and 19.22)
10. Lymphadenectomy of groups 11d and 10 (Figs. 19.23 and 19.24)
11. Operative field before reconstruction (Figs. 19.25, 19.26, and 19.27)

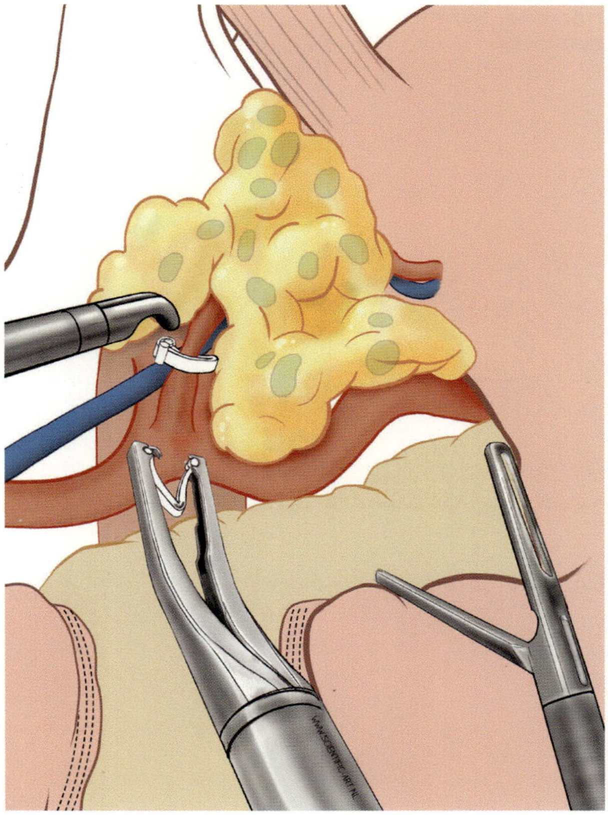

Fig. 19.16 Lymphadenectomy celiac trunk and division of left gastric artery

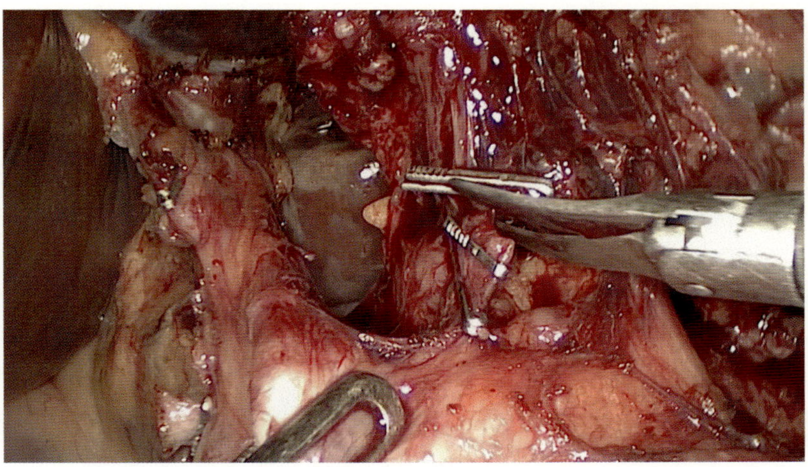

Fig. 19.17 Lymphadenectomy stations 7, 9 and 11p

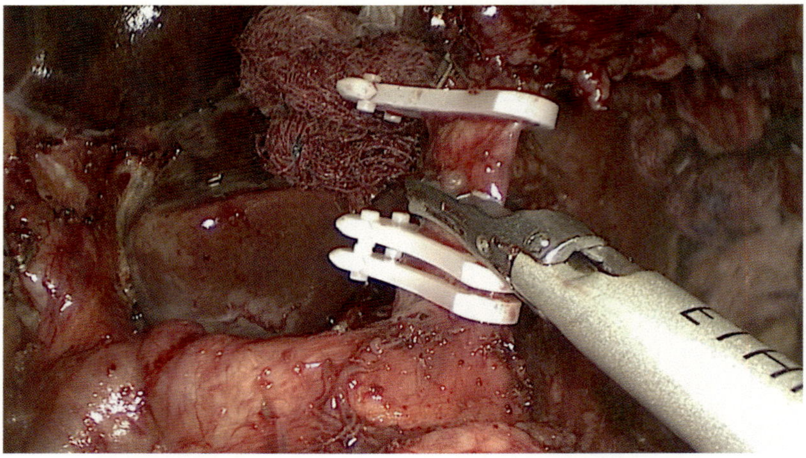

Fig. 19.18 Division left gastric artery

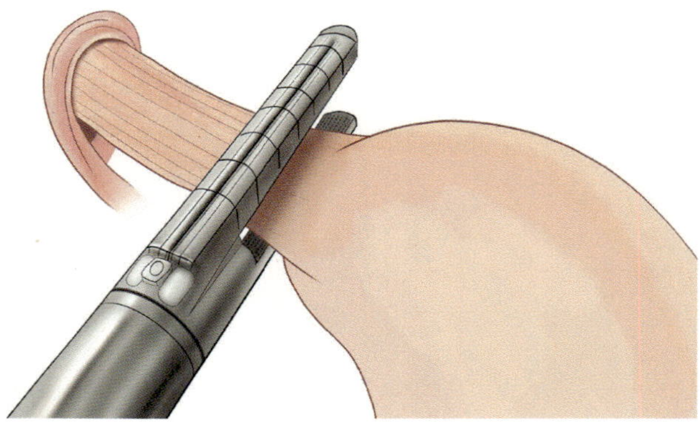

Fig. 19.19 Division distal esophagus

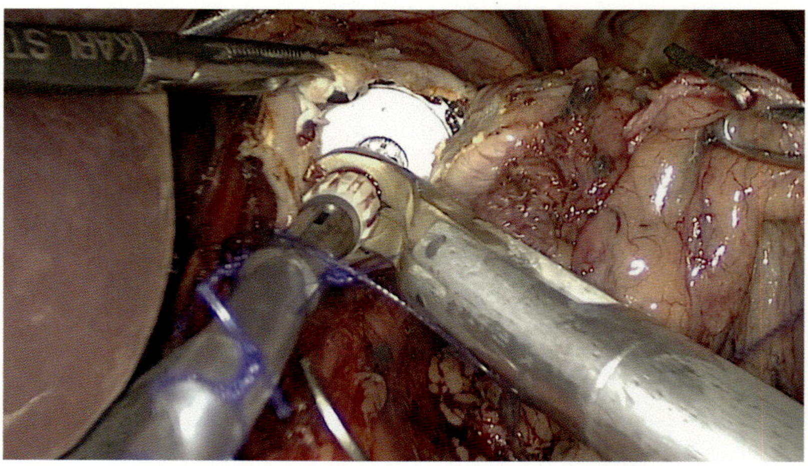

Fig. 19.20 Introduction anvil in the esophagus

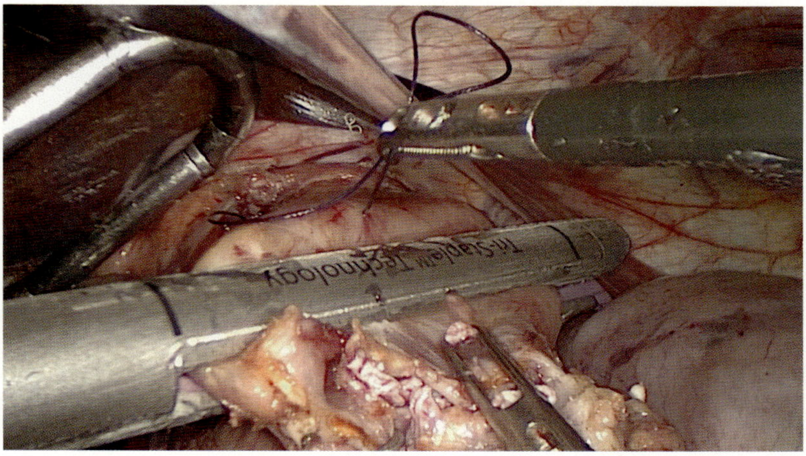

Fig. 19.21 Division of esophagus

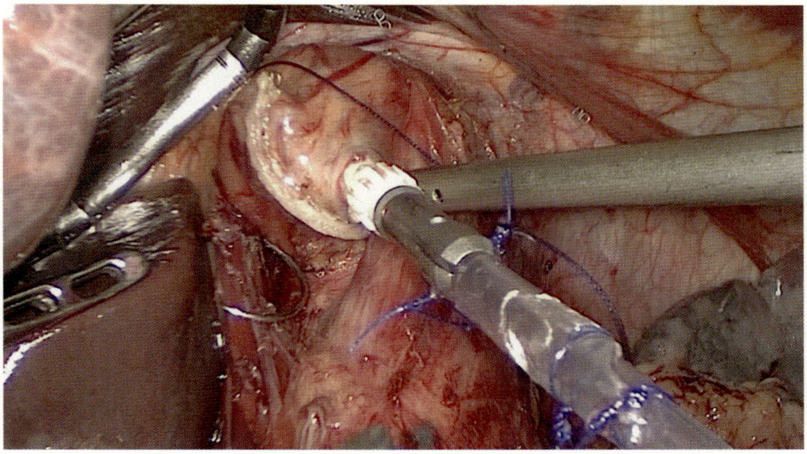

Fig. 19.22 Anvil in place

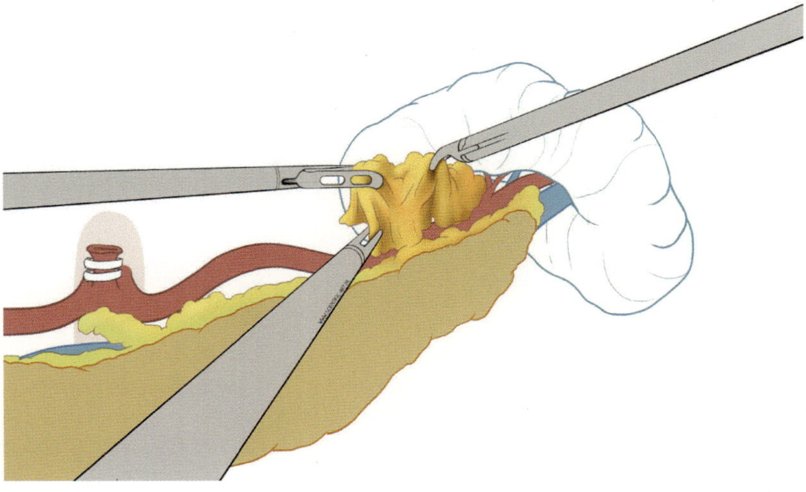

Fig. 19.23 Lymphadenectomy along splenic artery

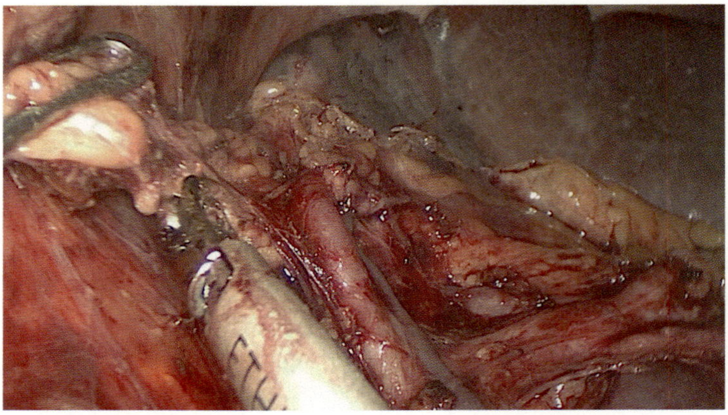

Fig. 19.24 Lymphadenectomy stations 11d and 10

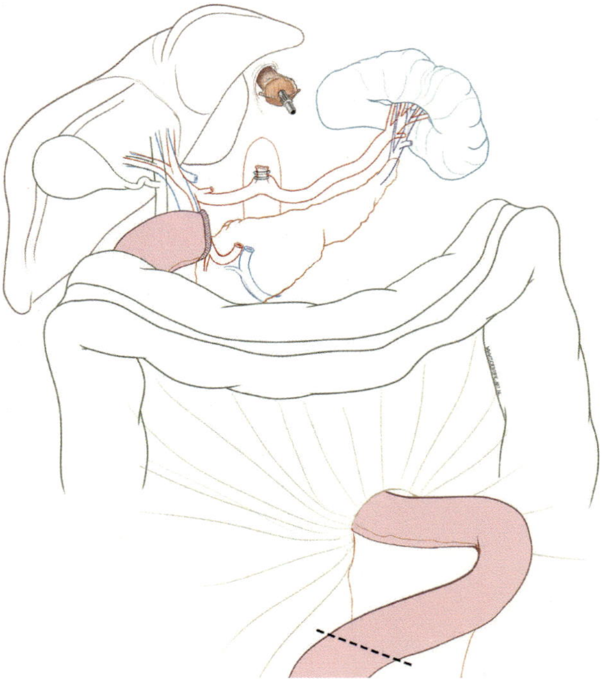

Fig. 19.25 Operative field after total gastrectomy

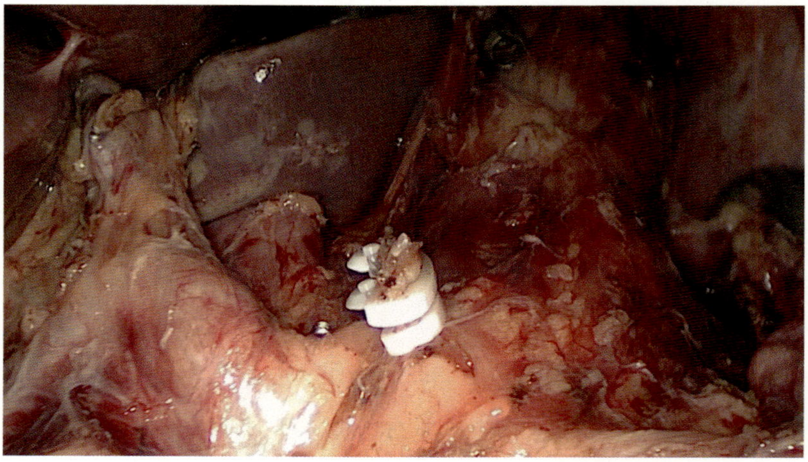

Fig. 19.26 General view lymphadenectomy hepatoduodenal ligament and celiac trunk

12. Opening a hole in the mesocolon. Dividing the proximal jejunum by stapler and placing the distal part through the mesocolon
13. Opening de jejunum and introducing the circular stapler 25 mm
14. End-to-side esophago-jejunostomy (Figs. 19.28, 19.29, 19.30, and 19.31)
15. Side-to-side jejuno-jejunostomy by stapler and closure of the opening (Figs. 19.32, 19.33, and 19.34)
16. Final situation after reconstruction (Fig. 19.35)
17. Retrieval of the specimen
18. Placing of drains

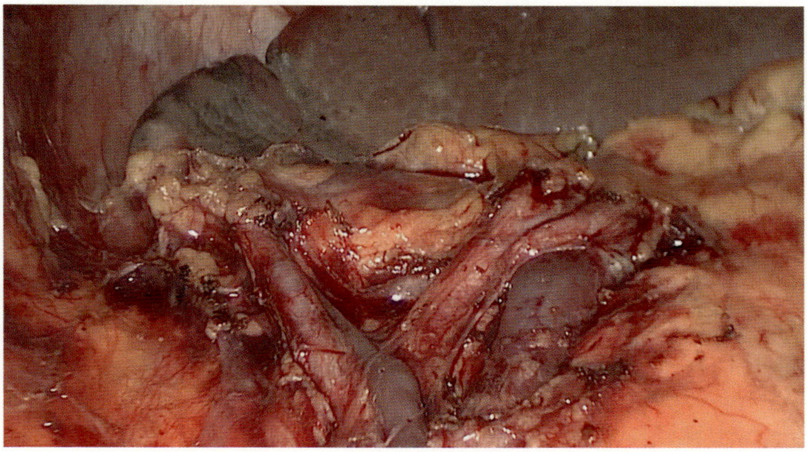

Fig. 19.27 View of lymphadenectomy splenic hilum

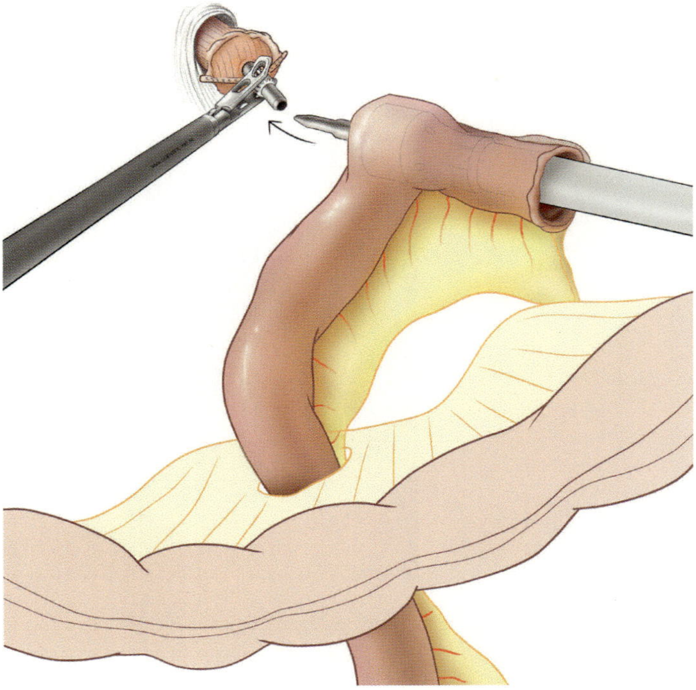

Fig. 19.28 End-to-side esophago-jejunostomy

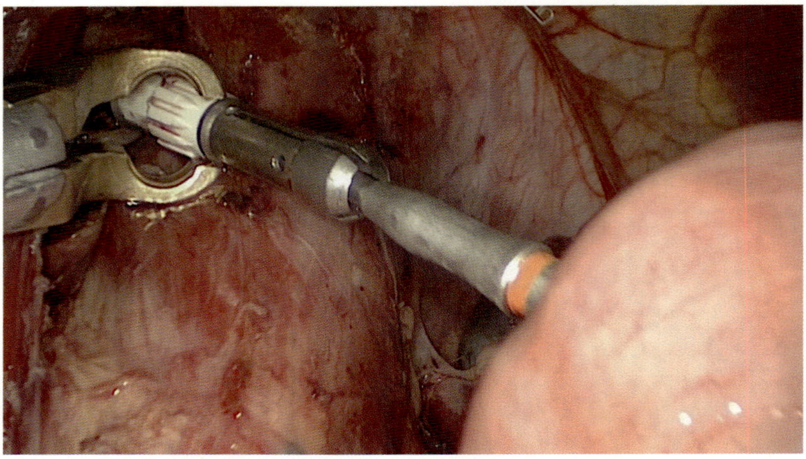

Fig. 19.29 Esophago-jejunostomy 1

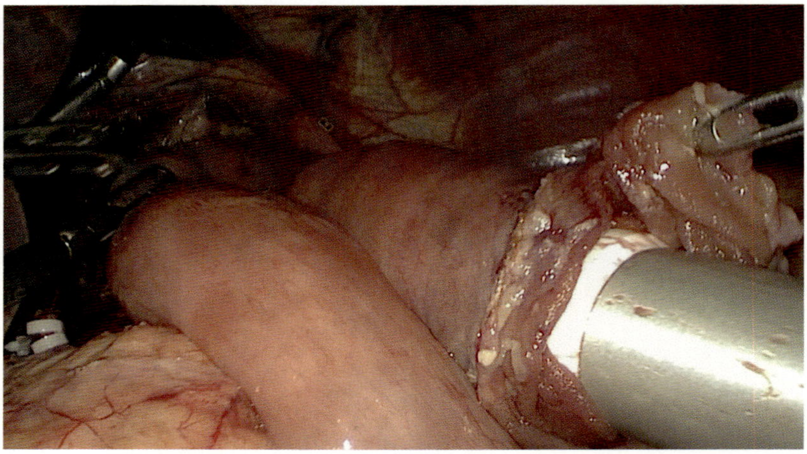

Fig. 19.30 Esophago-jejunostomy 2

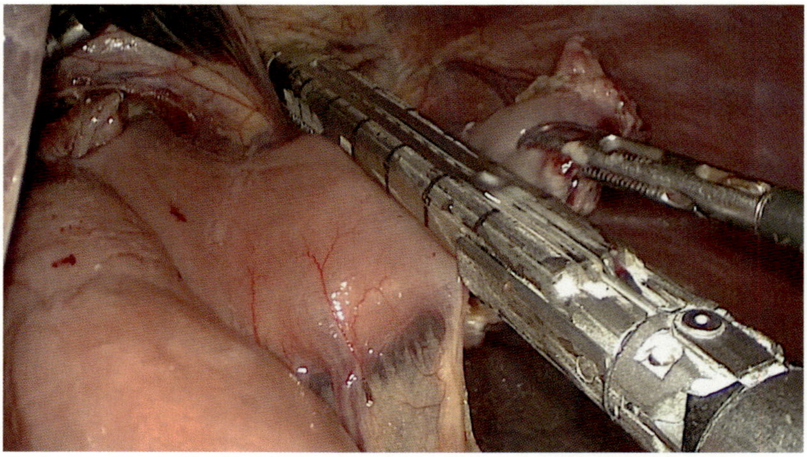

Fig. 19.31 Resection of lateral jejunum loop

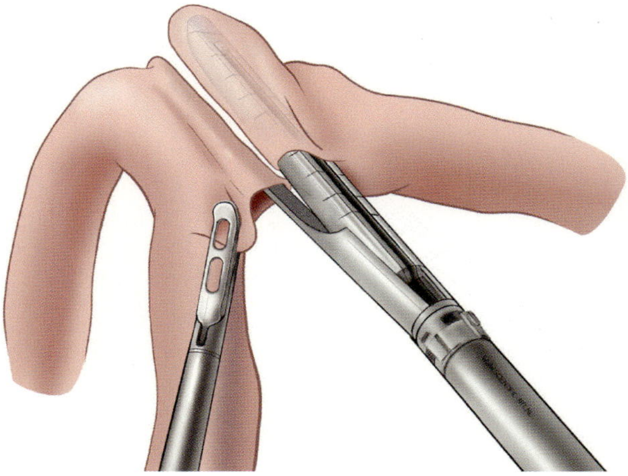

Fig. 19.32 Side-to-side jejuno-jejunostomy

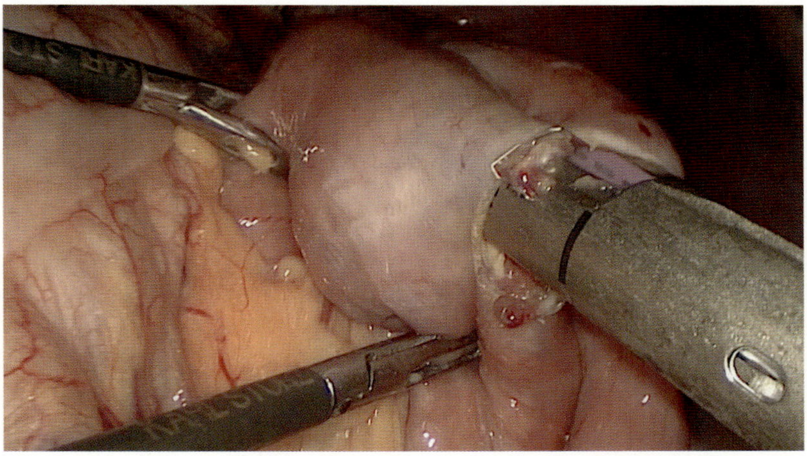

Fig. 19.33 Jejuno-jejunostomy

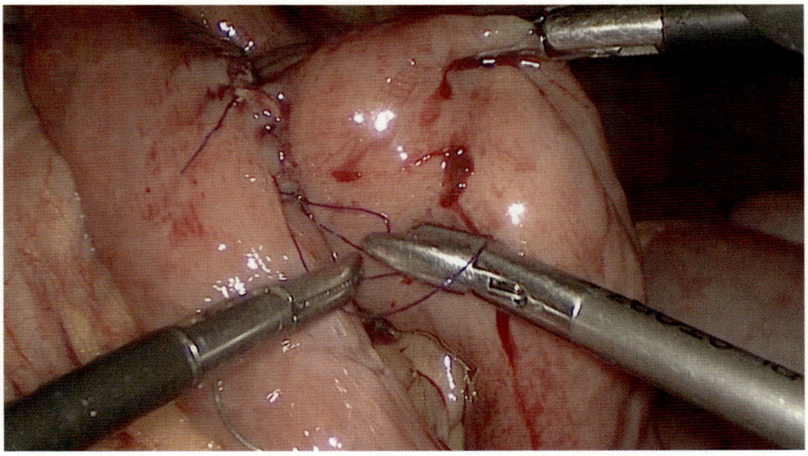

Fig. 19.34 Closure of defect after jejuno-jejunostomy

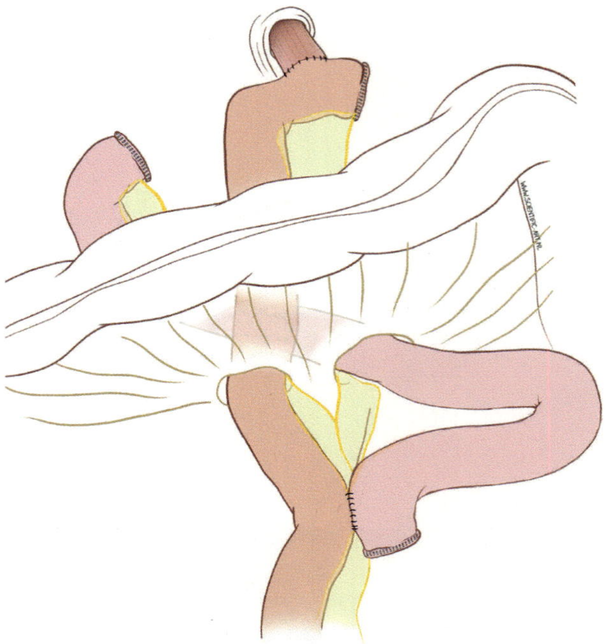

Fig. 19.35 Final view after reconstruction

19.2 Step by Step: Laparoscopic Subtotal Gastrectomy (Video 19.2)

1. Positioning of patient and placement of trocars (Fig. 19.36)
2. Omentectomy from the transverse colon to the left up to the level of the gastric resection (Figs. 19.37, 19.38, and 19.39). Lymphadenectomy station 4sb (Fig. 19.40)
3. Dissection of omentum to the right up to hepatic flexure
4. Dissection, lymphadenectomy and division of the right gastroepiploic vessels at the level of the pancreas (station 6) (Fig. 19.41)
5. Dissection of the common hepatic artery and lymphadenectomy of stations 8a and 12a in the hepatoduodenal ligament along the portal vein. Ligation of the right gastric artery (Figs. 19.42 and 19.43)
6. Dissection and division of the proximal duodenum by staplers (Fig. 19.44)
7. Lymphadenectomy along the celiac trunk, left gastric vein (Fig. 19.45) and artery (with division of the vein and artery). Lymphadenectomy along the splenic artery (stations 7, 9 and 11p) (Figs. 19.46, 19.47, 19.48, 19.49, and 19.50)
8. Lymphadenectomy along the lesser curvature from the esophagus up to the level of gastric resection (stations 1 and 3) (Figs. 19.51 and 19.52). This lymph nodes are included in the specimen.
9. Division of the stomach at the proper level by staplers (from left to right) (Figs. 19.53, 19.54, and 19.55)
10. Opening a hole in the mesocolon
11. Division of a loop of the proximal jejunum (Fig. 19.56)
12. Distal jejunum up through mesocolon hole (Fig. 19.57)

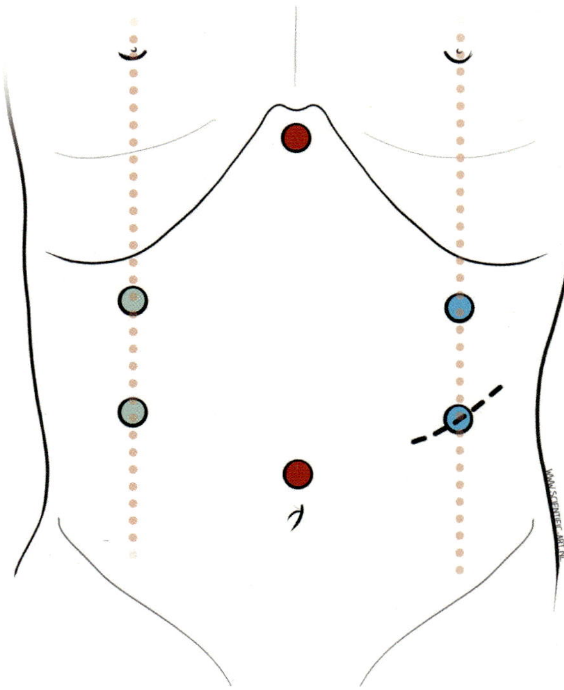

Fig. 19.36 Trocars and help incision in subtotal gastrectomy

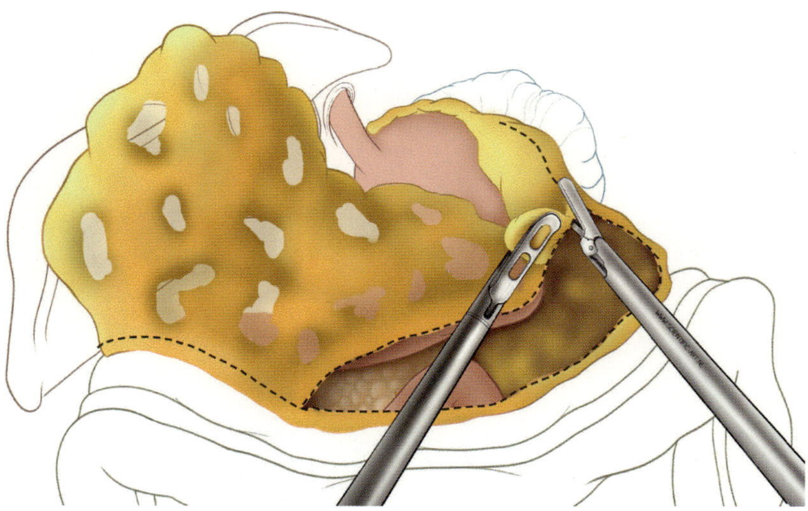

Fig. 19.37 Omentectomy in subtotal gastrectomy

13. Side-to-side gastro-jejunostomy by longitudinal stapler from the right followed by closure of the defect (Figs. 19.58, 19.59, 19.60, and 19.61)
14. Side-to-side jejuno-jejunostomy anastomosis by stapler followed by closure of the defect (Figs. 19.62 and 19.63)
15. Placing this anastomosis at the inframesocolic level and fixing it to the mesocolon (Fig. 19.64)
16. Retrieval of specimen
17. Placing of drains

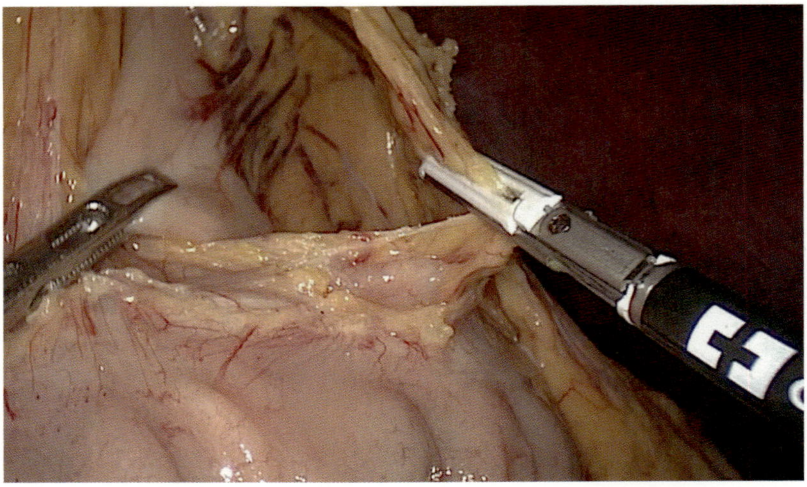

Fig. 19.38 Omentectomy

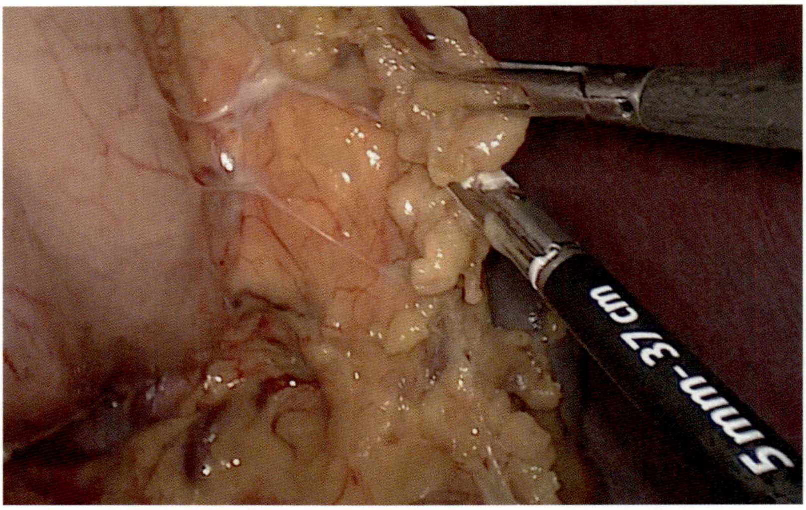

Fig. 19.39 Dissection of omentum up to short gastric vessels

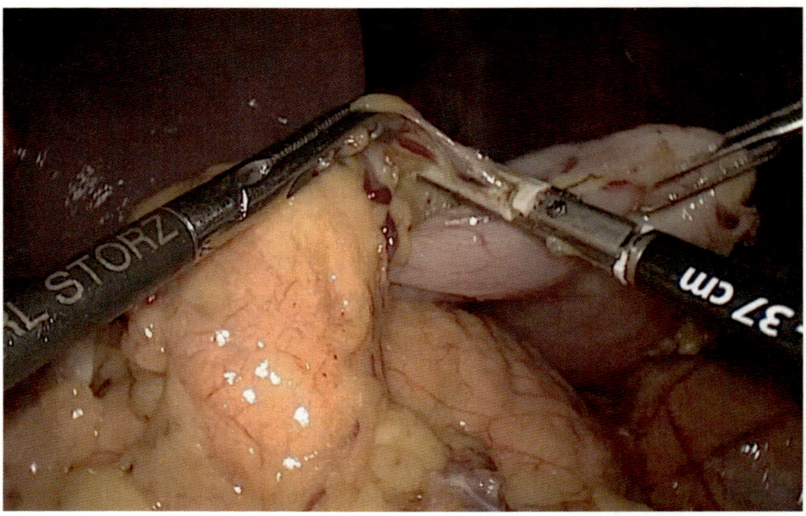

Fig. 19.40 Lymphadenectomy 4sb

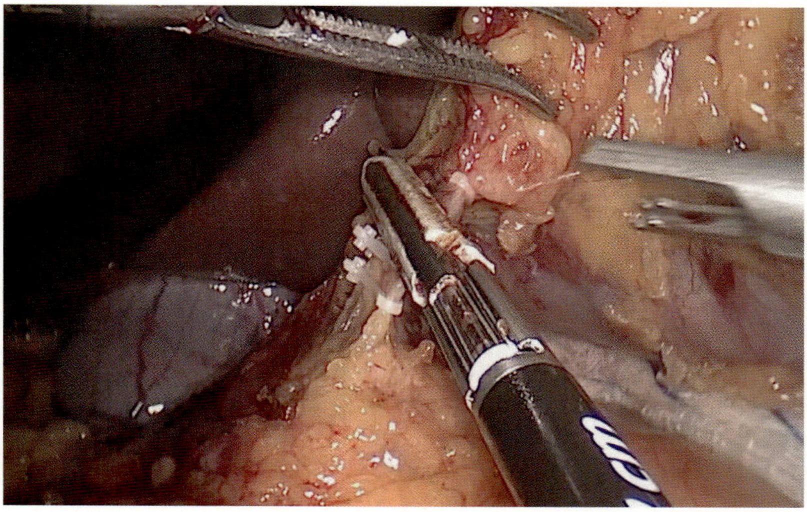

Fig. 19.41 Lymphadenectomy station 6

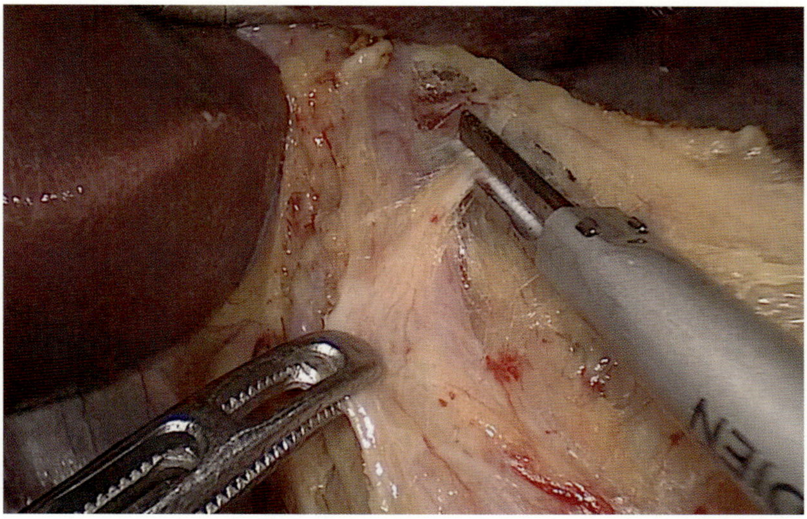

Fig. 19.42 Dissection hepatoduodenal ligament

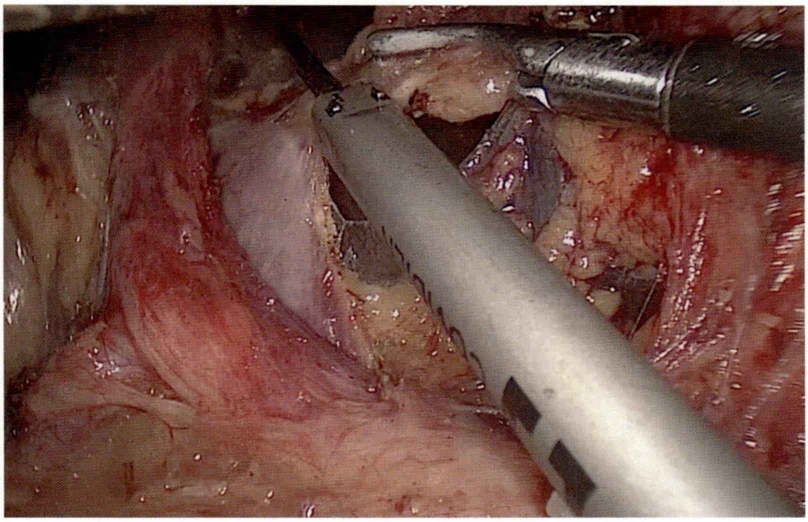

Fig. 19.43 Lymphadenectomy stations 8a and 12a

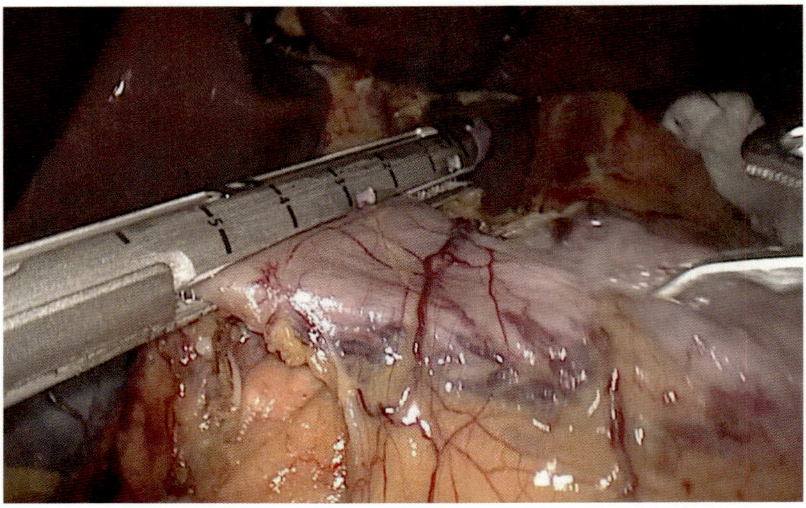

Fig. 19.44 Section duodenum

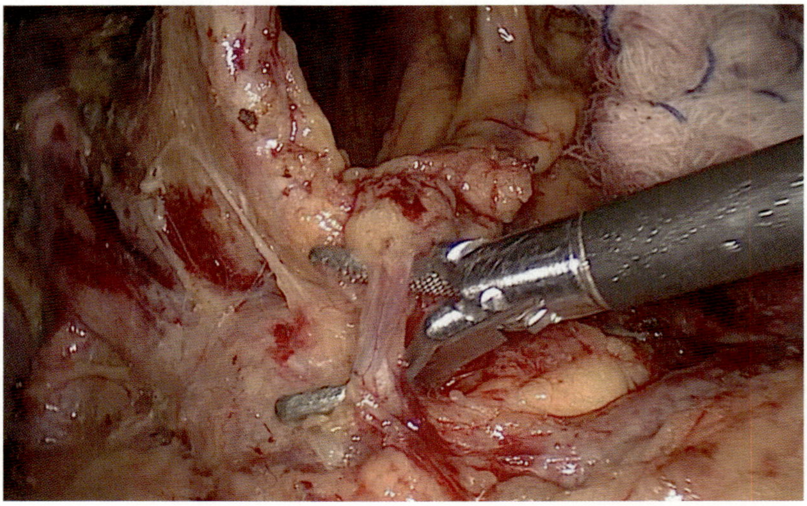

Fig. 19.45 Dissection right gastric vein

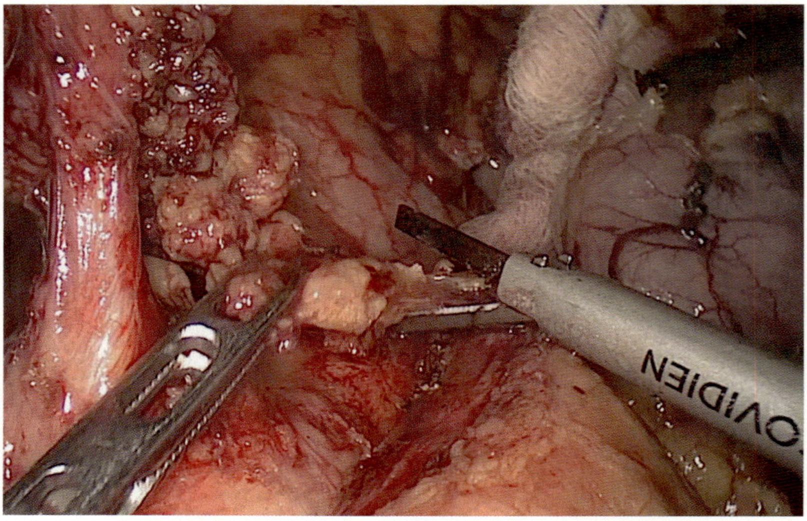

Fig. 19.46 Lymphadenectomy stations 7, 9 and 11p

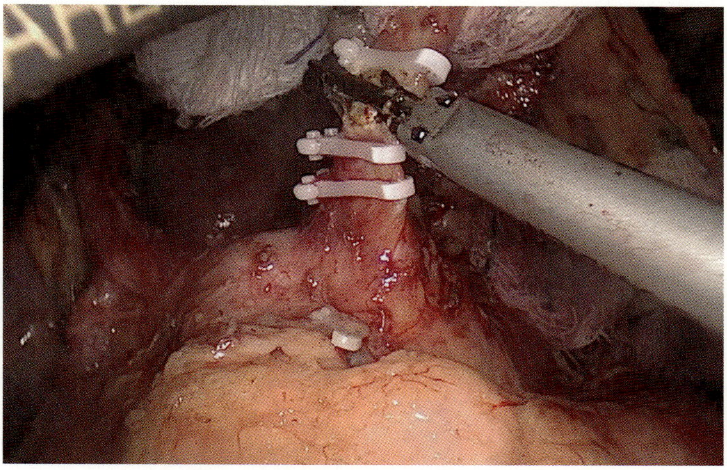

Fig. 19.47 Division left gastric artery

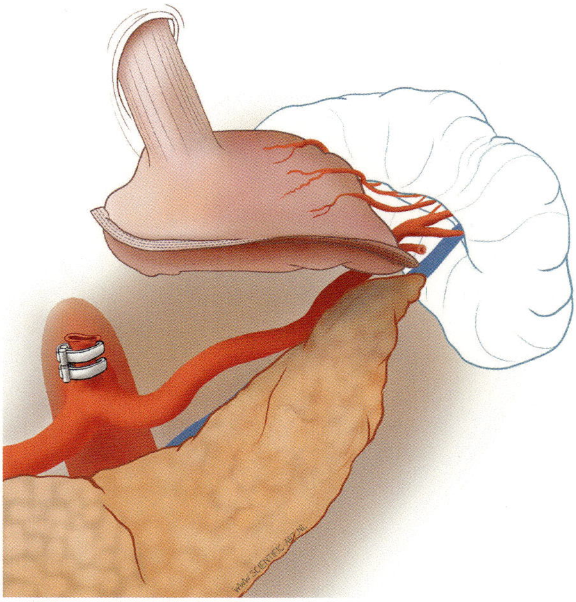

Fig. 19.48 D2 lymphadenectomy stations of celiac trunk and along the splenic artery

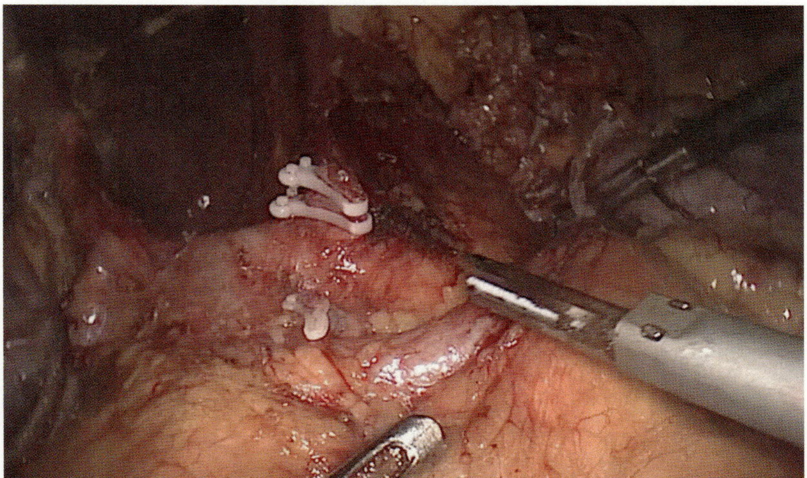

Fig. 19.49 General view lymphadenectomy celiac trunk

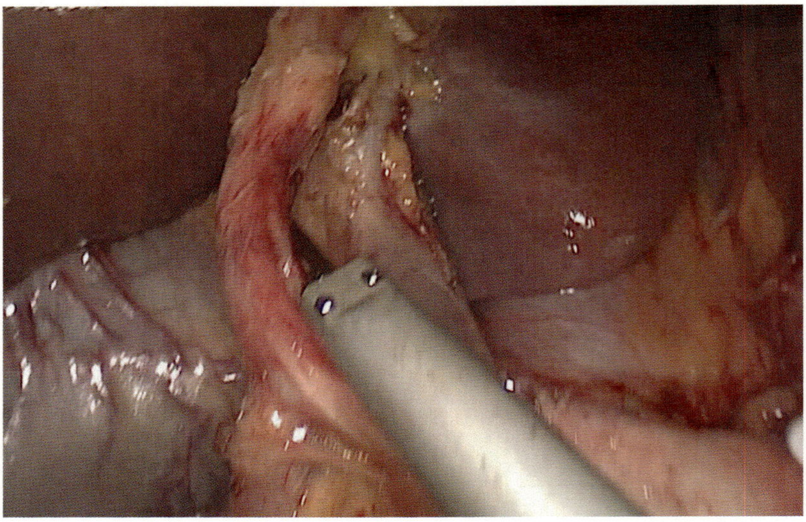

Fig. 19.50 View lymphadenectomy hepatoduodenal ligament

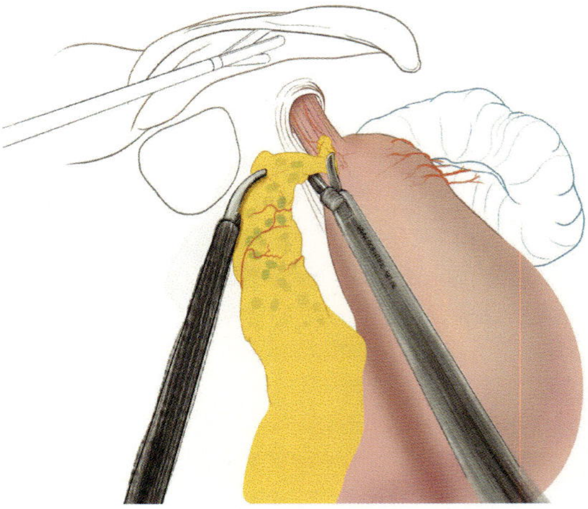

Fig. 19.51 Lymphadenectomy stations 1 and 3

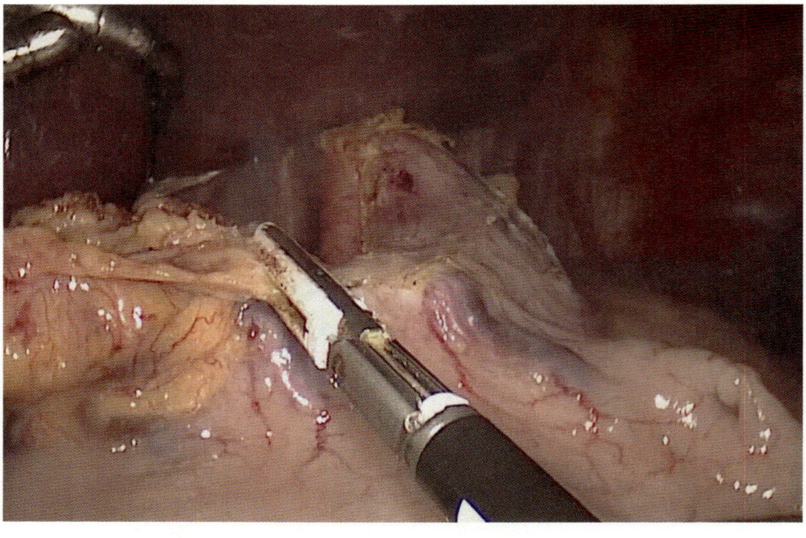

Fig. 19.52 Lymphadenectomy stations 1 and 3 along small gastric curvature

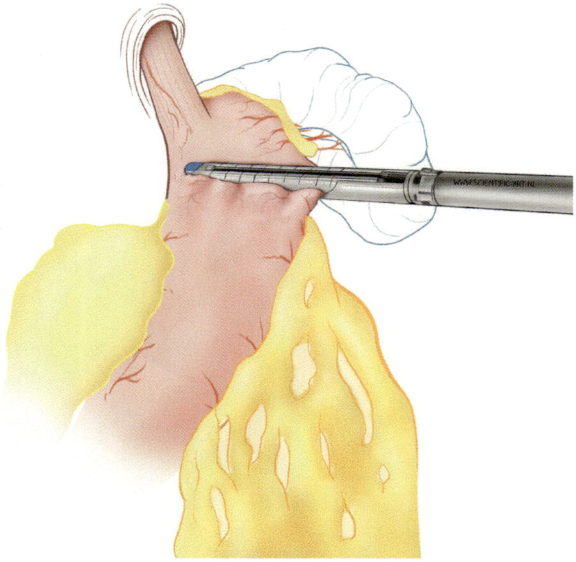

Fig. 19.53 Division of the proximal stomach by staplers

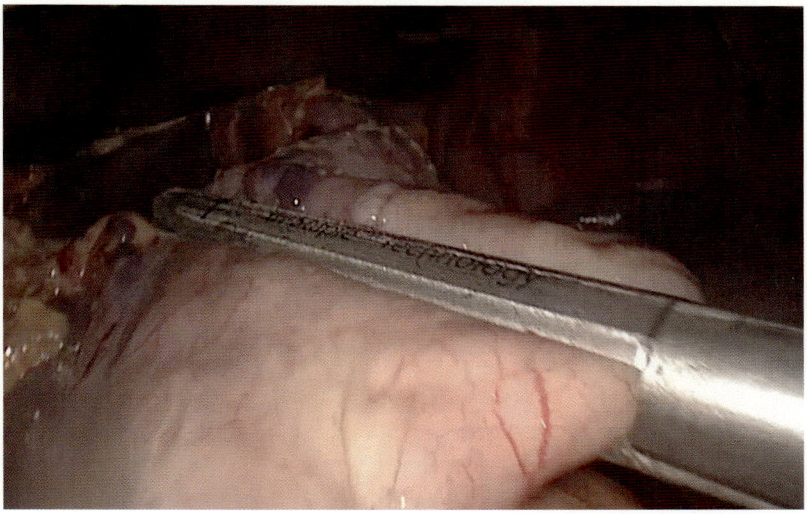

Fig. 19.54 Division of the stomach

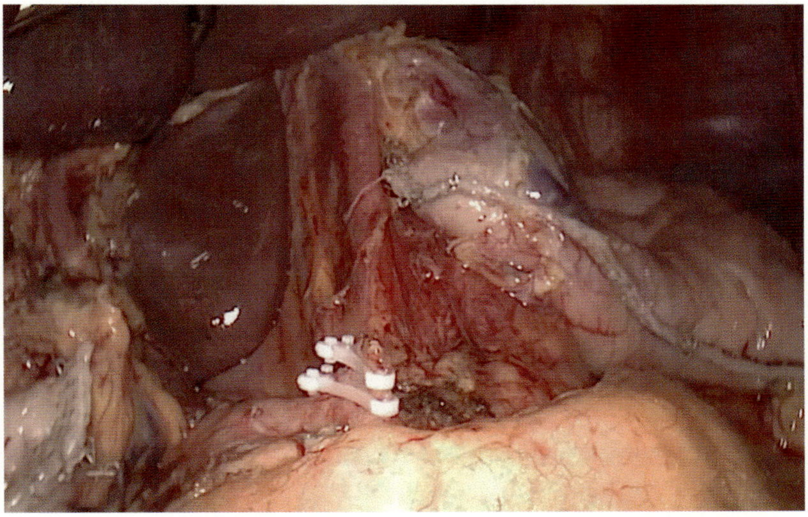

Fig. 19.55 Stomach is divided

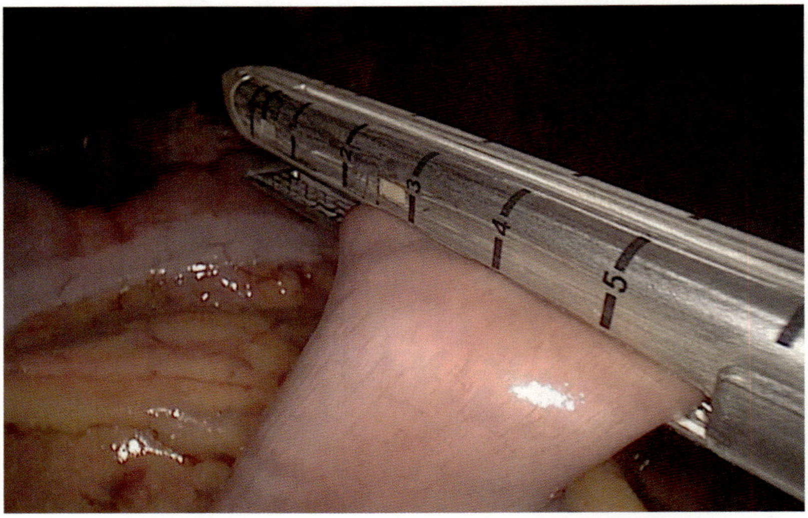

Fig. 19.56 Division by staplers of proximal jejunum

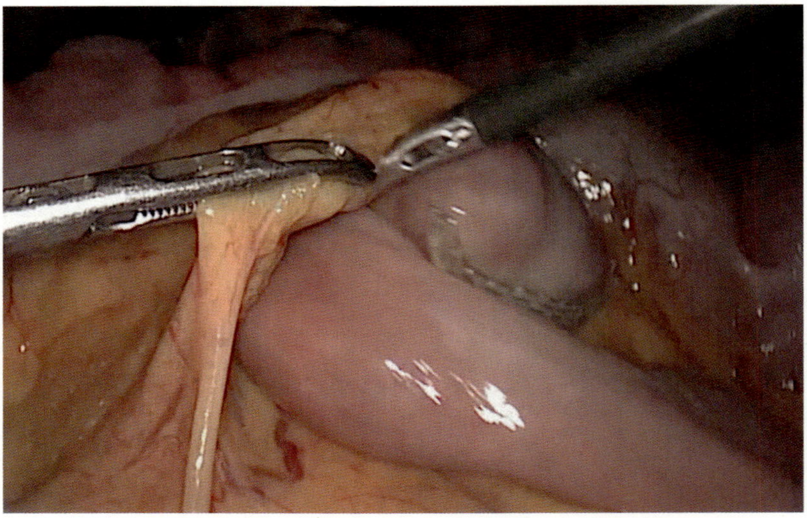

Fig. 19.57 Jejunum loop transmesocolic to upper abdomen

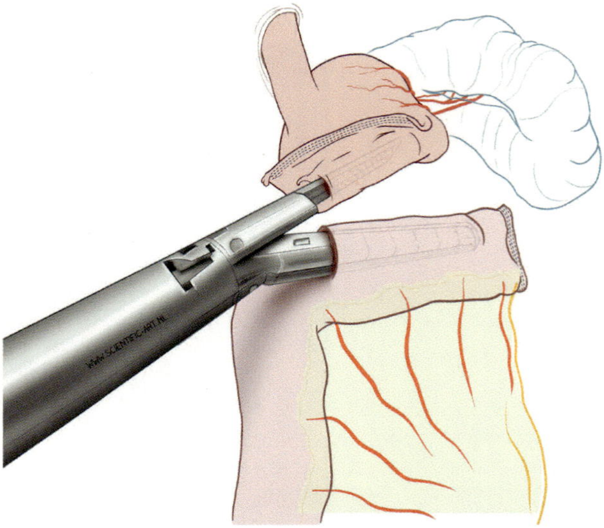

Fig. 19.58 Side-to-side gastro-jejunostomy anastomosis

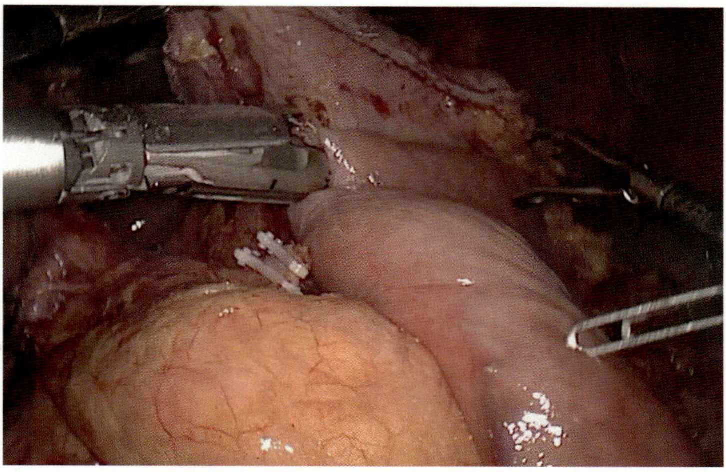

Fig. 19.59 Gastro-jejunostomy

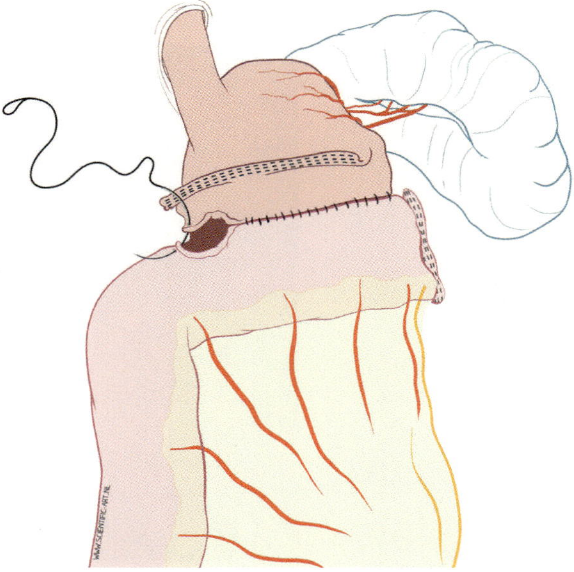

Fig. 19.60 Closure defect of gastro-jejunostomy

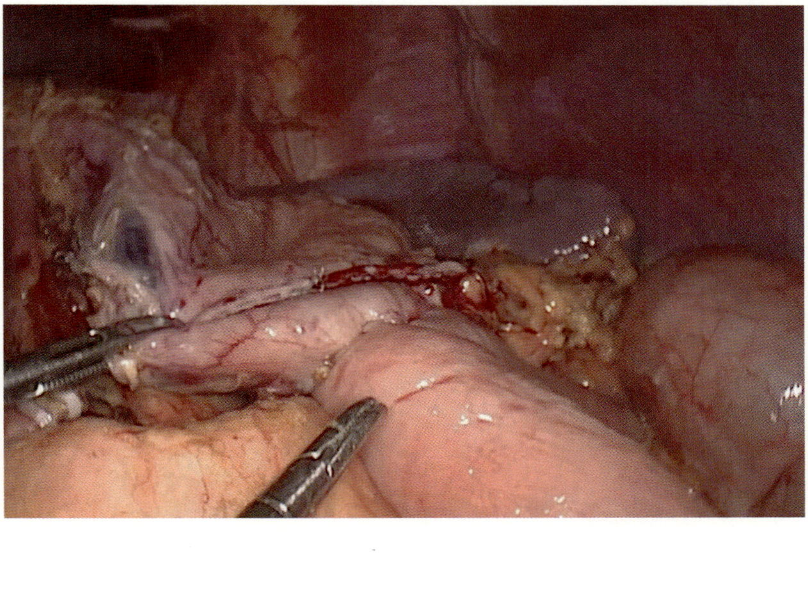

Fig. 19.61 Gastro-jejunostomy

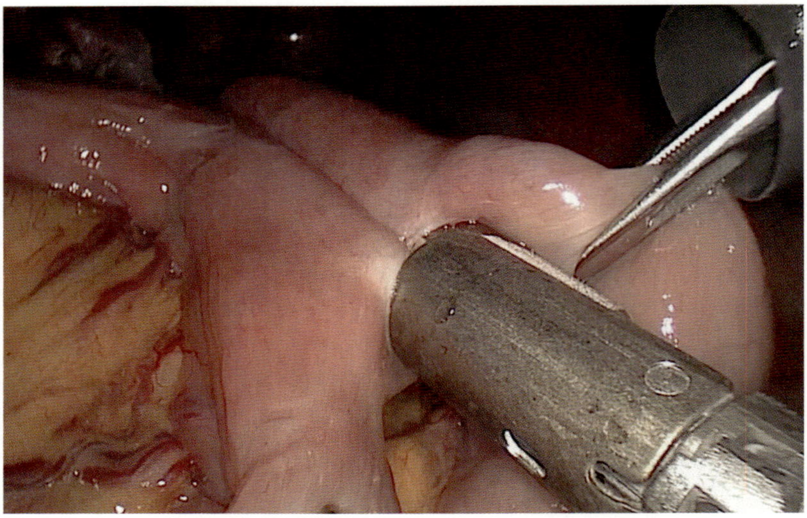

Fig. 19.62 Side-to-side jejuno-jejunostomy

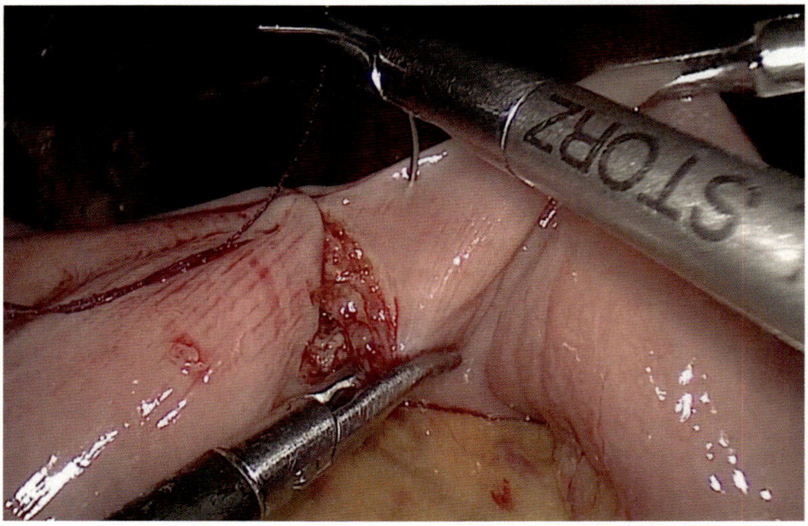

Fig. 19.63 Closure of the opening of the jejuno-jejunostomy

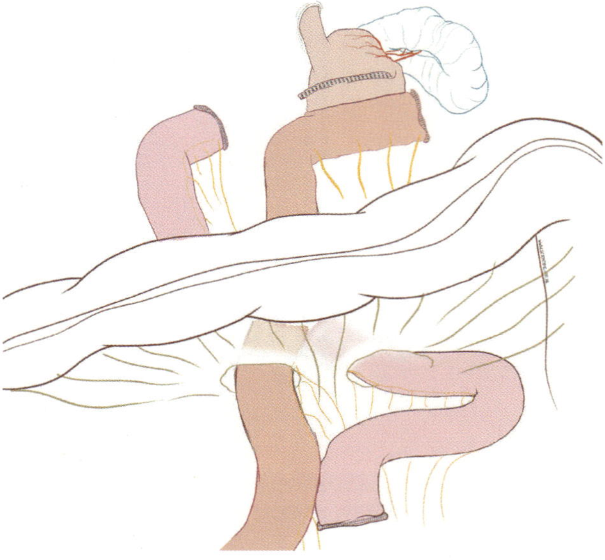

Fig. 19.64 Final aspect of the reconstruction after subtotal gastrectomy

Part IV

Duodenum-Pancreas Tumors

Pancreatic Resection After Neoadjuvant Treatment

20

Mustafa Suker and Casper H.J. van Eijck

20.1 Introduction

Pancreatic cancer has a very poor prognosis, with the projection to be the second leading cancer-related death in 2020 [1]. Pancreatic cancer can be divided in three stages: resectable (15%), locally advanced (35%) and metastatic disease (50%) [2]. The diagnosis of resectable and locally advanced pancreatic cancer is determined by the tumor invasion of critical structures, in particular the portal vein, superior mesenteric vein, coeliac artery and superior mesenteric artery. This tumor invasion is usually assessed by contrast enhanced computed tomography (CT). There are several definitions for resectable and locally advanced disease, usually based on the tumor burden of the surrounding major vessels. This tumor burden can be defined as no invasion at all to the surrounding structures (resectable disease) and too much invasion in the surrounding structures to be deemed resectable (locally advanced disease). In between these two extremes there is a diagnostic gap where a tumor has some vessel involvement but is still resectable, this gap is called borderline resectable disease. The two most commonly used definitions for (borderline) resectable disease and locally advanced disease are that of National Comprehensive Cancer (NCCN) and the combined definition of Americas Hepato-Pancreato-Biliary Association (AHPBA), the Society of Surgical Oncology (SSO), and the Society for Surgery of the Alimentary Tract (SSAT) [3, 4]. Both the definitions of NCCN and AHPBA/SSO/SSAT for borderline resectable and locally advanced disease are summarized in Table 20.1. For decades, the primary treatment for borderline resectable pancreatic cancer was upfront surgery. However, neoadjuvant therapy is becoming more and more a valuable upfront therapy for borderline resectable disease. Although there is no clear level I evidence for this treatment [5]. The main purpose of neoadjuvant treatment are threefold: (1) improve probability of radical resection, (2) patient selection of patients with rapid disease progression that will undergo unnecessary surgery, (3) early treatment of occult metastasis and finally more patients receiving systemic treatment since a significant portion of patient do not come to adjuvant therapy after surgical resection due to morbidity [6]. In contrary, locally advanced pancreatic cancer is conventionally treated with induction chemotherapy and sometimes followed by local therapy such as (chemo)radiotherapy or local ablation. Surgery is not recommended as an upfront treatment in locally advanced unresectable pancreatic cancer and is only reserved for patients with disease response and after tumor downstaging with chemotherapy and or (chemo)

M. Suker • C.H.J. van Eijck (✉)
Department of Surgery, Erasmus Medical Center, Rotterdam, The Netherlands
e-mail: c.vaneijck@erasmusmc.nl

M.A. Cuesta (ed.), *Minimally Invasive Surgery for Upper Abdominal Cancer*,
DOI 10.1007/978-3-319-54301-7_20

radiotherapy [7]. In this chapter, an overview will be given of studies that examined the effect of neoadjuvant treatment on surgical outcomes in borderline resectable and locally advanced unresectable pancreatic cancer. Lastly, an illustrative case report will be presented of a patient with locally advanced unresectable pancreatic cancer.

20.2 Borderline Resectable Pancreatic Cancer

The diagnosis of borderline resectable pancreatic cancer remains difficult. There are some consensus definitions (Table 20.1), but bottom line, borderline resectable pancreatic cancer is diagnosed by the surgeon if he deems the tumor resectable despite vascular encasement on CT with a possibility that the resection is radical and resected vascular structures are reconstructable [6]. Neoadjuvant treatment is emerging as a new and valuable addition to resection. When considering neoadjuvant treatment, tissue diagnosis is mandatory to avoid unnecessary adverse events of the neoadjuvant treatment. This is usually performed by endoscopic ultrasound guided (EUS) biopsy. Furthermore, if (chemo)radiotherapy is included in the neoadjuvant regimen, preferably patients should undergo a staging laparoscopy to exclude occult metastasis. Finally, a restaging CT should be performed after neoadjuvant treatment to avoid unnecessary laparotomies [4].

There are several studies published on the effect of neoadjuvant treatment and surgical outcomes [6]. In 2010, Chun et al. described in a retrospective study that 74 patients received neoadjuvant treatment versus 35 patients that received upfront surgery [8]. There were two different neoadjuvant treatments given: 5-Fluorouracil (5-FU) based chemoradiation and gemcitabine-based chemoradiation. All patients underwent a resection and the number of radical resections (R0) was much higher in the neoadjuvant treated patients then in the upfront surgery patients (59% vs. 11%, $p = <0.0001$). In addition, the overall survival of the neoadjuvant group was 23 months versus 15 months in surgery group ($p = 0.001$). There was no difference in surgical morbidity or mortality between both groups. Stokes et al. published in 2011 a prospectively maintained database study that compared borderline resectable pancreatic cancer patients whom received neoadjuvant

Table 20.1 NCCN and AHPBA/SSO/SSAT definitions of borderline resectable and locally advanced pancreatic cancer

	NCCN	AHPBA/SSO/SSAT
Borderline resectable	No distant metastases	No distant metastasis
	Solid tumor contact with SMA <180°	Solid tumor contact with SMA <180°
	Solid tumor contact with GA and/or CHA without involvement of CA	Solid tumor contact with GA and/or CHA without involvement of CA
	Reconstructable SMV and/or PV despite tumor involvement or occlusion	Reconstructable SMV and/or PV despite tumor involvement or occlusion without tumor contact with surrounding arteries
Locally advanced	No distant metastasis	No distant metastasis
	Solid tumor contact with SMA and/or CA >180°	Circumferential encasement of SMA and/or CHA
	Solid tumor contact with the first jejunal SMA branch and/or aortic involvement	Abutment of CA due to tumor involvement
	Unreconstructable SMV and/or PV due to tumor involvement or occlusion	Unreconstructable SMV and/or PV due to tumor involvement or occlusion
	Contact with most proximal draining jenjunal branch in to SMV	

SMA superior mesenteric artery, *GA* gastroduodenal artery, *CA* coeliac axis, *CHA* common hepatic artery, *SMV* superior mesenteric vein, *PV* portal vein capecitabine-based chemoradiation (n = 40) with resectable patients whom underwent surgery first (n = 75) [9]. Of the neoadjuvant group 40% underwent a resection with 75% being an R0 resection versus 68% resection rate without reporting the R0 resection rate in the surgery first group. The patients with borderline resectable disease had a median overall survival (OS) of 12 months, patients that eventually underwent a resection reached a median OS of 20 months. Median OS did not differ for patients that underwent a resection in the neoadjuvant group or the surgery first group. Similarly, Kang et al. showed in a retrospective study that borderline resectable patients (N = 32) receiving neoadjuvant gemcitabine with or without cisplatin-based radiotherapy have the same overall survival as the patient with resectable disease that underwent surgery first (N = 104) (median OS 31 vs. 26 months, $p = 0.709$) [10]. Accordingly all patients in both group underwent a resection and there were no differences in the radical resection rate (88% vs. 88%, $p = 0.272$). This high radical resection rate was seen as well by Lee et al., where 18 patients received neoadjuvant gemcitabine and capecitabine which resulted in 61% resections and 82% R0 resection [11]. In a prospective phase 2 trial Kim et al. included 39 patients with borderline resectable disease that received gemcitabine-oxaliplatin-based radiotherapy. The same neoadjuvant treatment was given to 23 patients with resectable disease [12]. Similar results were found as 62% were resected in the borderline resectable groups and 57% in the resectable group (p = not reported). Median OS were comparable as well with 18 versus 27 months (p = not reported). Another prospective phase 2 study by Takahashi et al. used gemcitabine-based radiotherapy as neoadjuvant treatment in 80 patients with borderline resectable disease and 188 patients with resectable disease [13]. There was a difference in the number of patients that underwent a resection with 54% in the borderline resectable compared to 87% in the resectable group ($p < 0.001$). The study showed that both groups that did not underwent a resection did not differ in median overall survival (11 months vs. 15 months, $p = 0.06$). However, the 5-years survival rate in the patients with borderline disease was lower than patients with resectable disease (34% vs. 57%, $p = 0.029$). The most recent phase 2 trial on this topic was conducted by Katz et al. where 22 borderline resectable patients received neoadjuvant leucovorin, 5-fluorouracil, irinotecan and oxaliplatin (FOLFIRINOX) followed by capecitabine-based radiotherapy [14]. This study showed a 68% resection rate with 93% being an R0 resection and a favorable median OS of 22 months in all included patients. All these studies are summarized in Table 20.2 with their main surgical and oncological outcomes. Although all these results are supportive for neoadjuvant treatment in borderline resectable pancreatic cancer, the conclusions

Table 20.2 Overview of the biggest neoadjuvant treatment studies for borderline resectable pancreatic cancer in the past 6 years

Author, year	N	Neoadjuvant regimen	% Resected	% R0 resection	Median OS, months
Chun, 2010	74	5-FU-RT	100	59	23
		Gem-RT			
Stokes, 2011	40	Cap-RT	40	75	12
Kang, 2012	32	Gem ± Cis-RT	100	88	32
Lee, 2012	18	Gem-Cap	61	82	NR
Kim, 2013	39	Gem-Ox-RT	62	NR	18
Takahashi, 2013	80	Gem-RT	54	98	NR
Katz, 2016	22	FOLFIRINOX, then Cap-RT	68	93	22

5-FU 5-flouraucil, *Gem* gemcitabine, *Cap* capecitabine, *Cis* cisplatin, *Ox* oxaliplatin, *FOLFIRINOX* leucovorin, 5-fluorouracil, irinotecan and oxaliplatin, *RT* radiotherapy, *NR* not reported should be drawn with caution. First of all, most studies are retrospective studies with a small sample size. Furthermore, most studies compare borderline resectable pancreatic cancer with resectable pancreatic cancer and one could argue whether these are two different patient populations. A patient with resectable pancreatic cancer was diagnosed before any vascular invasive components were found, while borderline resectable could invade major vessels before giving any symptoms. Last but not least, all the studies gave different neoadjuvant regimens, which make comparisons of these studies very difficult. However, there is some consensus that the postoperative mortality and morbidity rate in neoadjuvant treated patients does not differ from upfront surgery [15]. Moreover, there is some data suggesting that neoadjuvant treatment in borderline resectable pancreatic cancer gives better survival at a lower cost than upfront surgery (23.4 Quality adjusted life months (QALM) at $ 45.673 versus 18.8 QALM at $46.830) [15]. This was also seen in a Markov decision model of de Geus et al. which showed that the life expectancy of patients with borderline resectable pancreatic cancer that received neoadjuvant treatment (n = 871) was higher than patients receiving upfront surgery (n = 789) (32 vs. 27 months) [16]. In addition, the quality adjusted life expectancy was 26 month in the neoadjuvant groups versus 21 months in the upfront surgery group. In a recently published large propensity score matched analysis for patients (borderline) resectable pancreatic cancer by Mokdad et al. neoadjuvant treatment (n = 2005) showed a much higher median OS (26 vs. 21 months, $p < 0.01$) than upfront surgery matched group (n = 6015) [17]. In conclusion, there is some data suggesting that neoadjuvant treatment could be the new standard therapy for borderline resectable pancreatic cancer. However, there is no level I data from a large randomized controlled trial (RCT) which can give conclusive guidelines. Hopefully in the near future, a large Dutch RCT comparing upfront surgery followed by adjuvant gemcitabine with neoadjuvant gemcitabine-based radiotherapy followed by surgery and adjuvant gemcitabine (PREOPANC-trial) can give decisive conclusions on this hot topic [18].

20.3 Locally Advanced Pancreatic Cancer

The diagnosis of locally advanced pancreatic cancer (LAPC) is a more defined diagnosis. The tumor has a vascular invasive aspect on CT that makes it unresectable due to the high probability of micro- or macroscopically irradical resection. Unfortunately, there is no worldwide consensus on how much the vascular involvement should be to deem the tumor unresectable (Table 20.1). The diagnostic approach consists of a CT-scan of chest, abdomen and pelvis to exclude metastatic disease [6]. If in any phase of the treatment a local therapy is considered (i.e. radiotherapy or surgery), a staging laparoscopy is recommended [4]. A staging laparoscopy has shown to upstage around one third of the patients with LAPC on CT to a metastatic disease. Conventionally, LAPC is treated like metastatic disease with induction systemic chemotherapy. For decades fluorouracil was the standard first-line treatment for LAPC. This changed after an RCT in 1997 including patients with metastatic and locally advanced pancreatic cancer showed a median OS of 5.6 months in the gemcitabine arm while fluorouracil arm gave a median OS of 4.4 months ($p = 0.0025$) [19]. More recently, in 2011 an RCT was conducted by Conroy et al. with FOLFIRINOX versus gemcitabine for patients with metastatic [20]. The median OS in the FOLFIRINOX group was 11.1 vs. 6.8 months in gemcitabine group ($p < 0.001$). Since this revolutionary paper was published many case series with first-line FOLFIRINOX for LAPC are published. A recently published patient-level meta-analysis of 11 studies, showed that patients with LAPC (n = 315) treated with first-line FOLFIRINOX had a median OS of 24 months. (Chemo)radiotherapy was given following the FOLFIRINOX treatment in 57% of the patients. Eventually, 28% underwent a resection with 74% being an R0 resection. Resection rates and the addition of (chemo)radiotherapy were not based on patient-level data. Nevertheless, these subsequent treatments did not show a significant correlation with survival [21]. The survival and surgical data of these included 11 studies are

Table 20.3 Studies describing surgical data after first-line FOLFIRINOX treatment in LAPC

Author, year	N	% Resected	% R0 resection	Median OS, months
Conroy, 2011	11	0	NA	15,7
Hosein, 2012	14	43	83	32,7
Peddi, 2012	19	21	NR	Not reached
Boone, 2013	10	20	50	NR
Faris, 2013	22	23	100	24,7
Gunturu, 2013	16	13	NR	25,3
Mahaseteth, 2013	20	20	75	21,2
Hohla, 2014	6	33	NR	10,0
Moorcraft, 2014	8	25	NR	18,4
Marthey, 2015	77	36	89	21,1
Mellon, 2015	21	24	100	24,0
Sadot, 2015	101	31	52	26,0
Stein, 2016	31	42	100	26,6

Data adapted from Suker et al. and Stein et al. [21, 22]

shown in Table 20.3. Recently, a phase II trial endorsed these findings including 31 patients with LAPC that received first-line FOLFIRINOX. The median OS was 26.6 months, with 42% of the patients underwent a resection, which resulted in an R0 resection in all of these patients [22]. Another systemic chemotherapy regimen is nab-paclitaxel–gemcitabine examined in a recent RCT from Von Hoff et al., although including only patients with metastatic pancreatic cancer showed a survival benefit for nab-paclitaxel–gemcitabine versus gemcitabine alone (median OS 8.5 vs. 6.7 months, $p < 0.001$) [23]. The benefit of systematic therapy above surgery-first approach in patients with LAPC was further underlined in an American nationwide database set which showed a median OS of 21 months (n = 377) versus 14 months (n = 216) in favor of the neoadjuvant group ($p < 0.001$) [24].

Additional treatment after first-line chemotherapy is only advised if there is no clinical tumor progression. The optimal subsequent regimen has yet to be established, due to contradicting results. In the last decade there were three randomized trials that evaluated the effect of (chemo)radiotherapy versus chemotherapy alone in LAPC [6]. One study randomized gemcitabine (n = 60) versus fluorouracil-cisplatin-radiotherapy followed by gemcitabine (n = 59), which showed a median OS of 14.3 months versus 8.4 months in favor of gemcitabine alone arm ($p = 0.014$). In the contrary, another study randomized between gemcitabine versus gemcitabine-radiotherapy, which showed a median OS 9.2 months versus 11.1 months in favor of gemcitabine-radiotherapy arm ($p = 0.017$). The most recent study that was published showed no difference in subsequent treatment with radiotherapy. The study enrolled patients with LAPC for 4 months of gemcitabine with or without erlotinib and if no progression was seen the patients were randomized between 2 months extension (n = 136) of the chemotherapy or capecitabine-radiotherapy (n = 133) (median OS 15.2 vs. 16.5, $p = 0.83$). Little is known about the survival benefit of resection after induction chemotherapy and radiotherapy. There is no consensus in the literature on selection of patients with LAPC for resection after induction therapy [25]. After first-line FOLFIRINOX it seems that the resection rates do not influence the median OS [21]. Some studies conclude that there is a significant better survival of resected patients after induction therapy. These conclusions should be taken with much caution, as there are no randomized trials examining the role of surgery in the non-progressive or responsive LAPC. Therefore, if patients with LAPC have much better survival after induction therapy followed by resection this could merely rely on the fact that these patients are the good responders and therefore the long survivors.

20.4 Pancreatic Resection After Neoadjuvant Treatment

There is limited data on the surgical morbidity and mortality of surgery after induction therapy. One review showed that after induction FOLFIRINOX the surgical morbidity is reported to be as high as 60% with the surgical mortality being around 3% [26]. These mortality and morbidity rates were similarly found by Cooper et al. were retrospectively 1562 patients were identified that underwent pancreatic resection [27]. The neoadjuvant chemo(radio)therapy group (n = 199) were compared to the upfront surgery group (n = 1363). The 30-day mortality and postoperative morbidity rates were similar between both groups. Of note, there were fewer organ space infections (3% vs. 10%, p = 0.001) and fewer pancreatic fistula (7% vs. 15%, p = 0.03) in the neoadjuvant group. Another study showed in a group of 45 patients with borderline and locally advanced pancreatic cancer that the 90-days mortality was around 7% and the overall morbidity was as low as 33% [28]. These results were underlined by a retrospective study which identified 56 patients with borderline resectable and five patients with LAPC that received neoadjuvant treatment before undergoing a pancreatic resection and compared the perioperative results to 241 with resectable disease that underwent upfront surgery [29]. The 90-days mortality (2% vs. 4%, p = 0.69) and postoperative morbidity (39% vs. 31%, p = 0.23) were the same between the two groups while the R0 resection (97% vs. 84%, p < 0.001) was a lot higher in the neoadjuvant group. This higher R0 resection rate was also seen in a large nationwide database with (borderline) resectable pancreatic cancer (n = 7881) where 1188 patients received neoadjuvant treatment. The R0 resection rate was 80% in the neoadjuvant group versus 73% in the upfront surgery group (p < 0.01), where the 30-days readmission and 90-day mortality were not different in both groups. Because of these and other studies the American Society of Clinical Oncology (ASCO) advices in the most recent guideline to offer patients with (borderline) resectable neoadjuvant treatment as an alternative to upfront surgery [30]. Also, the most recent ASCO guideline advices that all patients with LAPC should receive first-line chemotherapy with or without radiotherapy and surgery should be only considered if dramatic response to induction therapy was achieved [7]. Of note, there is no data supporting survival benefit or disadvantage of resection after systematic therapy in patients with LAPC. There are much more prospective studies needed to help understand which treatment regimens are effective for patients with LAPC [7]. A large RCT is being conducted at the moment in France to compare gemcitabine with FOLFIRINOX to give definitive a conclusion on which regimen is the better (PRODIGE 29-NEOPAN, NCT02539537). Furthermore, a prospective phase 2 study in the Netherlands is enrolling patients with LAPC to receive stereotactic body radiotherapy (SBRT) after first-line FOLFIRINOX to assess feasibility and efficacy of this treatment regimen (LAPC-1, NCT02292745). Another worldwide multicenter phase 2 study is enrolling the same patient population to examine the efficacy of nab-paclitaxel–gemcitabine (LAPACT, NCT02301143).

20.5 Case Report

A 40-year old mother of two children without any relevant medical history presents with jaundice. On CT-scan a mass of 4.7 cm in the pancreatic head is seen with encasement of more than 270° and total occlusion of the superior mesenteric vein (SMV) (Fig. 20.1a). Some periumbilical collateral veins are seen, no metastatic suspected lesions were seen on the chest or pelvis CT-scan. The patient underwent an EUS with biopsy of the pancreatic mass and an endoscopic retrograde cholangiopancreatography without the possibility to place a stent in the common bile duct. By a percutaneous transhepatic cholangiography the bile drainage was secured and eventually a covered self-expandable biliary stent was placed. After the biopsy has shown adenocarcinoma, the patient underwent a staging laparoscopy which did not

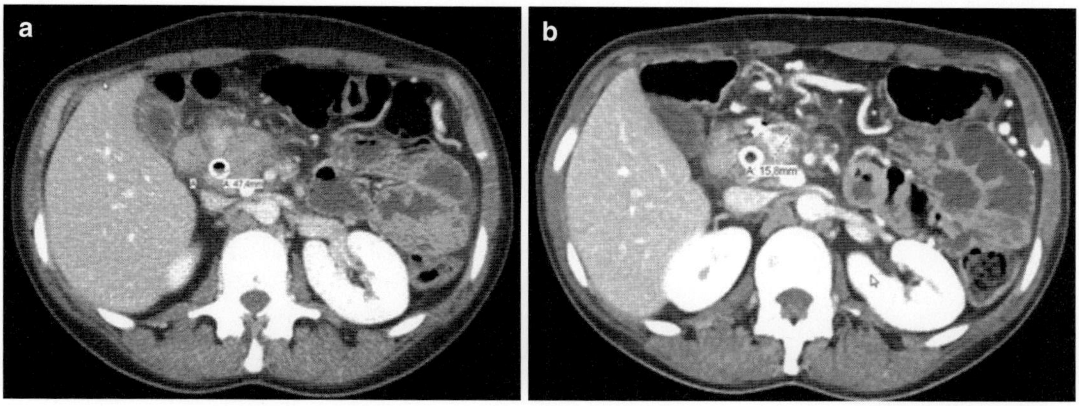

Fig. 20.1 (**a**) Baseline CT scan with pancreatic tumor of 4.7 cm. (**b**) CT scan with pancreatic tumor shrunk to 1.6 cm after 8 cycles of FOLFIRINOX and 40 Gray of SBRT

show any metastatic lesion. The patient was included in the LAPC-1 study (NCT02292745) and received a first block of 4 cycles of FOLFIRINOX. A restaging CT-scan showed a decrease in size of the tumor (4.1 cm) and furthermore a stable disease. After another block of 4 cycles of FOLFIRINOX a restaging CT-scan showed no alterations in size of tumor or metastatic suspected lesions. The patient was referred for SBRT and underwent EUS for fiducial markers to help guide the SBRT. The patient received 5 times 8 Gray SBRT (total 40 Gray in 5 days). The fist follow-up CT-scan after 3 months showed a significant response with tumor being shrunk to 1.6 cm with less than 90° encasement left of the SMV, however the occlusion was still present (Fig. 20.1b). This made the tumor borderline resectable and therefore the patient underwent a Whipple resection with SMV short segment resection and reconstruction (Fig. 20.2a). Histopathology showed a minimal rest of adenocarcinoma of the pancreas in an area of 1.5 cm and extensive tumor response in the form of fibrosis (Fig. 20.2b). Also in the lumen of the resected SMV adenocarcinoma was found. All resection margins were radical and staging given this information was ypT3N0M0 R0. The patient was discharges after 10 days in good condition and is being followed-up in the out-patient clinic. No additional CT-scan will be made until clinical symptoms will be present.

Conclusion

Pancreatic cancer has a very poor prognosis. There are trials being conducted to hopefully improve the survival in pancreatic cancer. In the recent years neoadjuvant treatment is being examined as possible upfront therapy for borderline resectable instead of the surgery first approach. There is some data suggesting that this could be a fruitful approach. At the moment, these neoadjuvant treatments should be only given in prospective trials to help establish a consensus on the efficacy of neoadjuvant treatment and the standard regimen. In case of locally advanced unresectable pancreatic cancer, there is some consensus for the treatment approach. The treatment should start with systemic chemotherapy, with FOLFIRINOX the first choice if the patient has an acceptable condition to undergo this highly active chemotherapy. Otherwise first-line nab-paclitaxel–gemcitabine can be considered but this should be only given in a prospective study. If these regimens are not feasible, the standard first-line chemotherapy is still gemcitabine. If subsequent local treatment is considered external beam or stereotactic body radiotherapy seem promising, but there is no level 1 evidence on which subsequent treatment is the best choice. Resection should only be considered if there is a good response on the prior treatment, i.e. the tumor has become a (borderline) resectable tumor.

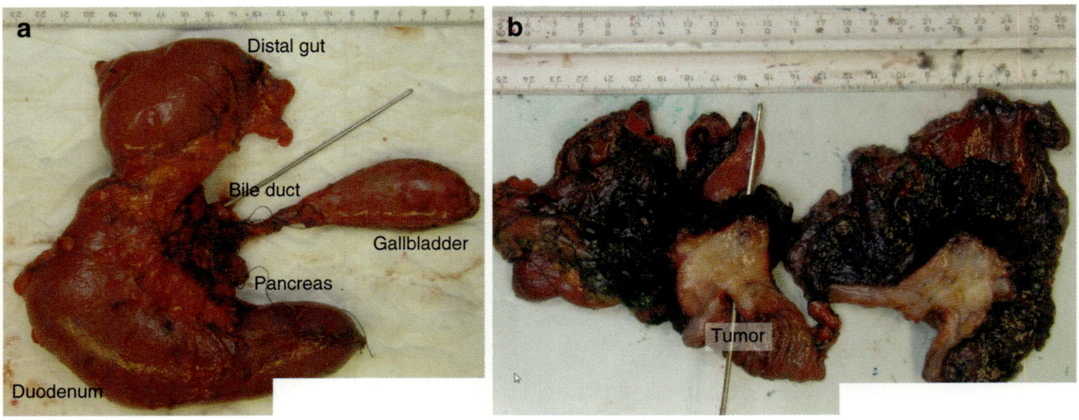

Fig. 20.2 (**a**) Whipple resection specimen. (**b**) Pancreatic tumor with rest active tumor and fibrosis

Of note is that there is no evidence at all for survival benefit of surgical resection after induction therapy. Hopefully, in the near future with high impact prospective studies there is more consensus on the role of neoadjuvant treatment for borderline resectable pancreatic cancer and on the treatment regimen for locally advanced pancreatic cancer.

References

1. Rahib L, Smith BD, Aizenberg R, Rosenzweig AB, Fleshman JM, Matrisian LM. Projecting cancer incidence and deaths to 2030: the unexpected burden of thyroid, liver, and pancreas cancers in the United States. Cancer Res. 2014;74(11):2913–21.
2. Stathis A, Moore MJ. Advanced pancreatic carcinoma: current treatment and future challenges. Nat Rev Clin Oncol. 2010;7(3):163–72.
3. Network. NCC. Pancreatic adenocarcinoma (version: 2.2015): NCCN. 2015. http://www.nccn.org/professionals/physician_gls/pdf/pancreatic.pdf.
4. Callery MP, Chang KJ, Fishman EK, Talamonti MS, William Traverso L, Linehan DC. Pretreatment assessment of resectable and borderline resectable pancreatic cancer: expert consensus statement. Ann Surg Oncol. 2009;16(7):1727–33.
5. Heinemann V, Haas M, Boeck S. Neoadjuvant treatment of borderline resectable and non-resectable pancreatic cancer. Ann Oncol. 2013;24(10):2484–92.
6. David P, Ryan HM. Initial chemotherapy and radiation for nonmetastatic locally advanced unresectable and borderline resectable exocrine pancreatic cancer. In: Post TW, editor. UpToDate. Waltham: UpToDate.
7. Balaban EP, Mangu PB, Khorana AA, Shah MA, Mukherjee S, Crane CH, et al. Locally advanced, unresectable pancreatic cancer: American Society of Clinical Oncology clinical practice guideline. J Clin Oncol. 2016;34(22):2654–68.
8. Chun YS, Milestone BN, Watson JC, Cohen SJ, Burtness B, Engstrom PF, et al. Defining venous involvement in borderline resectable pancreatic cancer. Ann Surg Oncol. 2010;17(11):2832–8.
9. Stokes JB, Nolan NJ, Stelow EB, Walters DM, Weiss GR, de Lange EE, et al. Preoperative capecitabine and concurrent radiation for borderline resectable pancreatic cancer. Ann Surg Oncol. 2011;18(3):619–27.
10. Kang CM, Chung YE, Park JY, Sung JS, Hwang HK, Choi HJ, et al. Potential contribution of preoperative neoadjuvant concurrent chemoradiation therapy on margin-negative resection in borderline resectable pancreatic cancer. J Gastrointest Surg. 2012;16(3):509–17.
11. Lee JL, Kim SC, Kim JH, Lee SS, Kim TW, Park DH, et al. Prospective efficacy and safety study of neoadjuvant gemcitabine with capecitabine combination chemotherapy for borderline-resectable or unresectable locally advanced pancreatic adenocarcinoma. Surgery. 2012;152(5):851–62.
12. Kim EJ, Ben-Josef E, Herman JM, Bekaii-Saab T, Dawson LA, Griffith KA, et al. A multi-institutional phase 2 study of neoadjuvant gemcitabine and oxaliplatin with radiation therapy in patients with pancreatic cancer. Cancer. 2013;119(15):2692–700.
13. Takahashi H, Ohigashi H, Gotoh K, Marubashi S, Yamada T, Murata M, et al. Preoperative gemcitabine-based chemoradiation therapy for resectable and borderline resectable pancreatic cancer. Ann Surg. 2013;258(6):1040–50.
14. Katz MH, Shi Q, Ahmad SA, Herman JM, Marsh Rde W, Collisson E, et al. Preoperative modified FOLFIRINOX treatment followed by capecitabine-based chemoradiation for borderline resectable pancreatic cancer: alliance for clinical trials in oncology trial A021101. JAMA Surg. 2016;151(8):e161137.
15. Asare EA, Evans DB, Erickson BA, Aburajab M, Tolat P, Tsai S. Neoadjuvant treatment sequencing

adds value to the care of patients with operable pancreatic cancer. J Surg Oncol. 2016;114(3):291–5.
16. de Geus SW, Evans DB, Bliss LA, Eskander MF, Smith JK, Wolff RA, et al. Neoadjuvant therapy versus upfront surgical strategies in resectable pancreatic cancer: a Markov decision analysis. Eur J Surg Oncol. 2016;42(10):1552–60.
17. Mokdad AA, Minter RM, Zhu H, Augustine MM, Porembka MR, Wang SC, et al. Neoadjuvant therapy followed by resection versus upfront resection for resectable pancreatic cancer: a propensity score matched analysis. J Clin Oncol. 2017;35(5):515–23.
18. Versteijne E, van Eijck CH, Punt CJ, Suker M, Zwinderman AH, Dohmen MA, et al. Preoperative radiochemotherapy versus immediate surgery for resectable and borderline resectable pancreatic cancer (PREOPANC trial): study protocol for a multicentre randomized controlled trial. Trials. 2016;17(1):127.
19. Burris 3rd HA, Moore MJ, Andersen J, Green MR, Rothenberg ML, Modiano MR, et al. Improvements in survival and clinical benefit with gemcitabine as first-line therapy for patients with advanced pancreas cancer: a randomized trial. J Clin Oncol. 1997;15(6):2403–13.
20. Conroy T, Desseigne F, Ychou M, Bouche O, Guimbaud R, Becouarn Y, et al. FOLFIRINOX versus gemcitabine for metastatic pancreatic cancer. N Engl J Med. 2011;364(19):1817–25.
21. Suker M, Beumer BR, Sadot E, Marthey L, Faris JE, Mellon EA, et al. FOLFIRINOX for locally advanced pancreatic cancer: a systematic review and patient-level meta-analysis. Lancet Oncol. 2016;17(6):801–10.
22. Stein SM, James ES, Deng Y, Cong X, Kortmansky JS, Li J, et al. Final analysis of a phase II study of modified FOLFIRINOX in locally advanced and metastatic pancreatic cancer. Br J Cancer. 2016; 114(7):737–43.
23. Von Hoff DD, Ervin T, Arena FP, Chiorean EG, Infante J, Moore M, et al. Increased survival in pancreatic cancer with nab-paclitaxel plus gemcitabine. N Engl J Med. 2013;369(18):1691–703.
24. Shubert CR, Bergquist JR, Groeschl RT, Habermann EB, Wilson PM, Truty MJ, et al. Overall survival is increased among stage III pancreatic adenocarcinoma patients receiving neoadjuvant chemotherapy compared to surgery first and adjuvant chemotherapy: an intention to treat analysis of the National Cancer Database. Surgery. 2016;160(4):1080–96.
25. Evans DB, George B, Tsai S. Non-metastatic pancreatic cancer: resectable, borderline resectable, and locally advanced-definitions of increasing importance for the optimal delivery of multimodality therapy. Ann Surg Oncol. 2015;22(11):3409–13.
26. Rombouts SJ, Walma MS, Vogel JA, van Rijssen LB, Wilmink JW, Mohammad NH, et al. Systematic review of resection rates and clinical outcomes after FOLFIRINOX-based treatment in patients with locally advanced pancreatic cancer. Ann Surg Oncol. 2016;23(13):4352–60.
27. Cooper AB, Parmar AD, Riall TS, Hall BL, Katz MH, Aloia TA, et al. Does the use of neoadjuvant therapy for pancreatic adenocarcinoma increase postoperative morbidity and mortality rates? J Gastrointest Surg. 2015;19(1):80–6. discussion 6–7.
28. Addeo P, Rosso E, Fuchshuber P, Oussoultzoglou E, De Blasi V, Simone G, et al. Resection of borderline resectable and locally advanced pancreatic adenocarcinomas after neoadjuvant chemotherapy. Oncology. 2015;89(1):37–46.
29. Mellon EA, Strom TJ, Hoffe SE, Frakes JM, Springett GM, Hodul PJ, et al. Favorable perioperative outcomes after resection of borderline resectable pancreatic cancer treated with neoadjuvant stereotactic radiation and chemotherapy compared with upfront pancreatectomy for resectable cancer. J Gastrointest Oncol. 2016;7(4):547–55.
30. Khorana AA, Mangu PB, Berlin J, Engebretson A, Hong TS, Maitra A, et al. Potentially curable pancreatic cancer: American Society of Clinical Oncology clinical practice guideline. J Clin Oncol. 2016; 34(21):2541–56.

Open or Minimally Invasive Pancreatic Surgery?

21

Robert J. Torphy and Barish H. Edil

21.1 Introduction

Laparoscopic surgery has become the standard of care for several abdominal operations. Minimally invasive pancreas surgery has been slower to gain acceptance because of the inherent challenges, including the retroperitoneal location of the pancreas, proximity to the superior mesenteric artery and vein, portal vein, hepatic arteries, and high complication rates. However, this is an emerging field that continues to gain acceptance and in the appropriate clinical scenario can minimize operative morbidity and blood loss while improving quality of life.

The indications for pancreatic resection are broad and include cystic neoplasms, chronic pancreatitis, neuroendocrine tumors, periampullary adenocarcinoma, and pancreatic ductal adenocarcinoma (PDAC). Options for pancreatic resection include enucleation, distal pancreatectomy with or without splenic preservation, pancreaticoduodenectomy and total pancreatectomy depending on the pathology being treated and its anatomic location.

Since the first reported cases of a laparoscopic distal pancreatectomy and a laparoscopic pancreaticoduodenectomy in the 1990s, the acceptance and adoption of these complex minimally invasive operations has increased [1, 2]. There is also a continually growing body of literature that demonstrates that these minimally invasive procedures can have benefits when compared to their open counterparts. While initial reports argued these operations should be reserved for benign surgical indications, there is now increasing evidence that minimally invasive resections for malignancies are not only feasible but may reduce morbidity and improve subsequent delivery of adjuvant therapy. This is an area that deserves significant attention, as PDAC is the 12th most common cancer in the world, with 338,000 new cases diagnosed in 2012, and surgical resection remains the only potentially curative therapy [3].

21.2 Laparoscopic Distal Pancreatectomy

Laparoscopic distal pancreatectomy emerged in the 1990s and was initially reported for the treatment of chronic pancreatitis and its application has since rapidly expanded over the subsequent

R.J. Torphy
Department of General Surgery,
University of Colorado School of Medicine,
Aurora, CO 80045, USA
e-mail: ROBERT.TORPHY@UCDENVER.EDU

B.H. Edil, M.D., F.A.C.S. (✉)
Department of Surgical Oncology, Pancreas and Biliary, University of Colorado School of Medicine,
1665 Aurora Court 5th Floor Room 5309, Aurora,
CO 80045, USA
e-mail: BARISH.EDIL@UCDENVER.EDU

M.A. Cuesta (ed.), *Minimally Invasive Surgery for Upper Abdominal Cancer*,
DOI 10.1007/978-3-319-54301-7_21

decade [1]. This technique has been shown to be a safe and feasible. In a meta-analysis of over 1800 patients who underwent laparoscopic distal pancreatectomy and open distal pancreatectomy for benign and malignant indications, patients who underwent laparoscopic distal pancreatectomy had lower blood loss, shortened hospital length of stay, and fewer overall complications. Hospital length of stay was reduced by 4 days in the laparoscopic group. The overall incidence of complications was 33.9% in the laparoscopic group vs. 44.2% in the open group. Patients in the laparoscopic group had significantly fewer surgical site infections (2.9% vs. 8.1%) and a lower hospital readmission rate (12.6% vs. 17.7%). Importantly, there was no difference in pancreatic fistula rate or operative mortality [4].

There have been no randomized controlled trials comparing laparoscopic to open distal pancreatectomy for PDAC. The literature is limited to a few retrospective series. In the United States, a retrospective study using the National Cancer Database compared 145 patients who underwent a laparoscopic distal pancreatectomy to 625 patients who underwent open distal pancreatectomy for PDAC between 2010 and 2011. A higher percentage of patients undergoing laparoscopic distal pancreatectomy were treated at academic or research institutions (70% vs. 59%). Patients in the open group also had slightly larger tumors (4.2 cm vs. 3.7 cm). Importantly, there was no difference between the two groups with regards to the number of lymph nodes harvested and the number of positive lymph nodes harvested. Furthermore, fewer patients undergoing laparoscopic resection had positive margins (12% vs. 20%). As shown in prior studies, the length of stay was shorter in the laparoscopic group and the 30-day mortality was equivalent. This study was limited by its retrospective nature and likely selection bias with smaller tumors being removed laparoscopically. Also, morbidity was not captured in the National Cancer Database so no comparisons could be made regarding post-operative complications [5]. A nationwide retrospective observational study was also recently performed in France which showed laparoscopic distal pancreatectomy was independently associated with reduced pulmonary complications, reduced blood transfusions, shorter hospital length of stay with no increase in severe abdominal complications when compared to the open approach [6]. In conjunction, these two studies show that laparoscopic distal pancreatectomy for PDAC has equivalent oncologic outcomes to open distal pancreatectomy in terms of margin positivity and lymph node harvest with reduced operative morbidity.

21.3 Laparoscopic Pancreaticoduodenectomy

The first laparoscopic pancreaticoduodenectomy was reported in 1996 and has been slow to gain popularity [2]. A recent review of the literature shows that laparoscopic pancreaticoduodenectomy can be performed safely and with acceptable complication rates [7]. Several retrospective studies have also attempted to compare laparoscopic vs. open pancreaticoduodenectomy. Asbun et al. compared a cohort from 2005 to 2011 of 53 laparoscopic pancreaticoduodenectomies vs. 215 open procedures. In this cohort of patients, the laparoscopic group had significantly less blood loss (195 mL vs. 1032 mL), fewer transfusions (0.64 units vs. 4.7 units), shorter intensive care unit stays (1.1 days vs 3 days) and shorter overall hospital stays (8 days vs. 12.4 days). Complication rates were similar between the two groups. Oncologically, the number of lymph nodes removed was greater for the laparoscopic group (23.44 nodes vs 16.83 nodes) and margin status was equivalent. Operating time was significantly longer in the laparoscopic group (541 min vs 401 min). While the cohorts in this study were well matched, if major vascular resection was required open surgery was performed adding some selection bias [8].

A subsequent study addressed this selection bias by comparing 31 laparoscopic and 58 open cases with equivalent vascular resections. As with prior studies, blood loss and length of hospital stay was shorter in the laparoscopic group. Oncologically, the laparoscopic patients had significantly more lymph nodes harvested (20 nodes vs 15.9 nodes) and more R0 resections (93.5% vs. 75.9%) [9].

Croom et al. went on to look specifically at patients undergoing resection for PDAC and compared 108 laparoscopic pancreaticoduodenectomies for PDAC to 214 open cases. Importantly, these two groups were equivalent with regards to tumor size, T-stage, and tumor grade. When comparing the two approaches they found similar node resection rates, margin status, and post-operative complications. Notably, they showed the laparoscopic cohort required fewer blood transfusions (19% vs. 33%), had a shorter time to initiation of adjuvant therapy (48 days vs 59 days), and there was a significantly higher proportion of patients in the open cohort (12%) who had a delay of over 90 days or who did not receive adjuvant chemotherapy at all compared to the laparoscopic cohort (5%). There was no overall survival difference between the two groups after a median follow up of 16 months but there was a significant improvement in progression free survival in the laparoscopic group [10]. This study clearly illustrates that in an experienced center, laparoscopic pancreaticoduodenectomy can be safely performed for PDAC with comparable oncologic resections. Laparoscopic resection may also improve outcomes by reducing transfusion burden and increasing successful delivery of adjuvant therapy, which may have long term implications in cancer outcomes.

21.4 Laparoscopic Total Pancreatectomy

While laparoscopic distal pancreatectomy and laparoscopic pancreaticoduodenectomy are reported widely in the literature, laparoscopic total pancreatectomy is rarely reported and mainly in small case series. There are indications that necessitate total pancreatectomy at the time of resection of precancerous or cancerous lesions, or in the setting of intractable chronic pancreatitis. Chapman et al. reported a case report with accompanying video of spleen-preserving laparoscopic total pancreatectomy for a main-duct IPMN in a patient with a diffusely dilated pancreatic duct and an associated mural nodule. This case report demonstrated this procedure could be completed efficiently (surgical time 270 min), with minimal blood loss (150 mL), and a hospital length of stay of only 7 days [11].

21.5 Robotic Pancreatic Surgery

Robotic pancreatic surgery is another area of growing interest that has not been studied yet in as much depth as laparoscopic pancreatic surgery. The first robotic distal pancreatectomy was described in 2003 [12]. This was shortly thereafter followed by the first description of a robot-assisted pancreaticoduodenectomy in which laparoscopy was used for pancreatic resection and the robot was used to perform intracorporeal biliojejunal and gastrojejunal anastomoses [13]. Subsequent refinements of the robotic technique have resulted in complete robotic pancreaticoduodenectomies.

The largest series studying robotic distal pancreatectomies and pancreaticoduodenectomies originate from the University of Pittsburgh. Shakir et al. reported a series of the first 100 laparoscopic distal pancreatectomies performed from 2008 to 2013 at the University of Pittsburgh. In this study they identified a learning curve of 40 cases, after which the operative time (331–210 min) and readmission rates (28% vs. 20%) were significantly reduced [14]. Boone et al. from this same group reported a series of 200 consecutive robotic pancreaticoduodenectomies from 2008 to 2014. In this study a significant learning curve was again reported with improvements in blood loss and conversion to open surgery after 20 cases (600 mL vs. 250 mL and 35% vs. 3.3%), reduction in incidence of pancreatic fistula after 40 cases (27.5% vs. 14.4%), and reduction in operative time after 80 cases (581 min vs. 417 min) [15]. In both of these series, they demonstrate that after optimization beyond the learning curve, robotic distal pancreatectomies and pancreaticoduodenectomies can be performed with longer operative times but with similar mortality and morbidity rates compared to historical open standards.

To more directly compare robotic vs. open pancreaticoduodenectomy, a multicentre study was recently completed comparing perioperative data for patient who underwent robotic (211 patients) vs. open (817 patients) pancreaticoduodenectomies. The robotic procedures were performed at centers within the United States that perform a large number of these procedures annually, and only operations performed "postlearning curve" were analysed. The robotic procedure was found to have longer operative times by 75 min, reduced blood loss, and an overall reduction in major complications [16]. However, hospital lengths of stay and readmission rates were equivalent. Future analysis of robotic pancreatic resection that critically appraises the cost-benefit analysis of the robotic platform, quality of life, and long term outcomes will be important in understanding the future role of robotics in pancreatic surgery.

References

1. Cuschieri A, Jakimowicz JJ, van Spreeuwel J. Laparoscopic distal 70% pancreatectomy and splenectomy for chronic pancreatitis. Ann Surg. 1996;223(3):280–5.
2. Gagner M, Pompe A. Laparscopic pylorus-preserving pancreatoduodenectomy. Surg Endosc. 1994;8:408–10.
3. World Cancer Research Fund International. Pancreatic cancer statistics. http://www.wcrf.org/int/cancer-facts-figures/data-specific-cancers/pancreatic-cancer-statistics.
4. Venkat R, Edil BH, Schulick RD, Lidor AO, Makary MA, Wolfgang CL. Laparoscopic distal pancreatectomy is associated with significantly less overall morbidity compared to the open technique: a systematic review and meta-analysis. Ann Surg. 2012;255(6):1048–59.
5. Sharpe SM, Talamonti MS, Wang E, Bentrem DJ, Roggin KK, Prinz RA, Marsh RDW, Stocker SJ, Winchester DJ, Baker MS. The laparsocpic approach to distal pancreatectomy for ductal adenocarcinoma results in shorter lengths of stay without compromising oncologic outcomes. Am J Surg. 2015; 209:557–63.
6. Sulpice L, Farges O, Goutte N, Bendersky N, Dokmak S, Sauvanet A, Delpero JR. Laparscopic distal pancreatectomy for pancreatic ductal adenocarcinoma: time for a randomized controlled tril? Results of an all-inclusive national observational study. Ann Surg. 2016;262:868–74.
7. Merkow J, Paniccia A, Edil BH. Laparoscopic pancreaticoduodenectomy: a descriptive and comparative review. Chin J Cancer Res. 2015;27(4):368–75.
8. Asbun HJ, Stauffer JA. Laparoscopic vs. open pancreaticoduodenectomy: overall outcomes and severity of complications using the Accordion Severity Grading System. J Am Coll Surg. 2012;215:810–9.
9. Croom KP, Farnell MB, Que FG, Reid-Lombardo KM, et al. Pancreaticoduodenectomy with major vascular resection: a comparison of laparoscopic versus open approaches. J Gastrointest Surg. 2015;19: 189–94.
10. Croome KP, Farnell MB, Que FG, Reid-Lombardo KM, et al. Total laparoscopic pancreaticoduodenectomy for pancreatic ductal adenocarcinoma: oncologic advantages over open approaches. Ann Surg. 2014;260(4):633–40.
11. Chapman BC, Paniccia A, Ryan C, Schulick RD, Edil BH. Laparoscopic spleen-preserving total pancreatectomy for a main-duct intraductal papillary mucinous neoplasm. Ann Surg Oncol. 2016;24(2):560.
12. Melvin WS, Needleman BJ, Krause KR, Ellison EC. Robotic resection of pancreatic neuroendocrine tumor. J Laparoendosc Adv Surg Tech A. 2003; 13:33–6.
13. Giulianotti PC, Coratti A, Angelini M, Sbrana F, Cecconi S, Balestracci T, Caravaglios G. Robotics in general surgery: personal experience in a large community hospital. Arch Surg. 2003;138:777–84.
14. Shakir M, Boone BA, Polanco PM, Zenati MS, Hogg ME, Tsung A, Choudry HA, Moser AJ, Bartlett DL, Zeh HJ, Zureikat AH. The learning curve for robotic distal pancreatectomy: an analysis of outcomes of the first 100 consecutive cases at a high-volume pancreatic centre. HPB. 2015;17:580–6.
15. Boone BA, Zenati M, Hogg ME, Steve J, Moser AJ, Bartlett DL, Zeh HJ, Zureikat AH. Assessment of quality outcomes for robotic pancreaticoduodenectomy: identification of the learning curve. JAMA Surg. 2015;150:416–22.
16. Zureikat AH, Postlewait LM, Liu Y, Gillespie TW, et al. A multi-institutional comparison of perioperative outcomes of robotic and open pancreaticoduodenectomy. Ann Surg. 2016;264(4):640–9.

Laparoscopic Distal Pancreatectomy

22

Andrea Laurenzi, Daniel Pietrasz, Gabriella Pittau, and Antonio Sa Cunha

22.1 Introduction

Laparoscopic distal pancreatectomy (LDP) was firstly described by Gagner in 1996 [1]. Nevertheless 20 years have passed from the first resection, the rate of laparoscopic approach remains between 10–20% in national wide series [2–4]. Recently a Cochrane review has compared the open to the laparoscopic approach in the treatment of pancreatic cancer [5]. In such review there are no differences between the two groups in terms of post-operative mortality, morbidity, pancreatic fistula, resection margins and disease recurrence. The only statistically significant difference is the length of hospital stay, which is in favor of laparoscopic approach. Currently there is an ongoing randomized clinical trial comparing the open versus laparoscopic distal pancreatectomy (Leopard NTR 5188).

LDP can be realized with or without splenectomy, such difference mainly depends on surgical indication, malignant tumors in the first case while benign or borderline disease in the latter one.

In case of spleen preservation, the pancreatic resection can be performed either with splenic vessels conservation [6] or resection also known as the Warshaw's technique (WT) [7].

The main issue of LDP is the lack of standardization of the technique. Recently the French Association for Hepatobiliary Surgery and Liver Transplantation (ACHBT) has realized a review of the literature in order to recognize and standardize the different steps of LDP [8].

22.2 Patient's Position and Trocars' Placement

Patient is placed in supine position with the legs opened, the operator stands between the legs, while the first and second assistant on the left and right side of the patients respectively, the scrub nurse stands between the operator and the second assistant just next to the right leg of the patient. During the operation the patient is placed in a reverse Trendelenburg position with the table that can be partially rotated on the right side to facilitate the dissection of the pancreas' tail and the spleen.

Some papers from Asia propose a right lateral decubitus in order to perform a retrograde dissection; however such position is not utilized in our daily practice.

Electronic Supplementary Material The online version of this chapter (doi:10.1007/978-3-319-54301-7_22) contains supplementary material, which is available to authorized users. On http://springerlink.com enter the DOI number given above.

A. Laurenzi • D. Pietrasz • G. Pittau
A.S. Cunha (✉)
Hepatobiliary Center, Paul Brousse Hospital, University of Paris Sud, Villejuif, France
e-mail: andrea.laurenzi@aphp.fr; antonio.sacunha@aphp.fr

M.A. Cuesta (ed.), *Minimally Invasive Surgery for Upper Abdominal Cancer*, DOI 10.1007/978-3-319-54301-7_22

We normally use four trocars as showed in Fig. 22.1. The pneumoperitoneum is realized with the open laparoscopy technique 3 cm above the umbilicus and a 10–12 mm is inserted at this site with a 12-mmHg pressure. This port is used for the optical device insertion which is a 30-degree high definition camera. Two others 10–12 mm trocars are placed on the left and right mid-clavicular line respectively 1–2 cm cranial to the camera trocar close to the costal margin. Finally, a 5 mm epigastric port is placed under the xiphoid process. Accessorily another 5 mm trocar can be inserted in the left flank to facilitate the exposure. Currently, we use the AirSeal System (Conmed, Utica, NY, USA) to establish the pneumoperitoneum, such device allows a better surgical view since it removes the fog produced during dissection without reducing the inflation level.

22.3 Surgical Dissection

We will now describe the technique used for the spleno-pancreatectomy for ductal adenocarcinoma of the pancreas, while surgical variations such as spleen preservation will be discussed in another paragraph.

The procedure begins with a complete exploration of the abdominal cavity in order to exclude any possible contraindication such as liver metastasis, carcinosis and adjacent organs invasion. Once the surgical indication is confirmed, the operation is started by opening the gastro-colic ligament using an energy based device; during this maneuver a forceps is placed in the 5 mm subxyphoid trocar in order to pull up the stomach while the surgeon's left hand lowers the transverse colon. Gastroepiploic vessels should be manipulated with care in order to avoid injuries.

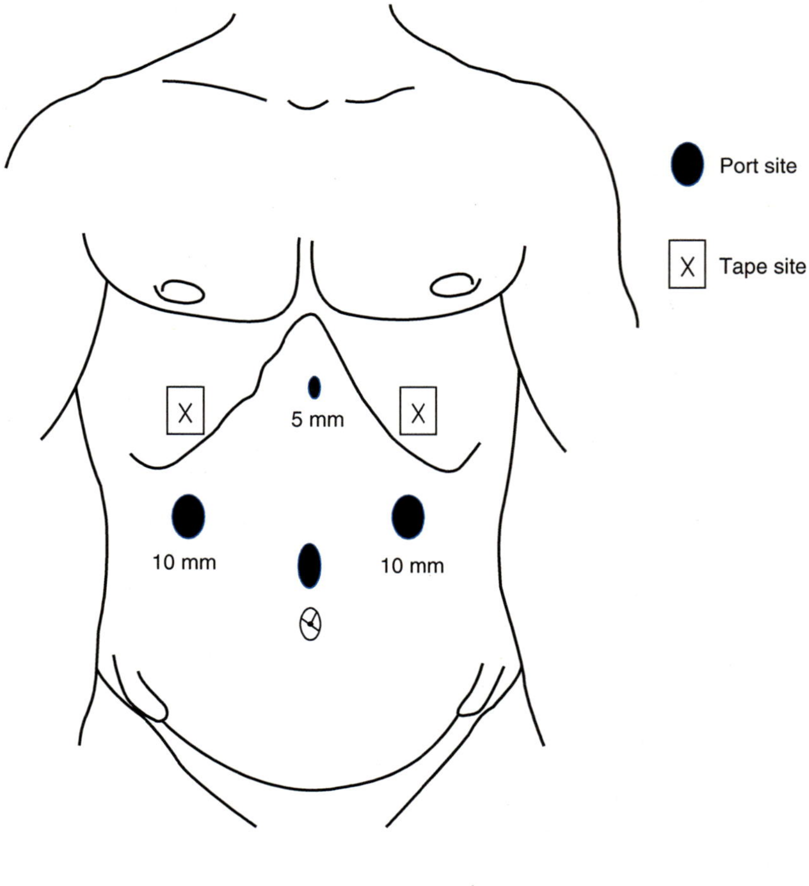

Fig. 22.1 Trocars' and tapes's position

Once the lesser sac is entered, we partially open the hepato-duodenal ligament in order to place two tapes around the stomach. The two tips of the tapes are pulled outside of the abdomen and secured with two forceps in the two subcostal regions (Fig. 22.1). Such technique allows retracting the stomach toward the anterior abdominal wall in a stable way, in order to better visualize the pancreas and free one of the assistant's hand (Fig. 22.2). At this time an intra-operative ultrasonography of the pancreas can be realized, if needed, to detect small lesions.

The dissection of the pancreas is then realized in an anterograde fashion; such approach reduces the tumor manipulation and allows an easier control of splenic vessels.

The first-step is a smooth dissection of the isthmic region in order to create a retro-pancreatic window. The neck is dissected with bipolar forceps, an energy based device and scissors. Once the superior mesenteric vein is identified the dissection is carried on following its anterior wall, once the window is created the dissection is continued on the superior border of the pancreas in order to identify the common hepatic artery (CHA). After having isolated the CHA a dissector is passed in the window behind the pancreas and a 5 cm tape is put around the neck. This tape allows a slight retraction of the pancreas in the caudal direction which facilitates the dissection of the superior border. The dissection is carried on from the right to the left in order to follow the CHA toward the celiac axis. Once the origin of the splenic artery is identified and dissected another 5 cm tape is passed around the vessel's wall to facilitate artery control before ligation. We normally use two or more 10 mm Hem-O-Lock (Teleflex, Athlone, Ireland) clips to control the artery 1–2 cm from its origin. The artery is then cut between clips.

The next step is the parenchymal section. After having pulled up the tape around the pancreas neck the stapler is inserted through one of the 10–12 mm trocars according to the best axis. The parenchymal section at the isthmic region has been shown to reduce the incidence of post-operative pancreatic fistula since the pancreas thickness is reduced if compared to the body or the tail (ref BJN).

The transection is usually achieved by using an Endo-GIA linear stapler (Medtronic Covidien, Minneapolis, MN, USA) with a medium/tick 45/60 mm recharge. This technique allows a faster and bloodless control of the two pancreatic stumps. The pancreas can be also divided using an energy based device and the Wirsung duct can be then sutured separately.

Once the parenchymal transection is realized, the splenic vein control is easier. After having dissected the origin of the splenic vein the vessel can be controlled either with clips or stapler, great attention must be taken in order to section the vein 1–2 cm far from the spleno-mesenteric confluence in order to avoid subsequent portal/superior mesenteric vein stenosis. In case of

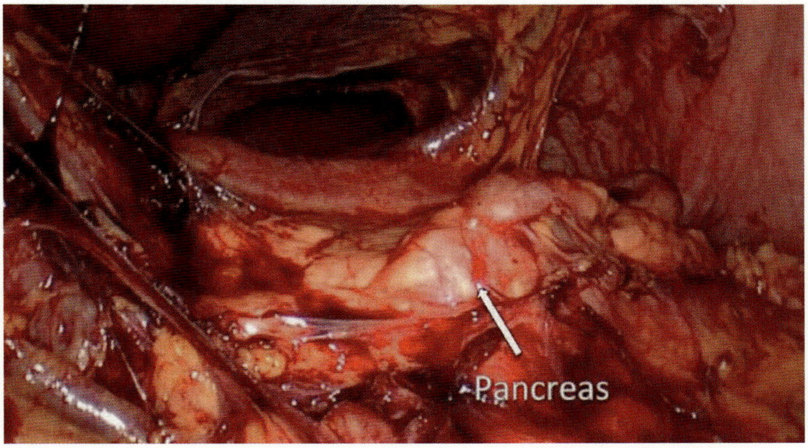

Fig. 22.2 Pancreas exposure after tape retraction

previous pancreatitis or obese patients, the control of pancreas and splenic vein separately is not always feasible. In such situation, the stapler section can include the parenchyma and the vein at the same time, however such approach is not utilized in our daily practice.

We recommend to routinely start from artery control, since an interruption of the vein before the artery can lead to an intra-operative development of portal hypertension that can increase bleeding and reduce the view on the surgical field.

The last step is the complete mobilization of the pancreas and the spleen. This dissection has two main objectives: (1) to complete the lymph-node dissection and (2) to achieve a wider posterior margin for oncological reasons. Such rules allow performing the radical antegrade modular pancreatosplenectomy (RAMPS) as proposed by Strasberg [9] (Fig. 22.3).

The dissection plane is carried on starting from the left side of superior mesenteric artery toward the spleen. The posterior and inferior limit of the dissection are the left renal vein and the transverse mesocolon, the Gerota's fascia must be resected together with the surgical specimen. The left adrenal gland can be resected or not according to its involvement with the tumor. The superior plane goes from the splenic artery stump until the gastro-splenic ligament with the division of all short gastric vessels. The resection ends up with the total liberation of the spleen with the lieno-phrenic ligament section.

Once the dissection is completed, a 15 cm endobag is inserted and the specimen is extracted through a Pfannestiel incision or enlarging the incision of the left mid-axillary line trocar.

The camera is then reinserted in order to verify the hemostasis and to place a suction drain next to the pancreatic stump.

Once the intervention is ended the surgical specimen is marked with paint in order to allow the pathologist a better understanding of the margins (Fig. 22.4).

22.4 Spleen Preservation

As mentioned above in case of benign or borderline tumors the spleen can be preserved. In such cases there are two main differences if compared to the above described splenopancreatectomy: (1) the site of parenchymal transection and (2) splenic vessel control.

The site of pancreas transection can be moved away from the pancreatic neck (i.e. pancreatic tail IPMN), the exact site of section can be decided either on the pre-operative imaging or with intra-operative ultrasounds. In such situation the parenchymal division is realized in the same fashion as previously described.

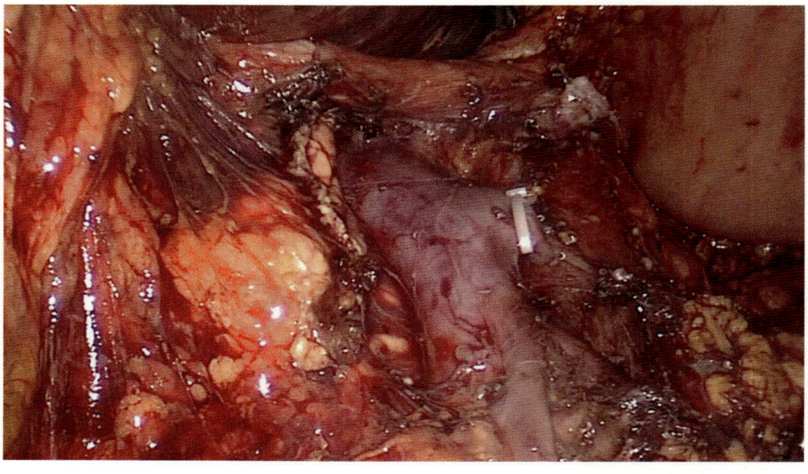

Fig. 22.3 Surgical field at the end of operation

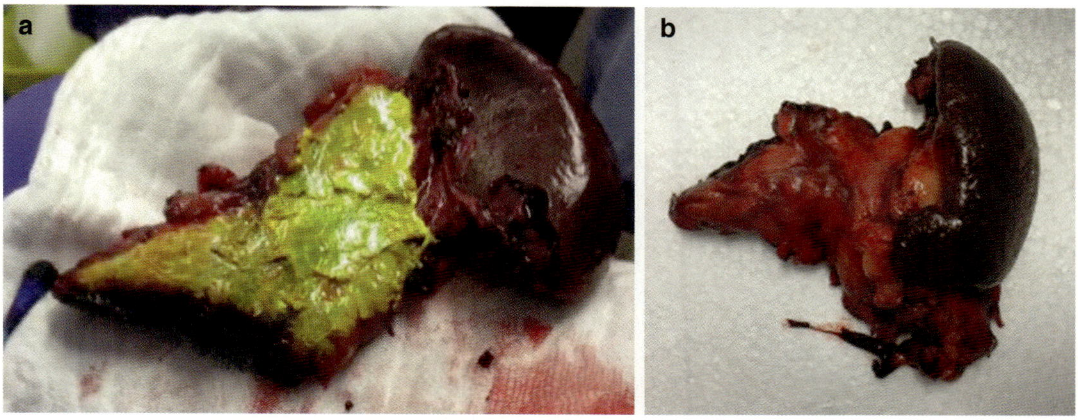

Fig. 22.4 (**a**) Surgical specimen is inked on the posterior margin (*yellow*) and on the transection line (*blue*); (**b**) the specimen is fixed on a hard surface in order to allow a better understanding of orientation

For what it concerns the splenic vessels management the artery and vein can be either resected with the specimen WT or preserved (Fig. 22.5).

In a recent meta-analysis comparing the two operations, there were no differences in terms of post-operative complications and incidence of pancreatic fistula between the two groups, however patients undergoing laparoscopic WT had statistically significant reduced blood loss but presented an increased rate of gastric varices and splenic infarction (Video 22.1).

In case of WT the artery is proximally controlled as mentioned before, the pancreas is then freed on is lower edge from the transverse mesocolon with an energy based device. The tail of the pancreas must be completely freed from the splenic hilum and the short gastric vessels must be identified at their origin. Such maneuver can be difficult and hemorrhagic if the tail is long. The artery is then sectioned before the origin of the first short gastric vessel. Once the arterial inflow is controlled the vein is sectioned proximally and distally and the specimen is freed from the surrounding tissue (Fig. 22.5a).

In case of splenic vessels preservation, the dissection must be carried on from the right to the left and the small arterial and venous branches going to the pancreas must be selectively controlled either with clips or coagulation (Fig. 22.5b).

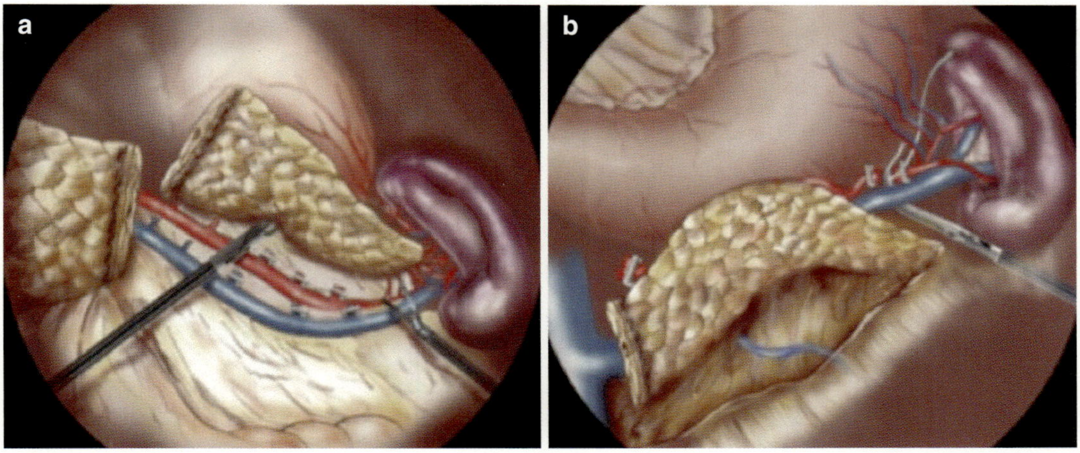

Fig. 22.5 Spleen preserving techniques: (**a**) Splenic vessels preservation; (**b**) Warshaw's technique with splenic vessels resection

References

1. Gagner M, Pomp A, Herrera MF. Early experience with laparoscopic resections of islet cell tumors. Surgery. 1996;120(6):1051–4.
2. de Rooij T, Jilesen AP, Boerma D, Bonsing BA, Bosscha K, Van Dam RM, et al. A nationwide comparison of laparoscopic and open distal pancreatectomy for benign and malignant disease. J Am Coll Surg. 2015;220(3):263–270.e1.
3. Sulpice L, Farges O, Goutte N, Bendersky N, Dokmak S, Sauvanet A, et al. Laparoscopic distal pancreatectomy for pancreatic ductal adenocarcinoma: time for a randomized controlled trial? Results of an all-inclusive national observational study. Ann Surg. 2015;262(5):868–73, discussion 873–4.
4. Balzano G, Bissolati M, Boggi U, Bassi C, Zerbi A, Falconi M, et al. A multicenter survey on distal pancreatectomy in Italy: results of minimally invasive technique and variability of perioperative pathways. Updat Surg. 2014;66(4):253–63.
5. Riviere D, Gurusamy KS, Kooby DA, Vollmer CM, Besselink MGH, Davidson BR, et al. Laparoscopic versus open distal pancreatectomy for pancreatic cancer. Cochrane Database Syst Rev. 2016;4:CD011391.
6. Kimura W, Inoue T, Futakawa N, Shinkai H, Han I, Muto T. Spleen-preserving distal pancreatectomy with conservation of the splenic artery and vein. Surgery. 1996;120(5):885–90.
7. Warshaw AL. Distal pancreatectomy with preservation of the spleen. J Hepatobiliary Pancreat Sci. 2010;17(6):808–12.
8. Mohkam K, Farges O, Pruvot FR, Muscari F, Régimbeau JM, Regenet N, et al. Toward a standard technique for laparoscopic distal pancreatectomy? Synthesis of the 2013 ACHBT Spring workshop. 2015. p.167–78.
9. Mitchem JB, Hamilton N, Gao F, Hawkins WG, Linehan DC, Strasberg SM. Long-term results of resection of adenocarcinoma of the body and tail of the pancreas using radical antegrade modular pancreatosplenectomy procedure. J Am Coll Surg. 2012; 214(1):46–52.

23 Hybrid Laparoscopic Duodenopancreatectomy

Ulrich Wellner, Kim Honselmann, and Tobias Keck

23.1 Introduction

Laparoscopic pancreatoduodenectomy is currently limited to a few tertiary centers worldwide. The slow distribution of this technique since its first description by Gagner and Pomp (Gagner 1994) more than twenty years ago is due to numerous reasons: (1) In contrast to laparoscopic distal pancreatectomy, the laparoscopic pancreatic head resection is characterized by a complex reconstruction involving the pancreatic anastomosis as well as the biliojejunal anastomosis. (2) The technical prerequisites for dissectors and instrumentation have only been developed during the past few years. (3) The combination of laparoscopic proficiency with profound expertise in pancreatic surgery has only just emerged in this new generation of surgeons. In summary, there has been a very dynamic development of the laparoscopic pancreatic head resection during the past few years. There have been published series with over 50 patients demonstrating the feasibility and safety of this technique in specialized centers. In highly specialized teams this technique is even advanced towards more complex surgeries including portal vein resection as well as laparoscopic portal vein reconstruction [1]. The rapid development of this field can be noted when highlighting the number of cases published between January 2012 and June 2013, which exceed the numbers of the 15 years prior [2].

In general, different techniques are differentiated by the nomenclature of the procedures: laparoscopic pancreatoduodenectomy with laparoscopic reconstruction, laparoscopic pancreatoduodenectomy with open reconstruction (Hybrid operation), hand-assisted laparoscopic pancreatoduodenectomy and telemetric -or robotic assisted pancreatoduodenectomy. We will be focusing on the first two techniques in this chapter. Of note, the results described in the following have been acquired in a few expert centers and are currently not recommended for common applicability.

23.2 Indication

Indications for minimal-invasive *pancreatoduodenectomy* are

- Cystic tumors
- Neuroendocrine tumors

U. Wellner • K. Honselmann • T. Keck, M.B.A. (✉)
Department of Surgery, University Medical Center Schleswig-Holstein, Campus Luebeck, Ratzeburger Allee 160, 23538 Luebeck, Germany
e-mail: Tobias.Keck@uksh.de

M.A. Cuesta (ed.), *Minimally Invasive Surgery for Upper Abdominal Cancer*,
DOI 10.1007/978-3-319-54301-7_23

The oncologic pancreatoduodenectomy is performed in

- Cystic tumors with malignant potential
- Neuroendocrine tumors with malignant potential
- Small malignant tumors

[3]. There have been studies describing experiences with complex operations with mesoenterico-portal vein reconstruction. The percentage of malignant tumors in these series represent up to 50% [2].

23.3 Specific Diagnostics

The computertomography with contrast (Angio-CT) is the gold standard diagnostic tool before surgical intervention of the pancreas. The MRI plus MRCP can give, especially in cystic lesions of the pancreas, additional information such as communication to the main duct or differentiation of serous or mucinous neoplasm. One of the most important details that must be obtained from imaging is the relationship to the mesenterico-portal axis, because an inflammatory contact or an invasive nature of the tumor into the mesenterico-portal vasculature often leads to conversion [4]. Detailed preoperative imaging can therefore assist with patient selection in order to reduce the conversion rate, especially in the beginning of the learning curve.

23.4 Consent

The current guidelines do not recommend the use of laparoscopic pancreatic head resection. Because lawsuits following complications from this procedure may result, extended consent must be obtained. Conversions are common even in large series and are reported to be around 15% [5, 6]. New studies from the American College of Surgeons National Surgical Quality Improvement Program demonstrate, that there is a highly relevant correlation between the number of laparoscopic pancreatic procedures in each center and their results. Centers with low expertise in pancreatic surgery in general had a highly significant increase in surgical mortality. So especially in low volume centers, this procedure can only be performed with a very detailed and extensive consent and cannot be recommended based on current knowledge [7]. The possible necessity to convert to an open procedure as well as injuries to the mesenterico-portal vasculature, the vessels of the celiac trunc and the mesenteric superior artery should be discussed. A common complication after open, but also laparoscopic pancreatic head resection is the pancreatic fistula (up to 20% in randomized control studies [8]). So far there is no evidence for a lower incidence of pancreatic fistulas in laparoscopic pancreatic head resections. Advantages are less hernias, shorter hospital and intensive care unit stays, less pain and less blood loss. Oncological advantages can be drawn from the conclusion that more patients are able to receive their adjuvant therapy faster [1]. Though, studies on this topic are not sufficient to draw real conclusions. General surgical complications result from the procedure itself and are described in commercially available consent forms. Complications include injuries to adjacent organs, acute hemorrhage, pancreatic fistulas, delayed hemorrhage (pseudoaneurysm), anastomotic leaks of the pancreatic-, the biliary- and the jejunal anastomoses.

23.5 Positioning

The patient is placed supine in a mildly reversed trendelenburg position with legs in abduction (modified beach chair position or French position). Both arms are tucked in order to avoid arm plexus lesions, the right arm can possibly be positioned out for better accessibility for the anesthesiologist.

Positioning aids are a footboard to lengthen the operating table, leg holders for variability of leg abduction, a detachable headrest, lateral retractors (especially on the right side of the patient), safety belt above both thighs. Also, the stabilizing positioning on a short vacuum mattress at the torso has been proven to be practical.

The safety belt is positioned above both upper thighs for fixation. Legs are abducted and are secured by elastic straps to the leg holders. The safety technology is of great importance, because in order to dissect the pancreatic tail to the left, the patient needs to be tilted far towards his right hand side. The neutral electrode is placed laterally on the left or right upper thigh. Possibly, the use of intermittent pneumatic compression can be considered for long procedures or risk patients.

The monitor is placed above the left shoulder of the patient, the surgeon stand on the right side, the (1) Assistant (camera) stands between the legs, the (2) assistant stands on the left side, if needed. The surgical nurse stands on the left leg of the patient (Fig. 23.1).

23.6 Technical Prerequisites

The following technical prerequisites should be present:

- Positioning table with the option of gravity displacement and leg abduction in order to establish the modified beach chair position or the French position.
- Dissection devices with bipolar coagulation (for example Ligasure Dolphin Tip, Fa. Covidien, Boulder, CO, USA), ultrasonic dissection device (for example Ultracision, Fa. J&J Ethicon, Cornelia, GA, USA) or combination devices (z.B. Thunderbeat, Olympus Tokyo Japan). Thermal effects on vessels (celiac trunk, superior mesenteric artery and the mesentericoportal vein axis (MPV)) and delicate dissection options should be considered when choosing a product.
- Regular instrumentation for laparoscopy, as well as laparoscopic bulldog vessel clamps (Aesculap), Goldfinger (OB Tech), bipolar

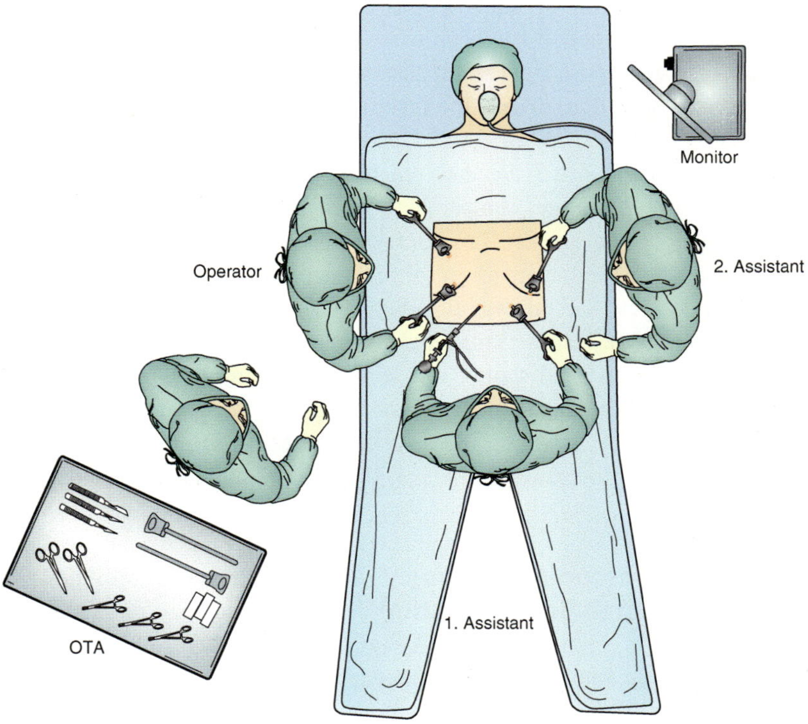

Fig. 23.1 Patient positioning in beach chair position. The surgeon is on the right hand side, the 1st assistant leading the camera between the patient's legs. The patient is half sitting, turned with raised trunk and slightly to the right

laparoscopic scissors and overholt (Aesculap), Endo Paddle Retract (Covidien), titan clips.
– Readily available operating instrumentation equipment for an open procedure in case of quick conversion for hemorrhage.

23.7 Thoughts on the Choice of Type of Procedure

23.7.1 Laparoscopic Resection and Open Reconstruction (Hybrid Operation)

There are multiple advantages pertaining to this procedure: (1) When combining the reconstruction via a retrieval incision in the upper abdomen with the laparoscopic resection, both the safe procedure of reconstruction and the good visibility of laparoscopy can be united in one procedure. (2) The incision for the reconstruction is not much bigger than the retrieval incision that is described in published series. (3) The learning curve for the complex and important reconstruction is avoided. (4) The combination of laparoscopic resection with open reconstruction has been used in other procedures (lap.- assist. right hemicolectomy, lap. assist. sigma resection). When the three types of procedures explained above (total laparoscopic, hybrid and robot- assisted) are analyzed, mortality and morbidity rates are comparable. In some series, laparoscopic assisted procedures showed the same advantages that are given for full laparoscopic procedures. And this was already present in the beginning of the learning curve and they sometimes even demonstrated shorter operating times and fewer complications. In most centers this procedure is seen as a 'Bridging' procedure for the full laparoscopic procedure.

23.7.2 Laparoscopic Resection and Open Reconstruction

Within this topic, most published series describe the laparoscopic resection with open reconstruction (see Table 3 in [2]). As it is common in open techniques, the pancreatojejunostomy as well as the pancreaticojejunostomy are used more often than the pancreatogastrostomy. The pancreatogastrostomy presents a simple and fast anastomosis, that especially in the laparoscopic setting can be simplified and therefore be advantageous. A randomized comparison between pancreatogastrostomy and pancreaticojejunostomy (RECOPANC) has meanwhile proven the safety of this reconstruction technique [8]. Biliary reconstruction can often be more difficult in the minimal invasive technique than the pancreatic anastomosis, because the angle for reconstruction is unfavorable via the ports placed for the resection. Cumulative studies of single series [9] demonstrate, that the average operating time of 422 min (7 h) for the preselected patients is still above the time for open procedures in centers with high pancreatic expertise. Morbidity (18–64%) and mortality (0–8%) are found within those of open procedures. This must be considered when looking at registry studies where a much higher mortality and morbidity is stated [10]. Single series might only publish the experience of experts and surgeons after the learning curve (Publication bias). In robotic reconstruction the advantages of angulation of the instruments are possibly leveled by the lack of haptic feedback in pancreatic surgery [9]. Long and shallow learning curves are often quoted as disadvantages of the laparoscopic pancreatic head resection. The usage of hybrid techniques has successfully been able to safely implement a laparoscopic pancreatic program [11]. Detailed studies of laparoscopic pancreatic surgery are suggesting 50 operations in order to be able to reach the advantages pertaining to OR time and reduced blood loss, where the ten first cases are the most relevant obstacles in implementing a program [11]. A cumulative sum analysis and a risk adjusted cumulative sum analysis is confirming these results [12].

For the dissection of small and multiple branches from the splenic vein and artery to the pancreas, dissection devices or metallic clips are technically suitable. In our experience, bipolar dissection devices are especially well suited. A critical point that diverges from the open technique is the transection of the pancreatic parenchyma on the mesenterico-portal axis. While the transection of the pancreatic neck in the open procedure is usually done with a scalpel and bleeding is avoided by putting holding sutures on the pancreatic arterial arcade, this technique cannot be advised in the laparoscopic setting due to high risk of hemorrhage. This is why the transection is usually performed using energy devices (often ultrasonic scissors) or staplers with reopening the pancreatic duct afterwards. Using ultrasonic scissors include the risk of thermic injuries to the organ [13, 14].

Practical tip
The transection of the pancreatic neck is especially challenging in the laparoscopic pancreatic head resection. Here staplers or ultrasonic dissection devices can be used.

Practical tip
In case of stapler use the pancreatic duct needs be reopened before anastomosis.

Practical tip
Transection with ultrasonic devices poses the risk of thermal injury to the pancreas and pancreatitis of the remnant.

23.8 Surgical Technique—How I Do It

23.8.1 Port Placement and Access to the Omental Bursa

During a laparoscopic pancreatoduodenectomy there are usually four working trocars and one camera trocar necessary (Fig. 23.2.). The camera trocar is placed 3 cm below the navel in the midline, the working ports are placed in the right upper abdomen, the left middle and lower abdomen in a semilunar line around the location of interest. The 5 mm ports on the right are placed a little bit more lateral than for a distal pancreatectomy in order to facilitate a full Kocher maneuver.

Practical tip
Extreme positioning is necessary for gravity displacement in laparoscopic pancreatic surgery. Lateral boards on the right hand side enable extreme positioning for the access to the pancreatic tail and allow for intraabdominal displacement of organs (colon and omentum).

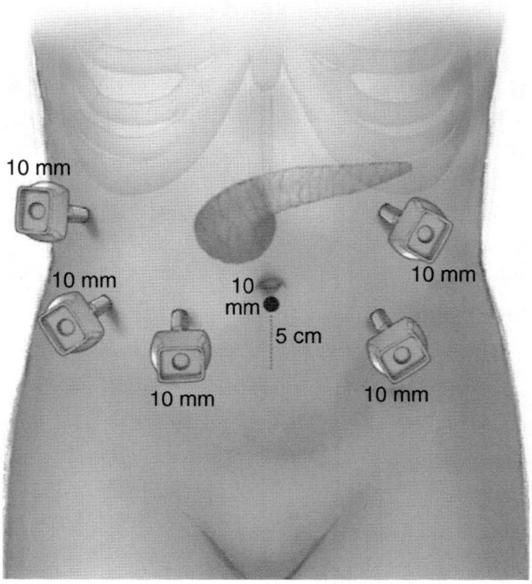

Fig. 23.2 Port placement for the laparoscopic pancreatic head resection in a five-trocar technique. The camera port must be introduced subumbilical or in the area of the right middle abdomen. The remaining trocars are placed in a semilunar line around the area of interest. The arms of the patient are tucked on both sides

Practical tip
The passive pulling of the omentum caudally by reverse Trendelenburg positioning can facilitate the transection of the omentum close to the gastroepiploic arcade instead of directly at the colon.

After abdominal exploration, the omental bursa is opened while conserving the gastroepiploic arcade. The omental bursa is entered close to the gastroepiploic arcade because then the major omentum can pull down the transverse colon by reverse Trendelenburg positioning.

The second assistant mostly has a static role. He or she stands on the left hand side of the patient and lifts up the stomach towards the abdominal wall with an atraumatic grasper.

23.8.2 Exploration and Laparoscopic Ultrasound

For small tumors, intraoperative ultrasound can be very helpful for localizing the tumor. Especially the relation to the mesenterico-portal axis and to the celiac trunk/superior mesenteric artery is crucial.

Practical tip

Sonographic information about the relation of the tumor to the mesenterico-portal axis can simplify further dissection and reduce the risk of vein injury.

In the following the right colic flexure is mobilized and the Kocher maneuver is performed, which in the laparoscopic setting is done past the inferior vena cava up to the origin of the superior mesenteric artery (mesenteric artery first Approach).

23.8.3 Mobilization of the Pancreas and Exposure of the Vessels (Fig. 23.3)

The exposure of the vessel starts from a caudal position. Structures of the gastrocolic trunk of Henle, especially the right gastroepiploic vein, serve as guiding structures. This vessel is ligated directly at the superior mesenteric vein (SMV), whereby a titan clip has proven its value. In bigger tumors dissection is performed closer to the duodenal knee by the mesenteric root. This dissection step (with circular exposure of the SMV) is quite demanding overall. After the circular exposure of the SMV, the dissection is carried on a few more centimeters along the lower pancreatic edge towards the pancreatic tail.

The right gastroepiploic artery is visualized and divided at the pancreatic head, the pylorus is

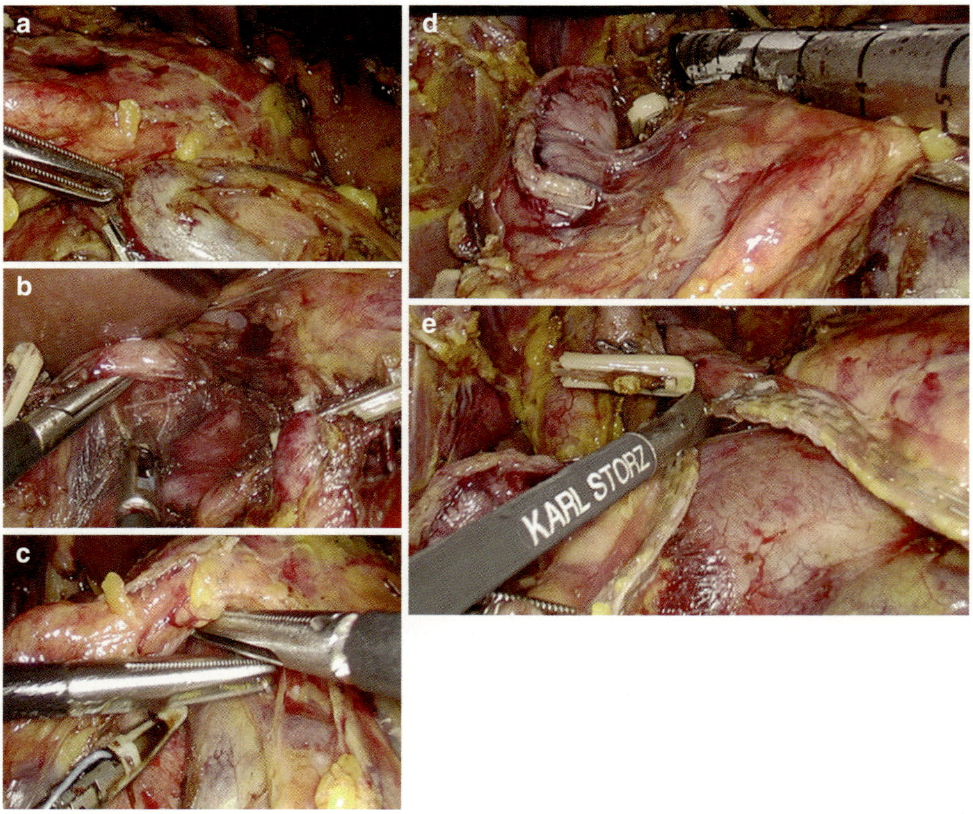

Fig. 23.3 Preparation and of the mesentericoportal axis and dissection of the pancreas. (**a**) Preparation of the inferior mesenteric vein on the lower border of the pancreas. (**b**) Preparation of the portal vein on the upper border of the pancreas. (**c**) Tunneling of the vein (**d**) Control of the tumor growth by endoscopic ultrasound. (**e**) Dissection of the pancreas on the mesentericoportal axis

dissected free in a circular fashion and the duodenum is transected via an endostapler 1 cm post pylorus, then the stomach is pushed into the left upper abdomen.

The hepatoduodenal ligament is visualized. Total lymphadenectomy is completed; visualization of the common, proper, right and left hepatic artery as well as the gastroduodenal artery (GDA) is completed. Before division of the bile duct, absence of a replaced or an additional right hepatic artery tangential to the bile duct has to be validated. Also, either antegrade or retrograde gallbladder dissection from the liver bed is achieved before bile duct division and while the gallbladder remains attached to the pancreatic side of the divided bile duct. After bile duct division, view on the GDA is facilitated for clipping it with PDS Clips. Lymphadenectomy is now completed at the upper pancreatic edge around the celiac trunk, the left gastric artery as well as circular exposure of the portal vein. From cranial and caudally the dissection levels at the pancreas will be combined and the organ will be undermined at the height of the mesenterico-portal axis.

23.8.4 Division of the Pancreas at the Neck and Dissection of the Mesopancreas Along the Superior Mesenteric Artery (Fig. 23.4)

After tunneling the pancreas at the mesenteric-portal axis, the parenchyma is divided at the pancreatic neck. The different techniques for this step are explained in 22.7.2. We prefer a

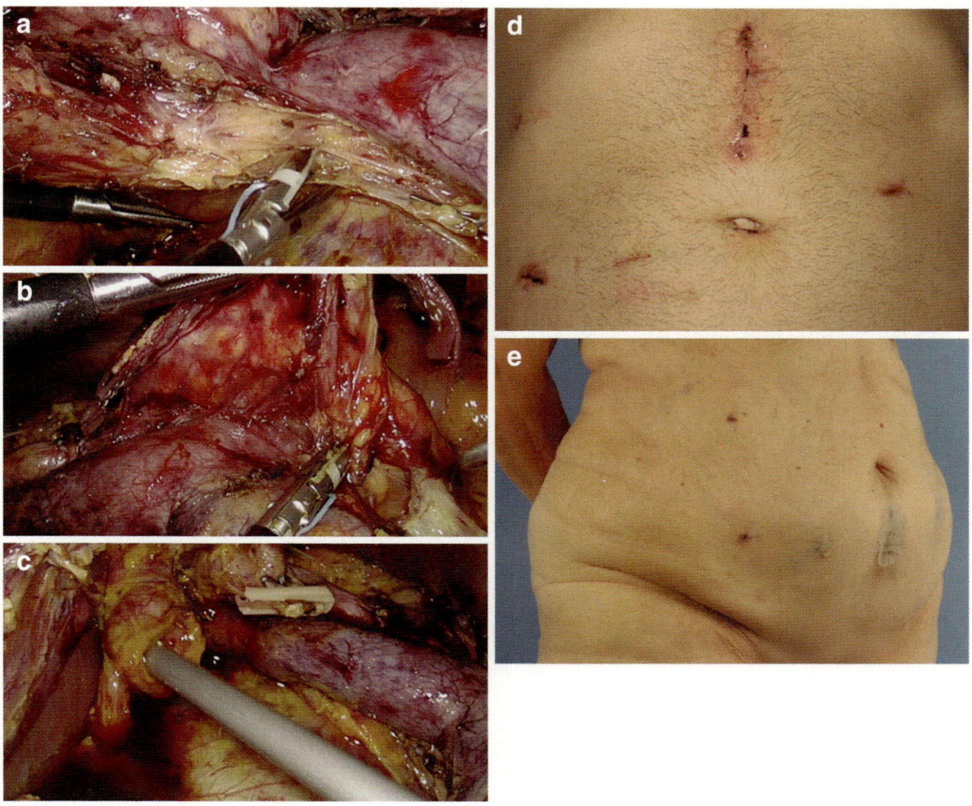

Fig. 23.4 Laparoscopic dissection of the mesenterico-portal axis. (**a**) Preparation of the uncinate process along the superior mesenteric artery. (**b**) Preparation remaining pancreatic tail in preparation of pancreatogastrostomy. (**c**) Situs after removal of the pancreatic head. (**d**) Cosmetic result after pancreastic head resection and hybrid/open reconstruction. (**e**) Cosmetic result after fully laparoscopic pancreatic head resection

linear endostapler with an articulation joint to reach good homeostasis. Before transection an ultrasound to judge localization of the tumor and distance to the transection margin is recommended.

Then the stapler row in the range of the pancreatic duct is selectively removed. Alternatively, the parenchyma can be divided stepwise with an ultrasonic dissector, but the main duct has to be identified and preserved. After organ division, the pancreas is mobilized leftward along the splenic vein over 3 cm in order to prepare the later step of the pancreatogastrostomy. Regularly, there are two small arterial branches coming off the superior mesenteric artery and splenic artery at the lower edge of the pancreas that have to be clipped via titan clips. In the next step the first jejunal loop is visualized underneath the mesocolon. For this, the second assistant raises the colon with an Endo-retractor (z.B. Endo Paddle Retract, Covidien Medtronic®). Further dissection is achieved towards the mesenteric root up to the fusion of the prior dissection plane from the Kocher maneuver. The jejunum is transected inframesocolic using a linear stapler and is placed into the right upper abdomen. Now the mesopancreas is transected stepwise along the first venous jejunal branches and later the superior mesenteric artery towards the head. To facilitate this process, the first assistant pushes the SMV with a 5 mm swab cranially and left laterally. The single branches of the SMA (inferior and superior pancreaticoduodenal artery) are secured with titanium clips and the dissection plane is again reconnected to the prior plane of the mesenteric artery first approach Kocher maneuver. Small venous branches from the pancreas into the mesenterico-portal axis are transected with an Energy Device.

Finally, the entire pancreatic head is mobilized. An endobag is introduced either via a Pfannenstiel incision or via a small epigastric median laparotomy and the specimen is removed from the abdomen. The epigastric median laparotomy can be used for the anastomoses (Hybrid Operation). A wound retractor (e.g. Alexis O Wound Retractor Applied®) can aid to keep the wound open.

23.8.5 Reconstruction and Anastomoses

23.8.5.1 Reconstruction Via Retrieval Incision (Hybrid Operation)

Especially in the initial phase of the learning curve, the reconstruction via the retrieval incision is a good method to reduce the risk of laparoscopic reconstruction as it has been shown in a few published reports. After the introduction of the wound retractor and the retractor system, the reconstruction is done typically via the retrieval incision. In our experience, a median epigastric laparotomy of about eight centimeter is sufficient. The retractor system conveys a pulling force into the right upper abdomen. The jejunal loop that has been pulled up retrocolically serves for the hepaticojejunostomy as an end-to-side anastomosis in single layer technique with 5-0 or 6-0 PDS C1. In our institution the pancreatic anastomosis is regularly done as a pancreatogastrostomy. Because the horizontal anastomosis as it is present in pancreato-or pancreaticojejunstomy is very challenging via this limited access. The pancreatogastrostomy is done as an invaginated anastomosis with a small dorsal gastrostomy and a larger ventral gastrostomy. A purse-string suture with 2-0 PDS SH will present the outer suture layer. The inner anastomosis is performed in single layer technique with 4-0 PDS SH in a circular manner. Also the duodenojejunostomy is made via the retrieval incision as an end-to-side anastomosis in a running fashion with 4-0 PDS. Easy-flow drains are placed via the trocar in the left and right lower abdomen to the pancreas and the biliary anastomosis. The fascia is closed with a running suture, subcutaneous sutures and intracutaneous sutures follow.

23.8.5.2 Laparoscopic Reconstruction (Pancreatogastrostomy, Hepatobiliary Anastomosis and Duodenojejunostomy)

Pancreatogastrostomy: In laparoscopic pancreatogastrostomy the incision is only made on the back wall of the stomach over a length of 2–3 cm. Two V-Loc® sutures (2-0) are placed at 6 and 12 o'clock around the dorsal incision of the stomach for later used purse-string sutures. The pancreatic invagination is achieved through two holding sutures at the lateral pancreas. These are marked with PDS Clips, which mark the height at which the stomach needs to be invaginated (usually around 2 cm). After invagination, the purse-string sutures are tightened and the pancreas is fixed into the stomach. Because randomized studies have shown more frequent hemorrhage from the transection site of the pancreas after open pancreatogastrostomies [8, 15], we close the pancreas with a stapler and only reopen the suture line in the area of the pancreatic duct. This must be done safely and the duct needs to be exposed. If unsure, intraoperative upper endoscopy can be of assistance.

Hepaticojejunal anastomosis: This anastomosis is the more difficult of the laparoscopic reconstruction anastomoses. Because the angle for this operation step is awkward, the surgeon moves in between the legs of the patient. The anastomosis is separated into two running sutures each running on one half of the circumference of the bile duct from 6 until 12 o'clock. This technique, where the sidewalls are sutured separately instead of the front and back wall has been a standard technique in laparoscopic surgery for better visibility. In case of a thick walled biliary duct, for example after preoperative stenting, the anastomosis can be done in a running fashion with self-holding sutures (Stratafix® 5-0 or V-Loc® 4-0 or Silk 5-0). For a thin biliary duct the suture is performed with a 5-0 or 6-0 PDS or Vicryl suture. PDS sutures are generally not suitable for a laparoscopic approach because the sutures can break when grabbed by the instruments.

Duodenojejunostomy: for this anastomosis, first an additional running suture fixes the stapler rows of the stomach and jejunum. Furthermore, the stapler rows are opened and the second row of the back wall suture as well as the front wall suture is performed as a running suture with 4-0 Vicryl. The drains of the anastomoses are placed as described above. The removal of the ports is done under visualization in order to detect hemorrhage from the abdominal wall. Trocar sites are closed by suture.

23.9 Distinct Intraoperative Complications and Their Management

Relevant intraoperative hemorrhage is often complicating a laparoscopic pancreatoduodenectomy. At the beginning of the surgery, the mesenterico-portal axis below the pancreas should be visualized to prepare for possible bleeding complications. Orientation is given by dissecting along the larger veins. Should a hemorrhage from the vein occur, bulldog clamps could be placed here laparoscopically. Portal vein hemorrhage appears less severe as during the open procedure because of the increased intra-abdominal pressure. Initially intra-abdominal pressure should be elevated (about 16 mm Hg). This helps with better visibility. Uncontrolled coagulation should be refrained from. Primary compression with a 10 mm pin should be accomplished first to get a clear view on the situation. A primary suture is rarely necessary.

Cave!

For venous hemorrhage, irrigation is more useful than suctioning for a better view. Suction reduces the intra-abdominal pressure and results in more bleeding.

As mentioned above, problems can occur when transecting the pancreas with a stapler. When bleeding occurs as the pancreas is divided, bipolar coagulation can be done carefully along the stapler suture line. Often the bleeding stops by applying pressure with a sterile compress. Thermal damage to the arteries can also present a danger near vascular preparation. We typically use titanium clips for clipping branches from the superior mesenteric artery to the pancreatic head or to the pancreatic body. A conversion is usually necessary when the arterial injury is more complex.

23.10 Evidence Based Evaluation

There are currently no prospective randomized trials comparing laparoscopic pancreatic head resections to open pancreatic head resections. In a systematic review of Boggi and co-authors [2] about 25 articles with 746 laparoscopic pancreatic head resection were evaluated. The majority of patients were operated completely laparoscopically (51.7%), followed by the robotically assisted pancreatic head resection (31.3%) and laparoscopically assisted surgery (Hybrid, 16.2%). For the operation generally 5–7 ports were used, where the camera was usually placed infraumbilically. In the above addressed issue of the transection of pancreas parenchyma, an ultrasonic dissector was used in most cases (55.9%). There was also disagreement regarding the extraction of the specimen after resection: here sub-umbilical, supra-pubic, supra-umbilical or subxyphoidal access is used. The most common anastomoses used in the literature were the Pancreato—or Pancreaticojejunostomy (84%) followed by Pancreatogastrostomy (9.8%), or the sole occlusion of the pancreatic duct (6.8%). The average operation time was over 7.5 h (338–710 min) and was significantly longer than for an open approach in most publications. The average hospital stay after surgery was dependent on the country in which the operation takes place (21.9 days Europe, 13.0 days Asia, 9.4 days United States) with a pancreatic fistula rate of an average of 22.3%. Taking this data into account safety benefits described above can currently not be assessed. Advantages of this procedure have been described regarding a reduction of blood loss and the time spent on the ICU. Even if current data from specialized centers show a very low mortality and similar morbidity rate, the learning curve and the need of sufficient caseload in the pancreatic center and of the surgeon must be noted. In a study by Adam et al. [7] 983 minimally invasive pancreatic resections showed that the mortality was increased with an odds ratio of 1.87 in the minimally invasive group. It is noteworthy that in this register study 92% of the participating hospitals performed less than 10 pancreatic resections in 2 years. Sharpe et al. [16] however, showed in a registry comparison of 4037 open against 284 laparoscopic pancreatic head resection, that this difference is not visible if the center performs more than 10 procedures per year. On the contrary, this study demonstrated shorter hospital stay (10 +/−8 vs. 12 +/−9.7 days, $p < 0.0001$) and less unplanned readmission (5% versus 9%; $p = 0.027$). In many centers as well as in our own experience about 30–40% of patients are operated laparoscopically producing a quorum of 40–50 pancreatic head resection in a center necessary to represent the learning curve. Kim et al. [17] indicated in a study, where the learning curve of 100 laparoscopic pancreatic head resections was analyzed, that improvement regarding the OR time, complications and length of stay still develop in between the middle and the last third of procedures. This makes the postulated learning curve of about 50 laparoscopic Whipple surgeries published in other publications likely (Table 23.1). In addition to patient-specific perioperative advantages arising from a laparoscopic pancreatic head resection, oncological aspects that are substantially more relevant should be considered. As most published series currently reflect strongly selected experiences, the perioperatively collected surrogate parameters of oncological radicality (R0 rate or LN rate) are only limited to answer this question. Interesting experiences from a highly specialized center for minimally invasive oncological pancreatic head resection come from the Mayo Clinic: a monocenter matched pair analysis of open against laparoscopic pancreatic head resection showed a longer progression-free survival in the laparoscopic group (Fig. 23.5).

At the same time a significantly lower rate of local recurrence was found there. In the experience of the Mayo clinic significantly more patients

Table 23.1 Learning curve of laparoscopic pancreatic head resection, adapted from Kim et al. [17]

	1. Third	3. Third
100 Operations		
OR time	9.8 h	6.6 h
Complications	33%	17%
Hospital length	20.4d	11.5d
Malignant 7%		
R0 100%		
LN 13 (median)		

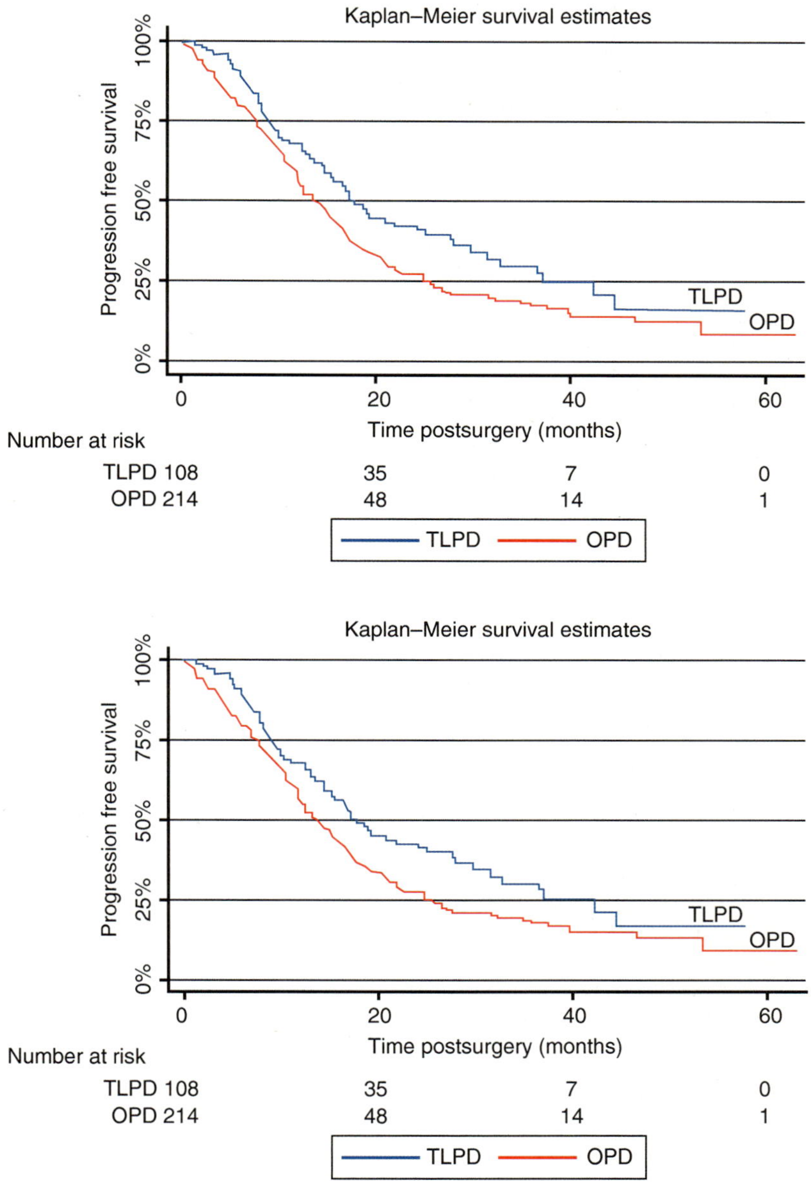

Fig. 23.5 Single series and expert results: No difference in overall survival but better progression-free survival after laparoscopic resection of the pancreatic head versus open pancreatic head resection (after Croome et al. [1])

received adjuvant therapy in less time after laparoscopic pancreatic head resection.

Single series and expert results: No difference in overall survival but better progression-free survival after laparoscopic resection of the pancreatic head versus open pancreatic head resection (after Croome et al. [1]).

So far this is a summary of the limited evidence for laparoscopic pancreatic head resection:

- Patient selection still necessary
- Feasibility demonstrated even for more complex operations
- Large case load necessary
- High hospital and high surgeon volume necessary
- Oncological quality equivalent in current data (cave: expert results)
- Registry studies required in the future

References

1. Croome KP, Farnell MB, Que FG, et al. Total laparoscopic pancreaticoduodenectomy for pancreatic ductal adenocarcinoma: oncologic advantages over open approaches? Ann Surg. 2014;260:633–40. doi:10.1097/SLA.0000000000000937.
2. Boggi U, Amorese G, Vistoli F, et al. Laparoscopic pancreaticoduodenectomy: a systematic literature review. Surg Endosc. 2015;29:9–23. doi:10.1007/s00464-014-3670-z.
3. Siech M, Bartsch D, Beger HG, et al. Indications for laparoscopic pancreas operations: results of a consensus conference and the previous laparoscopic pancreas register. Chirurg. 2012;83:247–53. doi:10.1007/s00104-011-2167-8.
4. Wellner UF, Küsters S, Sick O, et al. Hybrid laparoscopic versus open pylorus-preserving pancreatoduodenectomy: retrospective matched case comparison in 80 patients. Langenbeck's Arch Surg. 2014;399:849–56. doi:10.1007/s00423-014-1236-0.
5. Giulianotti PC, Sbrana F, Bianco FM, et al. Robot-assisted laparoscopic pancreatic surgery: single-surgeon experience. Surg Endosc. 2010;24:1646–57. doi:10.1007/s00464-009-0825-4.
6. Zeh HJ, Zureikat AH, Secrest A, et al. Outcomes after robot-assisted pancreaticoduodenectomy for periampullary lesions. Ann Surg Oncol. 2012;19:864–70. doi:10.1245/s10434-011-2045-0.
7. Adam MA, Choudhury K, Dinan MA, et al. Minimally invasive versus open pancreaticoduodenectomy for cancer: practice patterns and short-term outcomes among 7061 patients. Ann Surg. 2015;262:372–7. doi:10.1097/SLA.0000000000001055.
8. Keck T, Wellner UF, Bahra M, et al. Pancreatogastrostomy versus pancreatojejunostomy for RECOnstruction after PANCreatoduodenectomy (RECOPANC, DRKS 00000767). Ann Surg. 2016;263:440–9. doi:10.1097/SLA.0000000000001240.
9. Liao C-H, Wu Y-T, Liu Y-Y, et al. Systemic review of the feasibility and advantage of minimally invasive pancreaticoduodenectomy. World J Surg. 2016;40:1218–25. doi:10.1007/s00268-016-3433-1.
10. Adam U, Makowiec F, Riediger H, et al. Pancreatic leakage after pancreas resection. An analysis of 345 operated patients. Chirurg. 2002;73:466–73.
11. Speicher PJ, Nussbaum DP, White RR, et al. Defining the learning curve for team-based laparoscopic pancreaticoduodenectomy. Ann Surg Oncol. 2014; doi:10.1245/s10434-014-3839-7.
12. Wang M, Meng L, Cai Y, et al. Learning curve for laparoscopic pancreaticoduodenectomy: a CUSUM analysis. J Gastrointest Surg. 2016;20:924–35. doi:10.1007/s11605-016-3105-3.
13. Emam TA, Cuschieri A. How safe is high-power ultrasonic dissection? Ann Surg. 2003;237:186–91. doi:10.1097/01.SLA.0000048454.11276.62.
14. Lämsä T, Jin H-T, Nordback PH, et al. Pancreatic injury response is different depending on the method of resecting the parenchyma. J Surg Res. 2009;154:203–11. doi:10.1016/j.jss.2008.08.018.
15. Wellner UF, Sick O, Olschewski M, et al. Randomized controlled single-center trial comparing pancreatogastrostomy versus pancreaticojejunostomy after partial pancreatoduodenectomy. J Gastrointest Surg. 2012;16:1686–95. doi:10.1007/s11605-012-1940-4.
16. Sharpe SM, Talamonti MS, Wang CE, et al. Early national experience with laparoscopic pancreaticoduodenectomy for ductal adenocarcinoma: a comparison of laparoscopic pancreaticoduodenectomy and open pancreaticoduodenectomy from the National Cancer Data Base. J Am Coll Surg. 2015;221:175–84. doi:10.1016/j.jamcollsurg.2015.04.021.
17. Kim SC, Song KB, Jung YS, et al. Short-term clinical outcomes for 100 consecutive cases of laparoscopic pylorus-preserving pancreatoduodenectomy: improvement with surgical experience. Surg Endosc. 2013;27:95–103. doi:10.1007/s00464-012-2427-9.

Total Laparoscopic Pancreatoduodenectomy

24

Maurice J.W. Zwart, Thijs de Rooij, Olivier R.C. Busch, Michael F. Gerhards, Sebastiaan Festen, and Marc G.H. Besselink

24.1 Introduction

Pancreatoduodenectomy is the treatment of choice for pancreatic head and periampullary cancers and high-risk pancreatic cysts. Laparoscopic pancreatoduodenectomy, firstly performed in 1994 [1], has gained popularity only slowly, probably because of the required extensive laparoscopic dissection and the difficulty of the pancreatic and bile duct anastomoses. Improvements in surgical expertise, instrumentation and several cohort studies have apparently driven to the recent increased interest in laparoscopic pancreatoduodenectomy [2]. Nevertheless, only a few centers have acquired adequate experience with this complex procedure. A recent pan-European survey demonstrated that although 73% of pancreatic surgeons performed minimally invasive distal pancreatectomy, only 4.4% of surgeons had performed more than ten minimally invasive pancreatoduodenectomies [3]. A laparoscopic approach to pancreatic and periampullary lesions may enhance postoperative functional recovery and potentially shorten time to start with adjuvant chemotherapy. Naturally, a learning curve arises with the adaptation of a laparoscopic approach. This is reflected in reports on the laparoscopic pancreatoduodenectomy learning curve which is completed faster with extensive previous experience in laparoscopic surgery and adequate training in pancreatic surgery [4]. Additionally, high-quality surgical performance and low conversion rates are best achievable in high-volume centers [5].

24.2 Indications

Indications for laparoscopic pancreatoduodenectomy are similar to the open approach. The selection criteria for a laparoscopic approach depend mainly on the surgeon's experience with laparoscopic pancreatoduodenectomy. Less experienced surgeons are advised to perform laparoscopic resection only for small tumors without potential vascular involvement [6]. Ideal candidates are probably patients with a small periampullary mass with a 'double duct' sign, to facilitate safe anastomoses.

Electronic Supplementary Material The online version of this chapter (doi:10.1007/978-3-319-54301-7_24) contains supplementary material, which is available to authorized users. On http://springerlink.com enter the DOI number given above.

M.J.W. Zwart • T. de Rooij • O.R.C. Busch
M.G.H. Besselink (✉)
Department of Surgery, Academic Medical Center, Amsterdam, The Netherlands
e-mail: m.j.zwart@amc.uva.nl; m.g.besselink@amc.uva.nl

M.F. Gerhards • S. Festen
Department of Surgery, OLVG Hospital, Amsterdam, The Netherlands

M.A. Cuesta (ed.), *Minimally Invasive Surgery for Upper Abdominal Cancer*, DOI 10.1007/978-3-319-54301-7_24

24.3 Contraindications

Although vascular resection is technically possible in laparoscopic pancreatoduodenectomy in highly experienced hands, most authors advice to withhold from this approach until vast experience (*e.g.*, 40–80 procedures) has been obtained [7, 8]. Similarly, a laparoscopic approach is feasible after neoadjuvant radiotherapy, in case of chronic pancreatitis or in case of severe obesity (*i.e.*, body mass index beyond 30), but the general advice is to fully complete the learning curve before embarking on these challenging indications. Therefore, there are no strict contraindications except for technical limitations of the team.

24.4 Preoperative Investigations

As for all indications for pancreatic surgery, all patients require preoperative, high-quality, contrast-enhanced computed tomography within a dedicated pancreas protocol to assess tumor resectability with specific focus on aberrant vascularization (*e.g.*, right hepatic artery), and vascular involvement. Especially, aberrant vascularization should be recognized, since these variants may be difficult to detect early intra-operatively when operating laparoscopically. Preoperative procedures are exactly the same as for an open procedure. Endoscopic ultrasound (EUS) is indicated when computed tomography (CT) does not reveal a tumor mass. Preoperative biliary drainage (in the same procedure as EUS) using covered metal stents is helpful in jaundiced patients with a total serum bilirubin >250 mg/dL [9]. In case of lower bilirubin levels, early surgical exploration is advised [10]. Preoperative CA19-9 measurement is not mandatory for the diagnosis, but can be helpful in determining prognosis and in monitor the effectiveness of chemoradiotherapy [10].

24.5 Preoperative Preparation

Whether performing pancreatoduodenectomy open- or laparoscopic, preoperative preparations are identical. In both approaches, pancreatoduodenectomy carries a 40–50% risk of clinically relevant complications. Prophylactic measures include intra-operative antibiotics, glucose management, somatostatin analogues in high-risk patients, venous thromboprophylaxis with low molecular weight heparin, as well as compression stockings, when available with pneumatic compression [11, 12].

24.6 Anesthesia

Laparoscopic pancreatoduodenectomy is performed under general anesthesia. Epidural analgesia is not mandatory. Analgesic options that also may be considered are continuous wound infiltration and additional patient controlled analgesia [13]. Average operative times for laparoscopic pancreatoduodenectomy are considerably longer than with the open approach which can cause hypothermia in slender patients [2]. Therefore, careful temperature control is advised.

24.7 Positioning

The patient is fitted with a self-warming blanket and is placed in the French position with the right arm positioned to the patient's side and the left arm extended; or alternatively both arms extended. The surgeon stands between the patient's legs with the first assistant at the left and the second assistant at the right side of the patient.

24.8 Instrumentation

- Self-heating blanket and compression stockings
- Trocars: 3 × 12 mm and 3 × 5 mm
- High definition camera

(three-dimensional vision may be useful for the anastomotic phase)

- Tissue sealer (*e.g.*, Enseal®, which articulates or Ligasure® Maryland)
- Laparoscopic bipolar forceps
- Laparoscopic 90° forceps

- Laparoscopic needle drivers
- Laparoscopic hem-o-lok® clips and removal device
- Laparoscopic bulldogs clamps
- Laparoscopic ultrasonic dissector
- Vessel loops, ¼ length
- Endo clip 5 mm and 10 mm
- Endostapler (vascular vs. other)
- Endoscopic retrieval bag
- Small (6-8FR, 8 cm long) nasogastric tube
- Sutures: 6 × 3-0 barbed suture, 5-0 Vicryl® and a small, non-cutting needle
- Surgical non-suction drains

24.9 Procedure

After positioning and draping of the patient, and installment of all equipment, CO_2 insufflation through either a Veress needle (Palmer's point) or open introduction creates a 12 mmHg pneumoperitoneum. The first 12 mm trocar is placed infra-umbilical and in obese patients supra-umbilical. Two additional 12 mm trocars are placed laterally of the umbilicus. Laterally from these, two 5 mm trocars are placed approximately four fingerbreadths subcostally in the anterior axillary line, such that the trocars form a slight arc. Finally, a 5 mm trocar is placed just below the xiphoid, see Fig. 24.1.

A diagnostic laparoscopy is performed to rule out liver or peritoneal metastases. The teres ligament is slung using a transcutaneous straight needle which is placed in the epigastric region. Optionally, the liver can be retracted with a suture wire hanging method [14]. Furthermore, the cystic duct and artery are identified and transected before dissecting the lower one third of the gallbladder dissected. Next the gallbladder is sutured to the abdominal wall, thus further retracting the liver. A grasper is placed via the subxiphoid trocar until under segment one to lift the liver (Video 24.1).

The resection phase is then started by opening the lesser sac by dividing the gastrocolic ligament

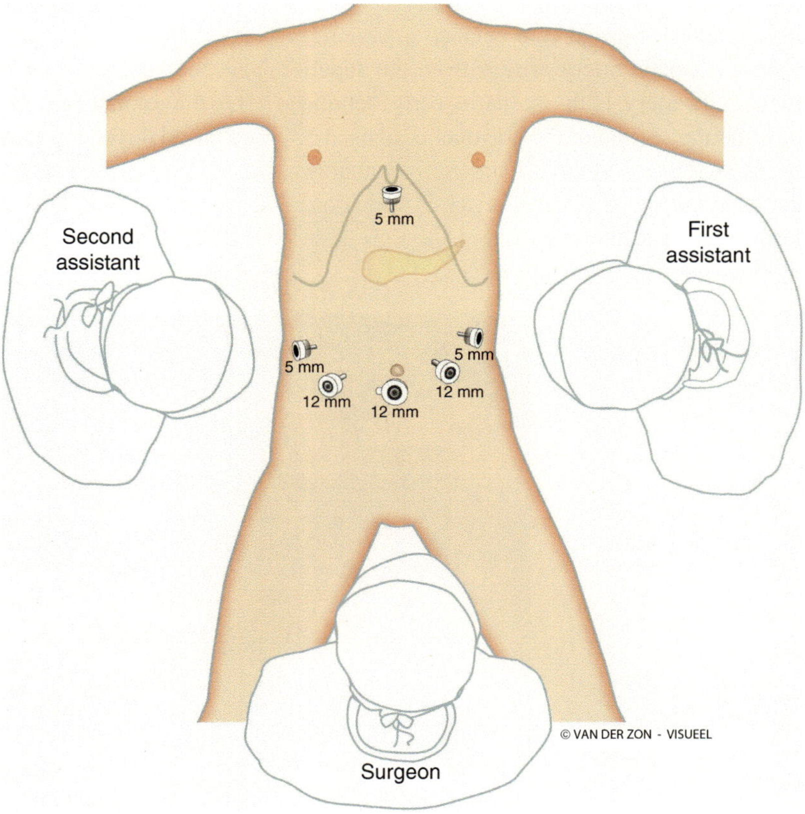

Fig. 24.1 Trocar placement for laparoscopic pancreatoduodenectomy

from the greater gastric curvature towards the hepatic flexure. The first assistant stretches the colon caudally whereas the second assistant lifts the stomach. Subsequently, the hepatic flexure is mobilized and the Kocher maneuver is completed until the left renal vein and the origin of the superior mesenteric artery are identified. During this phase the first assistant lifts the duodenum towards the patient's left side. The duodenum is further mobilized from the right side, potentially including Treitz' ligament. Once the superior mesenteric vein is identified, the right gastroepiploic vein is transected with a sealing device and vascular clips. The pancreas is now ready for tunneling from the inferior pancreatic border (see Fig. 24.2).

At the hepatic artery, lymph node station 8, is identified and removed for histopathological assessment. The portal vein and gastroduodenal artery are identified. After slinging the latter with a vessel loop, it is clamped with a grasper to detect whether arterial flow to the liver remains. Thereafter, the gastroduodenal artery is divided between vascular clips, aiming at a 10 mm stump for eventual coiling in case of bleeding. At least two vascular clips are advised at the side of the hepatic artery. Special care is taken in case of an aberrant hepatic artery arising from the superior mesenteric artery. In this scenario, early identification and transection of the bile duct is advised.

The nasogastric tube is temporarily withdrawn, the large curvature of the stomach is skeletonized just proximal to the pylorus and the right gastric artery is clipped. The stomach is transected using an endostapler just proximally from the pylorus (pylorus ring resection) and placed in the upper left abdomen until the start of the reconstruction phase. Alternatively, the first 2 cm of the duodenum are spared for a pylorus preserving procedure.

The jejunum is mobilized, either from the right or the left side of the mesenteric root, and divided with an endostapler. The duodenum is now entirely mobilized from the mesenteric root. When the jejunum is divided at the left of the mesenteric root, a suture is placed between both ends to facilitate rotation of the jejunal loop to the right side of the mesenteric root.

The uncinate process is then mobilized using a sealing device. The superior and inferior pancreaticoduodenal veins and arteries are divided using the tissue sealer. Care is taken not to injure the first jejunal venous branch of the superior mesenteric vein. The posteriorly tunneled pancreas is now transected with diathermy or ultrasonic dissector while using scissors in the vicinity of the main pancreatic duct to prevent unintentional closure of the duct. The retroperitoneal dissection is continued while working close to the superior mesenteric artery and flush on the portomesenteric vein. This is continued up to the insertion of the cystic duct into the common bile duct. The gallbladder is either removed direct or left in situ for liver hilum retraction and removed separately at the end of the procedure. A vessel loop is slung around the hepatic bile duct, a bulldog clamp is placed at the remnant

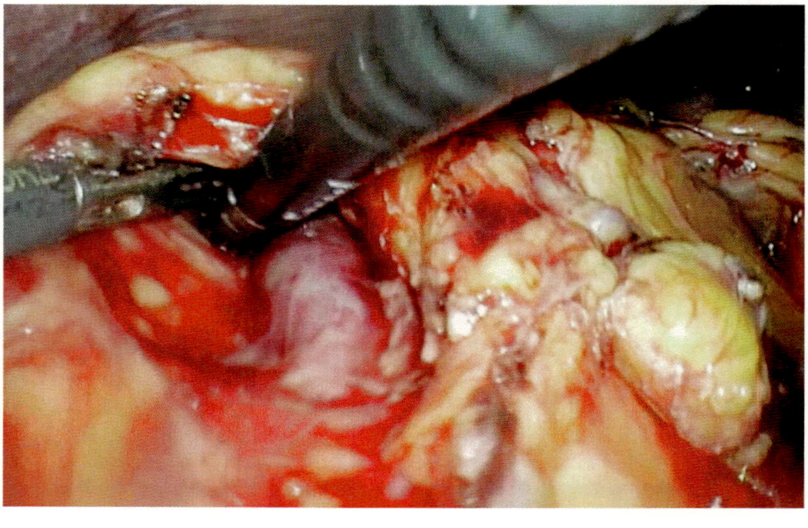

Fig. 24.2 Tunneling of the pancreas

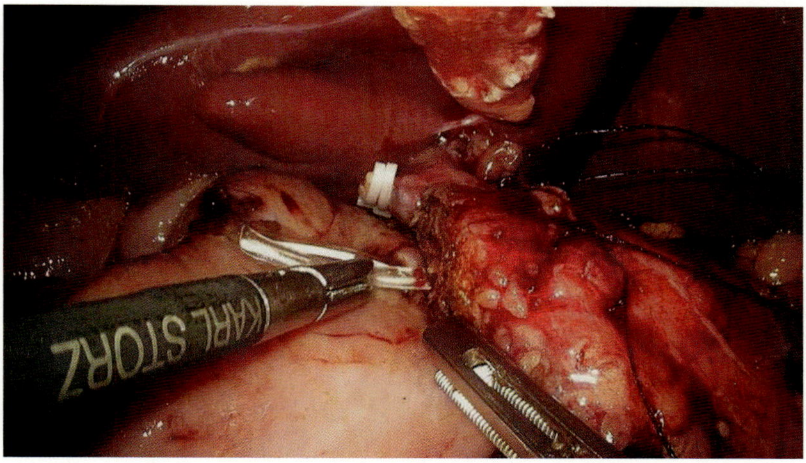

Fig. 24.3 Stent placement during in pancreatojejunostomy

bile duct, and a vascular clip at its distal end. Then, the bile duct is sharply divided. The specimen can now be collected in an endobag and removed through a Pfannenstiel incision. The Pfannenstiel incision is closed in layers of peritoneum, muscle, and fascia. When the gallbladder is temporarily left in place, alternatively, the specimen is placed in a internal collection bag so it can be removed at the end of the procedure together with the gallbladder.

At this stage, a short break is advised before starting the reconstruction.

24.9.1 Pancreaticojejunostomy

For the anastomotic phase three-dimensional vision may be useful. The jejunum is positioned close to the cut surface of the pancreas in order to create a modified Blumgart e/s pancreaticojeunostomy with an internal stent. Four barbed sutures (*e.g.* V-loc® 3/0, Medtronic inc., large needle) are placed anteroposterior through the pancreas, approximately 1 cm from the cut surface, through the jejunum and back through the pancreas. A small jejunotomy is made to enable the pancreatic duct-to-mucosa anastomosis with 5-0 Vicryl® and a small, non-cutting needle. After two sutures (*e.g.* at 5 and 8 o'clock) the pancreatic duct is stented with an 8 cm long 6-8FR stent with side holes at the pancreatic side and the final two sutures are placed (*e.g.,* at 11 and 2 o'clock) (Fig. 24.3). If feasible, more duct-to-mucosa sutures may be placed. The four barbed sutures are used again and placed through the jejunum and back on the anterior surface of the pancreas, hereby 'pulling' the jejunum over the pancreas to create an invagination. The barbed sutures are secured with clips closely to the outer layer of the pancreas after careful tightening. Alternatively, a pancreatogastrostomy can be performed [15].

24.9.2 Hepaticojejunostomy

The jejunum is then brought in position to the hepatic bile duct to determine the position of the hepatojejunostomy. For a non-dilated hepatic duct, Vicryl 5/0 standing sutures are advised. Running sutures Vicryl 5-0 or barbed sutures (*e.g.*, V-loc® V-20) can be used for a wider hepatic duct. When using barbed sutures, care must be taken to anchor the first suture on the bowel, lateral from the anastomosis since the 'loop' has no barbs. A back and front row is used for the running sutures, with the surgeon standing on the patients' left (or right) side. For the standing sutures, an approach can be used starting 6 o'clock on the bile duct to 12 o'clock on the bowel and thereafter both counterclockwise and clockwise on both sides going towards 12 o'clock on the bile duct (Fig. 24.4). To drain both the pancreatico- and hepatojejunostomy, a drain is placed, under the hepatojejunostomy, through the foramen of Winslow with the tip next to the pancreaticojejunostomy (drain 1). Optionally, a single suture between jejunal loop to the gallbladder bed may reduce tension on the anastomosis.

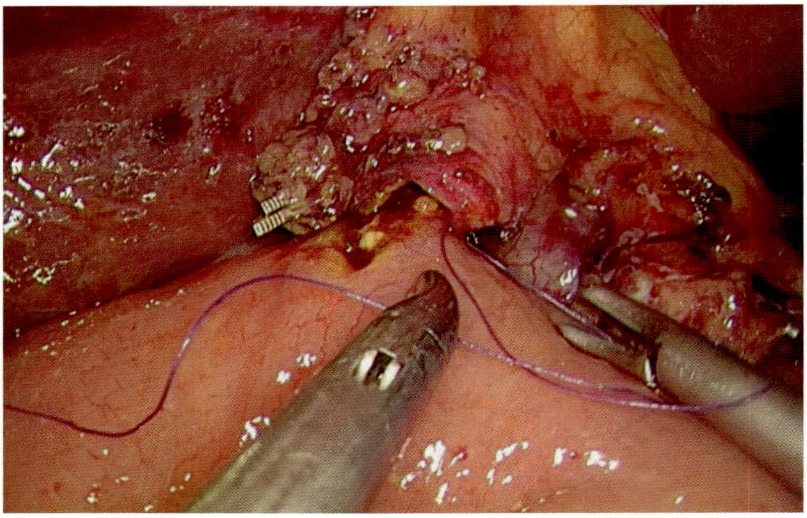

Fig. 24.4 Posterior suturing of the hepatojejunostomy

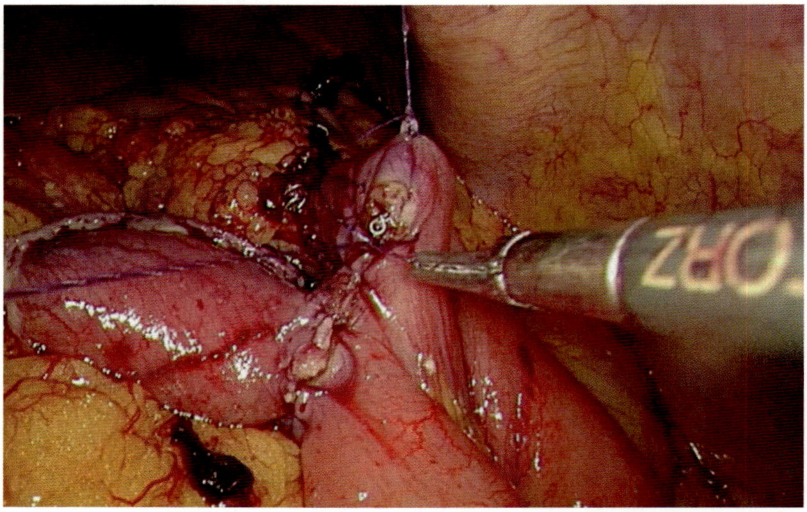

Fig. 24.5 Anterior suturing of the gastrojejunostomy

24.9.3 Gastrojejunostomy

The first jejunal loop is now identified, placed in an antecolic position, on the anterior wall of the stomach, and secured to the stomach with a single suture. Next, using diathermy, openings are made in the jejunal loop and on the anterior side of the stomach. A side-to-side gastrojejunostomy anastomosis is created using an endostapler. The anastomotic line of 4–5 cm is inspected for bleeding. A dot of ink may be placed in the efferent jejunal loop, thus facilitating later endoscopic feeding tube placement when required [16]. The remaining opening is closed using 3-0 barbed suture (Fig. 24.5) and finalized with two stitches between the efferent loop and the distal stomach to prevent torsion.

Alternatively, an end-to-side gastro- or duodenojejunostomy can be created. A second drain, entering via the most right-sided trocar is placed under this anastomosis such that it drains the caudal part of both the pancreaticojejunostomy and the gastrojejunostomy (drain 2). Omentum, is draped over the pancreaticojejunostomy.

After a final exploration for bleeding and leakage, drainage of CO_2 takes place and all trocars are removed under direct vision.

24.10 Tips and Comments

- After placing a suture at the stapler line of the jejunum and duodenum, the duodenum can be used to pull the jejunum through retrocolically towards the anastomosis sites.
- Conversion should not be perceived as a complication. Conversion is indicated in case of failure to progress, difficult dissection, resectable venous involvement or severe intraoperative bleeding.
- Doppler ultrasonography, regular probe, can be placed through the subxiphoid port to rule out insufficient hepatic flow after clamping the gastroduodenal artery.
- In case of a small bile duct diameter, temporary ductal stenting makes precise positioning of anastomotic standing sutures easier, as the ductal lumen orientation is apparent.
- In the reconstruction phase, three-dimensional vision facilitates laparoscopic suturing.

24.11 Follow-up

After the procedure, the patient is admitted to the postoperative care unit for pain control, blood glucose levels, and restoring fluid homeostasis. Patients are transferred to the surgical ward on day 1 with an enhanced recovery after surgery strategy [17]. Special attention is given to diabetes control, enzyme supplementation, and early mobilization. Drain amylase is checked on the third postoperative morning, so drains can be removed once amylase is lower than three times the upper limit of the normal amylase range.

Although preoperative evaluation aims to limit risk of intraoperative and postoperative complication, high morbidity rates are unfortunately common. For the best post-operative care, it is important to emphasize complication rescue and to aim for early detection of complications.

Adjuvant chemotherapy is advised within 12 weeks after resection of a pancreatic ductal adenocarcinoma.

24.12 Future

Pragmatic multicenter randomized controlled trials will have to demonstrate superiority of minimally invasive pancreatoduodenectomy. Currently, one monocenter trial was recently completed and two further trials are ongoing. The PLOT monocenter trial was performed in a highly experienced center in Coimbatore, India, and concluded that time to functional recovery is shorter after laparoscopic pancreatoduodenectomy after including 64 patients [18]. In Barcelona, the monocenter randomized PADULAP trial is ongoing [19], and in the Netherlands, the multicenter randomized controlled, patient blinded LEOPARD-2 trial [20].

During laparoscopic pancreatoduodenectomy, especially the anastomotic phase is challenging. Completing each anastomosis can take up to 40–50 min [21]. Robot-assisted surgery allows for wrist-like movements, potentially facilitating the anastomotic phase. Although good results with robot-assisted pancreatoduodenectomy have been reported, comparative studies are lacking and concerns about cost-effectiveness will have to be addressed [8, 22].

24.13 Summary

- In laparoscopic pancreatoduodenectomy, a body mass index exceeding 30 kg/m^2 is a relative contraindication.
- Patient specific anatomic understanding is essential as precautions are essential when undertaking laparoscopic pancreatoduodenectomy since anatomic variations are more difficult to detect intra-operatively when operating laparoscopically.
- Pancreatoduodenectomy with venous resection should not be attempted without conversion to open surgery until vast experience has been obtained.

References

1. Gagner M, Pomp A. Laparoscopic pylorus-preserving pancreatoduodenectomy. Surg Endosc. 1994;8:408–10.
2. Boggi U, Ugo B, Gabriella A, Fabio V, Fabio C, De Lio N, Vittorio P, Linda B, Mario B, Stefano S, Franco M. Laparoscopic pancreaticoduodenectomy: a systematic literature review. Surg Endosc. 2014;29:9–23.
3. De Rooij T, Besselink M, Shamali A, Butturini G, Busch O, Troisi R, Fernández-Cruz L, Topal B, Dagher I, Bassi C, Abu Hilal M. Pan-European survey on laparoscopic pancreatic surgery. HPB. 2016;18: e852–3.
4. de Rooij T, van Hilst J, Boerma D, Bonsing BA, Daams F, van Dam RM, Dijkgraaf MG, van Eijck CH, Festen S, Gerhards MF, Koerkamp BG, van der Harst E, de Hingh IH, Kazemier G, Klaase J, de Kleine RH, van Laarhoven CJ, Lips DJ, Luyer MD, Molenaar IQ, Patijn GA, Roos D, Scheepers JJ, van der Schelling GP, Steenvoorde P, Vriens MR, Wijsman JH, Gouma DJ, Busch OR, Abu Hilal M, Besselink MG. Dutch pancreatic cancer group: impact of a nationwide training program in minimally invasive distal pancreatectomy (LAELAPS). Ann Surg. 2016;264(5):754–62.
5. Sharpe SM, Talamonti MS, Wang CE, Prinz RA, Roggin KK, Bentrem DJ, Winchester DJ, Marsh RDW, Stocker SJ, Baker MS. Early national experience with laparoscopic pancreaticoduodenectomy for ductal adenocarcinoma: a comparison of laparoscopic pancreaticoduodenectomy and open pancreaticoduodenectomy from the National Cancer Data Base. J Am Coll Surg. 2015;221:175–84.
6. de Rooij T, Klompmaker S, Abu Hilal M, Kendrick ML, Busch OR, Besselink MG. Laparoscopic pancreatic surgery for benign and malignant disease. Nat Rev Gastroenterol Hepatol. 2016;13:227–38.
7. Wang M, Meng L, Cai Y, Li Y, Wang X, Zhang Z, Peng B. Learning curve for laparoscopic pancreaticoduodenectomy: a CUSUM analysis. J Gastrointest Surg. 2016;20:924–35.
8. Boone BA, Zenati M, Hogg ME, Steve J, Moser AJ, Bartlett DL, Zeh HJ, Zureikat AH. Assessment of quality outcomes for robotic pancreaticoduodenectomy: identification of the learning curve. JAMA Surg. 2015;150:416–22.
9. Tol JAMG, van Hooft JE, Timmer R, Kubben FJGM, van der Harst E, de Hingh IHJT, Vleggaar FP, Molenaar IQ, Keulemans YCA, Boerma D, Bruno MJ, Schoon, EJ, van der Gaag NA, Besselink MGH, Fockens P, van Gulik TM, Rauws EAJ, Busch ORC, Gouma DJ. Metal or plastic stents for preoperative biliary drainage in resectable pancreatic cancer. Gut. 2015; 65(12). gutjnl-2014-308762.
10. van der Gaag NA, de Castro SMM, Rauws EAJ, Bruno MJ, van Eijck CHJ, Kuipers EJ, Gerritsen JJ, Jan-Paul R, Greve JW, Hesselink EJ, Klinkenbijl JHG, Rinkes IHMB, Djamila B, Bonsing BA, van Laarhoven CJ, Kubben FJ, van der Harst E, Sosef MN, Koop B, de Hingh IH, de Wit LT, van Delden OM, Busch ORC, van Gulik TM, Bossuyt PMM, Gouma DJ. Preoperative biliary drainage for periampullary tumors causing obstructive jaundice; DR ainage vs. (direct) OP eration (DROP-trial). BMC Surg. 2007;7
11. Chew HK. Incidence of venous thromboembolism and its effect on survival among patients with common cancers. Arch Intern Med. 2006;166:458–64.
12. Keidar A, Andrei K. P102: high incidence of bleeding complications with preoperative administration of enoxaparine for venous thromboembolism prevention in bariatric patients. Surg Obes Relat Dis. 2008;4:350.
13. Mungroop TH, Veelo DP, Busch OR, van Dieren S, van Gulik TM, Karsten TM, de Castro SM, Godfried MB, Thiel B, Hollmann MW, Lirk P, Besselink MG. Continuous wound infiltration or epidural analgesia for pain prevention after hepato-pancreato-biliary surgery within an enhanced recovery program (POP-UP trial): study protocol for a randomized controlled trial. Trials. 2015;16:562.
14. Lee JS, Kim JJ, Park SM. A simple method of liver retraction for various types of laparoscopic upper gastrointestinal surgeries: the prolene hanging-up method. World J Surg. 2015;39:2362–6.
15. Topal B, Baki T, Steffen F, Raymond A, Joseph W, Tom F, Geert R, Claude B, Catherine H, Marc J, Jean C. Pancreaticojejunostomy versus pancreaticogastrostomy reconstruction after pancreaticoduodenectomy for pancreatic or periampullary tumours: a multicentre randomised trial. Lancet Oncol. 2013;14: 655–62.
16. Zonderhuis BM, van den Boom AL, de Graaf E, Meijer LL, Kazemier G, Scheepers JJ. Tattoo of scheepers. HPB. 2016;18:e597.
17. Dort JC, Farwell DG, Findlay M, Huber GF, Kerr P, Shea-Budgell MA, Simon C, Uppington J, Zygun D, Ljungqvist O, Harris J. Optimal perioperative care in major head and neck cancer surgery with free flap reconstruction: a consensus review and recommendations from the enhanced recovery after surgery society. JAMA Otolaryngol Head Neck Surg. 2016.
18. Pancreatic head and peri-ampullary cancer laparoscopic vs. open surgical treatment trial (PLOT). https://clinicaltrials.gov/ct2/show/NCT.
19. Poves Prim I. PADULAP study: to compare postoperative and pathologic results between open and laparoscopic approach for pancreaticoduodenectomy. http://www.isrctn.com/ISRCTN93168938.
20. Trial data. http://www.trialregister.nl/trialreg/admin/rctview.asp?TC=5689.
21. Rodríguez-Sanjuán JC. Laparoscopic and robot-assisted laparoscopic digestive surgery: present and future directions. World J Gastroenterol. 2016; 22:1975.
22. Napoli N, Niccolò N, Kauffmann EF, Francesca M, Perrone VG, Stefania B, Ugo B. Indications, technique, and results of robotic pancreatoduodenectomy. Updat Surg. 2016;68(3):295–305.

Robot Assisted Partial Pancreatectomy and Duodenopancreatectomy

25

Ugo Boggi and Carlo Lombardo

25.1 Introduction

Laparoscopy has revolutionized surgery, by showing that many abdominal operations can be performed safely and effectively despite minimally invasive access. Patients' demand for minimally invasive surgery, on one hand, and surgeons' motivation to pursue innovation and accept challenge, on the other, did the rest making laparoscopy an essential component of modern surgery. Laparoscopy, however, has intrinsic limitations, that are not completely overcome by expertise [1]. These limitations have made the outcome of laparoscopy highly operator dependent [2], and have restricted the range of complex operations that can be safely performed using this technique [3].

Robotic assistance enhances surgeon dexterity, and surpasses most of the limitations of conventional laparoscopy [2]. Further, while after more than two decades of continuous evolution in instruments and ancillary technologies, laparoscopy is likely to have reached a development plateau, robotic assistance is still in its infancy. As for other computer-controlled systems, robotic platforms are expected to evolve quickly. At the moment, only two robotic systems are commercially available. The most popular robotic system, is the Da Vinci Surgical System® (dVss) (Intuitive Surgical, Sunnyvale, CA, USA). Recently, another robotic platform was lunched, the TELELAP ALF-X (SOFAR S.p.A., ALF-X Surgical Robotics Department, Trezzano Rosa, Milan, Italy) [3]. Other robotic systems are under development [4, 5]. In this chapter only da Vinci surgery is addressed, because no data is available on the use of other robotic systems in pancreatic resections.

25.2 The da Vinci Surgical System

Four different models of dVss have been marketed since 1998. The basic components all dVss are similar [5].

In general, the dVss is a telemanipulator capable of transferring the movements of the hands of a remote surgeon to the tips of miniaturized intracorporeal instruments. The dVss is not capable of any programmed or autonomous action.

The dVss consists of three main components: the surgeon console, the patient side cart (PSC), and the vision cart.

1. The surgeon console is the remote working station from which the surgeon operates the robotic arms.

Electronic Supplementary Material The online version of this chapter (doi:10.1007/978-3-319-54301-7_25) contains supplementary material, which is available to authorized users. On http://springerlink.com enter the DOI number given above.

U. Boggi (✉) • C. Lombardo
Division of General and Transplant Surgery, University of Pisa, Pisa, Italy
e-mail: u.boggi@med.unipi.it; carlolombardomd@gmail.com

M.A. Cuesta (ed.), *Minimally Invasive Surgery for Upper Abdominal Cancer*, DOI 10.1007/978-3-319-54301-7_25

2. The PSC has three or four operative arms, holding the camera and the robotic instruments.
3. The vision cart contains all required complimentary technology.

25.3 Advantages and Disadvantages of Robotic Assitance as Compared with Laparoscopy

Robotic assistance enhances surgical dexterity by restoring hand–eye coordination and offering optimal working ergonomy. These improvements are made possible mainly thanks to:

1. The use of EndoWrist® instruments, having a very distal articulation allowing the tip of the instrument to achieve seven degrees of freedom. The shaft of robotic instruments is fully stationary, avoiding the "fulcrum effect" typical of conventional laparoscopic instruments, and causing no extra wear on the abdominal wall port.
2. The availability of a binocular endoscope offering high-quality, steady, stereoscopic vision with up to 15× magnification. Since the surgeon visualizes the stereoscopic images via a display located above his/her hands, and hand movements immediately and precisely corresponds to movements of the tips of intracorporeal instruments, the surgeon has the virtual sensation of operating within the patient's body. This type of vision is called "immersive vision", and is totally different from any HD and/or 3D vision provided by wall screens.
3. The availability of an additional robotic arm, that can be used either to provide steady and durable retraction or as an operative arm.

The dVss has also several limitations, that should be recognized to limit the risk of improper use of this very sophisticated technology:

1. The PSC is very bulky. Excluding the lastly released system (Xi), in pancreatic resections the PSC of all dVss is positioned over the head of the patient, limiting accessibility to patient's airways and infusion lines (Fig. 25.1).

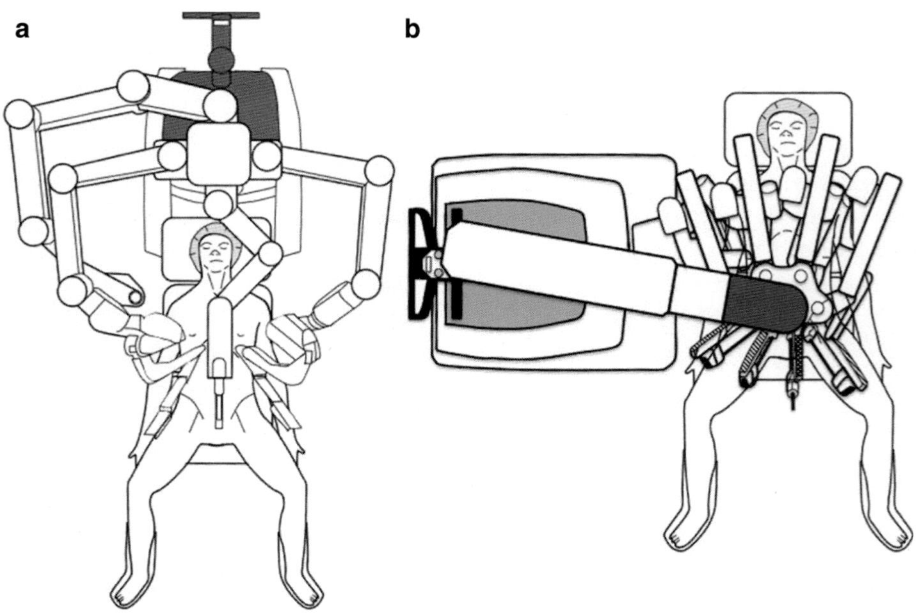

Fig. 25.1 Position of the PSC of the dVss for pancreatic resections. (**a**) With the dVss Si the PSC has to come from the head of the patient. Access to airways and infusion lines by the anesthesia team is limited. (**b**) The PSC of the dVss Xi can be positioned everywhere around the patient since the overhead boom, holding the robtic arms, rotates to reach optimal working position. Access to the patient is hence maintained 270° around the operating table

2. Careful set up of robotic arms is crucial to avoid internal and external collisions.
3. No haptic feedback is provided. Although some studies suggest the excellent quality of the vision the surgeon may provide virtual haptic sensations, lack of actual haptic feedback is known to cause tissue or suture damage, and does not allow tissue palpation.
4. When the instruments are not under direct visual control, the remote surgeon may lose the perception of their actual position. This limitation has been partially addressed in the dVXi, that provides visual signals at the boundaries of the screen showing were the tip of the instrument is located or from where it is reaching the field.
5. Despite the dVss is a robust and reliable platform, malfunction may occur [5].

Finally, costs are the major disadvantage of robotic assistance and the greatest barrier to further diffusion of this technology [6].

25.4 Rationale for the Use of Robotic Assistance in Pancreatic Resections

Nearly all surgical procedures are feasible using conventional laparoscopy, but adaptations from well-established open techniques are often required. Some of these adaptations have shown to be safe and have even led to changes in open procedures. Other variations, instead, have not been fully validated yet.

Robotic assistance allows to faithfully reproduce the open technique [2]. In pancreatic resections, the enhanced dexterity offered by robotic assistance is expected to be more rewarding in procedures including digestive reconstruction, such as pancreatoduodenectomy, than in straightforward resection only procedures, such as distal pancreatectomy with en-bloc splenectomy. The full range of pancreatic resections has been performed under robotic assistance [7].

25.5 Center and Surgeon Eligibility for Safe Implementation of a Program for Robotic Pancreatoduodenectomy

There are no currently agreed standards for surgeon training and credentialing as well as for Institution accreditation, but it is clear that these pathways are very much needed [8].

A program for robotic pancreatic resections is best developed at a high volume center, by proficient pancreatic surgeons with experience in advanced laparoscopic surgery. Robotic surgery reduces man power, in favor of team power. Two surgeons are needed, one operating from the console and the other accomplishing laparoscopic tasks at the table. An experienced scrub nurse is also required. The anesthetist must have extensive experience in both in laparoscopic surgery and pancreatic procedures. The entire team must familiarize with the system, and with the new operative conditions, in simple straightforward procedures. For the operating surgeon, preparatory surgeries could include simple operations that require intracorporeal sutures, such as repair of visceral aneurysms and pyeloplasty [11]. Distal pancreatectomy should be performed first. Pancreatoduodenectomy and central pancreatectomy should be implemented last. Proctor supervision is recommend, until the team feels confortable with the procedure.

The learning curve for distal pancreatectomy, with or without spleen preservation, includes approximately ten operations [9]. The learning curve for pancreatoduodenectomy includes between 40 and 80 procedures [10, 11]. For pancreatoduodenectomy, we recommend to select periampullary tumors and lean patients to learn about dissection of the posterior margin, and pancreatic cancer to learn about pancreatic reconstruction. Procedures should be learned stepwise and proficiency should be gained on each individual step before moving on to the next. During the initial phase of the learning curve the missed steps of the procedure (i.e. pancreatic anastomosis in periampullary tumors and dissection of the posterior margin in pancreatic cancer) should be performed by a proctor [12].

25.6 Selection Criteria for Robotic Pancreatic Resections

Patients must be eligible for laparoscopy. Selection criteria are expected to evolve with experience. Our current selection criteria, after nearly 300 robotic pancreatic resections, are reported in Table 25.1.

It is important that indications to surgery are not expanded because of the availability of robotic assistance. Likewise, cosmesis should play no role in the decision of surgical technique.

In patients with pancreatic head cancer and overt vein involvement (i.e. segmental occlusion, tumor abutment ≥180°) robotic resection should not be performed. In patients limited vein involvement (i.e. ≤180°), robotic resection can be considered, if the team is familiar with the corresponding open procedure, if all the oncologic principles can be respected, and if resection can be carried out with ease. Risk factors should not be cumulated, so that vein resection and reconstruction is best performed in patients in whom vein involvement is an isolated risk factor for troublesome resection or reconstruction. A low threshold for conversion should be maintained for all types of resection, especially when vascular procedures are required [13].

Table 25.1 Selection criteria for robot-assisted pancreatic resections

General criteria	Availability of robotic system
	Suitability for laparoscopy
Tumor enucleation	All patients eligible for open or laparoscopic surgery
Distal pancreatectomy	
≤10 procedures:	BMI: Males: ≤30 kg/m^2; Females: ≤35 kg/m^2
>10 procedures:	No specific BMI cutoff
With en-bloc splenectomy	
≤10 procedures:	No splenic vein occlusion
	No need for concurrent procedures
	No visceral involvement
>10 procedures:	Accept patients with splenic vein occlusion, if manageable
	Accept patients needing concurrent procedures, if manageable
	Accept patients needing visceral resections, if manageable
Pancreatic cancer	
≤10 procedures:	Do not accept
>10 procedures:	Accept if clear surgical margins can be defined
Other histology	
≤10 procedures:	Tumor diameter ≤ 5 cm
>10 procedures:	Accept all tumor sizes, if manageable
Modified Appleby	
≤10 procedures:	Do not accept
>10 procedures:	Accept if manageable
Spleen-preserving	
≤10 procedures:	Do not accept large tumors
	Do not accept tumors located within branched splenic vessels at the spleen hilum
>10 procedures:	Accept all tumor sizes and locations, if manageable
Central pancreatectomy	All patients eligible for open or laparoscopic surgery

Table 25.1 (continued)

Pancreatoduodenectomy	
≤40 procedures:	BMI: Males: ≤28 kg/m^2; Females: ≤30 kg/m^2
	No need for concurrent procedures
	No visceral involvement
	No vein involvement
41–80 procedures:	BMI: Males: ≤30 kg/m^2; Females: ≤35 kg/m^2
	Accept patients needing concurrent procedures, if manageable
	No vein involvement
	No visceral involvement
>80 procedures:	Do not accept patients with central obesity
	Accept patients needing concurrent procedures, if manageable
	Accept patients needing visceral resections, if manageable
	Accept patients needing vein resection, if manageable
Pancreatic cancer	
≤40 procedures:	Do not accept
41–80 procedures:	Accept if clear surgical margins can be defined. Be more selective for cancers in the uncinate process
>80 procedures:	Accept if clear surgical margins can be defined
Other histology	
≤40 procedures:	Do not accept large tumors
	Do not accept duodenal cancer
	Do not accept chronic pancreatitis
41–80 procedures:	Accept larger tumors
	Accept duodenal cancer, if no extravisceral growth
	Do not accept chronic pancreatitis
>80 procedures:	Accept all tumor sizes, if manageable
	Accept duodenal cancer, if manageable
	Accept chronic pancreatitis, if manageable
Total pancreatectomy	
≤20 procedures:	As for pancreatoduodenectomy ≤40 procedures
>20 procedures:	As for pancreatoduodenectomy >80 procedures
Tumor/disease type	
	Do not accept locally advanced tumors, of any histology
	Accept patients with multifocal PNET, IMPN, pancreatic metastasis and other tumors/diseases involving the entire pancreas

PNET pancreatic, neuroendocrine tumors; *IMPN* intraductal mucinous papillary neoplasm

25.7 Technique of Robotic Pancreatic Resections

There is no standardization of robotic techniques for pancreatic resections. The techniques presented herein are those developed at the University of Pisa [2, 7, 9, 10, 12–15].

Patient position on operative table, table orientation, and port placement are summarized in Fig. 25.2. It is worth noting that in pancreatoduodenectomy we prefer to place two robotic arms on the left side of the patient, while other teams prefer to have two robotic arm on the right side. The reason for having two robotic arms on the right side, is the use of one arm during dissection of the posterior margin to elevate the head of the pancreas. The same result can be achieved having the "fourth robotic arm" on the left side of the patient, and we prefer this configuration for port placement for several different reasons. First, robotic arms, placed to the left of the patient are operated by the surgeon at the console using the right hand (Fig. 25.3a). If the surgeon is right-handed, with this configuration, he or she has two right hands. Second, more room is left on the right side to place the camera port along the right pararectal line. Since one of the most challenging steps of pancreatoduodenectomy is dissection of the uncinate process and the posterior margin, looking at this hidden target slightly from the right improves vision as compared with looking at the same area from the midline because of the interposition of the superior mesenteric/portal vein (Fig. 25.3b).

The dVss Si requires a dedicated optic port, while with the dVss Xi all robotic ports can be used for the optic or the instruments (so called "port hopping"). In pancreatoduodenectomy the optic port is placed along the right pararectal line, to improve exposure of the uncinate process. In central pancreatectomy, total pancreatectomy, and distal pancreatectomy (for tumors located in the body) the optic port is placed just below or above the umbilicus. In distal pancreatectomies, performed for tumors located in the tail, the patient is placed on the right flank position and the optic port is inserted to the left of the umbilicus.

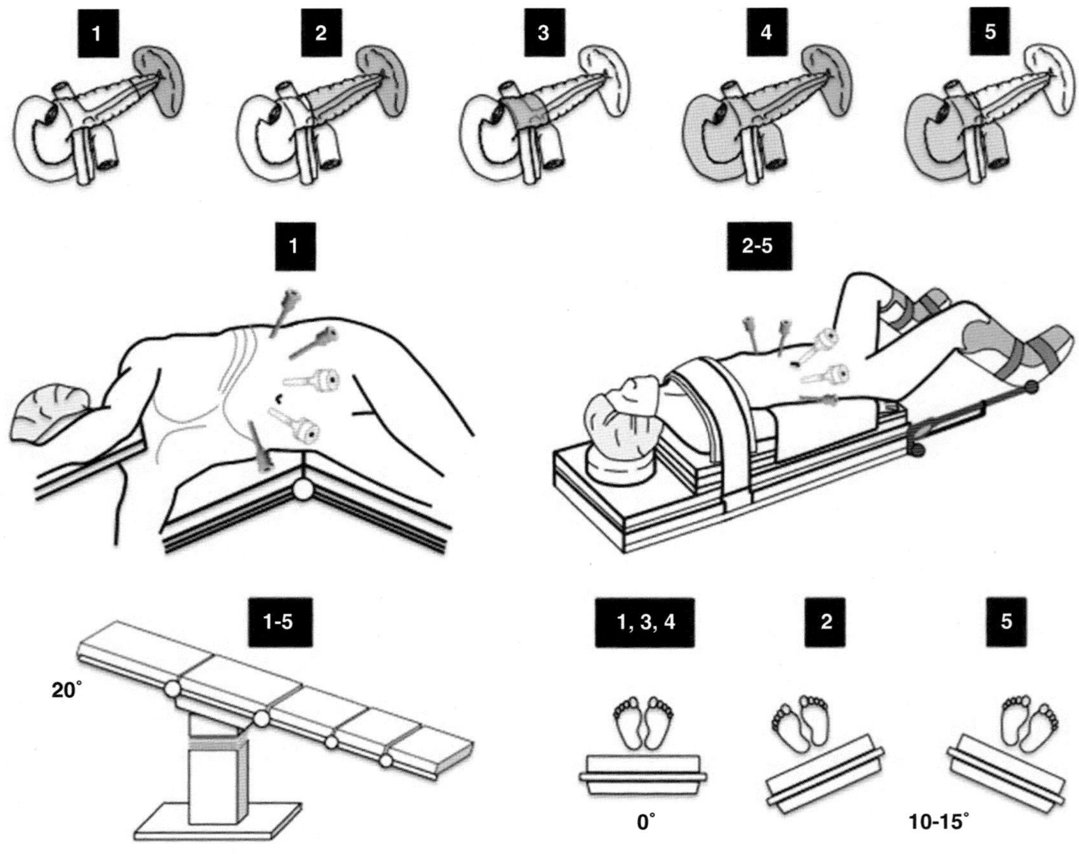

Fig. 25.2 The main types of pancreatic resections are numbered from 1 to 5 at the top of the figure. *1*: Resection of the pancreatic tail; *2*: Resection of the pancreatic body and tail; *3*: Central pancreatectomy; *4*: Total pancreatectomy; *5*: Pancreatoduodenectomy. Patient positions and operating table orientations are shown below and matched with procedure by numbers

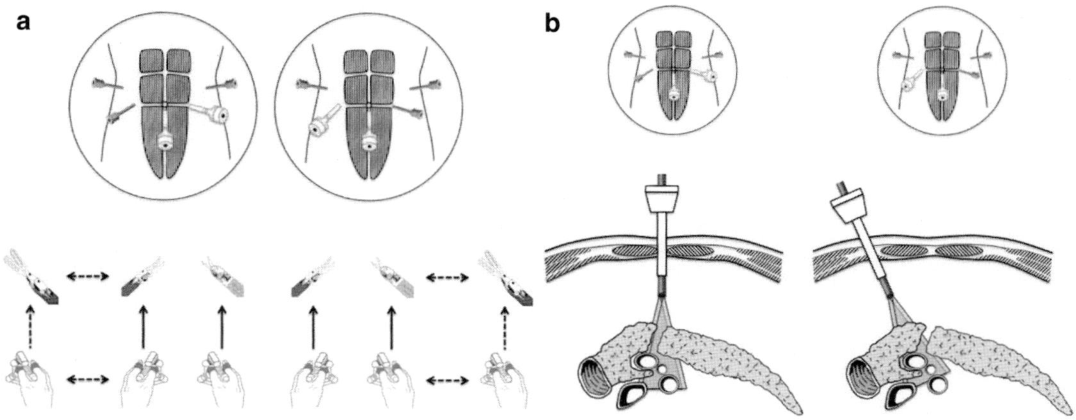

Fig. 25.3 Position of robotic arms and camera arm for pancreatoduodenectomy. (**a**) On the left hand side of this figure is shown the port configuration with "two robotic arms on the right side of the patient". As shown at the bottom of the figure the two right-sided robotic arms are operated by the surgeon's left hand. On the opposite side of the figure is shown the port configuration with "two robotic arms on the left side of the patient". The left-sided ports are operated by the surgeon's right hand. (**b**) On the left hand side of the figure the camera is placed in the umbilical port. From this observation point, the vision of posterior margin is covered by the overhead superior mesenteric/portal vein. On the opposite side of the figure, the camera is placed in the right para-rectal port. From this lateral perspective the posterior margin is seen more clearly

During robotic pancreatic resections, the fourth robotic arm is often used to achieve optimal exposure. The use of transparietal sutures may also be used to improve exposure, without the use of dedicated laparoscopic retractors. Using these sutures the fourth robotic arm becomes fully available as an additional operative arm. A summary of these maneuvres is presented in Fig. 25.4.

25.7.1 Distal Pancreatectomy

The procedure begins with mobilization of the splenic flexure of the colon. To avoid omental infarction, a potential complication when the gastrocolic ligament is divided [16], the lesser sac is entered by dividing the reflection of colon and omentum. The peritoneum along the inferior margin of the pancreas is incised and the distal pancreas is mobilized along the posterior avascular plane. The splenic vein is identified. The pancreas, at the level of intended resection, is elevated using stay sutures and divided using the harmonic scalpel and the robotic scissors. The duct is carefully identified, ligated or suture ligated, and the parenchyma is closed in a fish-mouth configuration using interrupted sutures of 4/0 polytetrafluoroethylene. The pancreas may also be transected using a laparoscopic stapler [9].

In case of splenectomy, the splenic artery is mobilized, doubly ligated, and divided at an early stage. If the splenic vein is thrombosed, and venous effluent is based on collateral circulation, the left gastroepiploic vessels and the short gastric vessels are left intact until the end of the operation. In the other patients, they are immediately divided using a combination of harmonic shears and clips. Division of the splenic vein, and mobilization of the spleen complete the operation. In patients diagnosed with pancreatic cancer, lymphadenectomy is performed, as required, from medial to lateral (Fig. 25.5). The specimen, placed in an endoscopic bag, is retrieved through a transverse suprapubic incision [9].

When the spleen is planned for preservation, the splenic artery and the splenic vein are dissected off the pancreas. Pancreatic veins are fixed using either energy devices or ligatures. Pancreatic arteries are preferentially ligated or suture ligated. The specimen, placed in an endoscopic bag, may be retrieved through

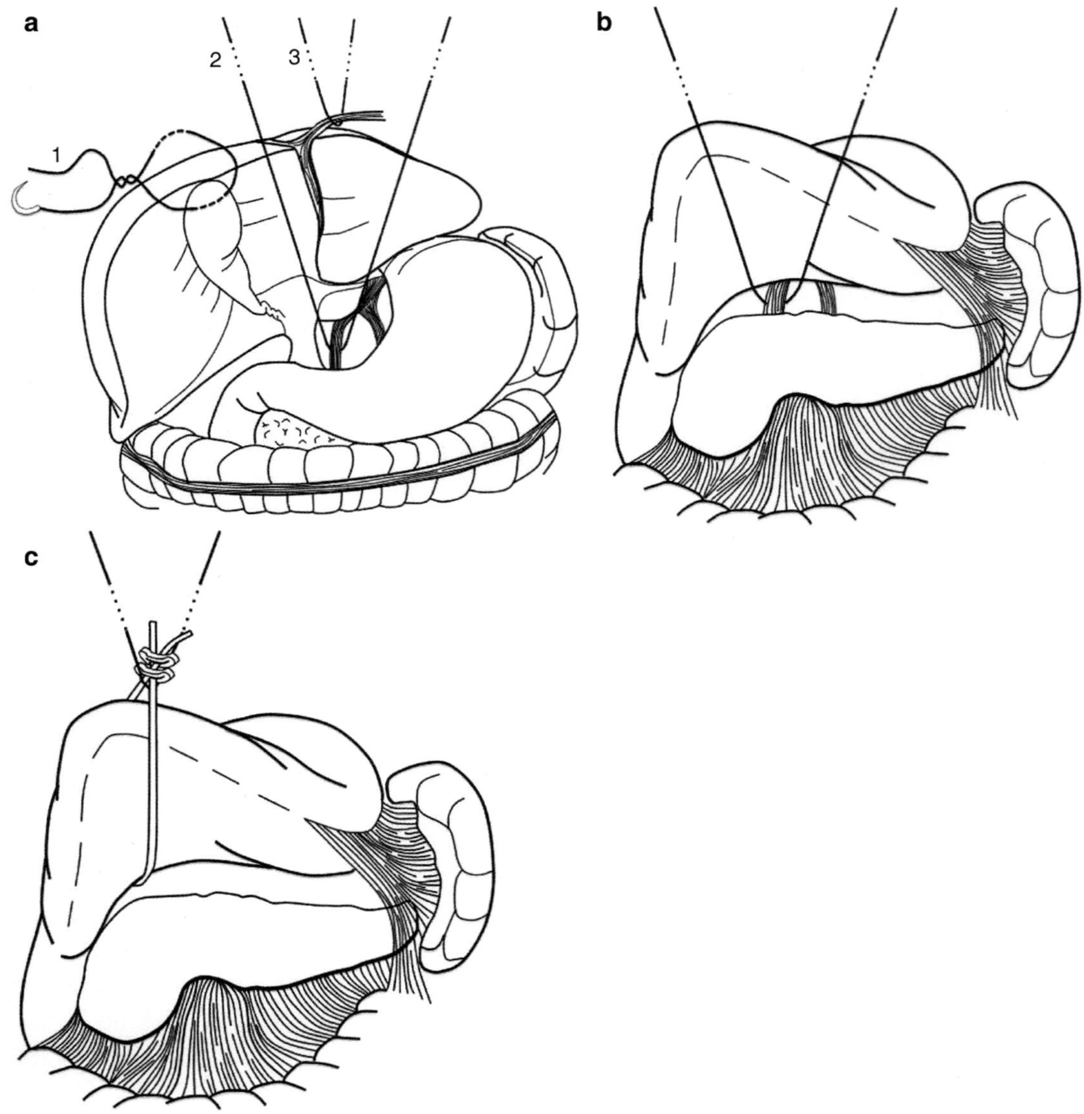

Fig. 25.4 Methods for instrumentless organ retraction during pancreatic resections. (**a**) Liver retraction during pancreatoduodenectomy. *1*. The fundus gallbladder is hanged to the right diaphragm using an intracorporeal suture. *2*. A V shaped sling is used to elevate left later segment of liver. Liver suspension is achieved using a transabdominal suture brought in at the level of the xiphoid, passed through the diaphragmatic crus, and brought out at the level of the right pararectal line, immediately below the costal margin. *3*. The round ligament of the liver is suspended using a transparietal suture. (**b**) Stomach retraction during distal pancreatectomy. A V-shaped transparietal suture, as described for liver retraction, elavates the stomach. (**c**) Stomach retraction during distal pancreatectomy. A vessel loop passed around the gastric antrum is closed using a Hem-o-lok® and hanged to the abdominal wall using a transparietal suture

either an enlarged port site or a transverse suprapubic incision. Two drains are left near the pancreatic transection margin. The round ligament of the liver is mobilized and used to cover the pancreatic stump [9].

25.7.2 Central Pancreatectomy

The lesser sac is entered by dividing the gastrocolic ligament, while preserving the gastroepiploic vessels. The neck of the pancreas and the

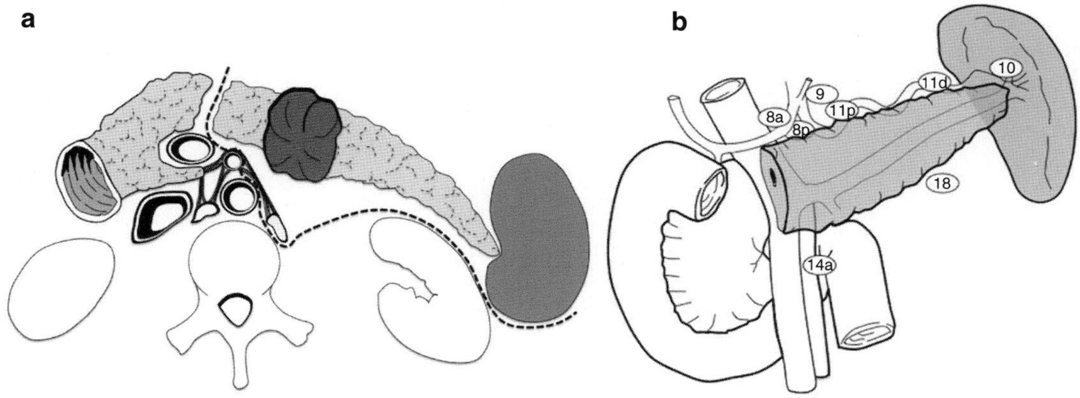

Fig. 25.5 Lymphatic clearance in robotic distal pancreatectomy for cancer. (**a**) The *dotted line* shows the posterior plane of dissection for radical distal pancreatectomy. The left-sided portion of the extrapancreatic nerve plexus is removed en-bloc with the specimen and the retroperitoneal tissues. (**b**) Lymph node stations removed during robotic distal pancreatectomy for cancer

distal portion of the body of the pancreas are dissected free. The pancreas is divided using a combination of harmonic scalpel and robotic scissors. The duct is identified on either sides, and one of the margins is tagged with a stitch for proper pathology orientation. If free margins are confirmed at frozen section histology, reconstruction can be performed using either a pancreatojejunostomy or a pancreatogastrostomy [14].

25.7.3 Pancreatoduodenectomy

After diagnostic laparoscopy, the gastrocolic ligament is opened and the right colonic flexure is mobilized, while the gastric antrum is gently elevated and retracted to the left, using the fourth robotic arm. The right gastroepiploic vessels are identified, dissected off, clipped by Hem-o- lok® (Teleflex Medical, Research Triangle Park, North Carolina, USA), and divided [2, 12].

During dissection of the hepatoduodenal ligament, exposure may be further improved by pulling upward and cephalad the gallbladder, using the fourth robotic arm. The right gastric vessels are divided between ligatures and the first part of the duodenum is divided with a laparoscopic stapler. The gastroduodenal artery is double-ligated proximally using 0 linen, and divided. The common bile duct is divided between ligatures or clips, to avoid bile spillage, and the duct margin is sent for frozen-section histology. Depending on tumor type, lymphadenectomy is performed as required. Lymph node 8a is always removed to facilitate exposure of the hepatic artery. In case of ductal adenocarcinoma, in addition to the lymph node included in a standard lymphadenectomy (i.e. 5, 6, 8a, 12b1, 12b2, 12c, 13a, 13b, 14a, 14b, 17a, and 17b), the following lymph nodes are removed: 8p, 9, 12a, 14c, 14d, and 14d) [17] (Fig. 25.6). The para-aortic nodes (station 16) are not removed [2, 12]. Attention is paid to remove en-bloc with the specimen the mesopancreas [13] (Fig. 25.7).

The pancreatic neck is elevated off the superior mesenteric/portal vein and stay sutures are placed at the inferior and superior border of the gland. The pancreas is divided using a combination of harmonic scalpel and robotic scissors and the pancreatic margin is sent for frozen-section histology. During division of the pancreas, attention is paid to identify the main pancreatic duct that is cut sharply a few mm to the right of the parenchymal transection to facilitate subsequent anastomosis [2, 12].

Following a complete Kocher manoeuvre, performed by retracting the duodenum to the left side, the first jejeunal loop is mobilized and brought to the right of the superior mesenteric vessels. The jejunal mesentery is divided using the harmonic scalpel, but the bowel is not divided at this stage, to facilitate rotation around mesenteric vessels at the time of reconstruction [2, 12].

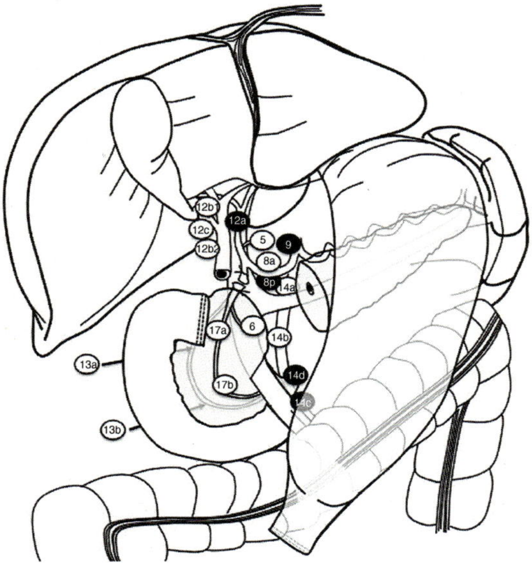

Fig. 25.6 Lymph node stations removed during robotic pancreatoduodenectomy for cancer. Within the *white ovoids* are depicted the lymph nodes usually removed en-bloc with the specimen. Within the *black ovoids* the additional lymph nodes removed when dealing with cancer

Dissection of the posterior margin is facilitated by hanging the duodenum using the fourth robotic arm. Dissection proceeds from bottom to up. The superior mesenteric artery is identified distally and dissection proceeds proximally along the periadventitial plane until the right diaphragmatic crus is reached. Pancreaticoduodenal arteries are ligated or clipped. Also large lymphatics are preferentially ligated or clipped. The use of energy devices is avoided as much as possible during this phase.

The specimen is eventually removed in an endoscopic bag through a small transverse suprapubic incision [2, 12].

In the presence of limited vein involvement, segmental resection and reconstruction of the superior mesenteric/portal vein may be performed. In these patients, the specimen is fully mobilized from the retroperitoneal margin without attempting any dissection in the area with suspected tumour abutment. In many patients an end-to-end reconstruction is not feasible, because a Cattell-Braasch maneuver cannot be performed and because of the reverse Trendelenburg position. In these patients we prefer to use the left internal jugular vein, as a jump graft. Additionally, when the spleno-mesenteric

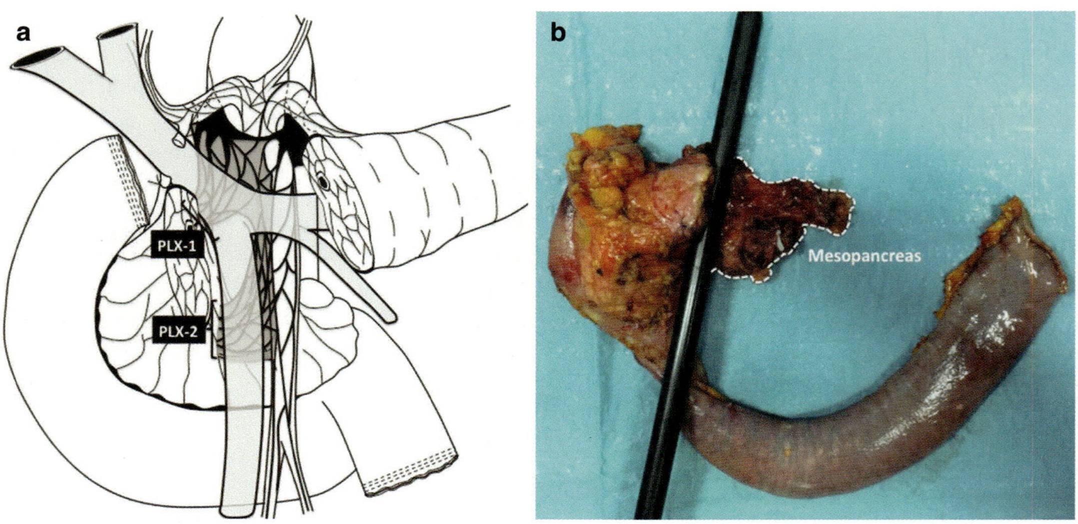

Fig. 25.7 Extrapancreatic nerve plexus and mesopancreas in resection of the head of the pancreas. (**a**) PLX1 and PLX2 depicts the two portions of the extrapancreatic nerve plexus that make up most of the mesopancreas. (**b**) Specimen from robotic pancreatoduodenecromy. The *black shaft* represents the superior mesenteric/portal vein. The margins of the mesopancreas, looping behind the superior mesenteric/portal vein, are highlighted by a *dotted line*

junction is included in the resection, we always prefer to reinsert the splenic vein. Once all the vessels are clearly exposed, the vessels are cross-clamped using laparoscopic bulldog clamps. The superior mesenteric artery is also crossclamped to reduce bowel congestion. No intravenous heparin is given. Reconstruction is carried out as in the open operation, but 6/0 expanded polytetrafluoroethylene is preferred to polypropylene because it is more resistant to robotic needle-driver manipulations. Two sutures of approximately 15 cm in length are used, and the posterior row of each anastomosis is sutured from within the lumen. When closing the sutures, attention is paid to avoid the "purse string effect", by leaving a small growth factor. Before the last suture is tied, the reconstructed vein segment is flushed with heparinized saline solution using a Bracci's catether. The clamp placed cranially on the portal vein is released first, so that the integrity of the vascular anastomoses can be checked at a lower pressure. Bleeding sites are addressed, as required, and all the clamps are released.

Each vascular anastomosis requires approximately 10 min. In order to minimize the time of complete cross-clamping of splancnic venous flow, the splenic vein and the portal vein are not occluded during the construction of the proximal anastomosis on the superior mesenteric vein. To avoid the obstacle of an additional bulldog clamp, we prefer to occlude the superior mesenteric vein distal to the anastomotic site using a Hem-o-lok® clip of appropriate size (Fig. 25.8) [13].

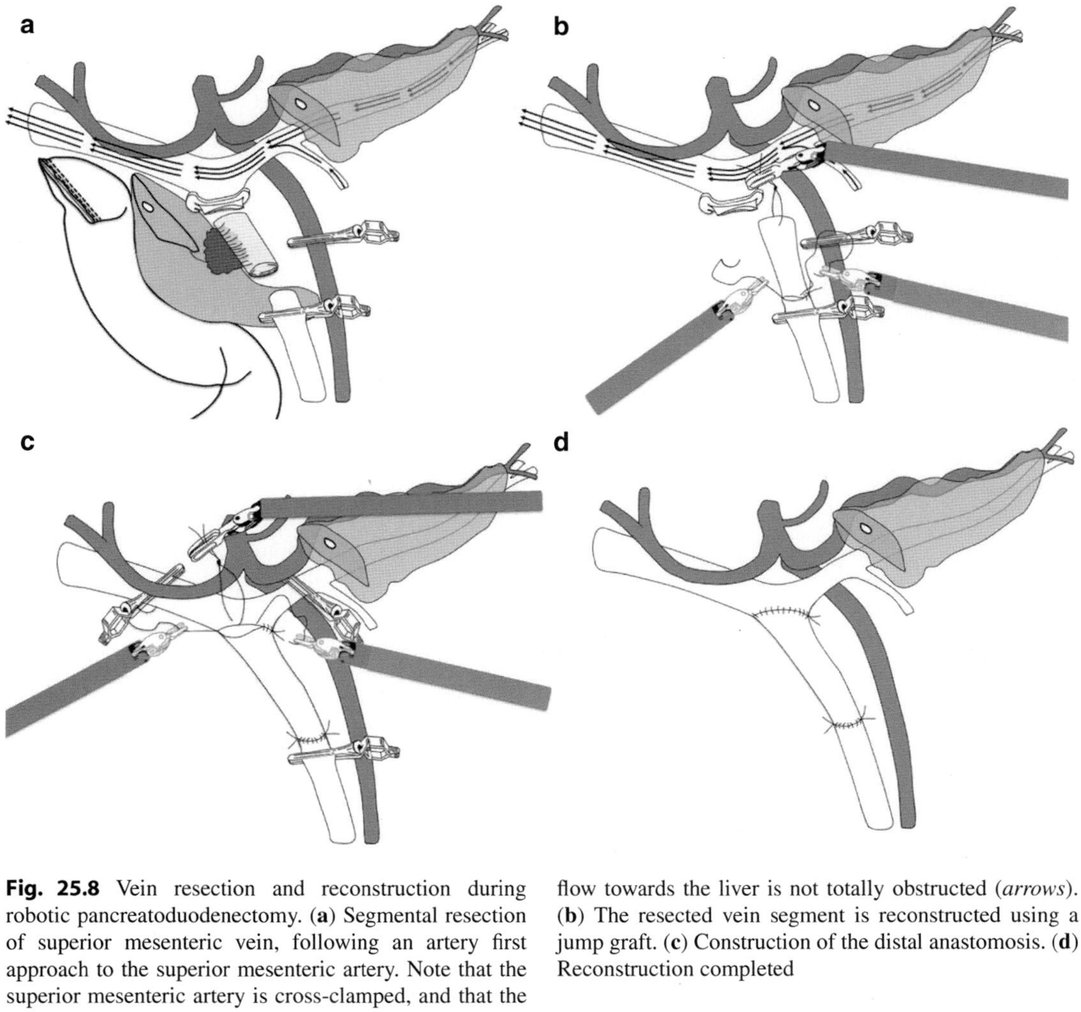

Fig. 25.8 Vein resection and reconstruction during robotic pancreatoduodenectomy. (**a**) Segmental resection of superior mesenteric vein, following an artery first approach to the superior mesenteric artery. Note that the superior mesenteric artery is cross-clamped, and that the flow towards the liver is not totally obstructed (*arrows*). (**b**) The resected vein segment is reconstructed using a jump graft. (**c**) Construction of the distal anastomosis. (**d**) Reconstruction completed

Reconstruction is performed on a single bowel loop. Before proceeding with anastomoses, the window behind the mesenteric vessels is closed by anchoring the jejunum and its mesentery to the peritoneum covering the infrarenal aorta. The pancreas stump is first anastomosed to the jejunum. In most patients we use a pancreatojejunostomy, but all types of reconstructions can be carried out under robotic assistance. The decision to perform an invaginating or a duct-to-mucosa anastomosis is taken as required in the individual patient. Recently, we have adopted a modified Blumbgart technique. If the duct is not large (i.e. ≤4 mm), we prefer to use an internal stent [2, 12].

When the pancreas is deemed at an exceedingly high risk for severe post-operative pancreatic fistula, especially if the patient is frail, we prefer to avoid the pancreatic anastomosis by creating a pancratico-cutaneous fistula, using a Bracci's catheter of suitable caliber threaded back into the Wirsung duct and brought outside through a small stab wound (Fig. 25.9). Finally, in the occasional patient with severe parenchymal atrophy of the pancreatic remnant the duct can be occluded without any type of drainage [12].

Hepaticojejunostomy is performed next end-to-side, approximately 7–10 cm downstream the pancreatojejunostomy, in a double layer, using half running sutures of 6/0 or 5/0 polydioxanone. The duodenojejunostomy or gastrojejunostomy is done in two layers 10–15 cm downstream from the hepaticojejunostomy [2, 12].

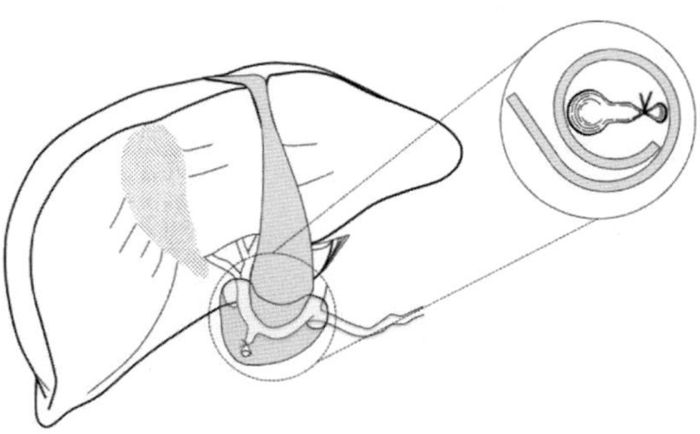

Fig. 25.9 Protection of the hepatic artery, and the stump of the gastroduodenal artery, with the round and falciform ligaments of the liver that are mobilized and wrapped around the artery (shown within the *circle*)

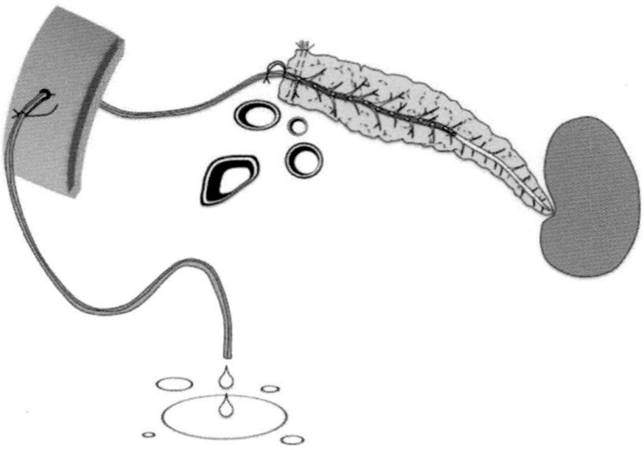

Fig. 25.10 Creation of a pancreatico-cutaneous fistula, in fragile patients with soft and fatty pancreas, and thin pancreatic duct. A catheter is threaded back into the main pancreatic duct and brought outside the abdominal wall through a small stab wound. Large vessels are protected using the round and falciform ligaments (not shown), and one or two drains are placed near the pancreatic stump (not shown)

At the end of the procedure the round ligament of the liver is mobilized and used to wrap the hepatic artery and to protect the stump of the gastroduodenal artery (Fig. 25.10) [12].

Three 14-Fr pig-tail catheters are placed and left to drain by gravity. One drain is placed in the Morrison's pouch, behind the hepaticojejunostomy. The other two drains are placed in front and behind the pancreato-jejunostomy, respectively. The drain running behind the pancreatojejunostomy is positioned through a small dedicated incision, placed between robotic ports 1 and 3 on the left flank. This drain is placed immediately after completion of the posterior layer of the pancreatojejunostomy, because at this stage it can be easily passed through the tunnel between the anastomosis and the superior mesenteric/portal vein [12].

25.7.4 Total Pancreatectomy

The technique for robotic total pancreatectomy merges the techniques described for pancreatoduodenectomy and distal pancreatectomy. In some patients, the operation begins as a pancreaticoduodenectomy, and is converted to total pancreatectomy because of intraoperative findings and/or of frozen section histology.

There are a couple of tips that can make this operation easier. First, when the spleen and the splenic vessels are planned for resection, the left gastric vein should be spared to avoid gastric venous ischaemia. Earlier identification of the left gastric vein is hence suggested. In some patients the course of the left gastric vein can be defined on preoperative computed tomography. The ideal configuration is a confluence into the portal vein (type 1 anatomy). When the confluence is in the splenic vein (type 2 anatomy), sparing the left gastric vein requires also preservation of a segment of splenic vein. Second, until the left pancreas is fully mobilized, the duodenum (or the stomach) should not be divided to avoid retraction of the stomach in the left upper quadrant, that complicates subsequent dissection of the distal pancreas.

It is also worth to note that despite the large operative field, spanning the entire upper abdomen, repositioning of the patient and redocking of the dVss is not usually required [14].

25.8 Results

Laparoscopy is increasingly used for resection of left-sided pancreatic tumors [18] and, after many years of gestation, is gaining momentum also for pancreatoduodenectomy [19].

At many high volume centers laparoscopy is conveniently employed in most patients undergoing distal pancreatectomy [7, 18]. Concerns on oncologic radicality, especially for pancreatic cancer, are also fading away although final undisputed evidence is not available yet [18]. In the setting of distal pancreatectomy the advantages of robotic assistance may be less immediately evident, because no reconstruction is needed. A recent meta-analysis showed that robotic distal pancreatectomy, when compared to laparoscopic distal pancreatectomy, is associated with longer operating time, lower estimated blood loss, a higher spleen-preservation rate, and shorter hospital stay. There was no difference between the procedures in transfusion, conversion to open surgery, R_0 resection rate, number of examined lymph nodes, overall complications, severe complications, pancreatic fistula, clinically relevant pancreatic fistula, stay in the intensive care unit, total cost, and 30-day mortality [20].

In robotic pancreatoduodenectomy the advantages of robotic assistance are expected to be more compelling, because of the more challenging dissection and the need for complex digestive reconstructions. So far, however, most information refer to laparoscopic pancreatoduodenectomy because this procedure was pioneered by laparoscopic surgeons [19]. Other factors that have limited a wider diffusion of robotic assistance in pancreatoduodenectomy are the higher costs of robotics [6] and the often limited accessibility to the system, that is typically used in busy urology and gynecology practice. The only comparative study between laparoscopic and robotic pancreatoduodenectomy was published very recently by Liu et al. [21]. In this study 27 patients underwent robotic pancreatoduodenectomy and 25 laparoscopic pancreatoduodenectomy. Patients were selected for the two approaches based on patient preference. The surgical team had completed the learning curve for both procedures and the two groups were comparable. The use of robotic assistance resulted in shorter operative time (387 ± 58 vs. 442 ± 96; $p = 0.015$), lower estimated blood loss (219 ± 126 vs. 334 ± 175; $p = 0.01$), and shorter length of hospital stay (17 ± 5 vs. 24 ± 13; $p = 0.012$) [21]. A summary of results achieved robotic pancreatoduodenectomy is provided in Table 25.2. Interpretation of these data is not always straightforward as not all authors used the same criteria to define and report outcome metrics.

In the author experience, the use of robotic assistance allowed pancreatoduodenectomy to be performed without any compromise on surgical technique. Indeed, the ability of throwing sutures and tying knots is unchanged from open surgery. Actually, when a suture has to be placed in a very deep and narrow space the use of a robotic arm may enhance precision and elegance, as demonstrated, for instance, by the excellent results achieved in urologic reconstruction after radical prostatectomy. In the most recently updates experience of the authors, only 3 of 112 consecutive robotic pancreatoduodenectomies (2.6%), including the learning curve, had to be converted to open surgery. None of these conversions was

Table 25.2 Reported outcomes for robotic pancreatoduodenectomy

Author	Year, [Ref.]	Cases	LOS[a] (days)	OR time[a] (min)	EBL[a] (mL)	Conversion (%)	POPF (%)	Morbidity (%)	Mortality[b] (%)
Giulianotti (Italy)	2010 [22]	36	28.7 (10–85)	400.5 (240–600)	250 (100–600)	25.0%	36.1%	NA	5.5%
Giulianotti (USA)	2010 [22]	24	12.5 (5–30)	452 (300–547)	433 (80–600)	8.3%	25.0%	NA	4.1%
Narula	2010 [23]	8	9.6	420.0 ± 360–510	NA	37.5%	NA	NA	NA
Zhou	2011 [24]	8	16.3 ± 4.1	718.7 ± 186.6	153.7 ± 43.4	0	25.0	25.0%	0
Chalikonda	2012 [25]	30	9.79	476	485	10%	6.6%	30.0%	3.3%
Lai	2012 [26]	20	13.7 ± 6.1	491.5 ± 94	247 (50–889)	5.0%	35.0%	50%	0
Zhan	2013 [27]	16	23.1	479.7 ± 111.5	633.8 ± 264.5	0	6.3%	37.5%	8
Zureikat	2013 [28]	132	10 (4–87)	527.0 ± 103.0	NA	6.0%	12.8%	66.6%	3.8%
Bao	2014 [29]	28	7.4 (5.5–17.1)	431 (340–628)±	100 (50–300)	14.2%	28.5%	NA	7.1%
Chen	2015 [30]	60	20 ± 7.4	410 ± 103	400	1.7%	13.3%	35.0%	1.7%
Liu	2016 [21]	27	17.0 ± 5.0	387.0 ± 58.0	219 ± 126	0	14.8%	29.6%	3.7%
Boggi	2016 [12]	112	22.0 ± 12.7	526.3 ± 102.4	NA	2.6%	33.0%	74.1%	3.6%
Total		501							

Series with ≥5 cases were considered. For each group only the most recent figures or the largest series were considered, to avoid duplication of data
Ref. reference, *LOS* length of hospital stay, *OR* operative room, *EBL* estimated blood loss, *POPF* post-operative pancreatic fistula, *NA* not available
[a]Mean or median
[b]Either 30- or 90-day mortality

caused by failure to progress or uncontrollable bleeding [12]. Robotic assistance was also used in 14 patients requiring simultaneous resection and reconstruction of the superior mesenteric/portal vein [13]. It is worth to note that in 13 of these 14 patients a segmental vein resection was carried out, and that an artery first approach was pursued in all patients. It may also be worth noting that the rate of margin negativity (R_0) in patients with ductal adenocarcinoma was 74%, in case of standard resection, and 83% in case of associated vein resection. These results were achieved despite six margins were assessed and a clearance of 1 mm was considered, further focusing on the importance of methodology when assessing outcome parameters. It is also interesting to note the mean number of examined lymph nodes, that was 44.6 ± 11 and 57.2 ± 14.6 in the two procedures, respectively [13].

Conclusions

Robotic pancreatic resections, including pancreatoduodenectomy, have a role in the future of pancreatic surgery. Safe implementation of a program for robotic pancreatic surgery requires dedication, caution, and high-volumes. Completion of a program of training and proctor supervision for the first cases, are both very much recommended (Video 25.1).

As newer robotic platforms are very close to marketing, it is hoped that competition will result in cost reduction and technology improvement.

References

1. Bonrath EM, Zevin B, Dedy NJ, Grantcharov TP. Error rating tool to identify and analyse technical errors and events in laparoscopic surgery. Br J Surg. 2013;100:1080–8. doi:10.1002/bjs.9168.
2. Boggi U, Signori S, De Lio N, Perrone VG, Vistoli F, Belluomini M, Cappelli C, Amorese G, Mosca F. Feasibility of robotic pancreaticoduodenectomy. Br J Surg. 2013;100:917–25. doi:10.1002/bjs.9135.
3. Stark M, Pomati S, D'Ambrosio A, Giraudi F, Gidaro S. A new telesurgical platform – preliminary clinical results. Minim Invasive Ther Allied Technol. 2015;24:31–6. doi:10.3109/13645706.2014.1003945.
4. Leal Ghezzi T, Campos CO. 30 Years of robotic surgery. World J Surg. 2016; doi:10.1007/s00268-016-3543-9.
5. Freschi C, Ferrari V, Melfi F, Ferrari M, Mosca F, Cuschieri A. Technical review of the da Vinci surgical telemanipulator. Int J Med Robot. 2013;9:396–406. doi:10.1002/rcs.1468.
6. Turchetti G, Palla I, Pierotti F, Cuschieri A. Economic evaluation of da Vinci-assisted robotic surgery: a systematic review. Surg Endosc. 2012;26:598–606. doi:10.1007/s00464-011-1936-2.
7. Boggi U, Napoli N, Costa F, Kauffmann EF, Menonna F, Iacopi S, Vistoli F, Amorese G. Robotic-assisted pancreatic resections. World J Surg. 2016; doi:10.1007/s00268-016-3565-3.
8. Szold A, Bergamaschi R, Broeders I, Dankelman J, Forgione A, Langø T, Melzer A, Mintz Y, Morales-Conde S, Rhodes M, Satava R, Tang CN, Vilallonga R, European Association of Endoscopic Surgeons. European Association of Endoscopic Surgeons (EAES) consensus statement on the use of robotics in general surgery. Surg Endosc. 2015;29:253–88. doi:10.1007/s00464-014-3916-9.
9. Napoli N, Kauffmann EF, Perrone VG, Miccoli M, Brozzetti S, Boggi U. The learning curve in robotic distal pancreatectomy. Updat Surg. 2015;67:257–64. doi:10.1007/s13304-015-0299-y.
10. Napoli N, Kauffmann EF, Palmeri M, Miccoli M, Costa F, Vistoli F, Amorese G, Boggi U. The learning curve in robotic pancreaticoduodenectomy. Dig Surg. 2016;33:299–307. doi:10.1159/000445015.
11. Boone BA, Zenati M, Hogg ME, Steve J, Moser AJ, Bartlett DL, Zeh HJ, Zureikat AH. Assessment of quality outcomes for robotic pancreaticoduodenectomy: identification of the learning curve. JAMA Surg. 2015;150:416–22. doi:10.1001/jamasurg.2015.17.
12. Napoli N, Kauffmann EF, Menonna F, Perrone VG, Brozzetti S, Boggi U. Indications, technique, and results of robotic pancreatoduodenectomy. Updat Surg. 2016;68(3):295–305. doi:10.1007/s13304-016-0387-7.
13. Kauffmann EF, Napoli N, Menonna F, Vistoli F, Amorese G, Campani D, Pollina LE, Funel N, Cappelli C, Caramella D, Boggi U. Robotic pancreatoduodenectomy with vascular resection. Langenbeck's Arch Surg. 2016;401(8):1111–22. doi:10.1007/s00423-016-1499-8.
14. Boggi U, Amorese G, De Lio N, Perrone V, D'Imporzano S, Croce C, Vistoli F, Signori S, Cappelli C, Mosca F. Central pancreatectomy with inframesocolic pancreatojejunostomy. Langenbeck's Arch Surg. 2012;397:1013–21. doi:10.1007/s00423-011-0895-3.
15. Boggi U, Palladino S, Massimetti G, Vistoli F, Caniglia F, De Lio N, Perrone V, Barbarello L, Belluomini M, Signori S, Amorese G, Mosca F. Laparoscopic robot-assisted versus open total pancreatectomy: a case-matched study. Surg Endosc. 2015;29:1425–32. doi:10.1007/s00464-014-3819-9.
16. Javed AA, Bagante F, Hruban RH, Weiss MJ, Makary MA, Hirose K, Cameron JL, Wolfgang CL, Fishman

EK. Postoperative omental infarct after distal pancreatectomy: appearance, etiology management, and review of literature. J Gastrointest Surg. 2015;19:2028–37. doi:10.1007/s11605-015-2920-2.
17. Tol JA, Gouma DJ, Bassi C, Dervenis C, Montorsi M, Adham M, Andrén-Sandberg A, Asbun HJ, Bockhorn M, Büchler MW, Conlon KC, Fernández-Cruz L, Fingerhut A, Friess H, Hartwig W, Izbicki JR, Lillemoe KD, Milicevic MN, Neoptolemos JP, Shrikhande SV, Vollmer CM, Yeo CJ, Charnley RM, International Study Group on Pancreatic Surgery. Definition of a standard lymphadenectomy in surgery for pancreatic ductal adenocarcinoma: a consensus statement by the International Study Group on Pancreatic Surgery (ISGPS). Surgery. 2014;156:591–600. doi:10.1016/j.surg.2014.06.016.
18. Wright GP, Zureikat H. Development of minimally invasive pancreatic surgery: an evidence-based systematic review of laparoscopic versus robotic approaches. J Gastrointest Surg. 2016;20:1658–65. doi:10.1007/s11605-016-3204-1.
19. Boggi U, Amorese G, Vistoli F, Caniglia F, De Lio N, Perrone V, Barbarello L, Belluomini M, Signori S, Mosca F. Laparoscopic pancreaticoduodenectomy: a systematic literature review. Surg Endosc. 2015;29:9–23. doi:10.1007/s00464-014-3670-z.
20. Zhou JY, Xin C, Mou YP, Xu XW, Zhang MZ, Zhou YC, Lu C, Chen RG. Robotic versus laparoscopic distal pancreatectomy: a meta-analysis of short-term outcomes. PLoS One. 2016;11:e0151189. doi:10.1371/journal.pone.0151189.
21. Liu R, Zhang T, Zhao ZM, Tan XL, Zhao GD, Zhang X, Xu Y. The surgical outcomes of robot-assisted laparoscopic pancreaticoduodenectomy versus laparoscopic pancreaticoduodenectomy for periampullary neoplasms: a comparative study of a single center. Surg Endosc. 2016; doi:10.1007/s00464-016-5238-6.
22. Giulianotti PC, Sbrana F, Bianco FM, Elli EF, Shah G, Addeo P, Caravaglios G, Coratti A. Robot-assisted laparoscopic pancreatic surgery: single-surgeon experience. Surg Endosc. 2010;24:1646–57. doi:10.1007/s00464-009-0825-4.
23. Narula VK, Mikami DJ, Melvin WS. Robotic and laparoscopic pancreaticoduodenectomy: a hybrid approach. Pancreas. 2010;39:160–4. doi:10.1097/MPA.0b013e3181bd604e.
24. Zhou NX, Chen JZ, Liu Q, Zhang X, Wang Z, Ren S, Chen XF. Outcomes of pancreatoduodenectomy with robotic surgery versus open surgery. Int J Med Robot. 2011;7:131–7. doi:10.1002/rcs.380.
25. Chalikonda S, Aguilar-Saavedra JR, Walsh RM. Laparoscopic robotic-assisted pancreaticoduodenectomy: a case-matched comparison with open resection. Surg Endosc. 2012;26:2397–402. doi:10.1007/s00464-012-2207-6.
26. Lai EC, Yang GP, Tang CN. Robot-assisted laparoscopic pancreaticoduodenectomy versus open pancreaticoduodenectomy – a comparative study. Int J Surg. 2012;10:475–9. doi:10.1016/j.ijsu.2012.06.003.
27. Zhan Q, Deng XX, Han B, Liu Q, Shen BY, Peng CH, Li HW. Robotic-assisted pancreatic resection: a report of 47 cases. Int J Med Robot. 2013;9:44–51. doi:10.1002/rcs.1475.
28. Zureikat AH, Moser AJ, Boone BA, Bartlett DL, Zenati M, Zeh 3rd HJ. 250 Robotic pancreatic resections: safety and feasibility. Ann Surg. 2013;258:554–9. doi:10.1097/SLA.0b013e3182a4e87c.
29. Bao PQ, Mazirka PO, Watkins KT. Retrospective comparison of robot-assisted minimally invasive versus open pancreaticoduodenectomy for periampullary neoplasms. J Gastrointest Surg. 2014;18:682–9. doi:10.1007/s11605-013-2410-3.
30. Chen S, Chen JZ, Zhan Q, Deng XX, Shen BY, Peng CH, Li HW. Robot-assisted laparoscopic versus open pancreaticoduodenectomy: a prospective, matched, mid-term follow-up study. Surg Endosc. 2015;29:3698–711. doi:10.1007/s00464-015-4140-y.

26 Laparoscopic Duodenopancreatectomy Step by Step: How I Do It

Antonio Talvane Torres de Oliveira,
Croider Franco Lacerda, Paulo A. Bertulucci,
and Miguel A. Cuesta

26.1 Step by Step: Laparoscopic Duodenopancreatectomy (Video 26.1)

1. Positioning of the patient and placement of trocars (Fig. 26.1)
2. Kocher manoeuvre (Figs. 26.2 and 26.3)
3. Dissection of the superior mesenteric vein and the portal vein under the neck of the pancreas by opening the infrapancreatic peritoneum (Figs. 26.4 and 26.5)
4. Opening the hepatoduodenal ligament
5. Dissection of the common bile duct. Section of the hepatic duct and cholecystectomy (Figs. 26.6 and 26.7)
6. Lymphadenectomy of the hepatic propria artery, dissection and ligation of the gastroduodenal artery and division of the right gastrica artery (Figs. 26.8 and 26.9)

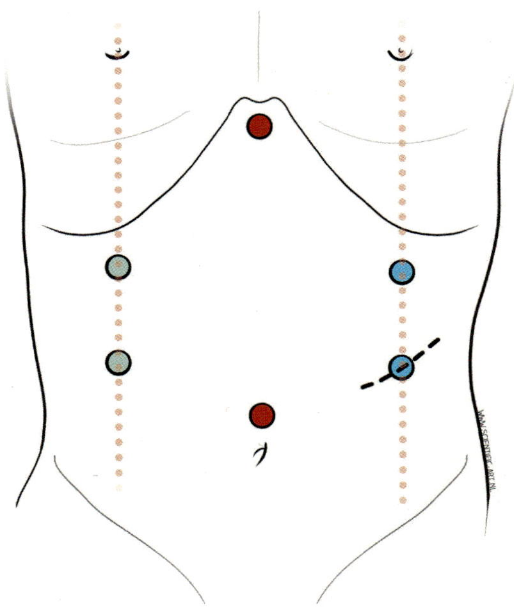

Fig. 26.1 Placement of trocars and help incision

7. Skeletonizing the distal stomach on both sides for distal gastrectomy (Fig. 26.10)
8. Completing the tunnel of the pancreas at the level of resection
9. Proximal jejunum (short segment) division and skeletonizing the short mesentery at the side of jejunum (Fig. 26.11)
10. Making a hole in the mesocolon, putting the jejunum up on the right side

Electronic Supplementary Material The online version of this chapter (doi:10.1007/978-3-319-54301-7_26) contains supplementary material, which is available to authorized users. On http://springerlink.com enter the DOI number given above.

A.T.T. de Oliveira • C.F. Lacerda • P.A. Bertulucci
Department of Upper GI Surgery, Americas Medical City Hospital, Rio de Janeiro, Brazil

M.A. Cuesta (✉)
Emeritus Professor of the Department of Surgery, VUmc, Amsterdam, The Netherlands
e-mail: ma.cuesta@vumc.nl

M.A. Cuesta (ed.), *Minimally Invasive Surgery for Upper Abdominal Cancer*,
DOI 10.1007/978-3-319-54301-7_26

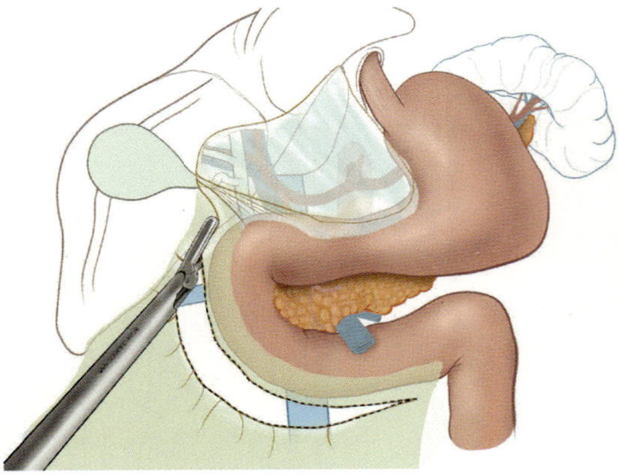

Fig. 26.2 Kocher maneuver

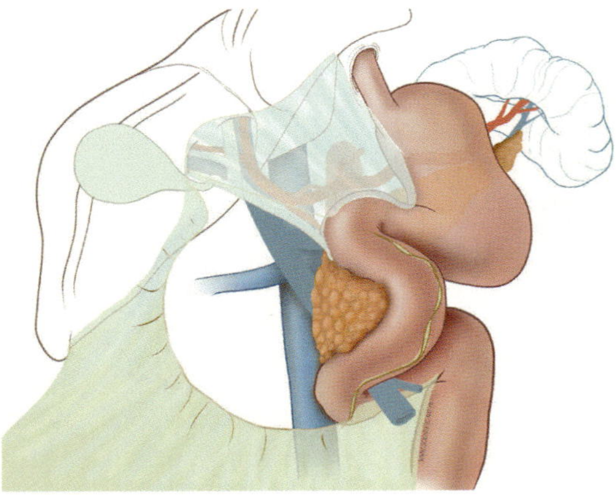

Fig. 26.3 Complete mobilization of duodeno-pancreas

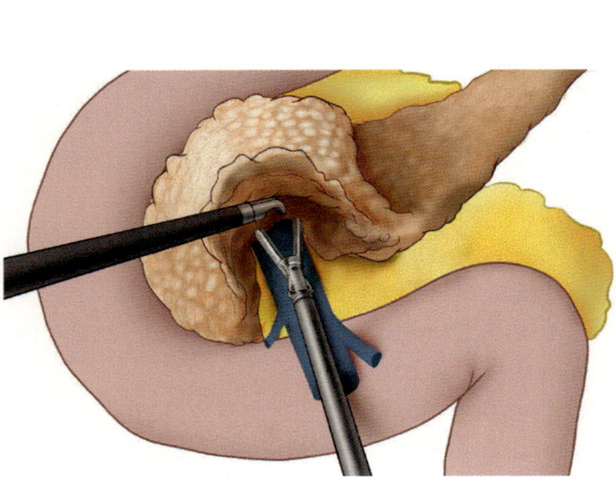

Fig. 26.4 Dissection of the superior mesenteric vein and portal vein, behind the pancreas

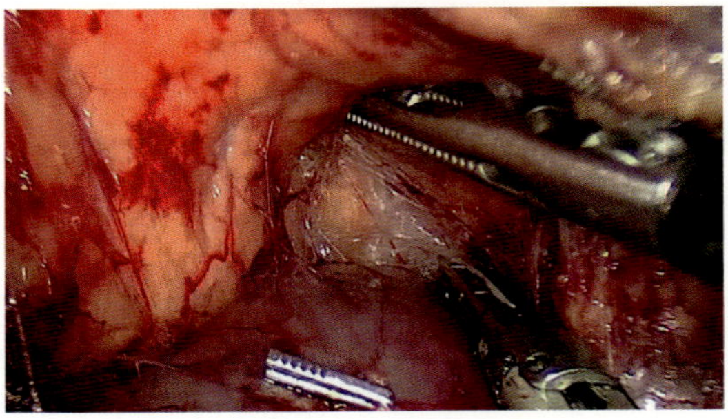

Fig. 26.5 Dissection of the SMV behind the pancreas

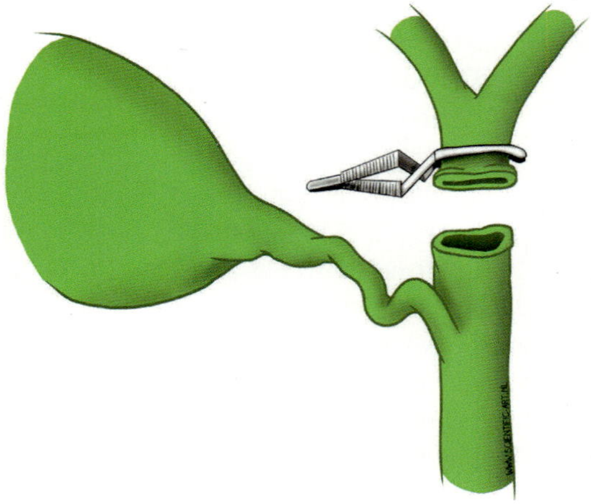

Fig. 26.6 Division of hepatic duct

11. Division of the pancreas with sealing device (Figs. 26.12 and 26.13)
12. Dissection of the uncinate process and attachments of pancreas to the Superior mesenteric vein and Portal vein (Figs. 26.14 and 26.15)
13. Resection is finished (Figs. 26.16, 26.17, 26.18, 26.19)
14. Starting the reconstruction (Fig. 26.20)
15. End-to-end pancreato-jejunostomy (Figs. 26.21, 26.22, 26.23)
16. End-to-side hepatico-jejunostomy (Figs. 26.24 and 26.25)
17. Inframesocolic end-to-side gastro-jejunostomy (Figs. 26.26 and 26.27)
18. Reconstruction is finished (Fig. 26.28). Retrieval of specimen
19. Placing of drains (Videos 26.1 and 26.2)

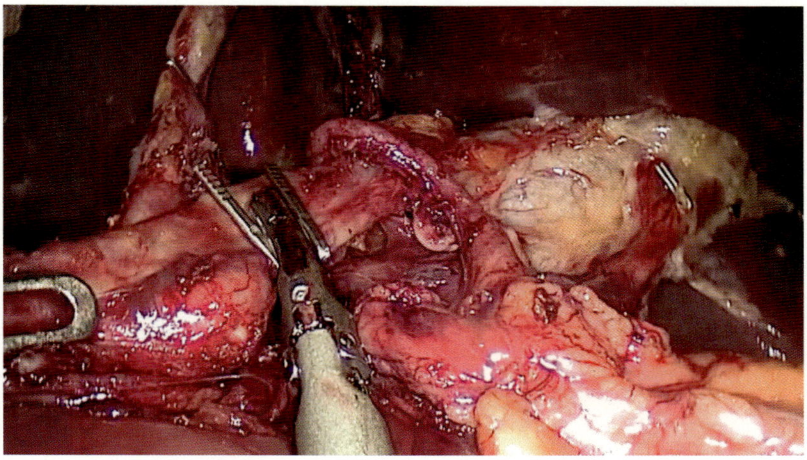

Fig. 26.7 Division of hepatic duct

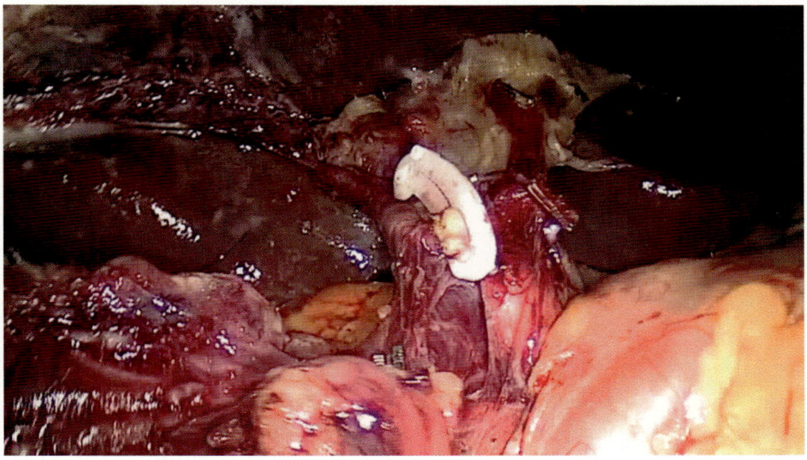

Fig. 26.8 Ligation of the gastroduodenal artery

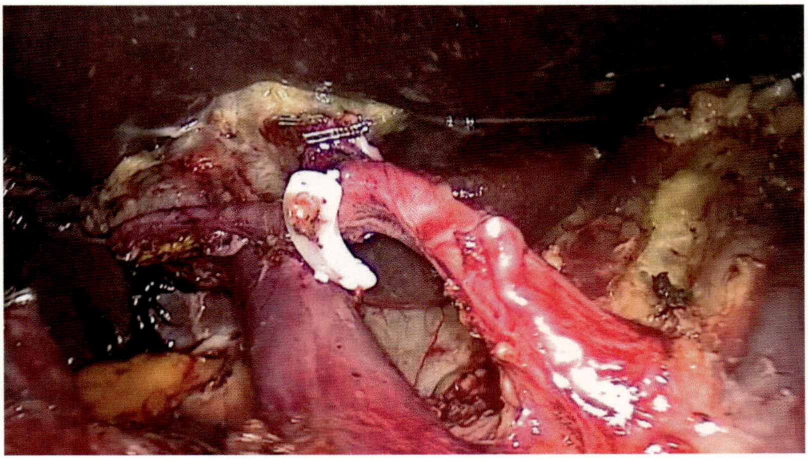

Fig. 26.9 Dissection of the hepatoduodenal ligament

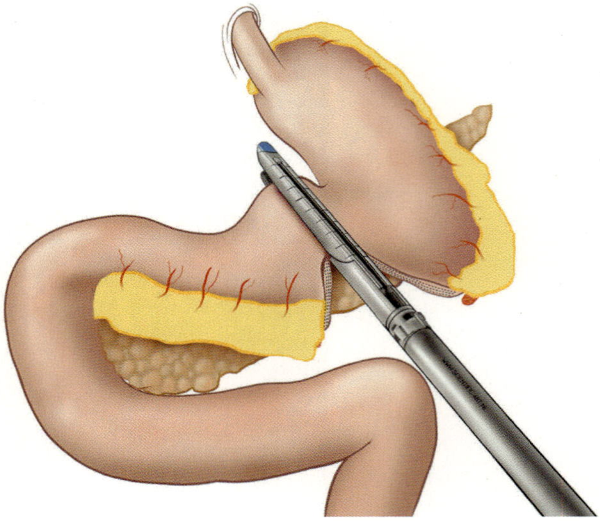

Fig. 26.10 Distal gastrectomy

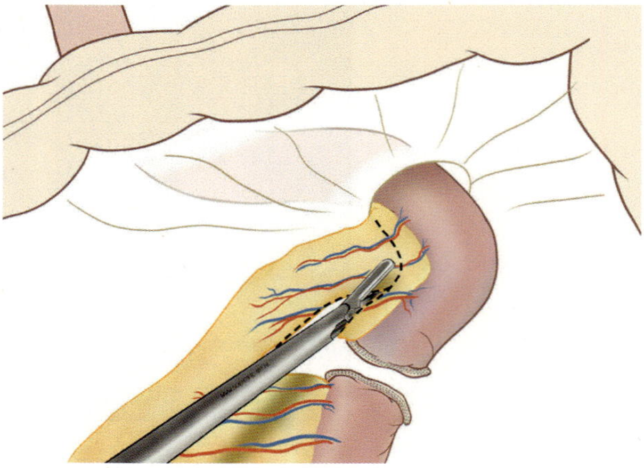

Fig. 26.11 Dissection and resection of proximal jejunum

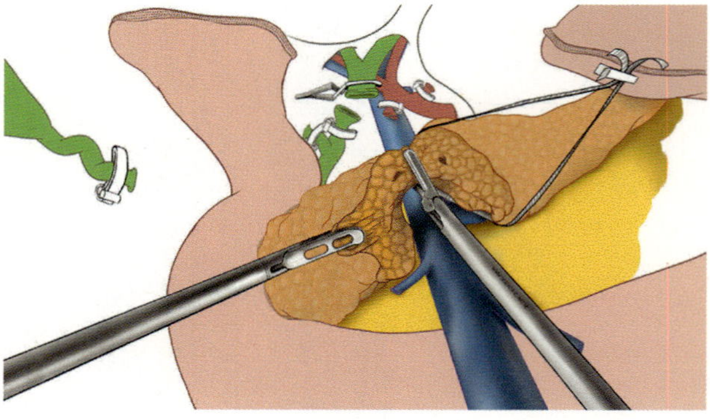

Fig. 26.12 Division of the pancreas

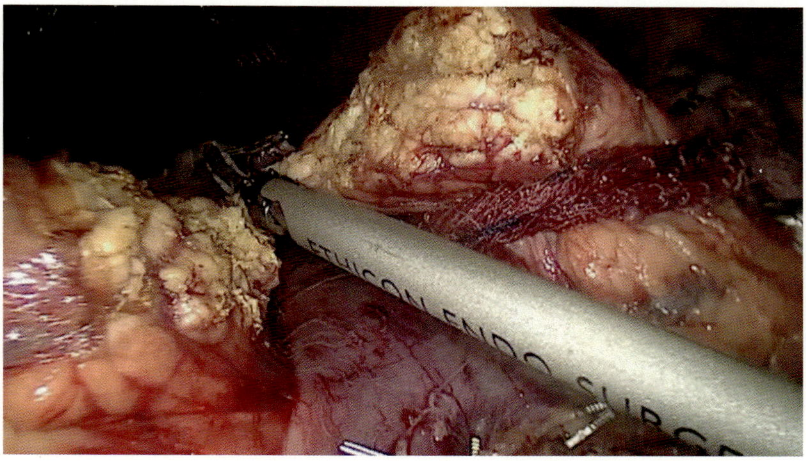

Fig. 26.13 Division of the pancreas

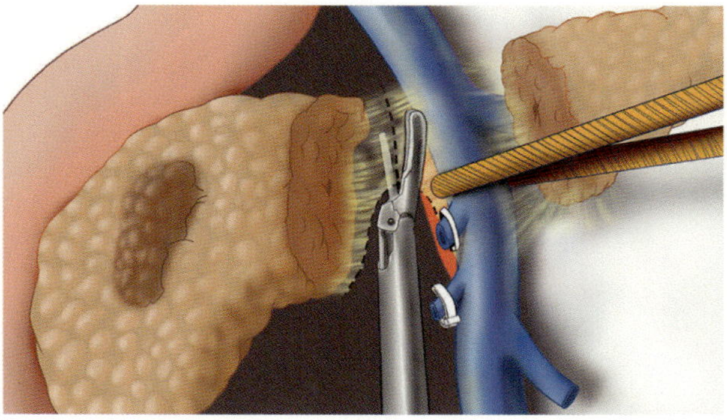

Fig. 26.14 Dissection of uncinate process and attachments of the head of the pancreas

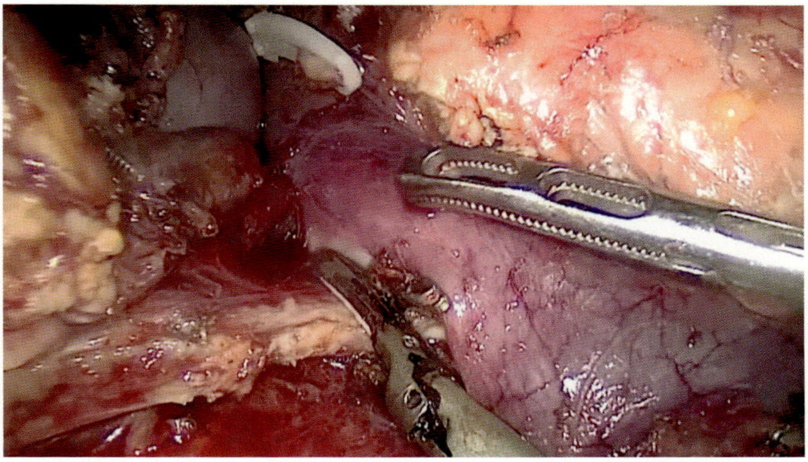

Fig. 26.15 Section of attachments of the head of the pancreas and portal vein

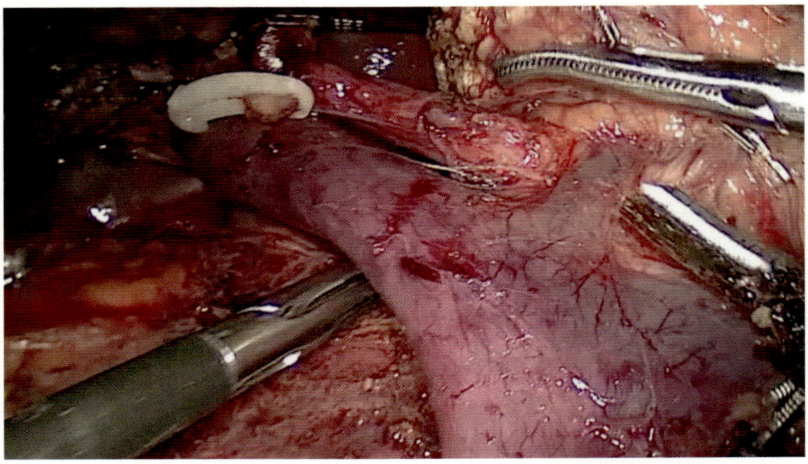

Fig. 26.16 View of the portal vein

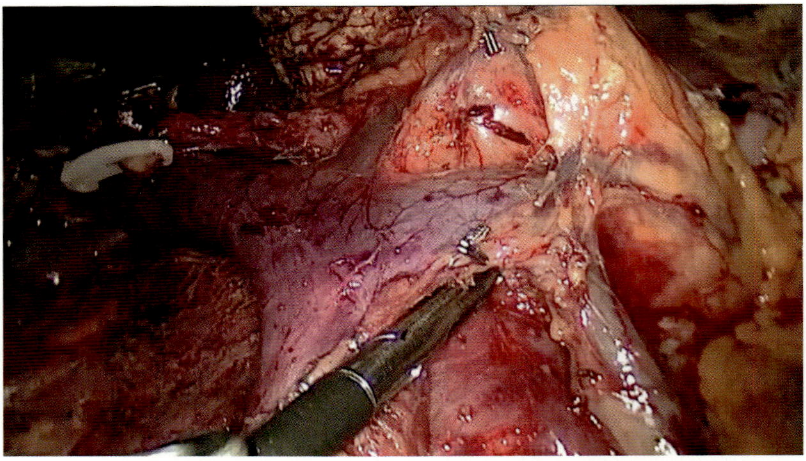

Fig. 26.17 View of the portal vein, left gastric vein, superior mesenteric vein and splenic vein

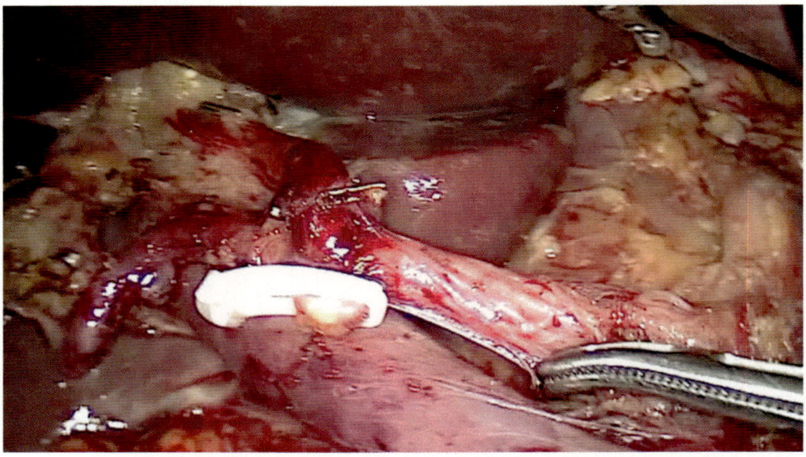

Fig. 26.18 View of the hepatoduodenal ligament

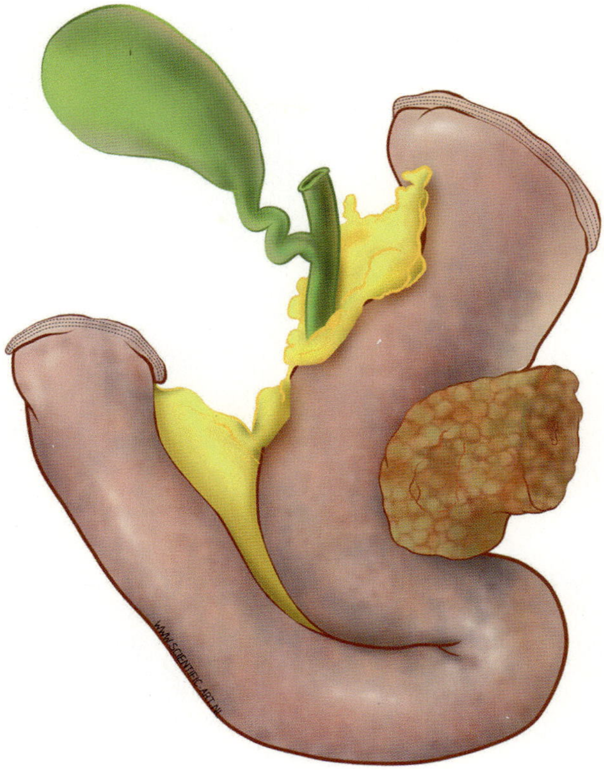

Fig. 26.19 Specimen

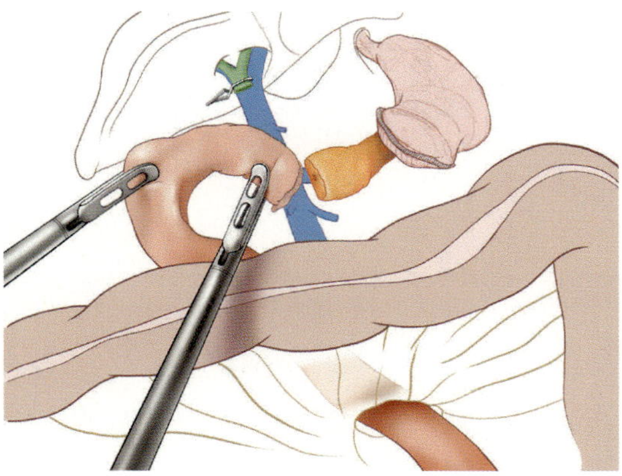

Fig. 26.20 Starting reconstruction

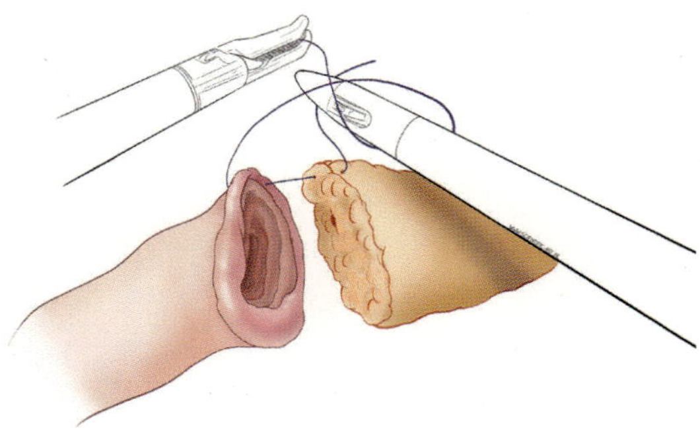

Fig. 26.21 End-to-end pancreato-jejunostomy

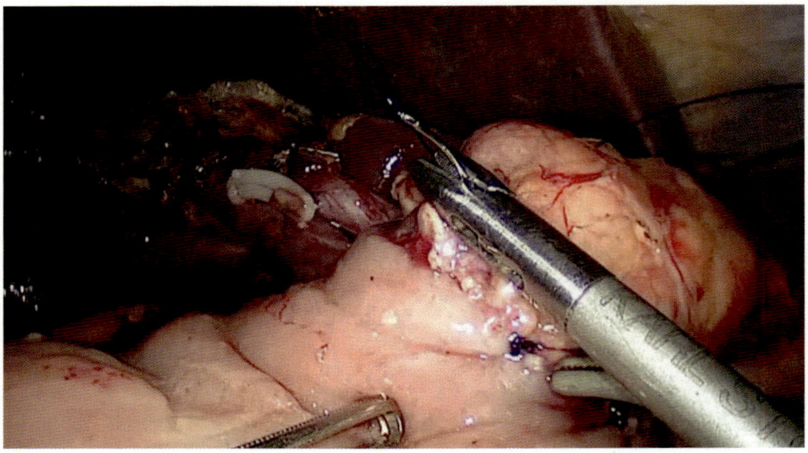

Fig. 26.22 Pancreato-jejunostomy

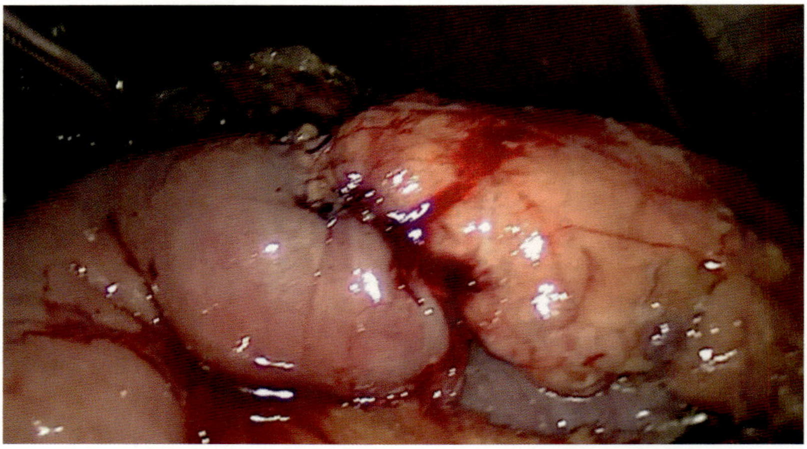

Fig. 26.23 Pancreato-jejunostomy

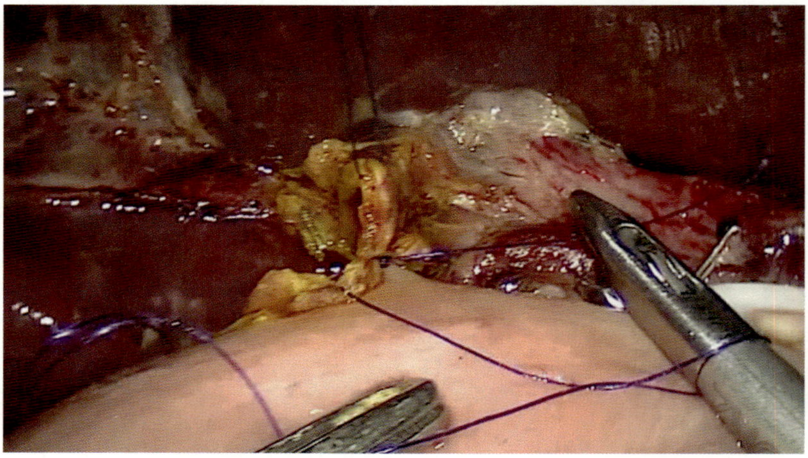

Fig. 26.24 Hepatico-jejunostomy

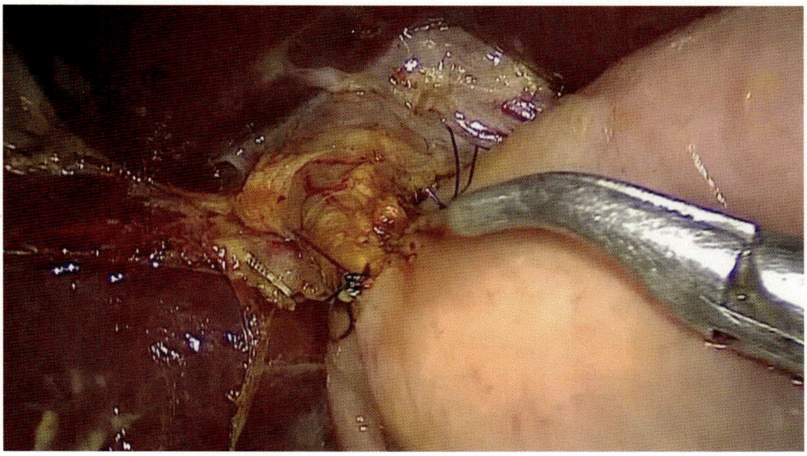

Fig. 26.25
Hepatico-jejunostomy

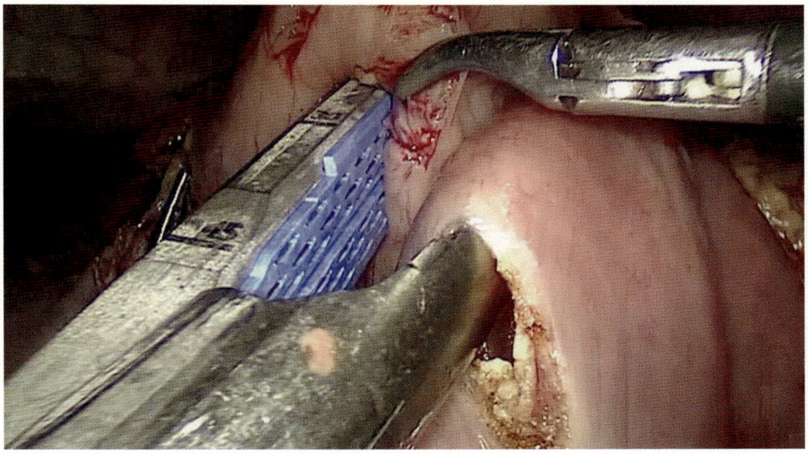

Fig. 26.26
Gastro-jejunostomy

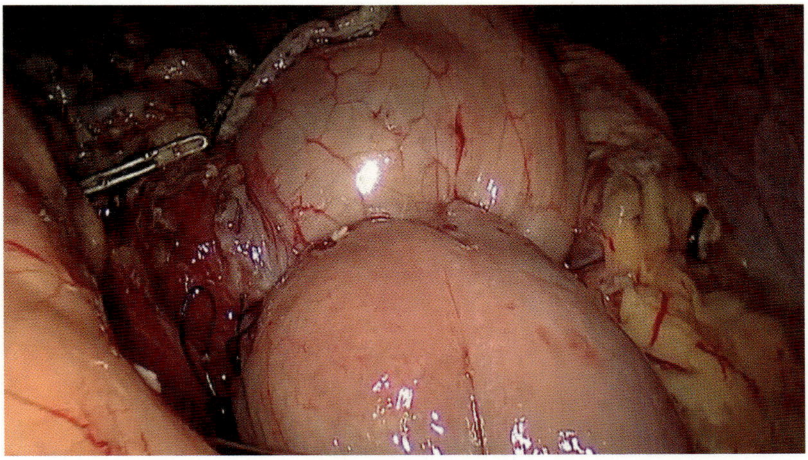

Fig. 26.27
Gastro-jejunostomy

Fig. 26.28 Final aspect of the reconstruction

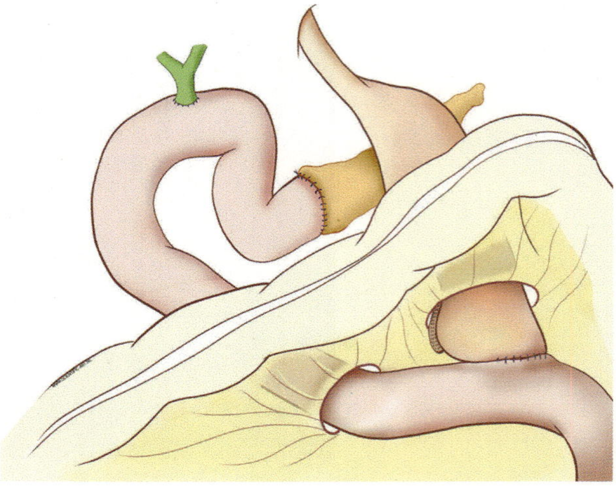

Part V

Liver Tumors

Open or Laparoscopic Liver Resection?

27

Rubén Ciria, Maria Dolores Ayllon, Irene Gómez-Luque, and Javier Briceño

27.1 Introduction

Liver surgery is complex and technically demanding. A teamwork consisting in experienced surgeons and well-trained anaesthesiologists is mandatory to achieve optimal results. Expertise teams have incorporated minimally invasive techniques to their liver surgery armamentarium and now, it is a well-established approach for several indications. Since the first laparoscopic left-lateral sectionectomies in 1996 [1, 2], the progression of laparoscopic liver resections has been exponential and now, complex liver resections, major hepatectomies, sequential procedures and even living donation are being performed laparoscopically. We will provide an overview of indications, advantages and technical considerations of this approach.

Electronic Supplementary Material The online version of this chapter (doi:10.1007/978-3-319-54301-7_27) contains supplementary material, which is available to authorized users. On http://springerlink.com enter the DOI number given above.

R. Ciria (✉) • M.D. Ayllon • I. Gómez-Luque
J. Briceño
Unit of Hepatobiliary Surgery and Liver Transplantation, IMIBIC, CIBERehd, University Hospital Reina Sofia, Córdoba, Spain
e-mail: rubenciria@gmail.com

27.2 Modalities of Minimally Invasive Liver Surgery

On November 2008, the first International Consensus Conference on Laparoscopic Liver Surgery was held in Louisville [3]. Forty-five experts in hepatobiliary surgery were invited to discuss the status of laparoscopic liver surgery. In this meeting, three modalities of laparoscopic liver procedures were defined: Pure Laparoscopy, Hand-assisted Laparoscopy and the Hybrid technique.

- **Pure Laparoscopy**. All the procedure is totally completed by laparoscopic approach. It involves a complete mobilization of the liver and the resection of the specimen under laparoscopy. Only a small incision for specimen extraction is performed. Although it was not commonly used at the beginning of minimally invasive liver procedures, it is the most commonly used approach nowadays.
- **Hand-Assisted Laparoscopy**. A hand port device is placed electively to introduce one hand into the abdominal cavity, for the purpose of assisting the laparoscopic procedure, either for mobilization or resection. This incision is also used for specimen extraction. Its advantages are: possibility to have tactile feedback, to facilitate mobilization or ability

M.A. Cuesta (ed.), *Minimally Invasive Surgery for Upper Abdominal Cancer*,
DOI 10.1007/978-3-319-54301-7_27

to compress liver in case of an eventual vascular injury. On the contrary, this approach requires a larger incision, higher risk of hand-port incisional hernia, greater postoperative pain and many times interferes with trocars. When the placement of a hand port is unplanned and occurs during a pure laparoscopic procedure, it should be called "pure laparoscopy with hand-port conversion". This could happen either because of a complication in the course of an operation, such as bleeding, or not technical progression.

- **Hybrid Laparoscopy**. It refers to a combined procedure, in which the operation starts as a laparoscopy, pure or hand-assisted, but the main procedure is completed through a mini-laparotomy incision. Generally, the mobilization is carried out using pure laparoscopic approach and then, the resection and extraction are performed through an abdominal incision that is smaller than the standard one used for conventional open hepatectomy [4].

Pure laparoscopy is the most commonly used technique worldwide, but there are geographical differences, and many centres use a combination of the previously reported variations in selected cases. There are no data that suggest the superiority of any to the others; however the two last techniques are claimed by their supporters to be beneficial for large and/or posterior lesions, donor hepatectomy and for the training of surgeons in major laparoscopic liver resections [4]. Another advantage is that, theoretically, these methods can decrease the frequency of conversion to a full open incision. These techniques have been attempted to bridge the gap between open and conventional total laparoscopic approach. The use of each modality seems to be at the preference of the surgeon with scarce data that directly compares the techniques in matched patients. Hand-assisted laparoscopy is used more commonly in EEUU, versus Europe or Asia, where pure laparoscopy is more frequent.

There are less common techniques, such as thoracoscopic approach, that may be a good option for tumours located in segments VII or VIII, especially those fully covered by the costal cage. In addition, all these techniques can be completed with robotic assistance. Robotic technology can overcome conventional laparoscopy, mainly in the most complex cases. This technique allows precise dissection, fine lymphadenectomy and biliary reconstruction even with small bile ducts and easier bleeding control [5]. It has been suggested that the learning curve of minimally invasive liver surgery is easier with the robotic approach, however is not widely utilized because of its high cost.

27.3 Technical Considerations in Minimally Invasive Liver Surgery

27.3.1 Anaesthesia

The technique for anaesthetic management during laparoscopic hepatectomy requires a strict and continuous monitoring. It is mandatory to keep central venous pressure (CVP) low (<5 mmHg) and maintain a urine output of 25 mL/h. One of the main advantages of laparoscopic liver surgery is the reduced amount of intraoperative blood loss and lower need of postoperative transfusions [6]. The main strategies to keep CVP low are strict fluid restriction, diuretics, the use of epidural anaesthesia (generating a splanchnic vasodilation, high doses of propofol and, less commonly, prostacyclin (0.05 mg/kg/min). After the specimen is removed, crystalloid fluids should be administered intravenously to achieve euvolemia [7]. The aggressive fluid restriction needed for liver surgery could be considered a risk factor for postoperative kidney dysfunction. However, a large analysis over more than 2000 cases, reported that biochemical alterations in eGFR are transient in the vast majority of patients after low-CVP-assisted hepatectomy and their clinical impact is limited. Less than 1% of the patients developed postoperative clinically relevant acute kidney injury [8].

It has been speculated that the risk of venous gas embolism is increased during liver parenchymal transection; furthermore, this risk may be increased with positive pressure carbon dioxide (CO2) pneumoperitoneum (PP) and exacerbated when low central venous pressure anaesthesia is used to minimize haemorrhage during liver resection. Very recently, Jayaraman et al. demonstrated on an experimental pigs model that Carbon dioxide embolism happened in about 75% of the cases. However, the majority of gas emboli were small gas bubbles associated with dissection of the major hepatic veins. Of the 19 animals, 18 experienced no significant hemodynamic changes, with only one pig in the positive gradient group experiencing hypotension in relation to gas embolism. The effects were only transient and did not preclude safe completion of the operation [9]. The largest published experience in humans demonstrated only one episode of CO2 embolism, which caused transient hemodynamic instability, in a series of 335 resections [10]. This is different to gas emboli with the use of argon plasma. By using argon, the risk of embolism is higher with a rapid increase in the intraperitoneal pressure because argon is 17 times less soluble than CO2 in the blood.

27.3.2 Surgical Strategies

Laparoscopic liver resections need to be carefully planned. Basic equipment for a proper minimally invasive liver surgery should include:

- Surgical surface coagulation device. High-energy fulguration should be avoided; instead, soft coagulation with saline to obtain a coagulation of the liver surface rather than a carbonization is strongly advisable
- Vessel sealing device. There are a several instruments available for this purpose. In our opinion, automated sealing devices are reliable for intrahepatic vessels.
- Staplers. Usually needed to section hilar plate, large hepatic veins or main portal vein branches.
- Dissection devices. Further than the first two superficial centimetres, careful dissection should be carried out to identify intrahepatic structures and avoid vessel damage or burn to bile ducts. Both traditional Kelly-clamp dissection and ultrasonic devices should be used.

Two main technical approaches may be considered in the laparoscopic surgery of the liver: the hilar or the Glissonian approach [11]. As reported in the Second International Consensus Conference in Laparoscopic Liver Resections that was held in Morioka in 2014 [4], "in the case of right or left hepatectomy, hilar dissection with individual vessel preparation is a standard practice". Although "the Glissonian approach serves as an important alternative when applied appropriately", potential complications regarding the risk of injury or stenosis to the contralateral hepatic duct were raised. Thus, it was agreed that "only surgeons experienced with this technique should use it". According to the recommendations from the Morioka Conference, our standard technical approach for major hepatectomies is the hilar approach (Table 27.1). Our standard approach for liver resections follows the positioning of patient and trocars in "Japanese position". They are depicted in Figs. 27.1 and 27.2. Our standard procedures for left lateral sectionectomy and left hepatectomy are described in Videos 27.1 and 27.2, respectively.

Table 27.1 Standard technical steps in most common laparoscopic liver resections

	Non-anatomical minor resection	Left lateral sectionectomy	Left hepatectomy	Right hepatectomy
Step 1	Mobilization of liver	Mobilization of left liver	Mobilization of left liver	Placing Pringle
Step 2	Placing Pringle	Placing Pringle	Left hanging maneuver	Cholecystectomy
Step 3	Surface transection with sealing device	Parenchymal transection to the left of falciform ligament	Section left hepatic artery	Section right hepatic artery
Step 4	Deep transection with dissection device	Identification space between left hilar plate and left hepatic vein	Section left portal vein (identify RPV)	Section right portal vein
Step 5		Stapling left hilar plate	Placing Pringle	Transection of segment I
Step 6		Stapling left hepatic vein	Section of left bile duct	Parenchymal transection above and below right bile duct
Step 7			Parenchymal transection	Section right bile duct
Step 8			Mobilization left lobe from segment I	Completion transection anterior to lower vena cava
Step 9			Section left hepatic vein.	Section right hepatic vein
Step 10				Mobilization right liver

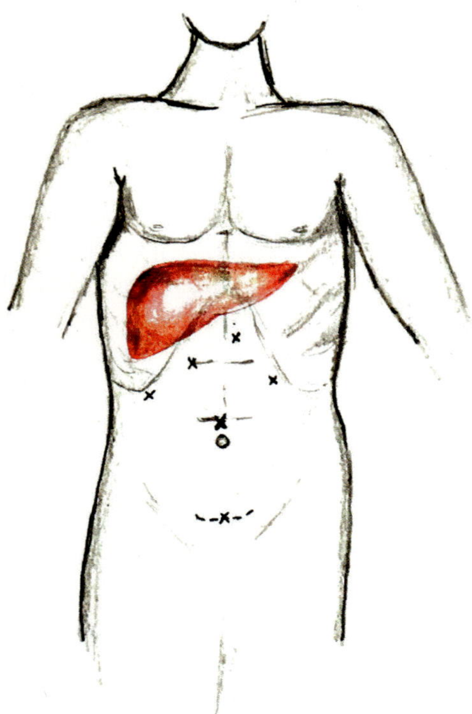

Fig. 27.1 Position of the patient and placement of the trocars in laparoscopic liver surgery for left and anterior segments

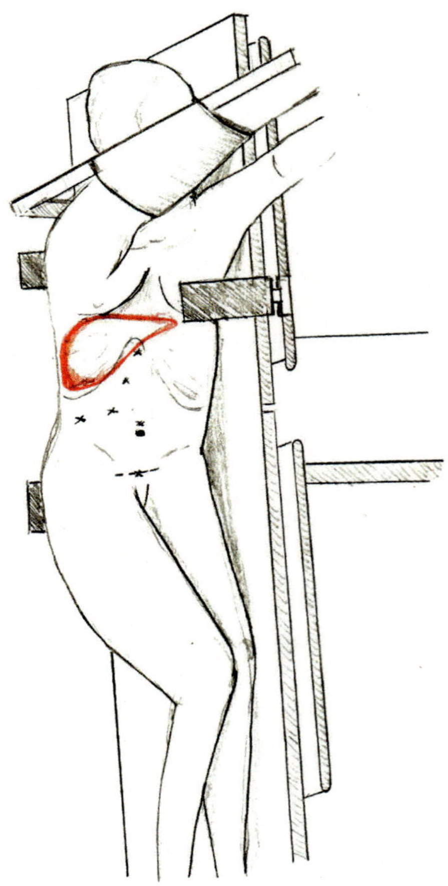

Fig. 27.2 Position of the patient and placement of the trocars in laparoscopic liver surgery for postero-superior segments

27.4 Current Status of Laparoscopic Versus Open Liver Surgery:

27.4.1 Hepatocellular Carcinoma

Hepatocellular Carcinoma (HCC) is the most common primary malignant liver lesion. HCC is the sixth most common malignancy worldwide and the third leading cause of death. Its incidence varies according to geographical areas and temporality. Risk factors associated with the development of HCC, besides the HCV and HBV infection, are alcohol abuse, Aflatoxin B1, smoking and excessive alcohol consumption among others [12].

Laparoscopic approach in liver resections for HCC has increased in recent years, thanks to the development and improvement in the learning curve and the advances of surgical devices and instruments. Laparoscopic left lateral sectionectomy and minor laparoscopic liver resection are now considered standard approaches, particularly for tumors located in the anterolateral segments of the liver. Xiao et al. reported, by a case control study, that laparoscopic resection for patients with HCC in posterosuperior segments may also offer the same oncologic outcomes than conventional procedures, being associated with advantages as lower blood loss, fewer complications and shorter hospital stay [13]. In a recent case control study with propensity score matching by Sposito et al. [14] over 269 patients undergoing minor liver resection, blood loss and need of transfusions was similar in patients undergoing laparoscopic and open liver resection. Postoperative morbidity was significantly lower in the laparoscopic group ($p = 0.004$) as less ascites, less infection, less chest complications, less pleural effusion and less abdominal wall complications. In general, patients in the open resection group had significantly longer hospital stay than laparoscopic patients ($p < 0.001$). Sposito reported that the use of laparoscopy was the only independent factor that reduced the risk of postoperative complications (OR = 0.12; [0.03–0.55] $p = 0.006$).

Regarding major hepatic resection (LMH) for HCC patients, there are several studies with a small number of patients. A recent case-control study from Komatsu et al. [15], on patients who underwent major liver resection, reports that the overall complication rates were significantly higher in the open group than in the laparoscopic group ($p = 0.011$). They did not find significant differences on intraoperative blood loss, blood transfusion and pedicle clamping rates. In the laparoscopic group the surgical time was significantly longer than in the open group ($p < 0.001$). Regarding hospital stay, the laparoscopic group showed a trend towards shorter, but it did not reach statistical significance. Komatsu concluded that the short-term results and oncological outcomes in the laparoscopic group are superior compared with the open group. The technical principles of LMH are based on the anterior approach of Liu et al., involving initial vascular inflow control, completion of parenchymal transection, and complete venous outflow control, before the liver is mobilized. This technique shows the effectiveness of LMH by an anterior approach for HCC cases due to meticulous dissection enabled by laparoscopic magnification and the excellent view of the retrohepatic to hepatocaval space.

Regarding long-term and oncological results, tumour margins are similar in both groups. In some studies it was significantly wider in LLR than OLR; this may be explained because tumour size in the OLR group tends to be larger and usually closer to vessels and hepatic pedicle. Overall survival and disease-free survival rates are similar in both groups. In different studies disease-free survival seems to be better in LLR group than in OLR. This may be because patients in LLR group have smaller tumour size and, thus, microscopic vascular invasion was more frequent in the OLR group. A selection bias may be present in these results, as all of them arise from non-randomized studies [16]. Major advantages of LLR are the rapid recovery and the shorter hospital stay, less postoperative pain, and lower incidence of postoperative liver failure and ascites (due to the maintenance of the parietal circulation and less liver manipulation). Long-term outcomes and survival and disease-free survival rates are similar in both groups. The last meta-analysis reported by Twaij et al. [17] suggests that LLR for HCC in cirrhotic patients is safe and may offer improved patient outcomes.

27.4.2 Colorectal Liver Metastases

The liver is the most common site of metastatic disease from various primary malignancies. The most frequent ones are liver metastases of colorectal origin (CRLM). Currently, liver resection is a treatment option with curative potential that may increase survival in these patients [18]. Although two-thirds of patients with CRLM have extrahepatic disease, some patients have liver-only limited disease. Among other potential treatment strategies, such as ablation therapies (alcoholic instillation, radiofrequency), intraarterial chemotherapy and radiotherapy, surgical resection is the only one that is associated with increased survival [19].

Metastatic liver disease can occur in two different moments, metachronous and synchronously. The development of high technology and new surgical instruments has allowed the implementation and progress of minimally invasive surgery in this disease. Open resection is an effective treatment for CRLM offering a 5-year survival between 16 and 74%. The CRLM resection by laparoscopic approach is proposed as a feasible and safe method carried out in specialized centers that could offer several advantages over the open approach.

Regarding the short-outcomes, a meta-analysis from Zhou et al. showed that rate of blood loss, need of transfusion and hospital stay were lower than in the laparoscopic group [20]. In this study, patients in laparoscopic group also had lower morbidity (21.1% vs 33.7%; p = 0.003). The postoperative mortality was not different. Luo et al. reported similar results [21] in a systematic review over 624 patients, detecting a lower incidence of postoperative complications (RR = 0.647[CI 0.477-0.877]; P = .005) and similar mortality (RR = 0.625[CI 0.12-3.25] P = .576). Less blood loss and less need for transfusion were also found in laparoscopic patients, whereas comparable operative time and length of hospital stay were reported in both groups.

From the oncological perspective, there are several studies that report wider surgical margins in the laparoscopic approach. Zhou et al. [20] showed higher rates of negative margin resection in the laparoscopic than in the open group (93.7% vs. 84.4%; P = 0.001). Luo et al. reported a lower incidence of R1 resection in the laparoscopic group (RR = 0.357 [0.180-0.708]; P = .003). The problem of not having the tactile sensation may be hypothesised as a risk in the laparoscopic approach. However, magnified view and the use of intraoperative ultrasound, equals or may even improve the resection margins in these patients.

No randomized studies have been published to date that may confirm comparable oncological outcomes between laparoscopic and open approach. Synchronous CRLM represent probably a more aggressive and worse prognosis tumour biology. The therapeutic strategy is determined by the symptoms that cause the primary tumour. At the moment, there is no consensus on whether simultaneous surgery could be considerer as a better strategy than the sequential approach, but it is an option that could provide better quality of life and lower costs. There are several recent main comparative reports [22–24] suggesting that simultaneous laparoscopic approach is technically feasible, safe and associated with similar short- and long-term outcomes compared to open surgery. Ratti et al. [23] reported a lower overall risk of complications, include anastomotic leak. In one recent study, Ferreti et al. [25] reported a case series with 142 patients who underwent laparoscopic combined resection in which Pringle's manoeuvre, length of hospital stay, ASA score and global operative time were independent predictors of postoperative morbidity.

27.4.3 Benign Tumours

It is well known that laparoscopic surgery offers many benefits with a direct impact on patient recovery. The inflammatory response following a laparoscopic procedure is less severe, allowing for faster healing, fewer complications, and a shorter hospital stay [6]. All these benefits are even higher in benign pathologies, since the other option through open surgery requires big incisions like Chevron, Mercedes or "in J" incision.

At the beginning of the minimally invasive liver surgery, up to 30–60% of resections in some series were for benign lesions. In 2007, a systematic review was published, where nearly half of surgeries were done for benign lesions [26]. After that, stabilization in the number of procedures for benign disease was observed. The experts agree that there is no reason to modify the management of patients with benign liver tumours based on the availability of minimally invasive surgery. Therefore, laparoscopy should not widen the indications for resection of benign lesions [10]. The most common benign liver tumours include haemangiomas, focal nodular hyperplasia and hepatocellular adenoma. These lesions are frequently found incidentally as a consequence of the widespread use of imaging test [27]. Their indications for surgery are limited, and they may be treated laparoscopically whenever possible by capable surgeons with adequate experience.

27.4.4 Living Donation

The most complex evolution of laparoscopic liver surgery is living donation. Although complex, the potential benefits to donors range from a faster recovery, as well as the almost absence of would complications and postoperative incisional hernias.

Two recent meta-analyses [28, 29] published in 2015 reported discordant results (but never favourable to open approach) regarding blood loss, hospital stay and operation time. In both of them, the rate of complications was lower in the laparoscopic approach. The statistics, methodology and bias assessment were excellent; however, there was a common bias in both of them, because the statistics were done using comparative series in which hybrid and pure laparoscopic procedures were combined and different grafts were mixed. Similarly, comparative studies and case series, had the same methodological problems, joining full laparoscopic and hybrid procedures, insufficient description of management of middle hepatic vein in left lobes, analyses of left lobes and left lateral sectors (LLS) together, cumulated experience biases, insufficient report of complications and satisfaction scales not validated.

Evidence regarding the use of left lateral sectors has two main comparative reports [30, 31] with 16 and 11 cases, respectively. Besides, recent series from [32–34], confirm the spread of this approach. The minimally invasive technique for the harvesting of LLS for LDLT seems feasible, has fewer complications than open approach and is safe. Troisi reported and interesting analysis of four cases using laparoscopic-harvested LLS for adult liver transplant (previously calculated small-for-size) [35].

Regarding left lobes, only Marubashi reported in 2013 a specific matched analysis of 31 hybrid cases versus 79 pure open cases [36]. An interesting CT scan "right portal vein" distance was reported as a risk factor of prolonged operating time. Physical recovery was improved in hybrid procedures versus open. In 2006, Kurosaki reported a "video-assisted" analysis in which most of the cases were left lobes and need of epidural analgesia was shorter [37]. Samstein reported a matched series of 22 laparoscopic (17 LLS and 5 Left lobes) versus 20 open cases showing equivalent results for both techniques [38].

Regarding right lobe grafts for LDLT, Makki and Zhang in 2014, Ha in 2013 and Baker in 2009 reported the best-matched and highest quality analyses [39–42]. All these comparative series were performed with hybrid procedures. All comparisons demonstrated similar results with no-inferiority results. Recent series show less postoperative pain and fewer incision-related complications. Besides, Makki reported improved quality of life in a well-assessed score. For full laparoscopic right lobe grafts, Takahara reported a comparative analysis in 2015 with six cases (three right lobes and three left lobes), showing its safety, increased operating time and significantly less blood loss [43]. Very recently, Rotellar has reported the first comparative analysis of 5 full laparoscopic right-lobe living donors compared with the previous 10 consecutive open cases [44]. In this study, Rotellar reported only two Clavien-Dindo Grade-I complications in the laparoscopic group, while open patients had ten Grade I, two Grade II and one Grade IIIa complications in the short-term period (<3 months). In the long-term setting (6–12 months follow-up), they also reported a significant benefit of laparoscopic approach (CCI: 1.74 vs 15.2; $p = 0.0059$).

27.5 Fast-Track and Enhanced Recovery After Surgery in Laparoscopic Approach Versus Open Liver Resection

Liver surgery has traditionally been considered as major surgery, and liver resections as high-risk procedures undertaken in specialist centres. There are few published data for intended enhanced recovery after liver resection. Recently, Schultz et al. reported excellent results in a prospective analysis of their fast-track program for liver resections including both open and laparoscopic approaches. Median length of stay for all patients was 5 days, with 2 days after laparoscopic versus 5 days following open resection [45]. The readmission rate was 6% and 30-day mortality was zero. In their study, all laparoscopic resections (N = 13) were minor ones. In our own experience, we have an aggressive fast-track program (discharge in less than 2 and 3 days for minor and major resections, respectively) and a super-fast track programme (discharge in less than 1 and 2 days for minor and major resections, respectively). From our analysis, almost 30% and 50% could be included in these super-fast-track and fast-track programs, respectively. Only two patients needed readmission due to non-biliary collections [46]. Our protocols are depicted in Tables 27.2 and 27.3.

Table 27.2 Fast-track perioperative protocol in minor liver resections and left lateral sectionectomy

Minor resections and left lateral sectionectomy. Perioperative protocol				
Day −1	Day 0 (presurgery)	Day 0 (postsurgery)	Day 0 (postsurgery)	Day +1
Admission	Surgery	Intermediate care unit	Ward	Ward
Furosemide 20 mg iv (11.00 pm)	Furosemide 40 mg iv (8.00 am)	Admission blood and gas analysis	Clear fluid +6 h	Blood + gas 7.00 am
Urinary Catheterization	Central venous and arterial lines	Continuous monitoring	Progression normal fluids and yoghourt	Start solid intake
Clear fluids	CVP < 5 mmHg	Lactate monitoring	Stand up and walk	Abd palpation
Stop oral intake 00.00	Epidural catheter	Water intake +2–3 h	Respiratory exercises	± Ultrasound
500 Saline iv during night	Propofol infusion	Removal epidural catheter	Family needed	**Discharge**
	Manitol iv	Discharge to Ward +3–5 h		

Table 27.3 Fast-track perioperative protocol in major liver resections

Major resections. Perioperative protocol					
Day −1	Day 0 (presurgery)	Day 0 (postsurgery)	Day 0 (postsurgery)	Day +1	Day +2
Admission	Surgery	Intermediate care unit	Ward	Ward	Ward
Furosemide 20 mg iv (11.00 pm)	Furosemide 40 mg iv (8.00 am)	Admission blood and gas analysis	Clear fluid +6 h	Blood + gas 7.00 am	Blood + gas 7.00 am
Urinary Catheterization	Central venous and arterial lines	Continuous monitoring	Progression normal fluids and yoghourt	Start solid intake	Full solid intake
Clear fluids	CVP < 5 mmHg	Lactate monitoring	Stand up and walk	Abd palpation	Abd palpation
Stop oral intake 00.00	Epidural catheter	Water intake +2–3 h	Respiratory exercises	± Ultrasound	± Ultrasound
500 Saline iv during night	Propofol infusion	Removal epidural catheter	Family needed	Blood + gas 6.00 pm	**Discharge**
	Manitol iv	Discharge to Ward +3–5 h	Blood + gas 10.00 pm		

Conclusions

Minimally invasive liver surgery can now be considered a standard of practice in several resections. It has clearly proven that, in experienced hands, may offer better short-term outcomes with similar long-term outcomes. However, surgeons who are willing to perform proper laparoscopic liver resections need full training in high-volume centers in which proper surgical technique may be learned. Minor resections are feasible and well standardized. Major resections are still under debate, although incoming series have reported excellent results. Regarding living donation, left lateral sectionectomy is close to be considered standard of practice. Few series on full-left and full-right lobes have been reported, but all of them report excellent safety with better perioperative outcomes. Laparoscopic liver surgery should not be considered anymore a secondary approach.

References

1. Azagra JS, Goergen M, Gilbart E, Jacobs D. Laparoscopic anatomical (hepatic) left lateral segmentectomy—technical aspects. Surg Endosc. 1996;10(7):758–61.
2. Kaneko H, Takagi S, Shiba T. Laparoscopic partial hepatectomy and left lateral segmentectomy: technique and results of a clinical series. Surgery. 1996;120(3):468–75.
3. Buell JF, Cherqui D, Geller DA, O'Rourke N, Iannitti D, Dagher I, et al. The international position on laparoscopic liver surgery: The Louisville Statement, 2008. Ann Surg. 2009;250:825–30.
4. Wakabayashi G, Cherqui D, Geller DA, Buell JF, Kaneko H, Han H-S, et al. Recommendations for laparoscopic liver resection: a report from the second international consensus conference held in Morioka. Ann Surg. 2015;261(4):619–29.
5. Montalti R, Berardi G, Patriti A, Vivarelli M, Troisi RI. Outcomes of robotic vs laparoscopic hepatectomy: a systematic review and meta-analysis. World J Gastroenterol. 2015;21(27):8441–51.
6. Ciria R, Cherqui D, Geller DA, Briceño J, Wakabayashi G. Comparative short-term benefits of laparoscopic liver resection: 9000 cases and climbing. Ann Surg. 2016;263(4):761–77.
7. Martin RCG, Scoggins CR, McMasters KM. Laparoscopic hepatic lobectomy: advantages of a minimally invasive approach. J Am Coll Surg. 2010;210(5):627–34, 634–6.
8. Correa-Gallego C, Berman A, Denis SC, Langdon-Embry L, O'Connor D, Arslan-Carlon V, et al. Renal function after low central venous pressure-assisted liver resection: assessment of 2116 cases. HPB (Oxford). 2015;17(3):258–64.
9. Jayaraman S, Khakhar A, Yang H, Bainbridge D, Quan D. The association between central venous pressure, pneumoperitoneum, and venous carbon dioxide embolism in laparoscopic hepatectomy. Surg Endosc. 2009;23(10):2369–73.
10. Koffron A, Geller D, Gamblin TC, Abecassis M. Laparoscopic liver surgery: shifting the management of liver tumors. Hepatology. 2006;44(6):1694–700.
11. Machado MAC, Makdissi FF, Surjan RC, Herman P, Teixeira AR, C Machado MC. Laparoscopic resection of left liver segments using the intrahepatic Glissonian approach. Surg Endosc. 2009;23(11):2615–9.
12. Kuper H, Tzonou A, Kaklamani E, Hsieh CC, Lagiou P, Adami HO, et al. Tobacco smoking, alcohol consumption and their interaction in the causation of hepatocellular carcinoma. Int J Cancer. 2000;85(4):498–502.
13. Xiao L, Xiang L-J, Li J-W, Chen J, Fan Y-D, Zheng S-G. Laparoscopic versus open liver resection for hepatocellular carcinoma in posterosuperior segments. Surg Endosc. 2015;29(10):2994–3001.
14. Sposito C, Battiston C, Facciorusso A, Mazzola M, Muscarà C, Scotti M, et al. Propensity score analysis of outcomes following laparoscopic or open liver resection for hepatocellular carcinoma. Br J Surg. 2016;103(7):871–80.
15. Komatsu S, Brustia R, Goumard C, Perdigao F, Soubrane O, Scatton O. Laparoscopic versus open major hepatectomy for hepatocellular carcinoma: a matched pair analysis. Surg Endosc. 2016;30(5):1965–74.
16. Chen J, Bai T, Zhang Y, Xie Z-B, Wang X-B, Wu F-X, et al. The safety and efficacy of laparoscopic and open hepatectomy in hepatocellular carcinoma patients with liver cirrhosis: a systematic review. Int J Clin Exp Med. 2015;8(11):20679–89.
17. Twaij A, Pucher PH, Sodergren MH, Gall T, Darzi A, Jiao LR. Laparoscopic vs open approach to resection of hepatocellular carcinoma in patients with known cirrhosis: systematic review and meta-analysis. World J Gastroenterol. 2014;20(25):8274–81.
18. Fong Y, Fortner J, Sun RL, Brennan MF, Blumgart LH. Clinical score for predicting recurrence after hepatic resection for metastatic colorectal cancer: analysis of 1001 consecutive cases. Ann Surg. 1999;230(3):309–18, discussion 318–21.
19. Adam R, De Gramont A, Figueras J, Guthrie A, Kokudo N, Kunstlinger F, et al. The oncosurgery approach to managing liver metastases from colorectal cancer: a multidisciplinary international consensus. Oncologist. 2012;17(10):1225–39.
20. Zhou Y, Xiao Y, Wu L, Li B, Li H. Laparoscopic liver resection as a safe and efficacious alternative to open resection for colorectal liver metastasis: a meta-analysis. BMC Surg. 2013;13:44.
21. Luo L-X, Yu Z-Y, Bai Y-N. Laparoscopic hepatectomy for liver metastases from colorectal cancer: a

meta-analysis. J Laparoendosc Adv Surg Tech. 2014;24(4):213–22.
22. Tranchart H, Fuks D, Viganò L, Ferretti S, Paye F, Wakabayashi G, et al. Laparoscopic simultaneous resection of colorectal primary tumor and liver metastases: a propensity score matching analysis. Surg Endosc. 2016;30(5):1853–62.
23. Ratti F, Catena M, Di Palo S, Staudacher C, Aldrighetti L. Impact of totally laparoscopic combined management of colorectal cancer with synchronous hepatic metastases on severity of complications: a propensity-score-based analysis. Surg Endosc. 2016;30(11):4934–45.
24. Lin Q, Ye Q, Zhu D, Wei Y, Ren L, Zheng P, et al. Comparison of minimally invasive and open colorectal resections for patients undergoing simultaneous R0 resection for liver metastases: a propensity score analysis. Int J Color Dis. 2015;30(3):385–95.
25. Ferretti S, Tranchart H, Buell JF, Eretta C, Patriti A, Spampinato MG, et al. Laparoscopic simultaneous resection of colorectal primary tumor and liver metastases: results of a multicenter international study. World J Surg. 2015;39(8):2052–60.
26. Laurence JM, Lam VWT, Langcake ME, Hollands MJ, Crawford MD, Pleass HCC. Laparoscopic hepatectomy, a systematic review. ANZ J Surg. 2007; 77(11):948–53.
27. European Association for the Study of the Liver (EASL). EASL Clinical Practice Guidelines on the management of benign liver tumours. J Hepatol. 2016;65(2):386–98. easloffice@easloffice.eu.
28. Bekheit M, Khafagy P-A, Bucur P, Katri K, Elgendi A, Abdel-salam WN, et al. Donor safety in live donor laparoscopic liver procurement: systematic review and meta-analysis. Surg Endosc. 2015;29(11):3047–64.
29. Berardi G, Tomassini F, Troisi RI. Comparison between minimally invasive and open living donor hepatectomy: a systematic review and meta-analysis. Liver Transpl. 2015;21(6):738–52.
30. Soubrane O, Cherqui D, Scatton O, Stenard F, Bernard D, Branchereau S, et al. Laparoscopic left lateral sectionectomy in living donors: safety and reproducibility of the technique in a single center. Ann Surg. 2006;244(5):815–20.
31. Kim KH, Jung DH, Park KM, Lee YJ, Kim DY, Kim KM, et al. Comparison of open and laparoscopic live donor left lateral sectionectomy. Br J Surg. 2011;98(9): 1302–8.
32. Soubrane O, De Rougemont O, Kim K-H, Samstein B, Mamode N, Boillot O, et al. Laparoscopic living donor left lateral sectionectomy: a new standard practice for donor hepatectomy. Ann Surg. 2015;262(5):757–61, discussion761–3.
33. Scatton O, Katsanos G, Boillot O, Goumard C, Bernard D, Stenard F, et al. Pure laparoscopic left lateral sectionectomy in living donors: from innovation to development in France. Ann Surg. 2015;261(3):506–12.
34. Yu Y-D, Kim K-H, Jung D-H, Lee S-G, Kim Y-G, Hwang G-S. Laparoscopic live donor left lateral sectionectomy is safe and feasible for pediatric living donor liver transplantation. Hepato-Gastroenterology. 2012;59(120):2445–9.
35. Troisi RI, Wojcicki M, Tomassini F, Houtmeyers P, Vanlander A, Berrevoet F, et al. Pure laparoscopic full-left living donor hepatectomy for calculated small-for-size LDLT in adults: proof of concept. Am J Transplant. 2013;13(9):2472–8.
36. Marubashi S, Wada H, Kawamoto K, Kobayashi S, Eguchi H, Doki Y, et al. Laparoscopy-assisted hybrid left-side donor hepatectomy. World J Surg. 2013;3 7(9):2202–10.
37. Kurosaki I, Yamamoto S, Kitami C, Yokoyama N, Nakatsuka H, Kobayashi T, et al. Video-assisted living donor hemihepatectomy through a 12-cm incision for adult-to-adult liver transplantation. Surgery. 2006; 139(5):695–703.
38. Samstein B, Griesemer A, Cherqui D, Mansour T, Pisa J, Yegiants A, et al. Fully laparoscopic left-sided donor hepatectomy is safe and associated with shorter hospital stay and earlier return to work: a comparative study. Liver Transpl. 2015;21(6):768–73.
39. Makki K, Chorasiya VK, Sood G, Srivastava PK, Dargan P, Vij V. Laparoscopy-assisted hepatectomy versus conventional (open) hepatectomy for living donors: when you know better, you do better. Liver Transpl. 2014;20(10):1229–36.
40. Zhang X, Yang J, Yan L, Li B, Wen T, Xu M, et al. Comparison of laparoscopy-assisted and open donor right hepatectomy: a prospective case-matched study from China. J Gastrointest Surg. 2014;18(4):744–50.
41. Ha TY, Hwang S, Ahn CS, Kim KH, Moon DB, Song GW, et al. Role of hand-assisted laparoscopic surgery in living-donor right liver harvest. Transplant Proc. 2013;45(8):2997–9.
42. Baker TB, Jay CL, Ladner DP, Preczewski LB, Clark L, Holl J, et al. Laparoscopy-assisted and open living donor right hepatectomy: a comparative study of outcomes. Surgery. 2009;146(4):817–23, discussion 823–5.
43. Takahara T, Wakabayashi G, Hasegawa Y, Nitta H. Minimally invasive donor hepatectomy: evolution from hybrid to pure laparoscopic techniques. Ann Surg. 2015;261(1):e3–4.
44. Rotellar F, Pardo F, Benito A, Zozaya G, Martí-Cruchaga P, Hidalgo F, et al. Totally laparoscopic right hepatectomy for living donor liver transplantation. Analysis of a preliminary experience on 5 consecutive cases. Transplantation. 2017;101(3):548–54.
45. Schultz NA, Larsen PN, Klarskov B, Plum LM, Frederiksen HJ, Christensen BM, et al. Evaluation of a fast-track programme for patients undergoing liver resection. Br J Surg. 2012;100(1):138–43.
46. Ciria R, Ayllon MD, Gomez I, Alconchel F, Moreno A, Luque A, et al. Aplicación de protocolos eras (early recovery after surgery) tras cirugia hepatica laparoscopica. Experiencia de una unidad de cirugia hepatica de alto volumen. Oral abstract. Spanish Meeting of Surgery. Congreso Nacional de Cirugía. October 2016.

Laparoscopic Left Lateral Sectionectomy

28

Marcel J. van der Poel, Pieter J. Tanis,
Dennis A. Wicherts, and Marc G.H. Besselink

28.1 Introduction

Since its first introduction in 1992 [1], the widespread implementation of laparoscopic liver surgery has been slow, in contrast to other laparoscopic abdominal procedures such as laparoscopic cholecystectomy and laparoscopic hernia repair. The need for advanced laparoscopic skills and several concerns have delayed the widespread adaptation of this technique. Most feared was the risk of uncontrollable intraoperative bleeding. The suggested poor visibility and poor ability to mobilize the liver caused doubts about oncological efficiency. Other concerns included the potential of gas embolism and tumor cell seeding at surgical ports during the extraction of the specimen. Furthermore, few surgeons felt comfortable with the idea of losing the ability to manually manipulate the liver and palpate liver lesions.

Initial reports and case-series demonstrated beneficial results including less pain, shorter hospital stay and faster recovery without compromising the efficiency of the procedure. After the publication by Cherqui et al. [2] of 30 laparoscopic liver resections, the feasibility of the technique was more widely acknowledged, leading to more and bigger series being reported.

In the early phases of laparoscopic liver surgery, the most performed resections were metastasectomies from anterior segments. The first report of laparoscopic left lateral sectionectomy (LLS) appeared in 1996, but this procedure was performed in 1993 [3]. This case-report was the first report of a formal, anatomical liver resection performed by laparoscopy. Nowadays, it is considered the most standardized laparoscopic liver resection and at the Louisville consensus conference in 2008 it was even declared standard of care over an open procedure in experienced hands [3]. In this chapter we will further discuss the standardized technique for this procedure and its advantages over open surgery.

28.2 Technique of Left Lateral Sectionectomy

28.2.1 Patient Selection

All patients with lesions in liver segments 2 and 3, with a 10–20 mm margin on the left hepatic vein origin are generally considered candidates for LLS. Routine work-up consists of bloodwork and imaging studies, usually consisting of contrast enhanced computed tomography (CT) scans

M.J. van der Poel • P.J. Tanis • D.A. Wicherts
M.G.H. Besselink (✉)
Department of Surgery, Academic Medical Center
Amsterdam, The Netherlands
e-mail: m.j.vanderpoel@amc.uva.nl;
m.g.besselink@amc.uva.nl

M.A. Cuesta (ed.), *Minimally Invasive Surgery for Upper Abdominal Cancer*,
DOI 10.1007/978-3-319-54301-7_28

and/or magnetic resonance imaging (MRI). The results of these studies are then discussed in a multi-disciplinary team including liver surgeons, medical oncologists, gastroenterologists, radiologists and pathologists. Treatment options depend on the patients performance status and resectability of the lesion(s). Depending on exact tumor location and size as well as histology, a more or less extensive resection (hemihepatectomy or non-anatomical wedge resection) or local ablative procedures might be considered more suitable. Left lateral sectionectomy might also be part of a two stage liver resection.

28.2.2 Positioning

Resections are performed under general anesthesia without epidural catheter. A supine position with legs spread (French position) is preferred when performing a laparoscopic left lateral sectionectomy, but the procedure can also be performed with the legs closed and the surgeon on the patient's right side [4]. Four ports are placed (Fig. 28.1). Care should be taken not to position the ports too low. Pneumoperitoneum is generally established around 12 mmHg.

28.2.3 Intraoperative Ultrasound

The use of ultrasound is generally advocated to evaluate the liver intraoperatively for any additional malignant lesions that were not seen on pre-operative imaging. For benign lesions this may only be indicated when the lesion is close to the resection margin. The resection line can be marked using a diathermic hook, which can then be seen on ultrasound as a hyperacoustic shadow over the liver parenchyma, ensuring enough distance between the resection line and the lesion(s). The typical resection line is 1 cm to the left of the falciform ligament.

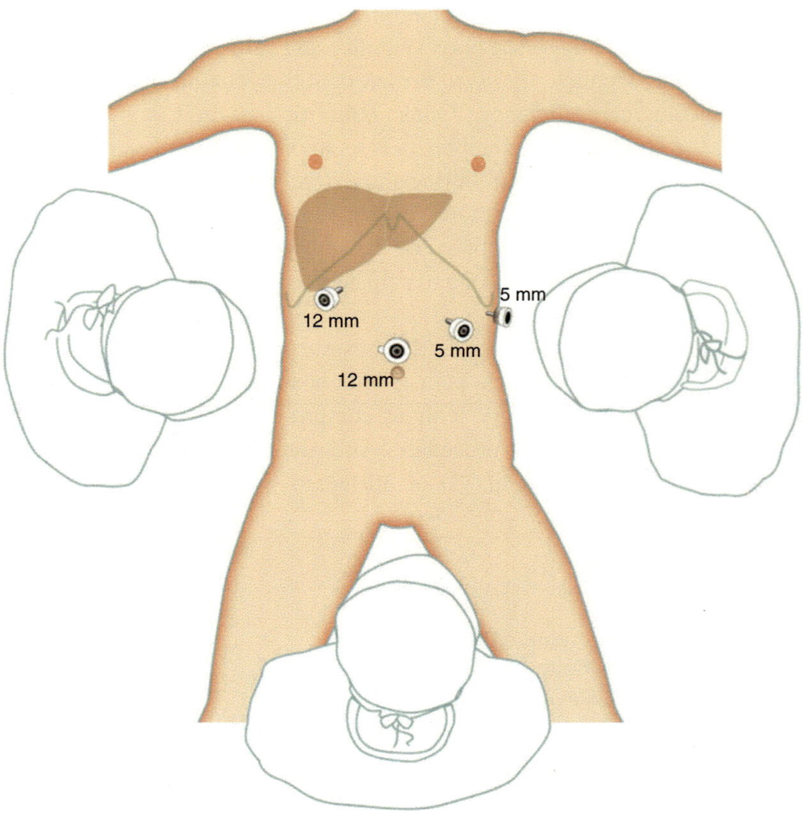

Fig. 28.1 Positioning and port placement

28.2.4 Control of Bleeding

An often-used method of extra-parenchymal bleeding control is the use of a Pringle-sling. Although not routinely required during LLS it can act as useful adjunct, for instance in patients with expected bleeding risk because of cirrhosis or chemotherapy associated 'blue liver'. A nylon tape is positioned around the portal triad and then passed through a 10–13 cm long surgical drain. The ends are extracted through the skin incision of a lateral port, but not through the port itself. Generally, an extra port placement is needed for this purpose, ideally 2 cm subcostally, right anterior axillary line. During parenchymal transection, the sling can be tightened by pulling at the ends and securing tension by clamping at the level of the skin. To reduce ischemic injury, one may decide to perform intermittent Pringle maneuvers (i.e. 10–20 min intervals). In the vast majority of procedures a Pringle sling/maneuver is not required.

28.2.5 Liver Mobilization

After diagnostic laparoscopy and intra-operative ultrasound, the left lobe of the liver is mobilized. The teres ligament is separated from the abdominal wall using the harmonic scalpel and is kept as long as possible so it can be used to retract and mobilize the liver. Using either the diathermic hook or ultrasonic shears the falciform, triangular and coronary ligament are divided up to the left hepatic vein. Care should be taken not to injure the left hepatic or diaphragmatic vein.

28.2.6 Parenchymal Transection

Routinely used equipment for superficial parenchymal transection is the harmonic scalpel. On indication the laparoscopic CUSA (cavitron ultrasonic surgical aspirator) may be used depending on the thickness of the parenchyma just lateral to the falciform ligament. This enables visualization of bigger vascular structures, but this is rarely needed for LLS. Transection is started on the upper liver surface, 1 cm to the left of the falciform ligament moving from front to back, taking small bites with slow closure of the ultrasonic shears until a 2 cm cut is completed. By going deeper into the liver parenchyma with the harmonic scalpel, the risk of significant bleeding increases. It is crucial to prevent tunneling, causing deep holes were visibility is compromised and bleeding can occur without noticing. Additional 1 cm parenchymal transection on the dorsal side is also optional.

Laparoscopic clips or hem-o-locks can be used to control bigger vascular structures, but this often needs dissection using a CUSA. One should also keep in mind that clips can interfere with future stapling.

When the remaining parenchyma is thin enough, the remaining parenchyma, which includes the 2/3 portal pedicle is transected using an endoscopic stapler that is passed along the groove between segments 2/3 and segment 1 (Fig. 28.2). The transection is finalized with one or two additional staplings. A 60 mm stapler with a wide opening and a medium height stapler size is typically ideal. A vascular stapler may be used when large vessels are clearly visible.

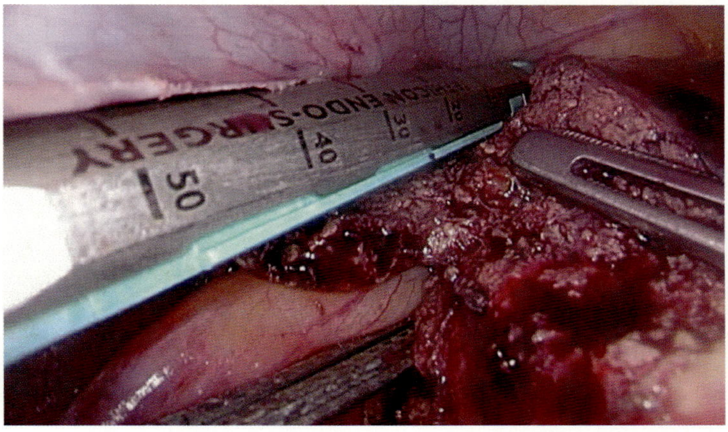

Fig. 28.2 Parenchymal transection using stapler

28.2.7 Treatment of the Parenchymal Transection Plane

When the transection is completed, the transection plane should be carefully examined for potential bile leak or hemorrhage. Bile leak can be managed using prolene sutures or clips. For the management of superficial bleeding, bipolar diathermy usually suffices. For more considerable bleeding prolene sutures and clips can be used. Haemostatic products such as fibrillar collagen or fibrin glue can be applied to the surface. A silicone drain can be left behind to drain any oozing that might occur but generally this is not necessary.

28.2.8 Removal of the Specimen

Once the dissection is completed, the specimen is placed in an impermeable bag that is introduced into the abdomen through a small suprapubical incision with transverse fascial incision and midline incision between the rectus muscles (Pfannenstiel incision). The bag with specimen is then extracted through this incision. Following removal of the specimen, the parenchymal transection plane is checked for hemorrhage for a final time.

28.3 Laparoscopic vs. Open

Initial reports and case series, as in other areas of abdominal surgery, demonstrated favorable outcomes of LLS, leading the way for further research. Throughout the years, multiple comparative studies have appeared, further evaluating the benefits of the laparoscopic approach. Overall conclusions have never differed much and have boosted the widespread implementation of this technique: LLS is feasible and safe with possible advantages over the open approach. These advantages are as can be expected from a minimally invasive approach: a decrease in intraoperative blood loss, shorter hospital stay and faster recovery, without compromising oncological efficiency or increasing the amount of complications. The only problem that remained was the increased operative difficulty that is inherent to a new technique, represented by an increase in operative time in early experiences [5, 6]. Hence, when in 2008 LLS was proposed as the standard of care, a side note mentioned for experienced surgeons only.

In the years thereafter, the learning curve of LLS was a much-debated subject. It was initially feared that patients were exposed to additional risks during early experience. Nevertheless, it appeared through further research that the learning curve of LLS is short and non clinical [7]. The only randomized trial on laparoscopic versus open LLS was stopped early because of slow accrual due to strong patient preference for the laparoscopic approach [8]. This further contributes to the statement that laparoscopy should be the standard approach for LLS.

References

1. Gagner M, Rheault M, Dubuc J. Laparoscopic partial hepatectomy for liver tumor. Surg Endosc. 1992;6:99.
2. Cherqui D, Husson E, Hammoud R, Malassagne B, Stéphan F, Bensaid S, Rotman N, Fagniez P. Laparoscopic liver resections: a feasibility study in 30 patients. Ann Surg. 2000;232:753–62.
3. Buell JF, Cherqui D, Geller DA, O'Rourke N, Iannitti D, Dagher I, Koffron AJ, Thomas M, Gayet B, Han HS, Wakabayashi G, Belli G, Kaneko H, Ker CG, Scatton O, Laurent A, Abdalla EK, Chaudhury P, Dutson E, Gamblin C, D'Angelica M, Nagorney D, Testa G, Labow D, Manas D, Poon RT, Nelson H, Martin R, Clary B, Pinson WC, Martinie J, Vauthey JN, Goldstein R, Roayaie S, Barlet D, Espat J, Abecassis M, Rees M, Fong Y, McMasters KM, Broelsch C, Busuttil R, Belghiti J, Strasberg S, Chari RS, World Consensus Conference on Laparoscopic Surgery. The international position on laparoscopic liver surgery: The Louisville Statement, 2008. Ann Surg. 2009;250:825–30.
4. Abu Hilal M, Pearce N. Laparoscopic left lateral liver sectionectomy: a safe, efficient, reproducible technique. Dig Surg. 2008;25:305–8.
5. Aldrighetti L, Pulitanò C, Catena M, Arru M, Guzzetti E, Casati M, Comotti L, Ferla G. A prospective evaluation of laparoscopic versus open left lateral hepatic sectionectomy. J Gastrointest Surg. 2008;12:457–62.
6. Abu Hilal M, McPhail M, Zeidan B, Zeidan S, Hallam M, Armstrong T, Primrose J, Pearce N. Laparoscopic versus open left lateral hepatic sectionectomy: a comparative study. Eur J Surg Oncol. 2008;34:1285–8.

7. Lesurtel M, Cherqui D, Laurent A, Tayar C, Fagniez P. Laparoscopic versus open left lateral hepatic lobectomy: a case-control study. J Am Coll Surg. 2003;196:236–42.
8. Wong-Lun-Hing EM, van Dam RM, van Breukelen GJ, Tanis PJ, Ratti F, van Hillegersberg R, Slooter GD, de Wilt JH, Liem MS, de Boer MT, Klaase JM, Neumann UP, Aldrighetti LA, Dejong CH; ORANGE II Collaborative Group. Randomized clinical trial of open versus laparoscopic left lateral hepatic sectionectomy within an enhanced recovery after surgery programme (ORANGE II study). Br J Surg. 2017;104:525–35.

29 Laparoscopic Techniques in Major Liver Resections

Mark Halls, David Martinez-Cecilia, Salvatore Barbaro, and Mohammad Abu Hilal

29.1 Introduction

Major laparoscopic liver resections represent the evolution of minimally invasive liver surgery from the initial non-anatomical wedge resections to left lateral sectionectomies and finally to major anatomical and major complex resections.

Traditionally, major liver resections have been defined as those requiring the resection of three or more contiguous Couinaud's liver segments [4]. However, with the introduction of the laparoscopic approach the concept of major technical resections has emerged. These resections do not have a requirement of size but instead refer to resections in difficult locations such as segment 1, 4a, 7 and 8 [8]. Regardless of the size of the resection and location of the lesion all laparoscopic liver surgery is complex and requires excellent anatomical knowledge and advanced laparoscopic skills. In addition, an experienced and well-coordinated team is essential when considering the important role played by the scrub nurse, theatre assistant and the anaesthetistic team [11].

The most common cause of conversion in laparoscopic surgery is bleeding; careful dissection and advanced skills in bleeding control are of paramount importance when it comes to laparoscopic liver resections [1]. During laparoscopic liver surgery, bleeding control can be achieved by a combination of three factors: inflow control, a low central venous pressure and local control of vessels during parenchymal dissection [14, 5, 1, 10]. Due to the absence of venous valves in the hepatic veins and inferior vena cava the venous pressure of the liver is directly related to the pressure within the right atrium. Therefore, the maintenance of a low central venous pressure is a fundamental requirement to performing a laparoscopic liver resection and this should be regulated by the anaesthetist throughout the operation.

Electronic Supplementary Material The online version of this chapter (doi:10.1007/978-3-319-54301-7_29) contains supplementary material, which is available to authorized users. On http://springerlink.com enter the DOI number given above.

M. Halls • S. Barbaro
M. Abu Hilal, MD, FRCS, FACS, PhD, DocEurp (✉)
Department of Hepatopancreatobiliary Surgery, University of Southampton, Level E, Tremona Road, Southampton, SO16 6YD, UK
e-mail: mark.halls@nhs.net; abuhilal9@gmail.com

D. Martinez-Cecilia (✉)
Servicio Cirugía General, Hospital Virgen de la Salud, Level E, Tremona Road, Toledo, Spain

29.2 General Guidance

Prior to starting any operation the patient's preoperative imaging must be reviewed to ensure a comprehensive knowledge of the patient's liver anatomy, the location of the tumour and its relation with the major vascular structures.

M.A. Cuesta (ed.), *Minimally Invasive Surgery for Upper Abdominal Cancer*,
DOI 10.1007/978-3-319-54301-7_29

Following careful preparation with disinfectant and draping, patients are placed in the supine position with reverse Trendelenburg table tilt. The position of the surgeon and laparoscopic stack are dependent on the resection to be performed. It is not uncommon that the surgeon has to move from the patients left to the patients right and vice versa during the procedure. Access to the abdomen is achieved using an Open Hasson Technique to place a 12 mm port. The pressure of the pneumoperitoneum is maintained between 12 and 14 mmHg whilst the central venous pressure (CVP) is maintained between 0 and 5 cmH_2O (0–4 mmHg). A wide differential between the two should be avoided as it can encourage CO_2 emboli (although the solubility of CO_2 in the blood makes this less concerning than an air emboli) [5]. Following the successful creation of a pneumoperitoneum all further ports are inserted under direct vision.

With the progression of laparoscopic liver surgery an initial concern for complex resections was access. Some centres have reported the use of thoracic trans-diaphragmatic ports and the semi-prone position in order to access the postero-superior segments [9] however in our experience a conventional set-up (as already highlighted) combined with full mobilisation allows for more than adequate access and reduces the complexity of set-up. The first step in any resection is to confirm the location of the lesion(s), which is performed using laparoscopic ultrasound. This permits the surgeon to assess the relation of the lesion(s) to the major vascular structures and to mark the resection lines on the surface of the parenchyma ensuring sufficient free margins will be achieved [3].

The next step is then mobilisation of the liver, freeing it from its ligaments. The round ligament and the falciform ligament are transected with an ultrasonic dissector. These divided structures then become useful as points of traction that can held by one of the assistants in order to manipulate the view and achieve better access. Further mobilisation of the liver is dependent upon the resection to be performed (Fig. 29.1).

29.2.1 Pringle's Manoeuvre

Pringle's manoeuvre is performed by retracting the liver caudally (either by the gallbladder or divided Falciform ligament) to allow access to the Foramen of Winslow. A grasper is passed through the Foramen of Winslow from a 5 mm port in the right upper quadrant (Fig. 29.2).

The left liver lobe is then lifted to permit a clear view of the hepato-gastric ligament (Fig. 29.3). This is opened using diathermy to allow a 5-mm nylon tape to be grasped by the forceps in the Foramen of Winslow and pulled around the portal triad. The nylon tape is then passed through a 10-cm silicon tube with an atraumatic tip so that the tube maybe snugged against the structures whilst the tape encircles them to provide control. The nylon tape is then exteriorised through a port that is then removed and replaced so the tape can be controlled externally without needing to pass through the lumen of a port.

29.2.2 Transection

Superficial parenchymal transection is achieved using a Torsional Ultrasound Device (LOTUS; S.R.A Devon, UK) or a harmonic scalpel (Ethicon ACE, Endo-Surgery; Johnson & Johnson) to dissect 2–3 mm of the superficial parenchyma along the intended resection lines.

For deep dissection, a Cavitron Ultrasonic Surgical Aspirator (CUSA) (Integra Lifesciences, New Jersey, USA) is used to transect the deeper parenchyma and to identify the deep/major vasculature and biliary structures. During parenchymal dissection it is important to avoid tunnelling and the creation of deep holes in which views are compromised and bleeding control is more difficult. Structures encountered during dissection should be carefully secured using laparoscopic clips (Hem-o-Lock clips, Weck Closure Systems, Research Triangle Park, USA) or vascular staplers depending on the size of the structure. Clips and haemolocks should be placed away from the transection line in order to avoid subsequent inclusion into endovascular stapler lines.

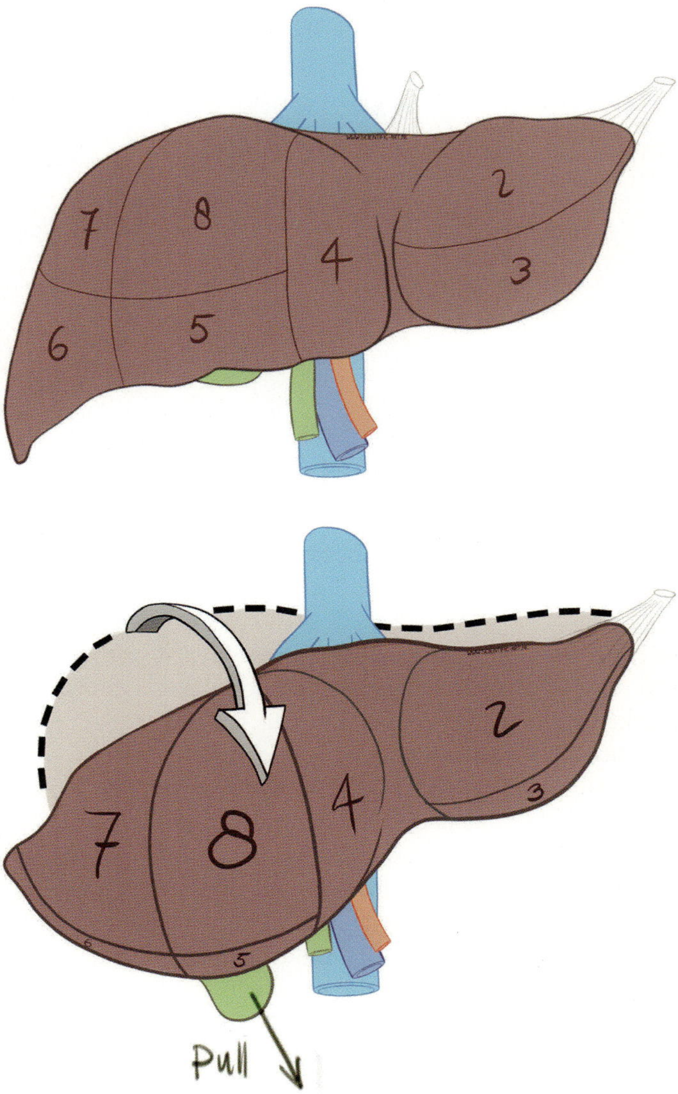

Fig. 29.1 Mobilization of the liver to visualize all hepatic segments

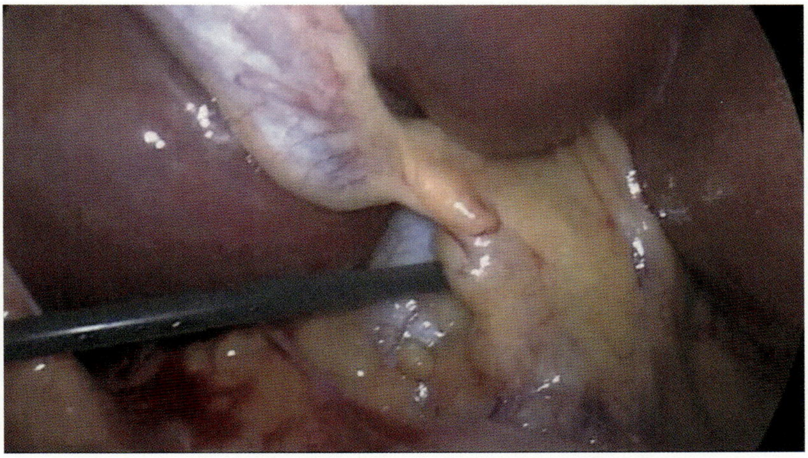

Fig. 29.2 The gallbladder is retracted caudally to allow access to the Foramen of Winslow from a port placed in the right upper quadrant

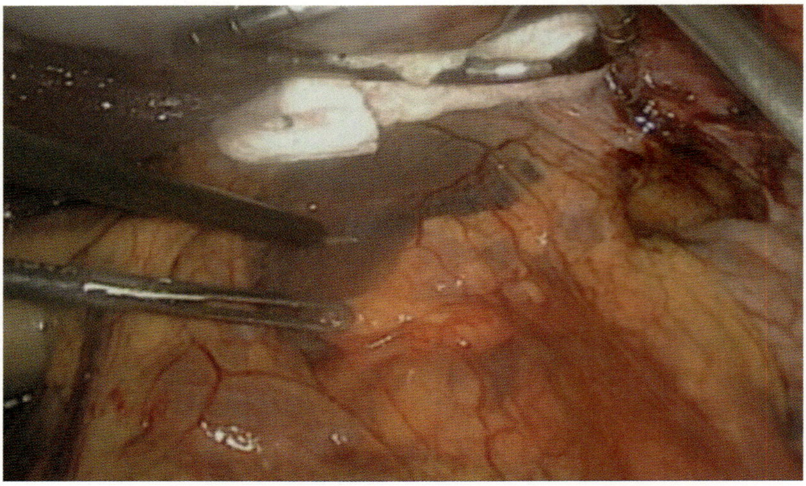

Fig. 29.3 The left lobe of the liver is retracted caudally using either the falciform ligament or a flexible retractor—this then demonstrates the lesser omentum that consists of the hepato-gastric ligament (indicated here with the diathermy hook) and laterally the hepato-duodenal ligament (containing the portal triad)

29.2.3 Revision of Transection Surface

Prior to the completion of the operation and removal of the laparoscopic ports haemostasis is checked with a restored central venous pressure provided by the anaesthetist with fluid replacement, vasopressors and the Valsalva Manoeuvre. The transection line is compressed with a clean gauze swab—this provides a tamponading effect and the presence of bile on the gauze highlights a bile leak. A Bile leak is controlled with Prolene 3-0/4-0 stitches or with clips if a pedicle is identified clearly. Haemostasis is obtained using monopolar diathermy (set to spray) for small bleeding points while clips and Prolene sutures are used for any substantive bleeding. Haemostatic products such as fibrin glue (Evicel; Johnson & Johnson Wound Management) and fibrillar Snow (Johnson & Johnson Wound Management) can be additionally used in areas of difficult access areas or close to hepatic veins. A 20-Fr tube drain is then positioned near each of the resection margins.

29.2.4 Removal of the Specimen

The specimen is removed in an impermeable bag (Endopouch retriever TM, Ethicon, Inc.) Introduced through a 15 mm supra-pubic port that is subsequently extended to a 4–6 cm Pfannenstiel incision. The incision should be as small as possible to minimise trauma, however it is important not to damage the specimen pulling it through a tight incision to permit an accurate histological examination and margin evaluation.

29.3 Left Hemihepatectomy [12]

Patients are positioned in the supine position. The surgeon stands to the patient's left for the hilar dissection and then moves to the patient's right for the parenchymal dissection. Five ports are necessary in this procedure (Fig. 29.4).

Port 1 (5 mm) is placed in the left upper quadrant to aid with the dissection of the left triangular/coronary ligament and allows the assistant to provide suction, manipulation of the liver via the movement of the round ligament.

Ports 2 and 3 (12 mm) accommodate the camera, instruments for dissection and endoscopic staplers. The camera can be switched between these ports in order to adequately expose the resection margin without the dissecting instruments obstructing the surgeon's view. The camera should be aligned parallel with the resection line; this can be facilitated with the use of a 30-degree scope. In patients with tumours less than 10 cm in diameter the ports should be placed in the epigastrium, one-third of the distance from the umbilicus to the costal margin. In patients with large tumours or hepatomegaly, it is necessary to place the ports at the

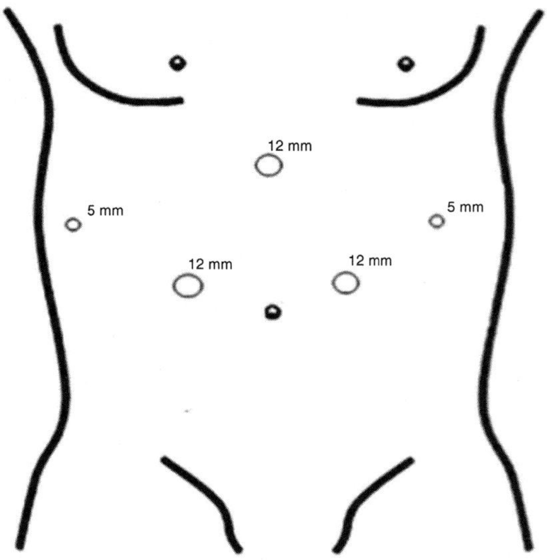

Fig. 29.4 The port placement for left hemihepatectomy

level of the umbilicus to facilitate access for the initial dissection.

Port 4 (5 mm) is for gallbladder retraction and to pass the tape for the Pringle's manoeuvre.

Port 5 (12 mm) is used to elevate the liver by retracting the falciform ligament or with the use of a 12-mm fan retractor. During initial transection an instrument placed through this port can be used to help open the transection line by moving the falciform ligament to the left. In large or obese patients it can also be useful for access of dissecting instruments during hilar dissection and for the last stages of the transection close to the left hepatic vein.

29.3.1 Liver Mobilization

After explorative laparoscopy and intraoperative ultrasonography, mobilisation is performed by dividing the round and falciform ligaments to the level of the hepatico-caval venous confluence, until the antero-lateral surface of the left and middle hepatic veins is identified and dissected free. This sequence of dissection helps to avoid accidental division of the middle hepatic vein in patients with a common hepatic venous confluence.

The triangular ligament is then divided using an ultrasonic dissector in port 1 while port 2 and 3 accommodate the camera and a soft grasper that allow the left lobe of the liver to be lifted and rotate it to the right. The line of dissection is extended medially along the anterior border of the left coronary ligament, keeping the left diaphragmatic vein in sight until the lateral border of the left hepatic vein is identified. The table can be tilted 30° left side up to facilitate this phase of the procedure. The left lobe is then lifted and moved to the right using a 10-mm articulating fan retractor to permit division of the lesser omentum (Fig. 29.3), the operator must be aware of the possibility of a replaced or accessory left hepatic artery originating from the left gastric artery or the celiac trunk, which requires formal control with Hem-o-lock clips before division.

29.3.2 Vascular Control

In this procedure, as for all major anatomic resections, inflow control is achieved by extra parenchymal techniques after a careful dissection of the hilar structures and a clear understanding of the hilar anatomy. In our opinion, the extra parenchymal approach, although technically more challenging, is safer and more efficient in a laparoscopic context. Special attention must be given to the arterial anatomy and the position of any aberrant or replaced vessels. Preoperative magnetic resonance cholangiopancreatography is routinely performed to exclude an aberrant insertion of the right-sided ducts into the left hepatic system, as these biliary anomalies are difficult to identify if encountered intraoperatively. The vascular control is of paramount importance and is technically demanding so good access is essential. Access to the portal structures can be obtained by elevating the liver using the gallbladder as a retractor via port 1 or 4 (Fig. 29.5), the falciform ligament through port 1 or by using a 10-mm articulating fan retractor through port 5 to lift the left lobe of the liver and expose the hilar structures.

The dissection starts with a superficial transverse incision of the hepato-duodenal ligament from left to right 1–2 cm below the hilar plate (Arantius' ligament). The neurolymphatic tissue is dissected carefully and divided with a diathermy hook and ultrasonic dissector, ensuring good haemostasis and avoiding damage to any hilar structures. The left hepatic artery is identified, slung and dissected using a diathermy hook, a non-traumatic grasper and a 10-mm right angle Gemini dissecting forceps (Elmed) (Fig. 29.6). The sling allows for gentle handling of the vessel to avoid causing damage to the arterial wall and also provides a means for rapid control should there be sudden, unexpected bleeding. A bulldog clip can be placed on the artery to produce temporary exclusion when an assessment of the anatomy and ischemic line is needed (Fig. 29.7).

Once the arterial anatomy is clear, the left hepatic artery is gently retracted laterally to allow for its ligation with three self-locking polymer Hem-o-lock clips (Fig. 29.8). Finally, the artery is divided leaving a minimum of 3-mm cuff beyond the clips. Division of the artery opens the plane, which allows for direct vision of the left hepatic duct and portal vein.

It is often easier to identify and divide the left portal vein before dissecting out the left hepatic duct, because the left portal vein is usually longer and more malleable than the adjacent left hepatic duct (Fig. 29.9). This then permits improved views of the left hepatic duct, which can then be dissected out in the

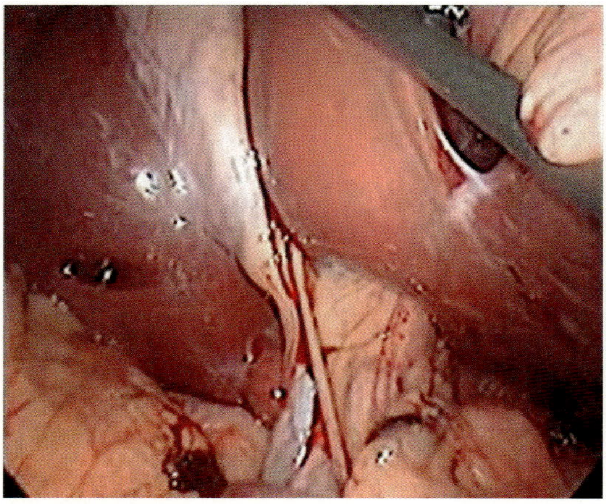

Fig. 29.5 The view obtained following mobilisation of the liver and its subsequent elevation using the gallbladder (retraction from non-traumatic grasper in port 1)

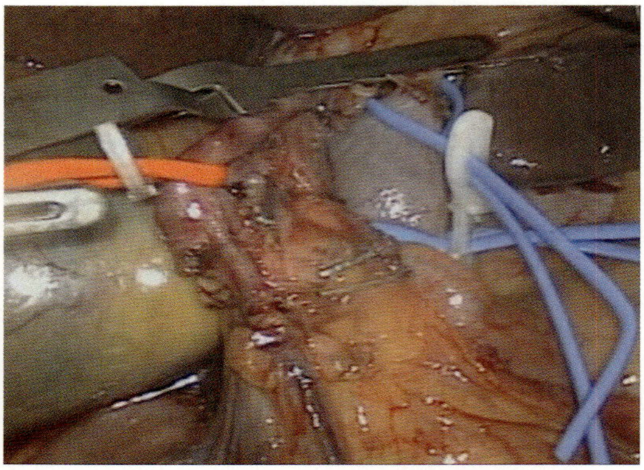

Fig. 29.7 The left hepatic artery is slung (*red sloop*) and the portal vein and left branch are slung (*blue sloop*). This allows for atraumatic manipulation of the vessels. A bulldog may be used to temporarily exclude flow to demonstrate the vascular anatomy prior to its ligation

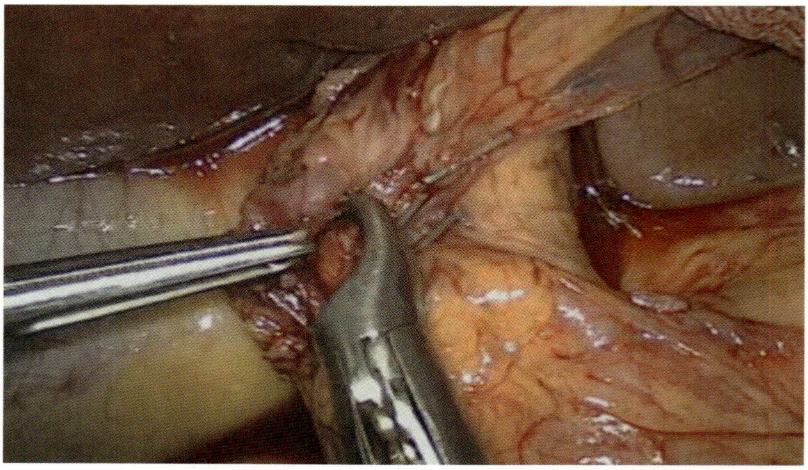

Fig. 29.6 Dissection if the hepato-duodenal ligament using atraumatic grasper and Gemini dissecting forceps

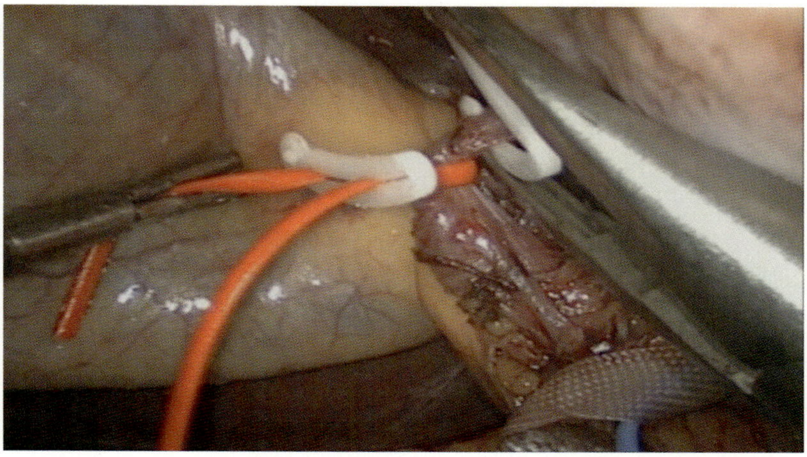

Fig. 29.8 Application of polymer clips to left hepatic artery

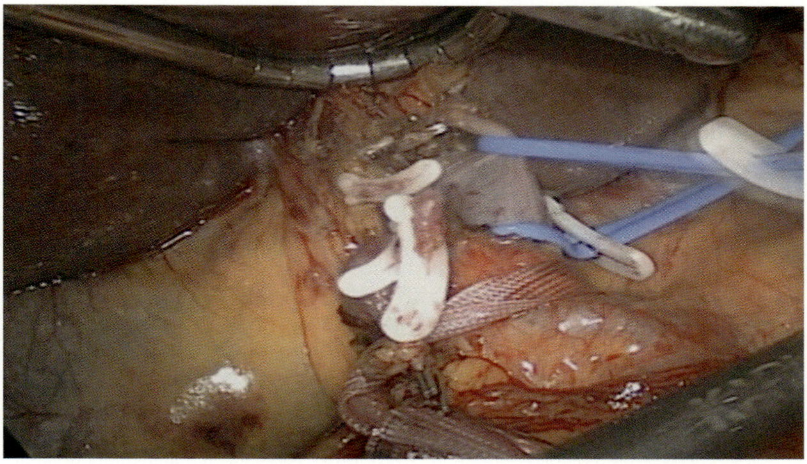

Fig. 29.9 The left hepatic artery has been divided and traction is applied to the sloop on the left portal vein. The lower sloop was placed on the main portal vein earlier in the procedure and remains in place until the anatomy is clarified

liver parenchyma away from the confluence or can be controlled intra-parenchymally if the lesion is not very near to the biliary bifurcation. The extra parenchymal ductal control is only performed for lesions very near to the bifurcation to ensure wider clear resection margins.

After clear identification of the anatomy, the left portal vein is dissected, slung and divided after the origin of the small caudate branches are identified. Small caudate branches can be spared or ligated with metal clips if needed.

The vein can be divided between Hem-o-Lock clips or with an endovascular stapler (Endoscopic Articulating Linear Cutter ETS 45 mm, Ethicon Endo-Surgery).

29.3.3 Intraoperative Ultrasonography

A second ultrasonographic scan is performed to confirm and mark the line of transection (Fig. 29.10). The transection line is marked with a diathermy hook 5 mm to the right of the line of demarcation, while taking care to ensure adequate clearance of all tumour deposits. This marked line is seen on ultrasound as a hyper-echoic line casting an acoustic shadow into the liver parenchyma in between the lesions and the demarcation line.

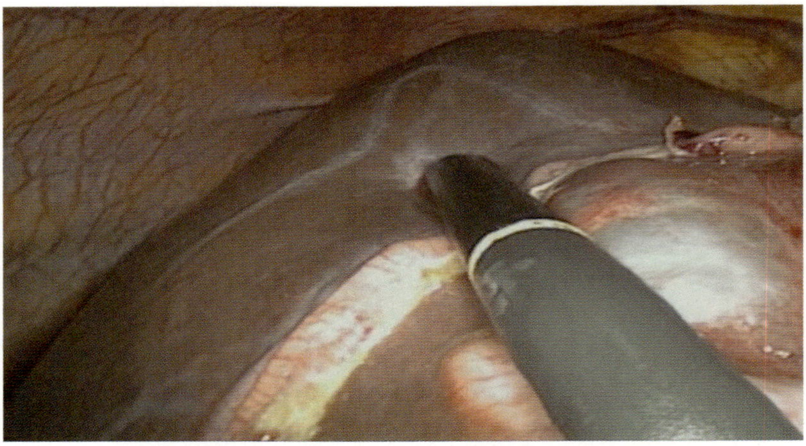

Fig. 29.10 Intra-operative endoscopic ultrasound to confirm the site of the lesion and planning of resection border

29.3.4 Parenchymal Dissection

Good views are an essential part of this procedure and are achieved by keeping both camera and operating instruments in the line of the transection. This requires use of a 30-degree scope and careful port positioning to ensure that ports 2 and 3 are low enough to offer a good view and access to the initial transection line, but high enough to allow access to the superior parts of the liver later in the procedure. The course of the middle hepatic vein is identified on intraoperative ultrasound and its relation to any tumour deposits is noted. The line of transection is then marked using the diathermy staying 5–10 mm to the left of the middle hepatic vein but providing adequate clear margins in malignant disease (Fig. 29.11).

When resection of the caudate lobe is also required, this is carried out alongside the dissection of the left liver. After lifting the left lobe and pushing it to the right with the aid of a 10-mm articulating fan retractor, the inferior part of the caudate lobe is dissected away from the vena cava using the harmonic scalpel and metallic clips for vascular branches as encountered. Next the left lobe of the liver is resected giving better exposure of the middle and posterior parts of the caudate lobe. This dissection is continued until large middle hepatic vein branches are encountered. In this stage, a two-handed technique can be adopted, using the CUSA in conjunction with the ultrasonic dissector to skeletalise vascular structures, allowing correct identification and control before division (Fig. 29.12).

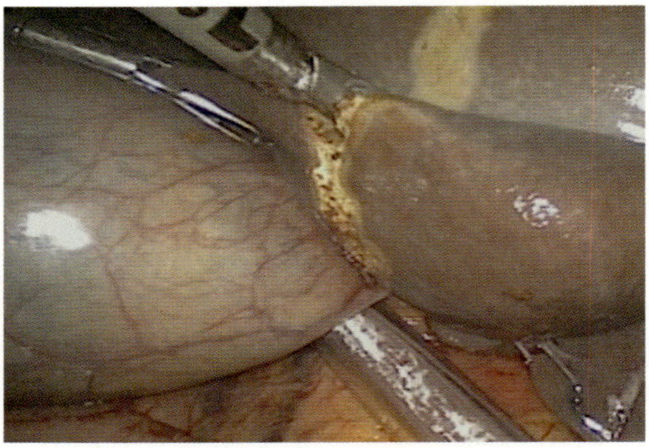

Fig. 29.11 Following USS guided marking of the surface of the liver superficial parenchymal dissection is performed using an ultrasonic dissector

A 60-mm Endoscopic Linear Cutter (Echelon flex, Ethicon Endo-Surgery) is used to transect the left hepatic duct and Glissonian sheath. When the left hepatic vein confluence is revealed the parenchyma is dissected to reveal the superior and medial surfaces over a 10-mm length of vein. The transection is then completed using a single firing of an endovascular stapler to divide the vein (Fig. 29.13) and any remaining adjacent parenchyma, taking care to avoid traction injury to the middle hepatic vein and the cava. Haemostatic products are used if bleeding is encountered especially in proximity to the middle hepatic vein.

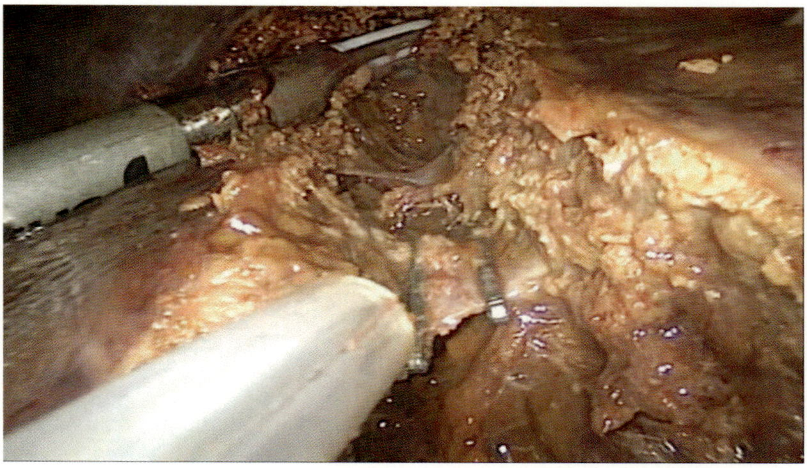

Fig. 29.12 Two-handed technique using an ultrasonic dissector and CUSA to dissect out vascular and biliary structures that are controlled prior to divided (control technique is dependent on size)

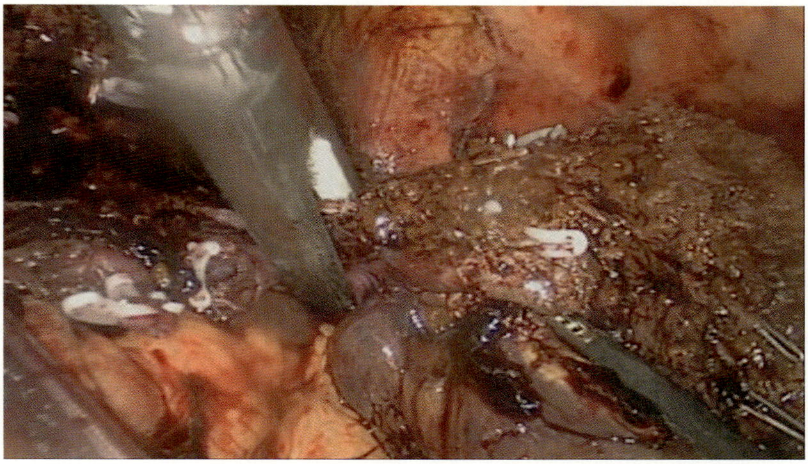

Fig. 29.13 Transection of the left hepatic vein using an endoscopic linear cutter

29.4 Right Hemihepatectomy [13]

The patient is placed in the supine position. The surgeon either stands between the patient's legs for the whole procedure or stands to the patient's right for the hilar dissection and then moves to the patient's left for the parenchymal dissection.

Five ports are necessary in this procedure (Fig. 29.14):

Port 1 (12 mm) is used for the dissection of the hepatic artery and portal vein, for division of the coronary ligament, for retraction of the falciform ligament and for elevation of the posterior surface of the right hemi-liver during dissection of the right triangular ligament.

Ports 2 and 3 (12 mm) accommodate the camera, instruments for dissection and endoscopic staplers. The camera can be switched between

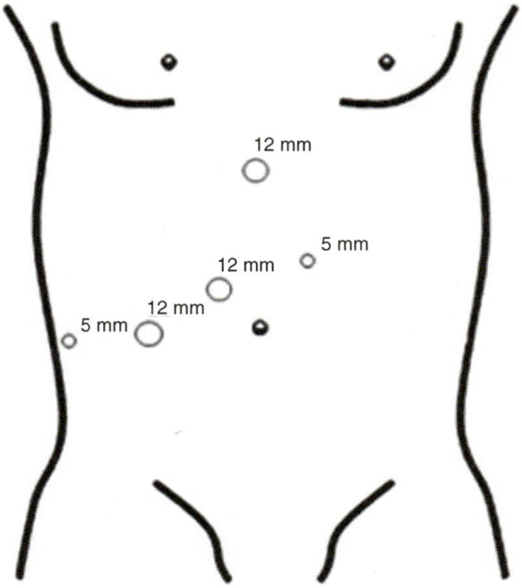

Fig. 29.14 The port placement for right hemihepatectomy

these ports in order to adequately expose the resection margin without the dissecting instruments obstructing the surgeon's view, thus it should be aligned parallel with the resection line; this can be facilitated with the use of a 30-degree scope.

Ports 4 and 5 (5 mm) are used for gallbladder retraction, dissection of the triangular ligament and serve to aid the assistant with suction, liver retraction, and elevation. To perform Pringle's manoeuvre the tape is held on an atraumatic grasper introduced through the right lateral port, passed in between the vena cava (posteriorly) and the portal vein (anteriorly) and then picked up and externalised with another grasper introduced through the left lateral port. Poor positioning of the ports will create angulations, which increase operative difficulty and risk for complications.

29.4.1 Liver Mobilization

After exploratory laparoscopy and intraoperative ultrasonography, the liver is mobilised by dividing the round and falciform ligaments up to the level of the hepatico-caval venous confluence. This is continued until the anterior surface of the right hepatic vein is identified and dissected free. This line of dissection is extended laterally along the anterior border of the right coronary ligament, as far as access permits (Fig. 29.15). The table is then tilted 30° right side up, and the surgeon moves to the left side of the patient. The liver is then lifted using a 10-mm articulating fan retractor to permit dissection of the relatively avascular planes in the retrocaval hepatic space. This is achieved using a combination of blunt dissection, ultrasonic dissectors and diathermy scissors down to the triangular ligament. Next, the hepatico-caval plane is gently dissected using a combination of scissors; hook diathermy, and blunt dissection. The short retro-hepatic veins draining directly into the inferior vena cava are skeletonized, clipped, and divided, leaving an adequate stump and two clips on the stay side. The dissection is continued superiorly as far as access permits to expose the right hepatic vein to facilitate the formal hepatectomy. The table is then levelled out for the hilar dissection. The medial aspect of the gallbladder is dissected from the liver bed and the cystic artery is divided. This allows elevation of the right liver and exposure of the portal triad for vascular dissection. The cystic duct is left in continuity at this stage, so the common hepatic duct can be lifted anteriorly by traction on the cystic duct. This opens up the posterior plane and gives access to the right hepatic artery. Counter traction can be provided by drawing down on the Pringle sling, putting tension on the hepato-duodenal ligament without constricting the vascular inflow to the liver.

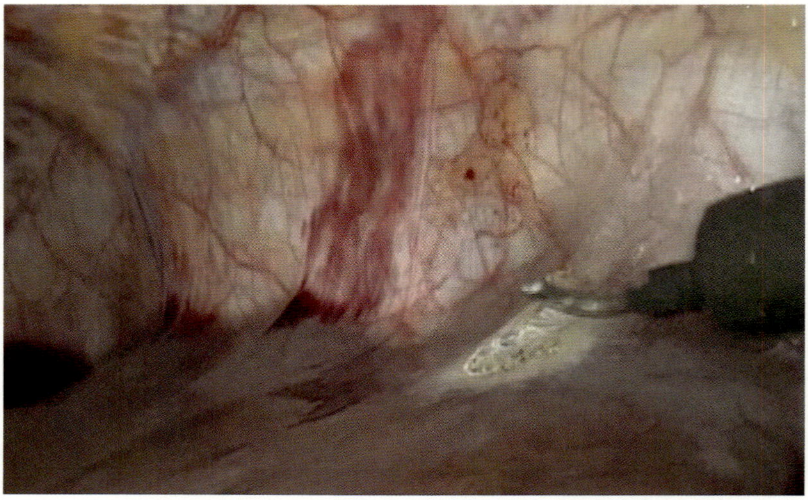

Fig. 29.15 Dissection of the postero-superior attachments of the liver from the diaphragm

29.4.2 Vascular Control

In this procedure, flow control is routinely achieved by extra-parenchymal means, which offers safe and haemostatic dissection of the parenchyma. Access to the portal structures can be obtained by lifting the liver via the gallbladder on one side and the falciform ligament on the other and then by gently retracting the cystic duct. Special attention must be paid to patient's arterial anatomy and the position of any aberrant or replaced vessels (Fig. 29.16).

The right hepatic artery is identified and dissected first, using a diathermy hook, a non-traumatic grasper and a laparoscopic 10-mm right-angle Gemini dissecting forceps (Fig. 29.17).

The right hepatic artery is then slung and gently retracted laterally to aid its ligation with three self-locking polymer Hem-o-lok clips. Finally, the artery is divided, leaving two clips on the proximal side and a minimum of 3 mm cuff beyond the clips. The division of the artery opens the plane, which enables the dissection of the right portal vein at the level of the bifurcation of the portal vein. After clear identification of the anatomy, the right portal vein is dissected out, and the caudate branches are identified and where necessary clipped or ligated and divided. The right portal vein is then controlled and divided in a similar fashion between Hem-o-lok clips (Fig. 29.18). The right hepatic duct is divided intra-hepatically during the parenchymal transection.

A second ultrasound scan is performed to confirm and mark the line of transection. The resection line is marked with a diathermy hook 5 mm to the right of the line of demarcation, while care is taken to ensure adequate clearance of all tumour deposits. This marked line is seen on ultrasound as a hyper-echoic line casting an acoustic shadow into the liver parenchyma in between the lesions and the demarcation line.

The parenchyma is dissected using a torsional ultrasonic device (LOTUS; S.R.A Devon, UK) or a harmonic scalpel (Ethicon ACE, Endo-Surgery; Johnson & Johnson) starting on the upper liver surface from front to the back, taking layers of 2–3 mm deep each time up to the level of the right hepatic vein. The dissection is continued in this way until large middle hepatic vein branches are encountered (Fig. 29.19).

At this stage, a two-handed technique is adopted using the CUSA in conjunction with the

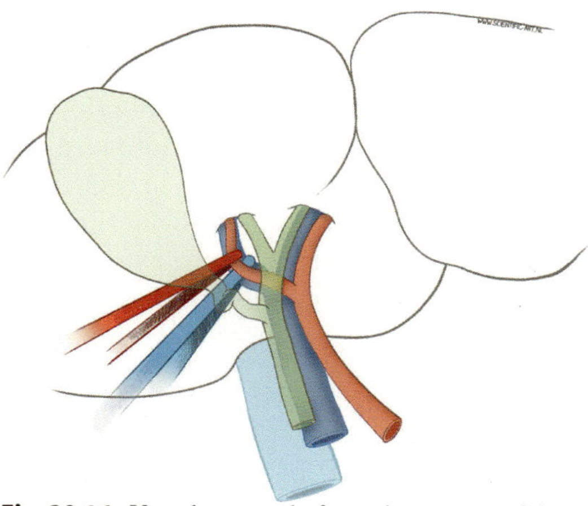

Fig. 29.16 Vascular control of portal structures of the right hepatic lobe

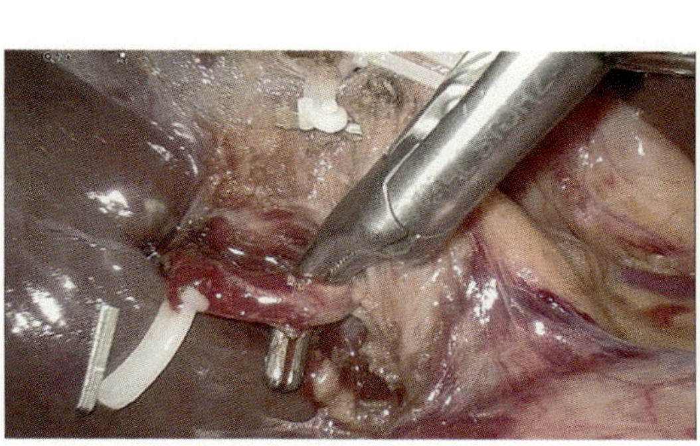

Fig. 29.17 Dissection of the hepato-duodenal ligament with Gemini forceps to isolate the right hepatic artery

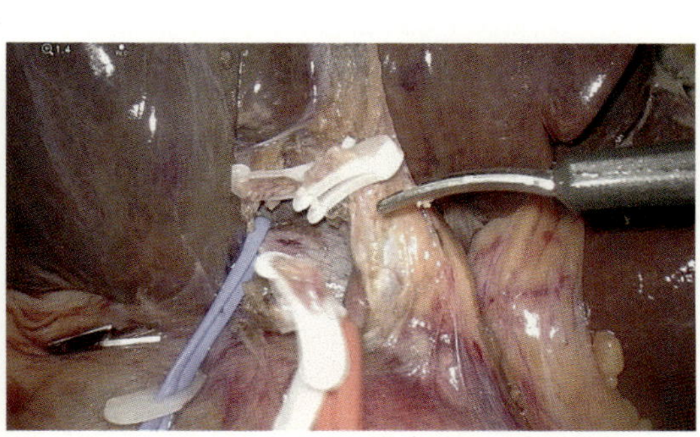

Fig. 29.18 The right hepatic artery has been divided and the right portal vein is slung in preparation for application of hem-o-lok clips

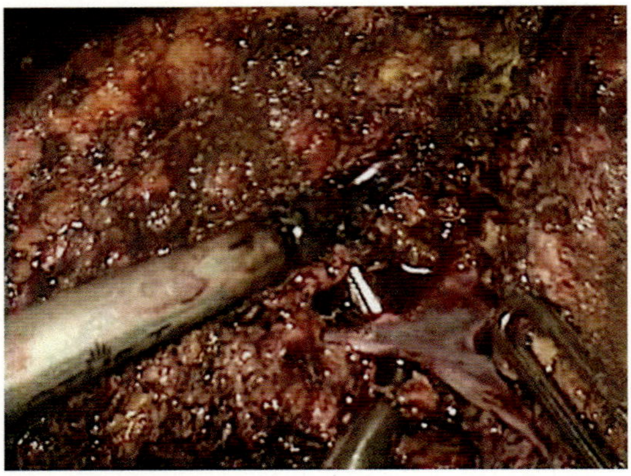

Fig. 29.19 The middle hepatic vein branches

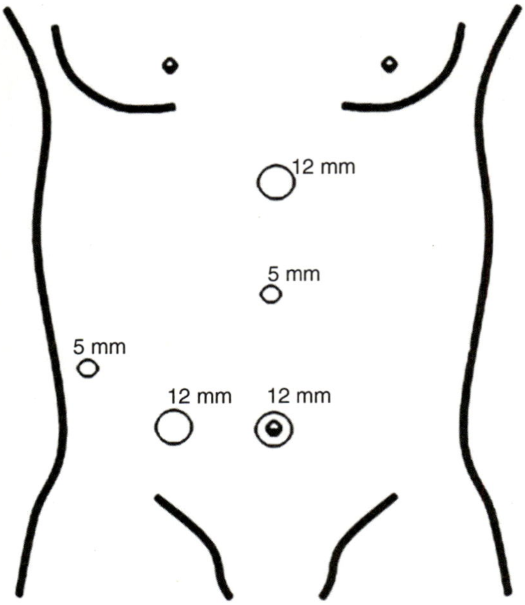

Fig. 29.20 Port placement for resection of lesions in segments 7 and 8

Lotus or Harmonic ACE to skeletonize vascular structures, allowing correct identification and control before dividing them. A 60-mm endoscopic linear cutter is used for division of the middle hepatic vein branches and broader and thicker pedicles of tissue (right hepatic duct and Glissonian sheath). After intrahepatic division of the right hepatic duct, the transection is continued posteriorly to the inferior vena cava. The right hepatic vein is identified at the superior margin of the transection, dissected out and divided either flush on the cava or intrahepatically with an endovascular stapler. The site of division is determined by the requirements of oncologic clearance and the degree of technical difficulty in approaching the vena cava.

29.5 Laparoscopic Parenchymal-Sparing Resections Lesion in the Posterior Segments (The Diamond Technique) [6, 7]

Laparoscopic resection of non-peripheral lesions and lesions in segments 7, 8 and 4a share some of the technical difficulties associated with a hemi-hepatectomy, specifically during the mobilization phase. Careful division of the triangular and the anterior and posterior right coronary ligaments to the level of the right hepatic vein insertion is usually required. This enables the surgeon to apply traction to the liver moving it down and rotating it to the left, offering better access to the posterior segments. This manoeuvre requires advanced laparoscopic skills and the ability to work in a small, deep, "distant" operative field. However, these operations do not require extra-hepatic hilar dissection or large parenchymal resection as in a formal hemi-hepatectomy. Therefore, these resections should be considered as a separate classification from minor resections and anatomically major resections—Technically major resections [8].

Initially, the right upper quadrant and epigastric ports are placed then laparoscopy is performed and the liver is inspected ultrasonographically, looking for unknown lesions and confirming the exact tumour size and location. This evaluation also helps to ensure correct placement of the remaining ports. A 4/5-port configuration in a reverse L-shape around the medial and inferior aspects of the tumour is recommended (Fig. 29.20).

This port placement is intended to facilitate four transection planes with good triangulation by running in parallel with the ports (Fig. 29.21).

The round and falciform ligaments must be divided unless the lesion is a diagnosed or suspected HCC. Unlike resections in segment 7 resections those undertaken for lesions in in segment 8 does not usually require mobilization of right liver as the anticlockwise rotation and caudal traction down of the liver is not usually required.

After insertion of all ports, ultrasonography is again performed for localisation of the lesion and its relationship with the major vessels and biliary drainage as well as assessing resection margins. In case of HCC, any satellite nodule must be comprehensively excluded. The resection margin is marked under direct ultrasonography view 2–3 cm away from the lesion.

Straight transection lines in a square shape are easier to follow, especially during dissection. The liver capsule is scored using the hook diathermy and these resection lines are seen ultrasonically as acoustic shadows allowing evaluation of the intended resection lines throughout their length (Fig. 29.22).

As previously, parenchymal transection is started with an ultrasonic dissector. Two or three

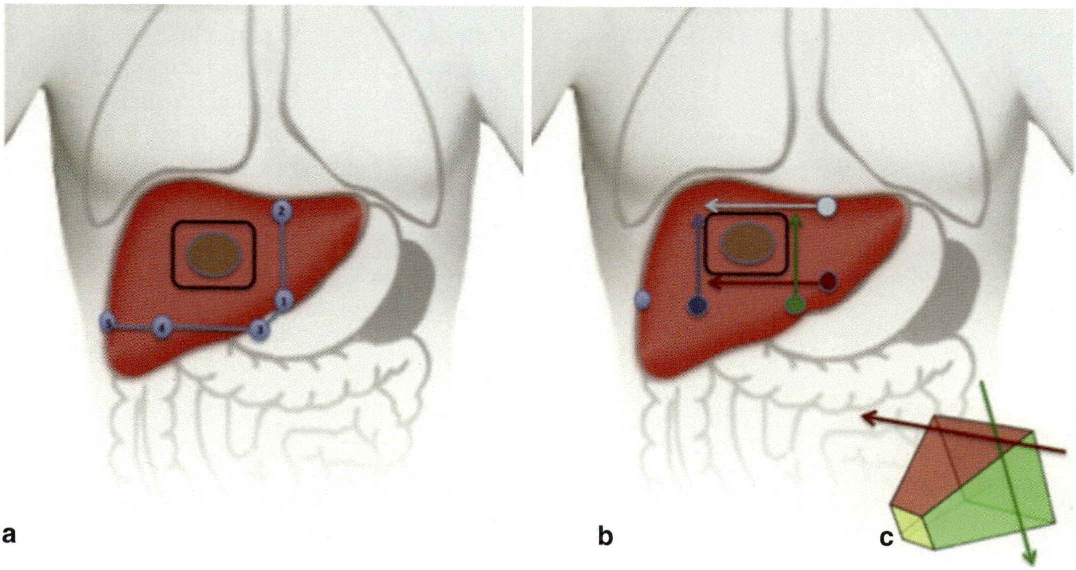

Fig. 29.21 (**a**) Indication of the port placement for "Diamond Technique" of lesions in segment 8. (**b**) Ports required to make each resection line to produce diamond. (**c**) The intended shape of resected tissue

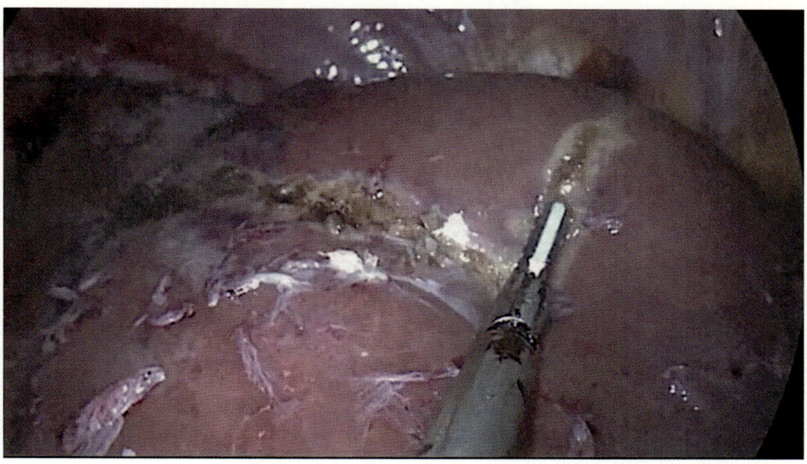

Fig. 29.22 Straight resection borders are marked on the surface of the liver and then superficial parenchyma resection occurs with an ultrasonic dissector

stitches may be placed at the edges of the specimen (away from the tumour) in order that the specimen can be manipulated in a non-touch technique to open the resection line and facilitate dissection (Fig. 29.23a, b). Care must be taken to avoid contacting the tumour in while positioning those stitches. The CUSA is the used to identify and dissect out the deep and major vascular and biliary structures. Millimetric readjustments of the dissection line can be performed on the basis of the ultrasonic findings.

Care must be taken to not progressively bear toward the centre of the specimen (a well-known risk in open surgery). In laparoscopy, this is magnified by the absence of tactile feedback. Although we conventionally call this the "diamond technique," due to the similarity of the final specimen to a diamond shape, we emphasize the need for continuous assessment and adjustment of the transection line aiming toward a semi-diamond "frustum-shaped" specimen, rather than a complete diamond or a cone (Figs. 29.21c and 29.24). This is essential for achieving adequate tumour-free margins on both the lateral and basal transection planes. Repeated ultrasound and CUSA dissection facilitate the development of millimetric readjustments of the dissection line. Although the lateral margins can be easily assessed, evaluation of the basal margin can be challenging. For this, ultrasonic measurement of the tumour location from the surface can estimate the depth of dissection needed, and the specimen can be scanned from the lateral side of the specimen. When the lower plane is reached, the tip of the laparoscopic grasper that has been placed below the specimen can be detected on ultrasound, permitting the evaluation of its relation with the inferior part of the tumour. Intermittent inflow control

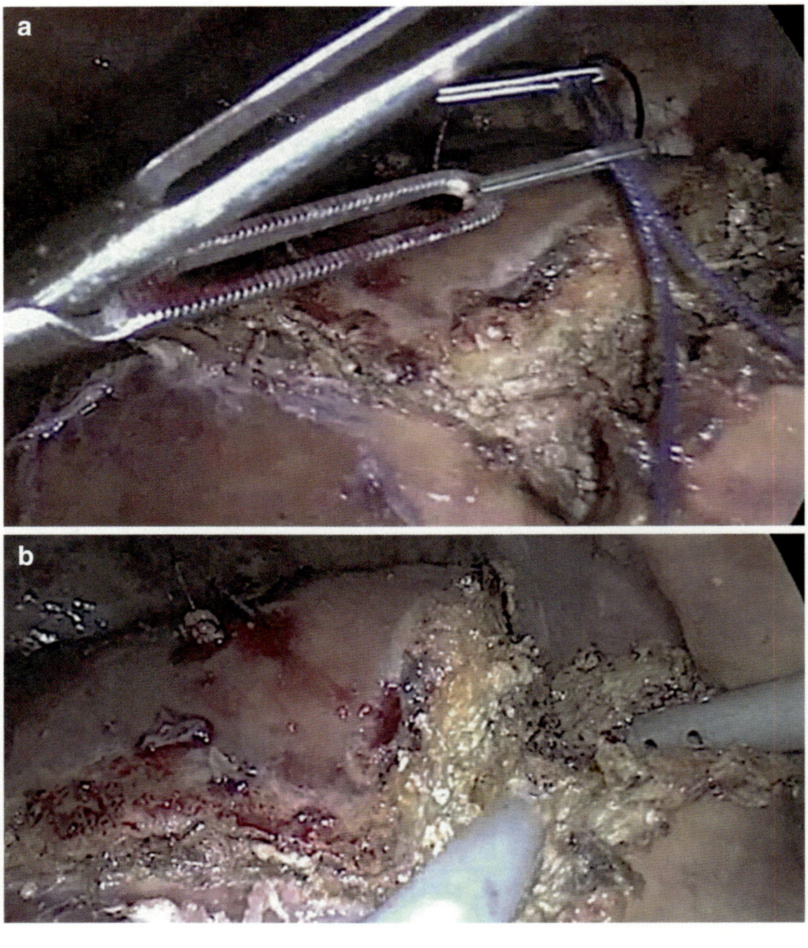

Fig. 29.23 (**a**, **b**) A stitch has been placed superficially in the specimen to allow for a "non-touch technique" and to provide retraction to open the resection plane

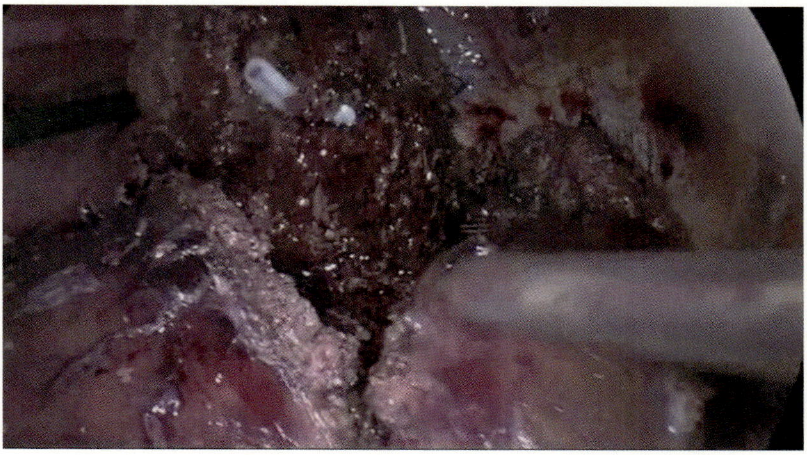

Fig. 29.24 Demonstration of the frustum-shaped specimen with straight resection lines

is performed during the dissection phase in the majority of cases, as described elsewhere.

In case of small specimens these can be removed from a slightly enlarged port site while a Pfannenstiel incision can be used for larger specimens. After closing this incision, and prior to completing the operation, haemostasis is again assessed under restored central venous pressure and Valsalva manoeuvre.

References

1. Abu Hila M, Unerwood T, Taylor MG, Hamdan K, Elberm H, Pearce NW. Bleeding and haemostasis in laparoscopic liver surgery. Surg Endosc. 2009; 24(3):572–7.
2. Abu Hilal M, van der Poel M, Samim M, Besselink MG, Flowers D, Stedman B, Pearce NW. Laparoscopic liver resection for lesions adjacent to major vasculature: feasibility, safety and oncological efficiency. J Gastrointest Surg. 2015;19(4):692–8.
3. Araki K, Conrad C, Ogiso S, Kuwano H, Gayet B. Intraoperative ultrasonography of laparoscopic hepatectomy: key technique for safe liver transection. J Am Coll Surg. 2014;218:e37–41.
4. Buell JF, Cherqui D, Geller DA, et al. The international position on laparoscopic liver surgery: The Louisville Statement, 2008. Ann Surg. 2009;250(5): 825–30.
5. Chouillard EK, Gumbs AA, Cherqui D. Vascular clamping in liver surgery: physiology, indications and techniques. Ann Surg Innov Res. 2010;4:2.
6. Cipriani F, Shelat VG, Rawashdeh M, Francone E, Aldrighetti L, Takhar A, Armstrong T, Pearce NW, Abu HM. Laparoscopic parenchymal-sparing resections for nonperipheral liver lesions, the diamond technique: technical aspects, clinical outcomes, and oncologic efficiency. J Am Coll Surg. 2015;221(2): 265–72.
7. Coles SR, Besselink MG, Serin KR, Alsaati H, Di Gioia P, Samim M, Pearce NW, Abu HM. Total laparoscopic management of lesions involving liver segment 7. Surg Endosc. 2015;29(11):3190–5.
8. Di Fabio F, Samim M, Di Gioia P, Godeseth R, Pearce NW, Abu HM. Laparoscopic major hepatectomies: clinical outcomes and classification. World J Surg. 2014;38:3169–74.
9. Ikeda T, Toshima T, Harimoto N, Yamashita Y, Ikegami T, Yoshizumi T, Soejima Y, Shirabe K, Maehara Y. Laparoscopic liver resection in the semiprone position for tumours in the anterosuperior and posterior segments, using a novel dual-handling technique and bipolar irrigation. Surg Endosc. 2014;28: 2484–92.
10. Jones M. and Hardy. Central venous pressure and its effect on blood loss during liver resection. Br J Surg. 1998;85(8):1058–60.
11. Kluger MD, Vigano L, Barroso R, Cherqui D. The learning curve in laparoscopic major liver resection. J Hepatobiliary Pancreat Sci. 2013;20(2):131–6.
12. Pearce NW, Di Fabio F, Teng MJ, Syed S, Primrose JN, Abu HM. Laparoscopic right hepatectomy: a challenging, but feasible, safe and efficient procedure. Am J Surg. 2011a;202:e52–8.
13. Pearce NW, Di Fabio F, Abu HM. Laparoscopic left hepatectomy with extraparenchymal inflow control. J Am Coll Surg. 2011b;213:e23–7.
14. Tranchart H, O'Rourke N, Van Dam R, Gaillard M, Lainas P, Sugioka A, Wakabayashi G, Dagher I. Bleeding control during laparoscopic liver resection: a review of literature. J Hepatobiliary Pancreat Sci. 2015;22(5):371–8.

Laparoscopic Liver Resection in Cirrhotic Patients

30

Tan To Cheung

30.1 Introduction

Laparoscopic liver resection has been considered an advanced operation in the field of hepatobiliary and pancreatic surgery. There are a lot of doubts and skepticism because even open liver resection alone is still considered a complex operation which requires a long period of training before a surgeon can master the skill [1–3].

Laparoscopic liver resection is becoming a standard practice as more and more centers are picking up this skill. Many reports have shown that it can be carried out with very low mortality and morbidity even in patients with liver cirrhosis [4–9]. After two very large-scale consensus meetings on laparoscopic liver resection, many doubts have been removed [2]. Laparoscopic liver resection remains a complex operation but, as long as the surgeons understand their own limits and carry out the procedure cautiously, the morbidity can be very low.

30.2 Problems of Liver Resection in Patients with Liver Cirrhosis

Liver cirrhosis and hepatocellular carcinoma usually present together. The presence of cirrhosis makes liver resection more difficult. Hepatocellular carcinoma has a highest incidence in Asia because many Asians have hepatitis B, and hepatitis-B-related hepatocellular carcinoma is usually associated with liver cirrhosis. Hepatectomy is more difficult in the presence of portal hypertension, splenomegaly, gastric or esophageal varices, or thrombocytopenia. Therefore, patients with liver cirrhosis have higher mortality and morbidity rates after hepatectomy. To overcome the difficulties, close cooperation with the anesthesiologist is very important. In the perioperative period, a very tight intravenous fluid administration is followed. During operation, a central venous line is inserted to monitor the central venous pressure, which should be maintained at 0–5 cmH2O. A head-up position, low tidal volume and low positive end-expiratory pressure can reduce the central venous pressure. Vasodilators and diuretics can be administrated during hepatic transection. All these are useful methods to reduce blood loss during liver transection [10].

Electronic Supplementary Material The online version of this chapter (doi:10.1007/978-3-319-54301-7_30) contains supplementary material, which is available to authorized users. On http://springerlink.com enter the DOI number given above.

T.T. Cheung
Hepatobiliary and Pancreatic Surgery, Department of Surgery, Queen Mary Hospital, The University of Hong Kong, 102 Pok Fu Lam Road, Hong Kong SAR, China
e-mail: tantocheung@hotmail.com

M.A. Cuesta (ed.), *Minimally Invasive Surgery for Upper Abdominal Cancer*,
DOI 10.1007/978-3-319-54301-7_30

Table 30.1 Selection criteria for laparoscopic liver resection for patients with hepatocellular carcinoma and cirrhosis

Inclusion	Exclusion
Can tolerate general anesthesia	Decompensated Child B or C liver cirrhosis
Child A liver cirrhosis	Diffuse hepatocellular carcinoma
For minor hepatectomy, platelet count $>40 \times 10^9$/L	Tumor invasion of the portal vein, hepatic vein or bile duct
For major hepatectomy, platelet count $>80 \times 10^9$/L	Vessel reconstruction would be required
Tumor smaller than 10 cm	Extrahepatic metastasis
Laparoscopic liver resection will be technically feasible	

30.3 Selection Criteria

Meticulous patient selection is important in preventing unexpected complications and outcomes. Special attention is needed if liver cirrhosis is present. Table 30.1 shows the selection criteria for laparoscopic liver resection for patients with hepatocellular carcinoma and cirrhosis.

It is always a good practice to start a new approach with easier procedures. Tumors located in the anterolateral position are easier lesions to start with. In general, minor liver resection, tumors smaller than 3 cm and tumors away from major vascular structures are good cases to start [11–16].

Laparoscopic left lateral sectionectomy is a good case to commence. The anatomy of laparoscopic left lateral sectionectomy is constant. There is only one hilar pedicle to control and only one left hepatic vein to divide [17].

30.4 Operation Equipment and Setup

The instruments used for laparoscopic liver resection are similar to other laparoscopic procedures. An additional endo-retractor or golden finger is required for hilum control. A laparoscopic ultrasonic dissector is another additional instrument that is required for liver parenchymal transection. A list of instruments required is shown in Table 30.2.

In the operation, the patient is usually placed in the French position. The surgeon stands between the legs of the patients. The display unit is positioned on the head side of the patient. The assistant sits next to the patient. A telescope is introduced after direct cut-down of the sub-umbilical port. Depending of the indication for the operation, usually 3–5 working ports are needed for laparoscopic hepatectomy. Fewer ports are required for minor hepatectomy. For major hepatectomy, usually four working ports are required. Figure 30.1 shows the placement of ports for laparoscopic major hepatectomy. Ultrasound examination is performed to confirm the location and size of the tumor and to check for additional lesions. An ultrasonic dissector is used for superficial liver parenchymal transection and a CUSA® is used for deep liver parenchymal transection. In major hepatectomy, the dissection method is the same as that used in the open approach. The intra-Glissonian approach is used for individual isolation of the liver inflow. The hepatic artery is doubly controlled by metal clips and the main branch of the portal vein is doubly controlled by a hemolock. The main bile duct is controlled by a stapler or a

Table 30.2 List of instruments required

Instrument	Quantity
30-degree Laparoscope	1
10-mm Telescope port	1
12-mm Working port	2–3
5-mm Working port	2–3
Laparoscopic ultrasound	1
Laparoscopic CUSA®	1
Energy source dissector (Olympus)/Sono Surg™ (Olympus)/Harmonic® scalpel (Ethicon)/Sonocision™ (Medtronic)	1
Stapling device with cartridge of 2.5–3 mm	1–2
Multi-firing metal clip	2–3
Hemolock	1–3
Laparoscopic argon bean coagulator	1
12-cm Endo Catch™	1
Laparoscopic bulldog clamp	1–2

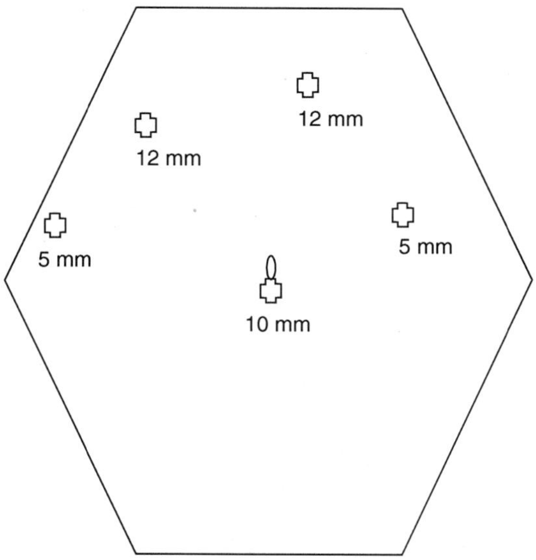

Fig. 30.1 Port placement for laparoscopic major right hepatectomy

hemolock. The major hepatic vein is controlled by an endovascular stapler. Hemostasis is performed with metal clips, diathermy and sutures as would be in the open approach. The liver specimen is delivered through a Pfannenstiel incision not larger than the largest diameter of the specimen [11–16]. Drainage tube is not routinely placed. Video 30.1 demonstrates a laparoscopic right hepatectomy in a patient with liver cirrhosis.

30.5 Setting Up of Pneumoperitoneal Pressure

Pneumoperitoneal pressure is the key to success in laparoscopic liver resection. In liver resection, bleeding occurs in vessels of the liver but not the liver parenchyma itself. The inflow of the liver is usually controlled when we are contemplating liver anatomical liver resection. Most of the bleeding actually comes from the hepatic vein and its tributaries. The hepatic venous pressure can be directly reflected by the central venous pressure which is kept at <5 cmH2O during the operation. The normal pressure set at 12 mmHg should be able to give a negative gradient to stop significant bleeding from the hepatic vein even when there is a small inadvertent venotomy. In case of a poorly controlled central venous pressure due to underlying cardiac conditions, we can temporarily increase the abdominal pressure up to 18 mmHg without serious consequences. The high solubility of carbon dioxide used for pneumoperitoneum will not cause any air-embolism effect during the operation. Subclinical CO2 embolism is possible but it seldom leads to hemodynamic disturbance [18–23].

30.6 Special Considerations in Laparoscopic Major Hepatectomy

30.6.1 Pringle Maneuver

In open liver resection, intermitted inflow control of the liver hilum is an important mean to reduce bleeding. This is particularly important as portal hypertension can be severe in patients with liver cirrhosis. Studies have shown that Pringle maneuver is effective in reducing the speed and the amount of bleeding and sometimes it could be life-saving. It is relatively easy to apply Pringle maneuver in open surgery but special technique is required in laparoscopic surgery.

In laparoscopic surgery, the ease of accessibility is limited by the number, size and location of the ports. In order to ensure smooth inflow control, the liver hilum has to be slung and controlled in advance. Controlling the liver hilum in case of bleeding will be chaotic. Figure 30.2 demonstrates the preparation for hilar control with vessel loops. If bleeding is anticipated, a bulldog clamp can be applied for 20 minutes without any disturbance to liver function.

30.6.2 Right Phrenic Vein—The North Star

In laparoscopic major hepatectomy, the transection starts at the inferior end of the liver and ends at the superior end. This South to North approach

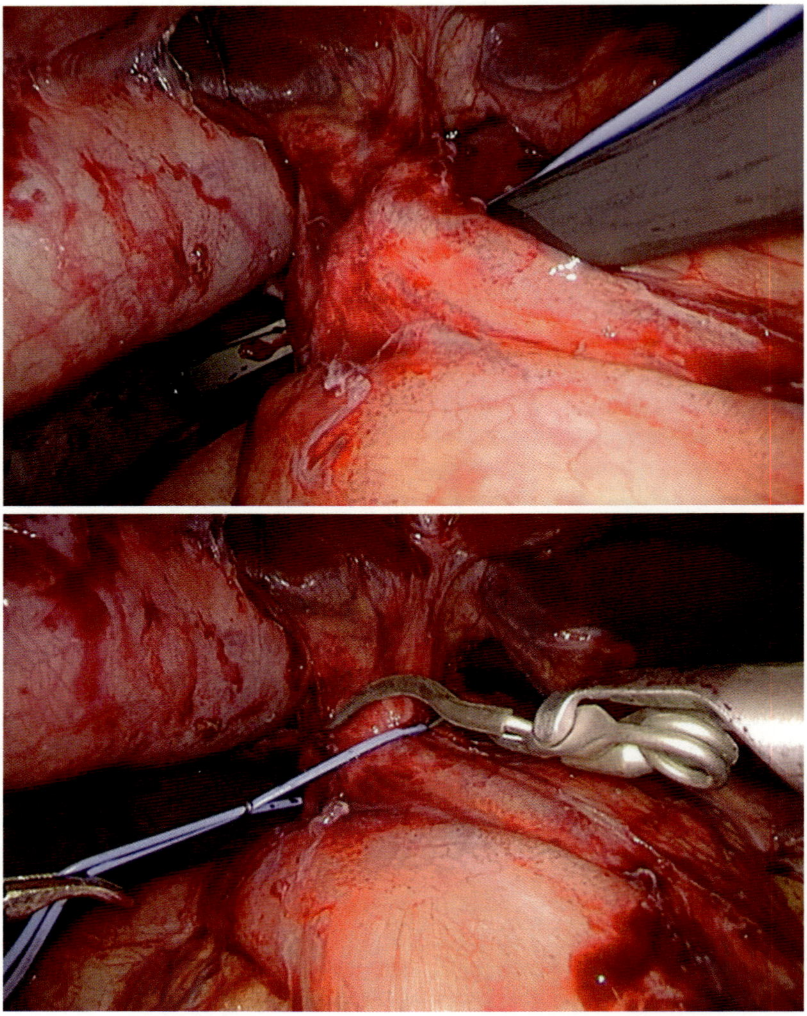

Fig. 30.2 Application of laparoscopic Pringle maneuver

is the only way a liver can be transected in a laparoscopic setting.

In laparoscopic liver surgery, the surgeon cannot feel or touch the liver. In addition, the angle of view is limited from the foot end of the patient most of the time. It may be difficult to determine the line of transection when the demarcation of the liver is not very obvious after hemi inflow control during major hepatectomy.

A high-definition video system allows very meticulous dissection of the liver hilum and liver parenchyma. The magnification can be more than ten times, with a crystal-clear image on the display unit. The right phrenic vein of the diaphragm can be shown very clearly.

The right phrenic vein serves as a very important landmark during laparoscopic hepatectomy. It drains constantly into the origin of the right hepatic vein (Fig. 30.3). Knowing the precise location of the right hepatic vein, an accurate transection line can be drawn between the gallbladder fossa. For major right hepatectomy, the Cantlie line will be from the gallbladder fossa to the medial of the right phrenic vein origin. For right posterior sectionectomy, the origin will be the right Glissonian groove to the lateral of the right phrenic vein origin.

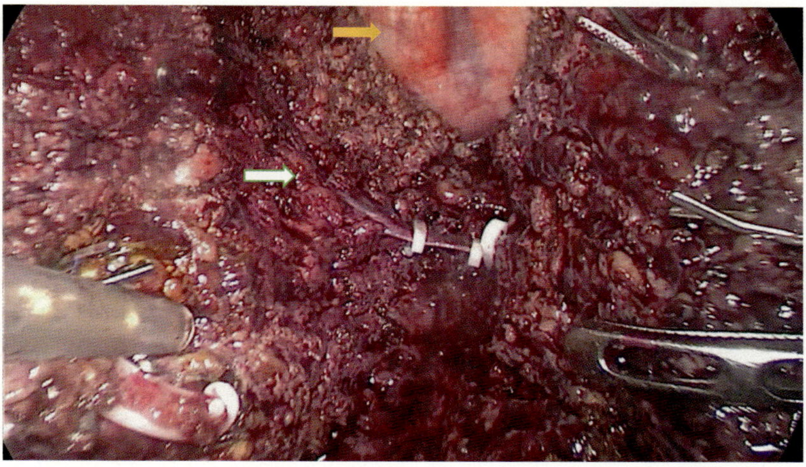

Fig. 30.3 The North Star. The right phrenic vein (*yellow arrow*) draining into the right hepatic vein (*white arrow*)

30.7 Benefits of Laparoscopic Hepatectomy for Patient with Liver Cirrhosis

Laparoscopic liver resection causes minimal invasive trauma to patients. In patients with liver cirrhosis, due to the presence of portal hypertension, there are a lot of varices and collateral developments in the abdominal wall. In open liver resection where a larger abdominal wound is created, there will be disruption of the liver blood flow. Patients will develop decompensation and ascites after laparotomy. This is evident not only in major hepatectomy but also in minor liver resection where a limited amount of liver has been sacrificed.

Although some surgeons advocate the use of a smaller wound in the upper abdomen for minor live resection, laparoscopic liver resection should still be a better option. In laparoscopic major liver resection, a larger wound is required for specimen retrieval, but the wound is usually placed as a horizontal wound in the suprapubic area. This type of wound usually only affects the dermatome and there will be minimal pain and minimal pulmonary complications.

30.8 Outcome of Laparoscopic Liver Resection

Up to date, there have been more than 10,000 cases of laparoscopic liver resection performed in the world and 2/3 of the cases involved cancer treatment.

Long-term outcomes have shown that laparoscopic liver resection can be safely performed in experienced centers. Laparoscopic liver resection is associated with less blood loss, shorter operation time, fewer pulmonary complications, and shorter hospital stay.

This approach has no oncological inferiority, and many major studies have shown that its results were comparable with those of open live resection.

In the study by Cheung et al. involving 440 patients with hepatocellular carcinoma and liver cirrhosis, patients having laparoscopic liver resection (110 cases) had better long-term outcomes. There is a possibility that laparoscopic live resection is associated with non-touch technique, less blood loss, and less inflammatory response. These are all good prognostic factors for survival of cancer patients.

Conclusion

With appropriate training and education, laparoscopic liver resection can be safely performed in patients with liver cirrhosis. The benefit of this approach is obvious and it is likely to become a mainstream because of its potential benefits.

References

1. Buell JF, Cherqui D, Geller DA, et al. The international position on laparoscopic liver surgery: The Louisville Statement, 2008. Ann Surg. 2009;250: 825–30.
2. Wakabayashi G, Cherqui D, Geller DA, et al. Recommendations for laparoscopic liver resection: a report from the second international consensus conference held in Morioka. Ann Surg. 2015;261:619–29.
3. Cheung TT, Dai WC, Tsang SH, et al. Pure laparoscopic hepatectomy versus open hepatectomy for hepatocellular carcinoma in 110 patients with liver cirrhosis: a propensity analysis at a single center. Ann Surg. 2016;264:612–20.
4. Yoon YI, Kim KH, Kang SH, et al. Pure laparoscopic versus open right hepatectomy for hepatocellular carcinoma in patients with cirrhosis: a propensity score matched analysis. Ann Surg. 2016.
5. Abu HM, Di FF, Syed S, et al. Assessment of the financial implications for laparoscopic liver surgery: a single-centre UK cost analysis for minor and major hepatectomy. Surg Endosc. 2013;27:2542–50.
6. Cai XJ, Wang YF, Liang YL, et al. Laparoscopic left hemihepatectomy: a safety and feasibility study of 19 cases. Surg Endosc. 2009;23:2556–62.
7. Martin RC, Scoggins CR, McMasters KM. Laparoscopic hepatic lobectomy: advantages of a minimally invasive approach. J Am Coll Surg. 2010;210:627–6.
8. Topal H, Tiek J, Aerts R, et al. Outcome of laparoscopic major liver resection for colorectal metastases. Surg Endosc. 2012;26:2451–5.
9. Medbery RL, Chadid TS, Sweeney JF, et al. Laparoscopic vs open right hepatectomy: a value-based analysis. J Am Coll Surg. 2014;218:929–39.
10. Cheung TT, Poon RT, Yuen WK, et al. Long-term survival analysis of pure laparoscopic versus open hepatectomy for hepatocellular carcinoma in patients with cirrhosis: a single-center experience. Ann Surg. 2013;257:506–11.
11. Cheung TT, Poon RT. Synchronous resections of primary colorectal tumor and liver metastasis by laparoscopic approach. World J Hepatol. 2013;5:298–301.
12. Nguyen KT, Marsh JW, Tsung A, et al. Comparative benefits of laparoscopic vs open hepatic resection: a critical appraisal. Arch Surg. 2011;146:348–56.
13. Ciria R, Cherqui D, Geller DA, et al. Comparative short-term benefits of laparoscopic liver resection: 9000 cases and climbing. Ann Surg. 2016;263:761–77.
14. Ban D, Tanabe M, Ito H, et al. A novel difficulty scoring system for laparoscopic liver resection. J Hepatobiliary Pancreat Sci. 2014;21:745–53.
15. Ban D, Kudo A, Ito H, et al. The difficulty of laparoscopic liver resection. Updat Surg. 2015;67:123–8.
16. Cheung TT, Ng KK, Poon RT, et al. A case of laparoscopic hepatectomy for recurrent hepatocellular carcinoma. World J Gastroenterol. 2010;16:526–30.
17. Cheung TT, Poon RT, Dai WC, et al. Pure laparoscopic versus open left lateral sectionectomy for hepatocellular carcinoma: a single-center experience. World J Surg. 2016;40:198–205.
18. Cheung TT, Dai WC, Tsang SH, et al. Pure laparoscopic hepatectomy versus open hepatectomy for hepatocellular carcinoma in 110 patients with liver cirrhosis: a propensity analysis at a single center. Ann Surg. 2016;264:612–20.
19. Cheung TT, Poon RT, Lo CM. Reply to letter: "Long-term survival analysis of pure laparoscopic versus open hepatectomy for hepatocellular carcinoma in patients with cirrhosis: a single-center experience". Ann Surg. 2015;262:e20–1.
20. Cheung TT, Lo CM. Laparoscopic liver resection for hepatocellular carcinoma in patients with cirrhosis. Hepatobiliary Surg Nutr. 2015;4:406–10.
21. Cheung TT, Poon RT, Yuen WK, et al. Long-term survival analysis of pure laparoscopic versus open hepatectomy for hepatocellular carcinoma in patients with cirrhosis: a single-center experience. Ann Surg. 2013;257:506–11.
22. Cheung TT, Poon RT. Synchronous resections of primary colorectal tumor and liver metastasis by laparoscopic approach. World J Hepatol. 2013;5: 298–301.
23. Cheung TT, Poon RT, Yuen WK, et al. Outcome of laparoscopic versus open hepatectomy for colorectal liver metastases. ANZ J Surg. 2013;83:847–52.

31 Robotic Liver Resection for Malignancies

Rachel E. Beard, Lee M. Ocuin, and Allan Tsung

31.1 Introduction

The benefits of minimally invasive surgery for quicker patient recovery with reduced complications are increasingly recognized, and laparoscopic abdominal surgery is now an integrated part of surgical training. Laparoscopic approaches to liver surgery have been widely adopted and are increasingly reported in the literature. Multiple studies have demonstrated the equivalency, and sometimes superiority, of perioperative parameters and short-term postoperative outcomes after laparoscopic liver surgery when compared to open liver resections, even for major hepatectomy [1–3]. A number of studies have largely allayed fears that oncologic outcomes would be compromised with a laparoscopic approach to liver surgery. Both meta-analyses and case-controlled series have shown similar rates of margin positivity, recurrence and survival when comparing laparoscopic and open liver resections for hepatocellular carcinoma (HCC) [4–6]. Likewise, laparoscopy has shown no disadvantages in regards to oncologic outcomes when used for colorectal carcinoma (CRC) liver metastases [2, 7–11]. In 2008 an international consensus conference on laparoscopic liver surgery composed the Louisville Statement, which was issued in 2009 [12]. They deduced that: (1) currently acceptable indications for laparoscopic liver surgery include solitary lesions of 5 cm or less that are located in segments 2–6, (2) laparoscopic left lateral sectionectomy should be considered standard of care, (3) major laparoscopic liver resections should be performed only by experienced surgeons, (4) conversion to open procedure should be readily considered for patient safety, long operative times and difficult resections, (5) a hand-assisted or hybrid approach may be beneficial. Importantly, however, a significant learning curve for laparoscopic liver surgery has been demonstrated, with a 45–75 cases needed for competency [13–17]. Though the feasibility, safety and oncologic efficacy of a laparoscopic approach to liver surgery are well established, the liver still presents significant technical challenges for larger anatomic resections, owing to the need for mobilization, limited space to maneuver and the complex and variant vascular and biliary anatomy.

The introduction of the da Vinci Surgical System (Intuitive Surgical, Inc., Sunnyvale, CA) aimed to address some of the technical shortcomings of laparoscopic surgery. Advantages of robotic-assisted surgery include full articulating motion that simulates the surgeon's wrist, an improved three-dimensional view of the surgical

R.E. Beard • L.M. Ocuin • A. Tsung (✉)
Division of Hepatobiliary and Pancreatic Surgery, University of Pittsburgh Medical Center, Kaufmann Medical Building, 3471 Fifth Ave., Suite 300, Pittsburgh, PA 15213, USA
e-mail: tsunga@upmc.edu

M.A. Cuesta (ed.), *Minimally Invasive Surgery for Upper Abdominal Cancer*,
DOI 10.1007/978-3-319-54301-7_31

field, elimination of the physiologic tremor and enhanced instrument dexterity for suturing and dissection. Disadvantages include the significant expense of purchasing and maintaining equipment, a significant learning curve and the loss of tactile feedback for the surgeon. Several early series demonstrated its safety and success when employed in abdominal surgery to treat a variety of diseases including antireflux operations, cholecystectomy, bariatric procedures, colon, gastric and adrenal resections [18–20]. Liver resections constituted a small minority of initial robotic surgeries—seven out of 153 procedures in one study and three of 207 in another [19, 20]. Over time, advances were made in the application of robotic liver surgery and it is now increasingly utilized with increased reports in the literature.

31.2 Robotic Liver Resection

There are now 19 major series (>9 patients) in the literature describing robotic hepatectomy, comprising 631 procedures and published between 2010 and 2016 [21–39] (Table 31.1).

31.2.1 Indication and Resection Type

Of the 631 robotic liver resections reported, the indication for 461 (73%) was malignancy (Table 31.1). All but three of the studies reported on specific pathologies and overall the most common malignancies were HCC (n = 205) and metastatic CRC (n = 136) (Table 31.3). Of the resections performed 139 (22%) were classified as major hepatectomy comprising a resection of at least three liver segments (Table 31.2).

31.2.2 Operative Time

All 19 series included data on operative times that ranged from 45 to 812 min (Table 31.2). Importantly a number of studies included procedures during which simultaneous other surgeries were performed, most frequently colectomies in the case of synchronous metastatic colorectal cancer [22, 26, 29–33, 36]. The shortest reported operative times were 163 minutes as reported by Kingham et al. with only 9% of resections in that series constituting major hepatectomies,

Table 31.1 Major series of robotic liver resections (≥9 patients)

Study	Center	Patients (n)	Malignant (%)	Reference
Giulianotti et al. (2011)	Chicago, USA	70	42 (60)	[29]
Lee et al. (2016)	Hong Kong, China	70	52 (74)	[37]
Kingham et al. (2016)	New York, USA	64	50 (78)	[36]
Tsung et al. (2014)	Pittsburgh, USA	57	40 (70)	[24]
Wu et al. (2014)	Taipei, Taiwan	52	39 (75)	[21]
Lai et al. (2013)	Hong Kong, China	41	41 (100)	[22]
Troisi et al. (2013)	Ghent, Belgium	40	28 (70)	[33]
Montalti et al. (2016)	Ghent, Belgium	36	26 (72%)	[38]
Choi et al. (2012)	Seoul, Korea	30	21 (70)	[28]
Tranchart et al. (2014)	Perugia, Italy	28	15 (54)	[32]
Chan et al. (2011)	Hong Kong, China	27	21 (78)	[27]
Spampinato et al. (2014)	Italy	25	17 (68)	[31]
Casciola et al. (2011)	Spoleto, Italy	23	19 (83)	[26]
Ji et al. (2011)	Beijing, China	13	8 (62)	[30]
Yu et al. (2014)	Seoul, Korea	13	10 (77)	[34]
Kim et al. (2016)	Seoul, Korea	12	7 (58)	[39]
Packiam et al. (2012)	Pittsburgh, USA	11	6 (55)	[23]
Croner et al. (2016)	Erlangen, Germany	10	10 (100)	[35]
Berber et al. (2010)	Cleveland, USA	9	9 (100)	[25]
Total		**631**		

Table 31.2 Patient demographics, operative variables, and postoperative outcomes

Study	Patients (n)	Age, years ± SD or (range)	Major hepatectomy (%)	Operative time, min ± SD or (range)	EBL (mL)	Transfusion (%)	Conversion (%)	Morbidity (%)	Median LOS (days)
Giulianotti et al. [29]	70	57 (21–84)	27 (39)	270 (90–660)	262	15 (21)	4 (6)	15 (21)	7
Lee et al. [37]	70	58 (20–82)	14 (20)	252 (97–620)	100	3 (4.3%)	4 (6)	8 (11)	5
Kingham et al. [36]	64	64 (40–91)	6 (9)	163 (56–480)	100	1 (1.6)	4 (6.3)	7 (11)	4
Tsung et al. [24]	57	58 ± 14.6	21 (37)	253 (180–355)	200	2 (3.8)	4 (7)	11 (19)	4
Wu et al. [21]	52	61 ± 14.9	20 (38)	380 ± 166	325	NR	2 (5)	3 (8)	NR
Lai et al. [22]	41	61 ± 10.9	10 (23)	229 ± 83	413	3 (7)	3 (7)	3 (7)	6
Troisi et al. [33]	40	65 ± 12.1	0 (0)	271 ± 100	330	NR	8 (20)	5 (13)	6
Montalti et al. [38]	36	62 (32–84)	0 (0)	306 ± 182 (53–790)	415	NR	5 (14)	7 (19)	6
Choi et al. [28]	30	52 (28–71)	20 (67)	507 (120–812)	343	4 (13)	2 (7)	13 (43)	12
Tranchart et al. [32]	28	67 (42–84)	0 (0)	210 (45–480)	200	4 (14)	4 (14)	5 (18)	6
Chan et al. [27]	27	61 (37–85)	1 (4)	200 (90–307)	50	NR	1 (4)	2 (7)	6
Spampinato et al. [31]	25	63 (32–80)	25 (100)	430 (24–725)	250	11 (44)	1 (4)	4 (16)	8
Casciola et al. [26]	23	66 ± 13.4	0 (0)	280 ± 101	245	NR	2 (9)	10 (43)	9
Ji et al. [30]	13	53 (39–79)	10 (77)	338	280	0 (0)	0 (0)	1 (8)	7
Yu et al. [34]	13	50 ± 12.2	3 (23)	292 ± 85	389	0 (0)	0 (0)	0 (0)	8
Kim et al. [39]	12	54 ± 12.2	0 (0)	404 ± 139	225	1 (8.3)	0 (0)	3 (25)	7
Packiam et al. [23]	11	57 ± 16	0 (0)	175 (156–253)	30	0 (0)	0 (0)	3 (27)	4
Croner et al. [35]	10	64 (45–76)	NR	321 (138–458)	306	NR	0 (0)	1 (10)	7
Berber et al. [25]	9	67 ± 6.4	0 (0)	259 ± 28	136	NR	1 (11)	1 (11)	NR

NR not reported, *EBL* estimated blood loss, *LOS* length of stay

Table 31.3 Oncologic outcomes

Study	Type of tumor (n)			Resection (%)		Pathology		Follow-up	
	CRC	HCC	Other	R0	R1	Tumor size, mm ± SD (range)	Margins, mm ± SD (range)	Follow-up, months ± SD (range)	Postoperative oncologic outcomes
Giulianotti et al. [29]	16	13	13	100	0	47 (11–110)	15 (1–70)	NR	NR
Lee et al. [37]	8	40	4	100	1	25 (10–120)	15 (0–60)	NR	NR
Kingham et al. [36]	NR	NR	NR	98	NR	25 (30–145)	NR	NR	NR
Tsung et al. [24]	21	7	12	100	0	32 (20–50)	NR	NR	NR
Wu et al. [21]	0	38	1	NR	NR	34 ± 17	NR	NR	NR
Lai et al. [22]	0	41	0	93	7	34 ± 1.9	NR	14	15% recurrence rate; 2 years OS/DFS: 94%/74%
Troisi et al. [33]	24	3	1	89	11	52 ± 38	NR	9.6 (CRC)	37% recurrence rate; 1/3 years DFS: 79%/62%
Montalti et al. [38]	21	3	2	NR	11	44 ± 31 (2–110)	NR	NR	OS for CRC 92, 65, 40% at 1, 3, 5 years
Choi et al. [28]	4	13	4	NR	NR	31 (8–50)	21 (1–35)	HCC: 11 (5–29) CRC: 12 (3–22) Other: 21 (3–22)	1 CRC recurrence at 5 mos
Tranchart et al. [32]	NR	NR	15	NR	NR	35 (6–115)	NR	NR	NR
Chan et al. [27]	7	13	1	NR	NR	NR	NR	NR	NR
Spampinato et al. [31]	11	2	3	100	0	NR	NR	NR	NR
Casciola et al. [26]	14	3	2	100	0	34 ± 18	15 ± 8	25 ± 12	1 HCC recurrence; 2 CRC recurrence
Ji et al. [30]	0	6	2	100	0	64 (18–120)	NR	NR	NR
Yu et al. [34]	0	10	0	NR	NR	31 ± 16	19 ± 10	NR	NR
Kim et al. [39]	1	6	0	100	0	23 (20–36)	18 (9–35)	NR	NR
Packiam et al. [23]	NR	NR	6	NR	NR	55 (24–65)	NR	NR	NR

Table 31.3 (continued)

Study	Type of tumor (n)			Resection (%)		Pathology		Follow-up	
	CRC	HCC	Other	R0	R1	Tumor size, mm ± SD (range)	Margins, mm ± SD (range)	Follow-up, months ± SD (range)	Postoperative oncologic outcomes
Croner et al. [35]	5	4	1	100	100	48 (29–105)	57 (10–150)	NR	NR
Berber et al. [25]	4	3	2	100	0	32 ± 13	NR	14	1 Distant and 1 local recurrence

NR not reported, *DFS* disease free survival, *OS* overall survival, *CRC* colorectal carcinoma, *HCC* hepatocellular carcinoma

and 175 minutes by Packiam et al. which reported exclusively on left lateral sectionectomies [23, 36]. In the 13 series that compared laparoscopic to open liver resections, 5 series reported significantly longer operative times with robotic resections [21, 24, 35, 37, 39].

31.2.3 Estimated Blood Loss and Transfusion Requirement

All series reported intraoperative estimated blood loss (EBL) and amounts ranged from 30 to 415 mL (Table 31.2). The lowest EBL of 30 mL was reported by Packiam et al. and all patients in that series underwent left lateral sectionectomy [23]. Spaminato et al. reported exclusively on major hepatectomies and reported an EBL value of 250 mL [31]. The highest EBL was 415 mL reported by Montali et al., however that series reported only on tumors located in the difficult to access posterosuperior liver segments [38].

31.2.4 Conversion Rate

Conversion rates ranged from 0 to 20% across series (Table 31.2). Of the 631 robotic procedures reported, 45 were converted to an open procedure for an overall conversion rate of 7.1%. Reasons for conversion included bleeding, concern for oncologic margins, adhesions and prolonged operatives times. The largest review laparoscopic liver resection by Nguyen et al. included 2804 patients and reports a conversion rate of 4% [1]. In the 13 series that compared laparoscopic and open robotic resections, only Troisi et al. reported a higher conversion rate with robotic procedures (20 vs. 7.6%; $p = 0.034$) [33] (Table 31.5).

31.2.5 Morbidity and Mortality

Of the 631 patients included across all major series, 102 suffered a complication for an overall rate of 16%, with a range of 0–43% (Table 31.2). The two series reporting a complication rate of 43% were among the earlier series published—Choi et al. (2012) and Casciola et al. (2011). Five studies reported complication rates of less than 10% [21, 22, 27, 30, 34]. By comparison Nguyen et al. reports a complication rate of 10.5% [1]. Of the 13 major series that compared laparoscopic to robotic procedures, only Packiam et al. reported a higher rate of minor complications with robotic approach (27 vs. 0%, $p = 0.019$) [23] (Table 31.5). Of the 631 patients included in the 19 major series there were three mortalities. Montalti et al. reported the death of one patient on postoperative day four from a myocardial infarction [38]. Kingham et al. reported the death of two patients at 90 days and the causes were not stated [36].

Table 31.4 Major series comparing robotic to open liver resections

Study	Open procedures (n)	Robotic procedures (n)	Significant cohort differences	Significant outcome differences
Kingham et al. [36]	64	64	• More hypertension with RR (42 vs. 0%; p < 0.001)	• Shorter operative time with RR (163 vs. 210 min; p = 0.017) • Higher EBL with OR (300 vs. 100 mL; p < 0.001) • Higher intraoperative transfusion with OR (14 vs. 1.6%; p < 0.03) • More need for Pringle with OR (75 vs. 9.4%, p < 0.001) • Shorter LOS with RR (4 vs. 7 days; p < 0.001) • More synchronous organ resection with OR (20 vs. 11%; p = 0.003)
Croner et al. [35]	53	10	• More previous abdominal surgery in open group (1.36 OR vs. 0.58 LR vs. 0.90 RR; p = 0.007)*	• Longer operative times with RR (186 OR vs. 242 LR vs. 321 RR; p = 0.001)* • Longer LOS with OR (10 OR vs. 8 LR vs. 7 days RR; p = 0.004)*
Ji et al. [30]	32	13	Statistical analysis not performed	

*P-values provided compare open, laparoscopic and robotic cohorts

OR open resection, *RR* robotic resection, *LR* laparoscopic resection, *EBL* estimated blood loss, *LOS* length of stay

Table 31.5 Major series comparing robotic to laparoscopic liver resections

Study	LR (n)	RR (n)	Significant cohort differences	Significant outcome differences
Lee et al. [37]	66	70	• More recurrent pyogenic cholangitis with RR (20 vs. 2%, p = 0.001) • More major hepatectomy with RR (20 vs. 3%, p = 0.002) • More wedge resection with LR (52 vs. 24%, p = 0.001)	• Longer operative time with RR (252 vs. 215 min, p = 0.008)
Montalti et al. [38]	72	36	None	• More frequent and longer Pringle with RR (56 vs. 22%; p = 0.001 and 77 vs. 25 min; p < 0.001)
Croner et al. [35]	19	10	• More previous abdominal surgery in open group (1.36 OR vs. 0.58 LR vs. 0.90 RR; p = 0.007)*	• Longer operative times with RR (186 OR vs. 242 LR vs. 321 RR; p = 0.001)* • Longer LOS with LR (10 OR vs. 8 LR vs. 7 days RR; p = 0.004)*
Kim et al. [39]	31	12	None	• Longer operative times for RR (337 vs. 216 min; p = 0.001)
Tsung et al. [24]	57	114	None	• Longer operative times for RR (253 vs. 199 min; p < 0.001) • Higher rates of purely MIS for major hepatectomy with RR (81 vs. 7%, p < 0.05)

Table 31.5 (continued)

Study	LR (n)	RR (n)	Significant cohort differences	Significant outcome differences
Tranchart et al. [32]	28	28	• More solitary tumors with LR (22 vs. 28; p = 0.02) • More superior/posterior segment tumors with RR (14 vs. 3; p = 0.003) • Higher number of lesions with RR (1, range 1–5 vs. 1; p = 0.03) • More associated procedures with RR (10 vs. 2; p = 0.02)	• More frequent Pringle with RR (12 vs. 0; p = 0.001)
Yu et al. [34]	17	13	None	None
Spampinato et al. [31]	25	25	• More neoadjuvant chemotherapy with LR (68 vs. 12%; p < 0.001)	• More frequent Pringle maneuver with LR (32 vs. 0%, p = 0.004)
Wu et al. [21]	69	52	• Older age for RR (61 vs. 54 years, p = 0.04) • Larger tumors size for RR (3.4 vs. 2.5 cm, p = 0.02) • More resection >2 segments for RR (78 vs. 37%, p = 0.04)	• Higher EBL with RR (325 vs. 173 mL, p = 0.03) • Longer operative time with RR (380 vs. 227 min, p = 0.04)
Troisi et al. [33]	223	40	• Older age in RR (65 vs. 55 years; p = 0.001) • More males in RR (68 vs. 44%; p = 0.01) • Previous abdominal surgery in LR (33 vs. 66%; p < 0.001) • Combined colorectal surgery in RR (25 vs. 2.7, p < 0.001) • More neoadjuvant chemotherapy in LR (13 vs. 38%, p < 0.004) • Higher mean lesion number in RR (1.97 vs. 1.57; p = 0.04) • More major hepatectomy in LR group (0 vs. 17%, p = 0.011) • More posterior, superior segment resections in RR (55 vs. 34%, p = 0.019)	• Higher EBL with RR (330 vs. 174 mL, p < 0.001) • More frequent Pringle maneuver with RR (45 vs. 3%, p < 0.001) • More frequent conversion with RR (20 vs. 7.6%, p = 0.034)
Packiam et al. [23]	18	11	None	• Higher rate of minor complications in RR (27 vs. 0%; p = 0.019) • Higher ICU admission rate with RR (46 vs. 6%; p = 0.01) • Longer LOS with RR (4 vs. 3; p = 0.031)
Ji et al. [30]	20	13	Statistical analysis not performed	
Berber et al. [25]	9	23	None	None

*P-values provided compare open, laparoscopic and robotic cohorts

LR laparoscopic resection, *RR* robotic resection, *OR* open resection, *EBL* estimated blood loss, *ICU* intensive care unit, *MIS* minimally invasive surgery, *LOS* length of stay

31.2.6 Length of Stay (LOS)

Median length-of-stay (LOS) was reported in 17 of the 19 series and ranged from four to 12 days (Table 31.2). In their review of laparoscopic liver resections, Nguyen et al. reported variability in regards to hospital stay based on country, with the shorter LOS in the USA and longer LOS in Asia and Europe [1]. Indeed, for robotic resections the three series reporting a median LOS of four days were American, whereas the series that reported 12 days originated from Korea [23, 24, 28, 36]. Both of the studies that compared open and robotic liver resections and performed statistical analysis reported significantly shorter LOS with robotic approach [24, 35] (Table 31.4). Two of the 13 studies comparing robotic and laparoscopic resections demonstrated a longer LOS with robotic approach [23].

31.2.7 Oncologic Outcomes

Oncologic outcomes were not consistently reported across studies (Table 31.3). R0 resection rate, when reported, was generally high ranging from 89 to 100%. Tumor size tended to be small ranging from 25 to 48 mm. Only a few series reported on margin status and even fewer reported any long-term follow-up or data on recurrence or survival.

31.3 Robotic Compared to Open Liver Resection

Three of the published major series compared robotic-assisted liver resection to open procedures [35, 36] (Table 31.4). The largest and most recent was reported by Kingham et al. and case-matched 64 robotic to 64 robotic hepatectomies at the same center [36]. Of their 64 robotic cases, 35 (55%) were for metastatic cancer and 13 (20%) were for primary liver cancer, though the specific pathologies were not specified. Another 13 (30%) were performed for benign pathology though seven of these tumors were found to be potentially premalignant gallbladder polyps or adenomas. The indications for surgery in the open resection cohort were not significantly different. They reported positive margins in 1.6% of robotic resections and 14% of open resections but this did not reach statistical significance ($p = 0.4\%$) and they did not differentiate between R1 and R2 resections. Patients were matched based on resection type and on benign or malignant pathology, and the only significant difference in the patient demographics was more hypertension in the robotic group (42 vs. 0%, $p < 0.001$). Intraoperatively the open cohort had longer median operative times (210 vs. 163 min, $p = 0.017$), higher median EBL (300 vs. 100 mL; $p < 0.001$), higher rate of intraoperative transfusion (14 vs. 1.6%; $p = 0.03$), greater need for Pringle maneuver (75 vs. 9.4%; $p < 0.001$) and more synchronous organ resections (20 vs. 11%; $p = 0.003$) than did the robotic cohort. Tumor number, size and margin positivity were not significantly different nor were postoperative complications, need for readmission or mortality (3% for robotic and 1.6% for open at 90 days; $p = 1.0$).

Croner et al. case-matched ten patients undergoing robotic resection to a control group of 53 contemporaneous open procedures at a single institution [35]. They also included a group of 19 patients undergoing laparoscopic resection so while statistical analysis was performed, p-values provided are derived from comparison amongst all three cohorts. The only statistically significant demographic difference between groups was a higher mean number of previous abdominal surgeries in the open group (1.36 open vs. 0.58 laparoscopic vs. 0.90 robotic; $p = 0.007$). The operative times were lower for the open group (186 open vs. 242 laparoscopic vs. 321 min robotic; $p = 0.001$). All other intraoperative parameters including EBL, tumor pathology characteristics and margin status were not significantly difference. Postoperatively the LOS was highest in the open group (10 open vs. 8 laparoscopic vs. 7 days robotic; $p = 0.004$), whereas morbidity, mortality and measures of postoperative pain were comparable between groups.

Ji et al. compared 13 consecutive robotic resections to a contemporary cohort-matched group of 32 open resections [30]. Though they reported and compared perioperative outcome parameters no statistical analysis was performed, making any true cohort comparison difficult. Mean operative times were longer for the robotic group (338 vs. 205 min) and mean EBL was higher in the open group (470 vs. 280 mL) as was transfusion requirement (4 vs. 0 units PRBC). LOS was longer for the open group (9.6 vs. 6.7 days).

31.4 Robotic Compared to Laparoscopic Liver Resection

Thirteen of the published major series compare laparoscopic and open liver resections [16, 21, 23–25, 31–35, 37–39] (Table 31.5). Most of the studies were retrospective and many reported on consecutive patients series, some with case matching. As of yet there are no randomized controlled trials comparing the two approaches.

Lee et al. retrospectively compared 66 laparoscopic to 70 robotic resections performed at a single institution [37]. There were more major hepatectomies performed in the robotic group (20 vs. 3%, $p = 0.002$) and longer operative times with robotic resections (252 vs. 215 min; $p = 0.008$). There were no differences in conversion rate, blood loss, hospital stay or morbidity. There was no mortality in either group. In a subgroup analysis looking solely at left lateral sectionectomies, all perioperative outcomes were statistically similar between the two groups.

Montalti et al. performed a 1:2 matched propensity score analysis between 36 robotic and 72 laparoscopic parenchymal-preserving liver resections of the posterosuperior segments performed at two institutions [38]. Patient demographics and disease characteristics were comparable. Intraoperative blood loss, conversion rate, and operative times were not significantly different but robotic procedures more often required a Pringle maneuver and for longer time periods (56 vs. 22%; $p = 0.001$ and 77 vs. 25 min; $p < 0.001$). Postoperatively the groups had identical complication rates (19.4%, $p = 1.0$) and though LOS was longer for the robotic group this did not reach statistical significance (6 ± 2.9 vs. 4.9 ± 2.95; $p = 0.07$).

Croner et al. included only minor resections and compared 10 robotic to 19 laparoscopic resections performed at a single institution [35]. They also compared these patients to a case-matched control group of 53 open resections done during the same time period, and statistical analysis reported provided p-values comparing all three groups. The only statistically significant demographic difference between groups was a higher mean number of previous abdominal surgeries in the open group (1.36 open vs. 0.58 laparoscopic vs. 0.90 robotic; $p = 0.007$). The operative times were lower for the open group (186 open vs. 242 laparoscopic vs. 321 min robotic; $p = 0.001$) with all other intraoperative measures including EBL, tumor pathology characteristics and margin status being comparable. The LOS was highest in the open group (10 open vs. 8 laparoscopic vs. 7 days robotic; $p = 0.004$), and morbidity, mortality and measures of postoperative pain were not significantly different.

Kim et al. retrospectively compared 12 robotic to 31 laparoscopic left lateral sectionectomies at a single institution [39]. There were no differences in the cohort demographics or in the tumor characteristics. The mean operation times were significantly longer for the robotic group (404 vs. 246 min; $p < 0.001$) but EBL was comparable. Postoperatively all of the reported parameters including LOS and rates of complication were comparable. There were also no significant differences in disease-free or overall survival between the two groups ($p = 0.462$ and 0.484, respectively).

Tsung et al. performed a 1:2 matched analysis between 57 robotic and 114 laparoscopic hepatic resections [24]. Demonstrated intraoperative differences included longer operative times for robotic cases (median 253 vs. 199 min; $p < 0.001$) and higher rates of purely minimally invasive major hepatectomies with a robotic approach (81 vs. 7%; $p < 0.05$). No differences were demonstrated in blood loss, transfusion, R0 resection, LOS, morbidity or mortality.

Tranchart et al. performed a case matched comparative study between 28 robotic liver resections performed at an Italian institution to 28 laparoscopic liver resections performed at a French center [32]. Patients in the robotic cohort had fewer solitary tumors, more tumors located in the superior/posterior segments, a higher number of lesions and more associated procedures, mostly colectomies, than did the laparoscopic cohort. Intraoperatively the robotic group more frequently required Pringle maneuver (12 vs. 0; p = 0.001) but otherwise EBL and conversion were comparable. Postoperatively none of the parameters including morbidity, mortality or LOS were significantly different.

Yu et al. included only patients undergoing left hemihepatectomy or left lateral sectionectomy and compared 13 robotic to 17 laparoscopic resections at a single center [34]. There were no differences in preoperative characteristics or tumor pathology. No intraoperative parameters or postoperative outcomes were significantly different between groups.

Spampinato et al. pooled data from four hepatobiliary centers and retrospectively compared 25 laparoscopic to 25 robotic major hepatectomies [31]. The only significant demographic difference was more neoadjuvant chemotherapy in the laparoscopic group (68 vs. 12%; p < 0.001). Intraoperatively the only difference was a greater need for Pringle maneuver with the laparoscopic group (32 vs. 0%; p = 0.004). Postoperatively there was a quicker return of bowel function with shorter reported time of first flatus (1 vs. 3 days; p = 0.023) and earlier tolerance of liquid diet (1 vs. 2 days; p = 0.001) with the laparoscopic group. Tumor margin status, morbidity, mortality, readmission and LOS were all comparable.

Wu et al. compared 52 robotic to 69 laparoscopic liver resections at a single institution [21]. The extent of the resections performed robotically was greater with 78% of patients having a resection of more than two segments compared to 37% of laparoscopic patients (p = 0.04). Operative times were longer for the robotic group (mean 380 vs. 227 min; p = 0.04) and EBL was higher (mean 325 vs. 173 mL; p = 0.03). There was no difference in conversion rate, length of stay or morbidity, and there was no mortality in either group.

Troisi et al. compared 223 consecutive laparoscopic liver resections performed at an institution in Ghent, Belgium to 40 consecutive robotic resections at an institution in Spoleto, Italy [33]. A number of differences in the cohort demographics were demonstrated with the robotic group being more elderly (65 vs. 55 years; p < 0.001) and more predominantly male (68 vs. 44%; p = 0.01). The laparoscopic group also had higher rates of previous abdominal surgery and neoadjuvant chemotherapy, whereas the robotic group had a higher percentage of combined colorectal procedures. Indication for surgery and mean tumor size were not significantly different, but the laparoscopic group had a higher mean lesion number (1.97 vs. 1.57; p = 0.04). More major hepatectomies were performed in the laparoscopic group and more posterior-superior segment resections were performed in the robotic group. Intraoperatively the robotic group had higher median EBL (330 vs. 174 mL; p < 0.001), more frequent need for Pringle maneuver (45 vs. 2.7%; p < 0.001), and higher conversion rates (20 vs. 7.6%; p = 0.034), most frequently due to bleeding. Postoperatively there were no significant differences in morbidity or mortality.

Packiam et al. retrospectively compared 11 robotic to 18 laparoscopic resections at a single center. Patients undergoing robotic resection had more intensive care unit (ICU) admissions (46 vs. 6%; p = 0.01), longer length of stay and increased rate of minor complication than the laparoscopic cohort [23]. There were no differences in major complications, conversion rate, EBL, transfusions or operative time. There was no mortality in either group.

Ji et al. compared 13 consecutive robotic resections to 20 laparoscopic hepatectomies that were contemporaneous and cohort-matched at a single institution [30]. In the laparoscopic group, mean operative times were shorter (130 vs. 338 min) and conversions were higher (2 vs. 0 conversions), however statistical analysis was not performed.

Berber et al. prospectively compared nine robotic resections performed over a 1-year period to 23 laparoscopic resections at the same institution [25]. One robotic case was converted to open whereas none were in the laparoscopic group, and one patient in the robotic group had a postoperative complication compared to four in the laparoscopic group. However no clinical, operative or postoperative parameters reached a clinically significant difference, likely in part due to small sample size.

31.5 Systematic Reviews and Meta-analyses

A number of meta-analyses have aimed to pool data to compare outcomes following robotic hepatectomy. Recently Nota et al. performed a review and meta-analysis of 12 studies with 363 patients with subgroup analyses of (i) minor resections of easily accessible segments (2/3, 4B, 5, 6), (ii) minor resections of difficult located segments (1, 4A, 7, 8), and (iii) major resections (≥4 segments) [40]. When surgical outcomes were pooled they reported a mean operative time of 300 min, mean EBL of 230 mL, conversion rate of 1% and mean LOS of 5 days for subgroup (i) and a mean operative time of 220 min, mean EBL of 170 mL, conversion rate of 0% and mean LOS of 5 days for subgroup (ii). All parameters were higher for major resections with mean operative time of 405 min, mean EBL of 380 mL, conversion rate of 8% and mean LOS of 11 days.

Meta-analyses have also been performed with studies comparing laparoscopic and robotic liver resections. Montalti et al. performed a meta-analysis of seven articles published between 2010 and 2014 encompassing 694 patients with 479 laparoscopic resections and 215 robotic resections [41]. After pooling data they demonstrated a significantly lower mean blood loss (mean difference = 83.96, 95%CI: 10.51–157.41, $p = 0.03$) and lower operative times (mean difference 68.43, 95%CI: 39.22–97.65, $P < 0.00001$) with the laparoscopic approach. No differences were demonstrated with regards to conversion rate, morbidity, hospital stay or R1 resections. Qiu et al. performed a meta-analysis of nine studies involving 774 patients comparing laparoscopic and robotic resections [42]. They also found longer operative time with robotic procedures (mean difference 48.49; 95% confidence interval (CI) 22.49–74.49 min; $p = 0.0003$) but no significant differences in EBL, LOS, morbidity or surgical margin.

Jackson et al. performed a systemic review and meta-analysis of articles comparing laparoscopic hepatectomy with both robotic and open resections [43]. They included 49 articles, three of which compared laparoscopic and robotic resections and 46 of which compared laparoscopic to open approaches, including 3702 patients comprising 1901 laparoscopic resections, 1741 open resections and 60 robotic procedures. Their outcomes were operative time, blood loss, LOS, resections margins, morbidity, mortality and cost. They found no difference in any of these outcomes between laparoscopic and robotic approaches, whereas open procedures had greater EBL, longer LOS and higher complications rates. Their operative cost analysis included three studies comparing laparoscopy to open surgery and one study comparing robotic and open surgery [23] and showed a non-significant trend towards higher total operative cost for minimally invasive approaches ($334, 95% CI, −$753.50 to $1421.60).

31.6 The Cost of Robotic Surgery

Seven of the major case series provided some degree of analysis on cost [23, 25, 29, 30, 34, 35, 39] (Table 31.6). Most of these studies provided numerical data on comparative costs with the exceptions of Berber et al., which roughly estimated that the robotic equipment added a $500 per case increase to the laparoscopic equipment cost, and Montalti et al., who reported the mean instrumentation costs of their laparoscopic procedures to be €1406 and then referenced the estimate by Berber et al. [25, 38]. Kim et al. reported a significantly higher total cost with their robotic compared to their laparoscopic procedures ($8183 vs. $5190; $p = 0.009$). They also looked at total costs amongst cancer patients compared to those with benign pathologies and found that only the cancer patients undergoing robotic surgery had a significantly

Table 31.6 Major studies including cost analysis

Study	Cost parameter reported	Robotic cases		Laparoscopic cases		Open cases		p-Value
		n	Cost	n	Cost	n	Cost	
Kim et al. [39]	Total cost	12	$8183	31	$5190	NA	NA	0.009
Croner et al. [35]	Perioperative costs	10	€8765	19	€3437	53	€2672	NR
Yu et al. [34]	Total medical cost	13	$11,475	17	$6762	NA	NA	<0.001
Packiam et al. [23]	Direct cost of operating room supplies	11	$5130	18	$4408	NA	NA	0.40
Ji et al. [30]	Hospital cost	13	$12,046	20	$7618	32	$10,548	NR

NR not reported, *NA* not applicable

higher cost ($8302 vs. $4535; p = 0.002), whereas for the benign patient cohort the costs were comparable ($8017 vs. $7437; p = 0.826) [39]. Croner et al. reported the highest perioperative cost with robotic surgery (€8765, 64% of the total surgical cost), followed by laparoscopic surgery (€3437, 42% of the total surgical cost), and lastly open surgery (€2672, 36% of the total surgical cost), however statistical analysis for this metric was not performed [35].

Yu et al. found that the total medical cost of robotic procedures was significantly higher than laparoscopic procedures ($11,475 vs. $6762; p < 0.001) despite a trend towards shorter hospital stay (7.8 vs. 9.5 days; p = 0.053) [34]. Packiam et al. compared the direct costs of operating room supplies and found that though the costs for their robotic procedures were higher than for laparoscopic, the difference did not reach statistical significance ($5130 vs. $4408; p = 0.4) [23]. Ji et al. found that total hospital cost of the robotic procedures ($12,046) exceeded the cost of both the laparoscopic ($7618) and open procedures ($10,548), however no statistical analysis was performed [30].

The cost of the da Vinci robotic surgical system was reported at $1.2 million US dollars with an annual of $138,000 for maintenance in 2009 [44, 45]. A number of studies have compared the expense of robotic liver resection to that of open and laparoscopic approaches. One recent single institution retrospective study from the University of Washington compared cost data for 71 robotic hepatectomies to 88 open procedures and found that despite higher perioperative costs for the robotic procedures, the postoperative costs and subsequent direct hospital costs were lower when compared with open procedures ($14,754 vs. $18,998; p = 0.001), perhaps owing to a 2 day shorter hospital stay on average after robotic procedures (4.2 vs. 6.5 days; p < 0.001) [46]. The increased cost of minimally invasive techniques is certainly significant, but data thus far is inconsistent and these parameters are likely to change as the market surrounding this technology evolves.

31.7 Current Status and Future Applications

Robotic liver surgery is increasingly gaining acceptance is it becomes more widespread and increasingly analyzed. Studies have shown that it is feasible for all kinds of liver resections, including difficult to access segments and major resections, and that it is well-tolerated with acceptable intraoperative and short-term postoperative outcomes, including EBL and conversion rate, which are largely comparable to those achieved with a laparoscopic approach. Some studies have demonstrated longer operative times with a robotic approach but as Tsung et al. demonstrated these times can decrease as experience is gained [24]. Though the data on oncologic outcomes is somewhat limited, parameters such as R0 resections and tumor margins do not appear to be compromised with robotic surgery.

As experience with robotic surgery is gained, both on an individual and institutional level, outcomes improve. King et al. describes the implementation of a robotics program over a 5-year period at a major academic center [47]. The study looked at 1236 robotic surgeries performed by 14 surgeons, 157 of which were liver procedures. From 2009 to 2014, operative volume increased (7 cases/month vs. 24 cases/month; $p < .001$), mean operative times decreased (471 vs. 211 min; $p < .001$), conversion rates decreased (12 vs. 1.7%; $p = .009$) and morbidity decreased (49 vs. 12%; $p < .001$).

Novel techniques in robotic liver surgery are increasingly reported as its applications continue to be expanded. In managing colorectal liver metastases, robotic resections are now combined with not only resection of the primary tumor but also with lung metastases [48, 49]. Small numbers of robotic resections for intrahepatic cholangiocarcinomas have been reported and radical resections for hilar cholangiocarcinomas are now described, though perioperative and oncologic outcomes have raised some concerns [50, 51]. An entirely robotic ALPPS (associating liver partition and portal vein ligation in staged hepatectomy) procedure has also been performed [52].

In moving forward, the challenge will also lie in clarifying the indications and optimal surgical approach for different liver lesions in order to optimize perioperative and oncologic outcomes and minimize healthcare costs. Factors specific to the patient and to individual tumors combined with surgeon expertise and institutional experience will drive these decisions. In a review specifically focused on the differentiating indications for laparoscopic versus robotic liver surgery, Bonapasta et al. noted that the use of robotic surgery has allowed for increasingly complex and parenchymal sparing resections, thereby expanding the number of patients who may benefit from a less invasive procedure. They also pointed out that long-term oncologic outcomes for these patients are not yet well established in the literature [53].

As experience is gained, applications for a robotic approach in liver surgery are expanding and outcomes, including operative times, continue to improve. There is also reason to believe that the costs associated with robotic approaches may decrease in the future as alternative robotic platforms are developed and introduced. It is a reasonable expectation that robotic liver surgery will become increasingly adopted in the future.

References

1. Nguyen KT, Gamblin TC, Geller DA. World review of laparoscopic liver resection-2,804 patients. Ann Surg. 2009;250(5):831–41.
2. Nguyen KT, Laurent A, Dagher I, Geller DA, Steel J, Thomas MT, et al. Minimally invasive liver resection for metastatic colorectal cancer: a multi-institutional, international report of safety, feasibility, and early outcomes. Ann Surg. 2009;250(5):842–8.
3. Dagher I, O'Rourke N, Geller DA, Cherqui D, Belli G, Gamblin TC, et al. Laparoscopic major hepatectomy: an evolution in standard of care. Ann Surg. 2009;250(5):856–60.
4. Xiong JJ, Altaf K, Javed MA, Huang W, Mukherjee R, Mai G, et al. Meta-analysis of laparoscopic vs open liver resection for hepatocellular carcinoma. World J Gastroenterol. 2012;18(45):6657–68.
5. Twaij A, Pucher PH, Sodergren MH, Gall T, Darzi A, Jiao LR. Laparoscopic vs open approach to resection of hepatocellular carcinoma in patients with known cirrhosis: systematic review and meta-analysis. World J Gastroenterol. 2014;20(25):8274–81.
6. Takahara T, Wakabayashi G, Beppu T, Aihara A, Hasegawa K, Gotohda N, et al. Long-term and perioperative outcomes of laparoscopic versus open liver resection for hepatocellular carcinoma with propensity score matching: a multi-institutional Japanese study. J Hepatobiliary Pancreat Sci. 2015;22(10):721–7.
7. Wei M, He Y, Wang J, Chen N, Zhou Z, Wang Z. Laparoscopic versus open hepatectomy with or without synchronous colectomy for colorectal liver metastasis: a meta-analysis. PLoS One. 2014;9(1):e87461.
8. Abu Hilal M, Di Fabio F, Abu Salameh M, Pearce NW. Oncological efficiency analysis of laparoscopic liver resection for primary and metastatic cancer: a single-center UK experience. Arch Surg. 2012; 147(1):42–8.
9. Kazaryan AM, Pavlik Marangos I, Rosseland AR, Rosok BI, Mala T, Villanger O, et al. Laparoscopic liver resection for malignant and benign lesions: ten-year Norwegian single-center experience. Arch Surg. 2010;145(1):34–40.

10. Castaing D, Vibert E, Ricca L, Azoulay D, Adam R, Gayet B. Oncologic results of laparoscopic versus open hepatectomy for colorectal liver metastases in two specialized centers. Ann Surg. 2009;250(5):849–55.
11. Cannon RM, Scoggins CR, Callender GG, McMasters KM, Martin 2nd RC. Laparoscopic versus open resection of hepatic colorectal metastases. Surgery. 2012;152(4):567–73, discussion 73–4.
12. Buell JF, Cherqui D, Geller DA, O'Rourke N, Iannitti D, Dagher I, et al. The international position on laparoscopic liver surgery: the Louisville Statement, 2008. Ann Surg. 2009;250(5):825–30.
13. Lin CW, Tsai TJ, Cheng TY, Wei HK, Hung CF, Chen YY, et al. The learning curve of laparoscopic liver resection after the Louisville statement 2008: will it be more effective and smooth? Surg Endosc. 2016;30(7):2895–903.
14. Kluger MD, Vigano L, Barroso R, Cherqui D. The learning curve in laparoscopic major liver resection. J Hepatobiliary Pancreat Sci. 2013;20(2):131–6.
15. Brown KM, Geller DA. What is the learning curve for laparoscopic major hepatectomy? J Gastrointest Surg. 2016;20(5):1065–71.
16. Vigano L, Laurent A, Tayar C, Tomatis M, Ponti A, Cherqui D. The learning curve in laparoscopic liver resection: improved feasibility and reproducibility. Ann Surg. 2009;250(5):772–82.
17. Nomi T, Fuks D, Kawaguchi Y, Mal F, Nakajima Y, Gayet B. Learning curve for laparoscopic major hepatectomy. Br J Surg. 2015;102(7):796–804.
18. Hanly EJ, Talamini MA. Robotic abdominal surgery. Am J Surg. 2004;188(4A Suppl):19S–26S.
19. Tomulescu V, Stanciulea O, Balescu I, Vasile S, Tudor S, Gheorghe C, et al. First year experience of robotic-assisted laparoscopic surgery with 153 cases in a general surgery department: indications, technique and results. Chirurgia (Bucur). 2009;104(2):141–50.
20. Giulianotti PC, Coratti A, Angelini M, Sbrana F, Cecconi S, Balestracci T, et al. Robotics in general surgery: personal experience in a large community hospital. Arch Surg. 2003;138(7):777–84.
21. Wu YM, Hu RH, Lai HS, Lee PH. Robotic-assisted minimally invasive liver resection. Asian J Surg. 2014;37(2):53–7.
22. Lai EC, Yang GP, Tang CN. Robot-assisted laparoscopic liver resection for hepatocellular carcinoma: short-term outcome. Am J Surg. 2013;205(6):697–702.
23. Packiam V, Bartlett DL, Tohme S, Reddy S, Marsh JW, Geller DA, et al. Minimally invasive liver resection: robotic versus laparoscopic left lateral sectionectomy. J Gastrointest Surg. 2012;16(12):2233–8.
24. Tsung A, Geller DA, Sukato DC, Sabbaghian S, Tohme S, Steel J, et al. Robotic versus laparoscopic hepatectomy: a matched comparison. Ann Surg. 2014;259(3):549–55.
25. Berber E, Akyildiz HY, Aucejo F, Gunasekaran G, Chalikonda S, Fung J. Robotic versus laparoscopic resection of liver tumours. HPB (Oxford). 2010;12(8):583–6.
26. Casciola L, Patriti A, Ceccarelli G, Bartoli A, Ceribelli C, Spaziani A. Robot-assisted parenchymal-sparing liver surgery including lesions located in the posterosuperior segments. Surg Endosc. 2011;25(12):3815–24.
27. Chan OC, Tang CN, Lai EC, Yang GP, Li MK. Robotic hepatobiliary and pancreatic surgery: a cohort study. J Hepatobiliary Pancreat Sci. 2011;18(4):471–80.
28. Choi GH, Choi SH, Kim SH, Hwang HK, Kang CM, Choi JS, et al. Robotic liver resection: technique and results of 30 consecutive procedures. Surg Endosc. 2012;26(8):2247–58.
29. Giulianotti PC, Coratti A, Sbrana F, Addeo P, Bianco FM, Buchs NC, et al. Robotic liver surgery: results for 70 resections. Surgery. 2011;149(1):29–39.
30. Ji WB, Wang HG, Zhao ZM, Duan WD, Lu F, Dong JH. Robotic-assisted laparoscopic anatomic hepatectomy in China: initial experience. Ann Surg. 2011;253(2):342–8.
31. Spampinato MG, Coratti A, Bianco L, Caniglia F, Laurenzi A, Puleo F, et al. Perioperative outcomes of laparoscopic and robot-assisted major hepatectomies: an Italian multi-institutional comparative study. Surg Endosc. 2014;28(10):2973–9.
32. Tranchart H, Ceribelli C, Ferretti S, Dagher I, Patriti A. Traditional versus robot-assisted full laparoscopic liver resection: a matched-pair comparative study. World J Surg. 2014;38(11):2904–9.
33. Troisi RI, Patriti A, Montalti R, Casciola L. Robot assistance in liver surgery: a real advantage over a fully laparoscopic approach? Results of a comparative bi-institutional analysis. Int J Med Robot. 2013;9(2):160–6.
34. Yu YD, Kim KH, Jung DH, Namkoong JM, Yoon SY, Jung SW, et al. Robotic versus laparoscopic liver resection: a comparative study from a single center. Langenbeck's Arch Surg. 2014;399(8):1039–45.
35. Croner RS, Perrakis A, Hohenberger W, Brunner M. Robotic liver surgery for minor hepatic resections: a comparison with laparoscopic and open standard procedures. Langenbeck's Arch Surg. 2016;401(5):707–14.
36. Kingham TP, Leung U, Kuk D, Gonen M, D'Angelica MI, Allen PJ, et al. Robotic liver resection: a case-matched comparison. World J Surg. 2016;40(6):1422–8.
37. Lee KF, Cheung YS, Chong CC, Wong J, Fong AK, Lai PB. Laparoscopic and robotic hepatectomy: experience from a single centre. ANZ J Surg. 2016;86(3):122–6.
38. Montalti R, Scuderi V, Patriti A, Vivarelli M, Troisi RI. Robotic versus laparoscopic resections of posterosuperior segments of the liver: a propensity score-matched comparison. Surg Endosc. 2016;30(3):1004–13.
39. Kim YS, Kim MJ, Park SC, Sohn DK, Kim DY, Chang HJ, et al. Robotic versus laparoscopic surgery for rectal cancer after preoperative chemoradiotherapy: case-matched study of short-term outcomes. Cancer Res Treat. 2016;48(1):225–31.
40. Nota CL, Rinkes IH, Molenaar IQ, van Santvoort HC, Fong Y, Hagendoorn J. Robot-assisted laparoscopic liver resection: a systematic review and pooled

analysis of minor and major hepatectomies. HPB (Oxford). 2016;18(2):113–20.
41. Montalti R, Berardi G, Patriti A, Vivarelli M, Troisi RI. Outcomes of robotic vs laparoscopic hepatectomy: a systematic review and meta-analysis. World J Gastroenterol. 2015;21(27):8441–51.
42. Qiu J, Chen S, Chengyou D. A systematic review of robotic-assisted liver resection and meta-analysis of robotic versus laparoscopic hepatectomy for hepatic neoplasms. Surg Endosc. 2016;30(3):862–75.
43. Jackson NR, Hauch A, Hu T, Buell JF, Slakey DP, Kandil E. The safety and efficacy of approaches to liver resection: a meta-analysis. JSLS. 2015;19(1): e2014.00186.
44. Amodeo A, Linares Quevedo A, Joseph JV, Belgrano E, Patel HR. Robotic laparoscopic surgery: cost and training. Minerva Urol Nefrol. 2009;61(2):121–8.
45. Patel HR, Linares A, Joseph JV. Robotic and laparoscopic surgery: cost and training. Surg Oncol. 2009;18(3):242–6.
46. Sham JG, Richards MK, Seo YD, Pillarisetty VG, Yeung RS, Park JO. Efficacy and cost of robotic hepatectomy: is the robot cost-prohibitive? J Robot Surg. 2016;10(4):307–13.
47. King JC, Zeh 3rd HJ, Zureikat AH, Celebrezze J, Holtzman MP, Stang ML, et al. Safety in numbers: progressive implementation of a robotics program in an academic surgical oncology practice. Surg Innov. 2016;23(4):407–14.
48. Garritano S, Selvaggi F, Spampinato MG. Simultaneous minimally invasive treatment of colorectal neoplasm with synchronous liver metastasis. Biomed Res Int. 2016;2016:9328250.
49. Xu JM, Wei Y, Wang XY, Fan H, Chang WJ, Ren L, et al. Robot-assisted one-stage resection of rectal cancer with liver and lung metastases. World J Gastroenterol. 2015;21(9):2848–53.
50. Ocuin LM, Tsung A. Robotic liver resection for malignancy: current status, oncologic outcomes, comparison to laparoscopy, and future applications. J Surg Oncol. 2015;112(3):295–301.
51. Xu Y, Wang H, Ji W, Tang M, Li H, Leng J, et al. Robotic radical resection for hilar cholangiocarcinoma: perioperative and long-term outcomes of an initial series. Surg Endosc. 2016;30(7):3060–70.
52. Vicente E, Quijano Y, Ielpo B, Fabra I. First ALPPS procedure using a total robotic approach. Surg Oncol. 2016;25(4):457.
53. Bonapasta SA, Bartolini I, Checcacci P, Guerra F, Coratti A. Indications for liver surgery: laparoscopic or robotic approach. Updat Surg. 2015;67(2):117–22.

Part VI

Spleen Malignancies

32 Minimally Invasive Splenectomy for Oncological Diseases of the Spleen

Julio Lopez Monclova, Carlos Rodriguez Luppi, and Eduardo Mª Targarona Soler

32.1 Introduction

Laparoscopic splenectomy (LS) has become the gold standard procedure for the treatment of benign hematological disorders not associated with splenomegaly, such as idiopathic thrombocytopenic purpura (ITP) [1, 2]. The great advances in minimally invasive surgery (MIS) that have been made over the last two decades did also benefit patients suffering from hematological malignant diseases However, this patients usually develop splenomegaly and the endoscopic manipulation of bulky organs is technically more challenging, and retrieval of the specimen may prove difficult. Splenomegaly was initially considered a contraindication for LS, thus, many malignant hematological diseases which are associated with an enlarged spleen were traditionally reserved for open splenectomy (OS) with its associated increased morbidity. Improvements and refinement of LS techniques have resulted in the ability to remove an enlarged spleen using the laparoscopic approach and preserving all the advantages of the MIS [3–5].

Hematological malignancies rarely require major surgical interventions. When needed, major surgery in this setting typically involves either splenectomy, removal of an intra-abdominal or retroperitoneal mass, or lymph node sampling for staging.

The advantages of MIS for cancer treatment are widely accepted these days. It should be kept in mind that patients requiring splenectomy are usually elderly and frail, so a less invasive approach to their treatment may be an advantage.

32.2 Overview of Primary Hematological Malignancies

32.2.1 Hodgkin's Lymphoma

Hodgkin's lymphoma (HL) is a curable malignancy that shows a bimodal curve in incidence in economically developed countries; there is a

Electronic Supplementary Material The online version of this chapter (doi:10.1007/978-3-319-54301-7_32) contains supplementary material, which is available to authorized users. On http://springerlink.com enter the DOI number given above.

J.L. Monclova (✉)
Universidad Autónoma de Barcelona, Servicio de Cirugía General y del Aparato Digestivo, Hospital de la Santa Creu i Santpau, P Claret 167, 08025 Barcelona, Spain

Mexican Institute for Social Security, HGZ 11, Delicias, Mexico

C.R. Luppi • E.Mª. Targarona Soler
Universidad Autónoma de Barcelona, Servicio de Cirugía General y del Aparato Digestivo, Hospital de la Santa Creu i Santpau, P Claret 167, 08025 Barcelona, Spain
e-mail: emtargarona@gmail.com; ETargarona@santpau.cat

M.A. Cuesta (ed.), *Minimally Invasive Surgery for Upper Abdominal Cancer*, DOI 10.1007/978-3-319-54301-7_32

putative association with Epstein–Barr virus. The incidence of HD in European countries is about 2.2/100,000/year. The World Health Organization 2008 classification schema recognizes two histological types of HL: the nodular lymphocyte predominant and the "classic" HL. The latter encompasses four entities: nodular sclerosis, mixed cellularity, lymphocyte depletion, and lymphocyte-rich [6]. Most patients with HL present with asymptomatic superficial lymphadenopathy. The most common sites of disease are the cervical, supraclavicular and mediastinal lymph nodes, while sub-diaphragmatic, bone marrow, and hepatic involvement are less common. Splenic involvement is usually concomitant with hepatic disease and systemic symptoms; extranodal presentations are quite rare. Systemic symptoms are present in ~35% of cases. The stage of disease is defined according to the Ann Arbor staging system or its Cotswolds variant, and staging work-up includes physical examination, chest X-rays, chest and abdominal CT scan, and bone marrow biopsy. 18FDG-PET (18fluordeoxyglucose positron emission tomography) plays a central role in staging, response assessment and prognosis definition [7]. The choice of chemotherapeutic regimen combined with radiation therapy of 30–36 Gy depends on the clinical stage. ABVD, using a combination of four drugs (**A**driamycin, **B**leomycin, **V**inblastine, **D**acarbazine), or BEACOPP for advanced stage, (**B**leomycin, **E**toposide, **A**driamycin, **C**yclophosphamide, Vincristin = **O**ncovine, **P**rocarbazine, **P**rednisone), are the two regimens most commonly used. Treatment for relapsing disease includes different drug combinations. Autologous stem cell transplantation after high-dose chemotherapy may be considered [8].

In our center, 439 patients underwent LS over a period of 23 years and malignancy was found in 126 patients (29%) (Table 32.1). LS was performed in eight patients suffering from HL (7.4%). These patients were younger, and the size of the spleen was generally normal. Indications for LS in this setting are clinical suspicion of lymphoma without evidence of peripheral disease, or patients requiring re-staging after completion of chemotherapy due to suspicion of residual disease on conventional imaging or PET-CT.

Table 32.1 Peri operative outcome after LS for malignancy, stratified by diagnosis (Authors' personal experience)

Malignant	126	28.7%	126 de 439
NHLs (non-Hodgkin lymphomas)	73	16.6%	
CLL (chronic lymphoid leukemia)	9	2.1%	
Hodgkin lymphoma	8	1.8%	
Myelofibrosis	8	1.8%	
Metastases	6	1.4%	
Hairy cell leukemia	4	0.9%	
CML (chronic myeloid leukemia)	4	0.9%	
Primary splenic lymphoma	2	0.5%	
Others	12	2.7%	

32.2.2 Non-Hodgkin's Lymphoma

Non-Hodgkin's lymphoma (NHL) is a group of lymphoid malignancies that rank fifth in cancer incidence and mortality in most countries. The incidence increased by 80% over the last 30 years. NHL presents as an indolent disease, mainly nodular or follicular variant or highly aggressive disease. B-cell lymphomas are more common than T-cell types. The most common B-cell lymphoma types are: Diffuse large B-cell (31%) and Follicular lymphomas (22%). Less common variants are: MALT lymphoma (8%), Peripheral T-cell (7%), Mantle cell lymphomas (6.9%), Chronic lymphocytic leukemia (5.5%) and other types (3%).

Conventional treatment is based on the natural history of the disease, and ranges from a "watch-and-see policy," to radiation therapy alone, chemotherapy alone or chemoradiation therapy. Single-agent alkylation therapy and the CVP regimen (**C**yclophosphamide, **V**incristine, and **P**rednisone) are the mainstay treatments available for low-grade NHL. High-intensity therapy usually involves the CHOP regimen (Doxorubicin, Cyclophosphamide, Vincristine and Prednisone and Fludarabine). Treatment for relapsing disease after first line therapy includes a number of drug combinations. In the setting of relapsing disease, the 5-year survival is reported to be below 50%. Monoclonal antibody treatment is currently in clinical trials and shows promising results as first line and salvage therapy. Initial results with Rituximab, a chimeric anti CD-20 monoclonal antibody, and Alemtuzumab, a CDR-grafted human IgG monoclonal antibody, have led to the development of new medications and alteration of current therapies. Both medications are directed against the CD52 antigens expressed in leukemic T lymphocytes, macrophages, and monocytes [9–11].

The most frequent indication for LS in our series was NHL (73/126, 60%). LS is only indicated in cases where a diagnosis cannot be established by obtaining peripheral tissue and the clinical suspicion remains, or when the patient experiences clinical symptoms related to massive splenomegaly or low platelet count. LS does not alter the natural history of the disease, but related thrombocytopenia may improve in up to 75% of patients. The patients with NHL were older when compared with patients undergoing LS for other indications. Enlargement of the spleen was moderate with a mean weight of 1200 g (range 140–6100 g) (Table 32.1).

Chronic lymphocytic leukemia (CLL) was diagnosed in 9 of 126 cases (7%), and splenomegaly was moderate with a spleen weight of 1094 g (range 440–2952 g). In our practice, LS was mainly indicated to treat cytopenias, massive spleen enlargement, or progressive splenomegaly refractory to medical treatment. Splenectomy did improve cytopenias in up to 90% of our patients. HALS was required in one patient and conversion in another.

32.2.3 Chronic Myeloid Leukemia

Chronic myeloid leukemia (CML) was one of the first hematological diseases to be linked to a chromosomal defect, the so-called Philadelphia chromosome. It is a rare disease with an incidence of 1–2/100,000/year. It is easily diagnosed by blood tests and confirmed by genetic analysis (Phi chromosome or BCR-ABL transcripts) of peripheral white blood cells or bone marrow. A number of hematological, cytogenetic and molecular markers can be used to predict a response to treatment or to identify a possible blast crisis. Treatment for CML has advanced considerably over the last 40 years due to improved understanding of the molecular and genetic basis of this disease. Treatment strategies evolved from using Hydroxyl Urea and Busulfan, to stem cell transplantation, alpha Interferon, and more recently to molecular targeted therapies such as the tyrosine kinase inhibitor Imatinib. Current treatment protocols for chronic disease generally include Imatinib or allogenic stem cell transplantation. The selection of any of those therapies will depend on the existence of clinical predictors of blast crisis or the individual risk factors for stem cell transplantation. Novel therapies under development include additional tyrosine kinase inhibitors (Dasatinib or Nilotinib), immunotherapy with vaccines (BCR-ABL peptide vaccine), and immunochemotherapy combining Imatinib and interferon [12, 13].

It was most common in males in their sixth decade of life. Splenomegaly develops in 55–70% of patients. The spleen is often massively enlarged with a median weight of 3675 g (range 3200–4500 g) (Fig. 32.1). If splenomegaly develops rapidly, it may be a predictor of a blast crisis.

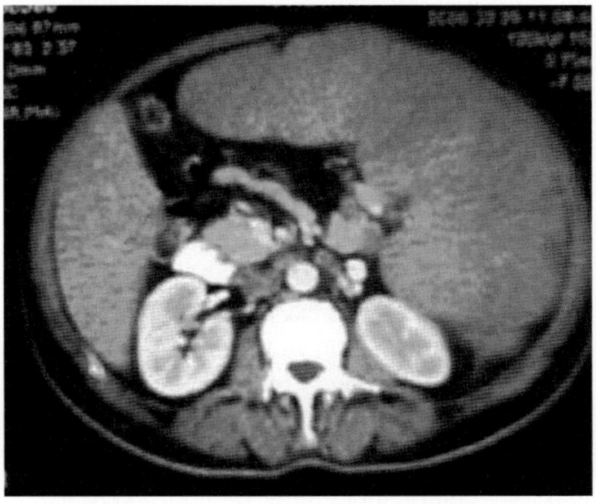

Fig. 32.1 CT scan of a patient with CML requiring splenectomy

CML was rarely an indication for LS. Splenectomy may be indicated in advanced disease and improves clinical symptoms in up to 15% of patients, but the risk to develop a blast crisis remains unchanged. Surgical risk in this subgroup is high because of associated coagulation disorders and platelet malfunction.

32.2.4 Myelofibrosis

Myeloid metaplasia with myelofibrosis is a chronic myeloproliferative disorder characterized by anemia, massive splenomegaly, extramedullar hepatosplenic hematopoiesis, stromal bone marrow reactions including fibrosis, osteosclerosis and angiogenesis.

Median survival is 5 years, ranging from 2 to 12 years, depending on the clinically defined prognostic factors. Clinical symptoms include portal hypertension, pulmonary hypertension, and leukemic changes and these patients often require blood transfusions. The only curative therapy is allogeneic bone marrow transplantation in younger, high-risk patients. Supportive therapy for clinically symptomatic anemia includes steroids, Danazol, EPO, Thalidomide, or a blood trans-fusion. In the event of splenomegaly Hydroxyl-urea, Busulfan, interferon, or surgery will be therapeutic options. Leukemic changes are associated with a grim prognosis. Evolving therapies include VEGF receptor inhibitors or a combination of therapies including Thalidomide or Etanercept [14, 15].

The third most frequent indication in our series was myelofibrosis (8/126, 11%), a malignant condition without definitive cure. The spleen, in this particular subgroup, was greatly enlarged with a median weight of 2700 g (range 300–3300 g). It is characterized by bone marrow fibrosis, pancytopenia, extramedullar hematopoiesis and hepatosplenomegaly and associated with massive spleen enlargement, requiring repeat transfusions. Surgery is mainly performed to palliate symptoms but is also indicated in cases of massive enlargement and portal hypertension, and to reduce transfusion requirements. The completion rate of LS was 87%. HALS was necessary in 50% of the patients. A well-known potential risk of LS, especially in this subgroup of patients, is development of postoperative portal vein thrombosis.

32.3 Primary Malignancies of the Spleen

Primary malignant tumors of the spleen are rare and include primary splenic lymphoma, angiosarcoma and Malignant fibrous histiocytoma.

Local symptoms are very unspecific. Currently available imaging techniques demonstrate only indirect signs. Surgery is usually warranted to confirm the diagnosis and will be performed with curative intent. Therapeutic LS may also be beneficial to patients in cases of a primary spleen lymphoma or splenic marginal zone lymphoma. A primary splenic lymphoma is a rare disorder and seen in less than 1% of NHL in our series.

32.4 Secondary Malignancies of the Spleen

The spleen is the second largest reticulum-endothelial organ. It is composed by large amounts of monocytes, synthesizes immunoglobulin and opsonins, and has a very efficient phagocytic activity, all of which seems to represent protection factors against malignant cell implantation and proliferation, and maybe these anatomic and immunologic features of the spleen account for the rather rare incidence of metastases to the spleen [16]. The most common primary cancers metastasizing to the spleen are: Melanoma, Breast, Lung, Colon, and Ovarian cancer. Splenectomy may be an option, if the spleen is the only site of disease and the primary tumor should have already been resected and well controlled. Therefore, surgery is planned with curative intent [17, 18].

Splenic metastases were found in 6/126 cases (4%). Metastases to the spleen are usually a sign of systemic disease and therefore rarely an indication for surgery [16]. Splenectomy may be performed, if it can be proven that the spleen is the

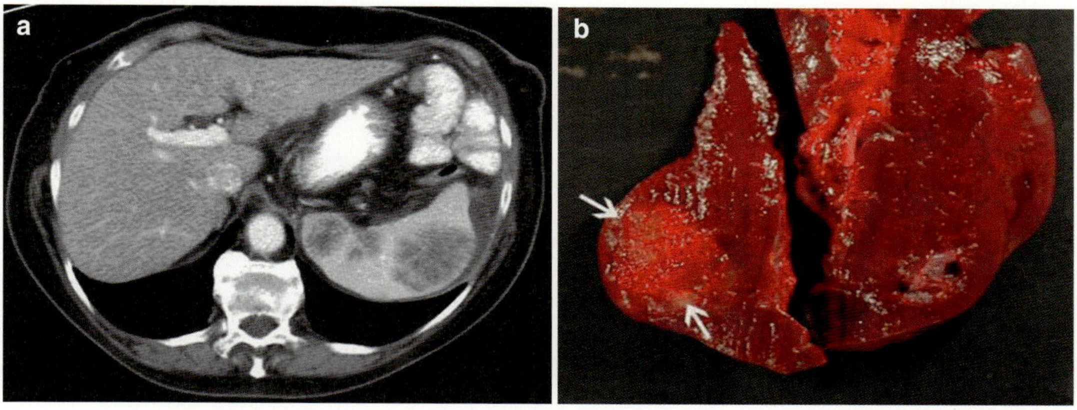

Fig. 32.2 Secondary splenic malignancy: Splenic metastasis from colon cancer. (**a**) CT scan, (**b**) macroscopic appearance

sole site of cancer spread. The six cases we treated included four patients with melanoma, one patient with sarcoma and one with colon cancer metastatic to the spleen (Fig. 32.2). Spleen enlargement was not excessive, and all six patients had an uneventful perioperative and postoperative outcome.

32.5 Surgical Approach to the Spleen

32.5.1 Indications for Splenectomy

LS is indicated in a variety of clinical situations, either for diagnostic, therapeutic, palliative, or staging purposes (Table 32.2).

32.5.2 Preoperative Evaluation

Patients undergoing elective LS for malignancy require careful preoperative evaluation. A thorough physical examination may enable the surgeon to get a rough estimate of the size of the spleen. Normal-sized spleens are usually not palpated below the costal margin. It is usually possible to palpate the lower pole of the spleen in the left upper quadrant of the abdomen in patients with moderate splenomegaly. Massive splenomegaly with spleen diameter ≥30 cm may occupy the entire abdominal cavity. Important findings during the abdominal exam includes mobility of the spleen and distensibility of the abdominal wall, both of which are important when planning the laparoscopic approach in order to assess the projection of the lower pole of the spleen towards the midline. All these pre-operatively collected data will determine if the laparoscopic approach is feasible or not, will help determine the best patient positioning on the operating table (supine, semi-supine or lateral), and guide the placement of a hand-assisted device, if needed. Preoperative blood transfusion should be considered depending on the results of blood tests, taking into account that an enlarged spleen pools a significant amount of blood. Coagulation profile is obtained, and the patient typed and cross-matched should the need for transfusion of the blood derivatives required perioperatively. All our patients get a polyvalent pneumococcal, meningococcal, and hemophilus vaccine in the preoperative period.

32.5.3 Preoperative Imaging

A preoperative computer tomogram (CT) or ultrasound (US) is recommended to evaluate the size and shape of the spleen. The shape of the spleen will influence operative planning and surgical strategy. Postoperative outcome is directly related to the shape of the spleen.

Table 32.2 Own experience with LS for splenic malignancies

	Hodgkin	Non-Hodgkin	CLL	CML	Myelofibrosis	Metastases
n	8	73	9	4	8	6
Age (years)	38 (27–49)	63 (32–84)	59 (40–72)	43 (22–54)	57 (48–72)	59 (25–81)
Spleen weight (g)	508 (250–1160)	1460 (140–6100)	1317 (410–2950)	3760 (3200–4500)	2296 (360–3300)	416 (162–640)
OR time (min)	101 (60–120)	129 (60–270)	140 (60–270)	180 (150–240)	188 (110–270)	144 (60–240)
HALS (n/%)	1 (12.5%)	33 (45.2%)	3 (33.3%)	3 (75%)	4 (50%)	0%
Conversion (n/%)	0%	11 (15.1%)	0%	1 (25%)	1 (12.5%)	1 (16.6%)
Morbidity (n/%)	2 (25%)	15 (20.6%)	2 (22.2%)	4 (100%)	4 (50%)	1 (16.6%)
Hospital stay (days)	5 (2–11)	6 (2–30)	5 (3–10)	15 (4–24)	9 (3–29)	4 (2–11)
Mortality (n/%)	0%	1 (1.4%)	0%	0%	1 (12.5%)	0%

CLL chronic lymphocytic leukemia, *CML* chronic myeloid leukemia

32.5.4 The Role of Preoperative Splenic Artery Embolization

Preoperative splenic artery embolization (SAE) has been considered to facilitate any splenectomy, not only laparoscopic splenectomy and serves three major purposes: to occlude terminal vascular branches, to diminish the risk of intraoperative bleeding and to reduce the spleen size.

Is considered that patients who underwent SAE showed 10% less intraoperative blood loss and subsequently a lower rate of emergency blood transfusions. However, SAE may be associated with other complications such as pain, hemorrhage, and hepatic or splenic abscesses. Preoperative SAE is not routinely recommended for LS but may play a role in spleens larger than 25 cm in maximum dimension [19].

32.5.5 Preoperative Platelet Transfusion

Although it was traditionally thought that severe coagulation alterations or platelet counts $<50 \times 10^9$/L were absolute contraindications for LS, several authors have found that platelet counts $<50 \times 10^9$/L, and even as low as 10×10^9/L, do not impede the performance of a safe LS. Moreover, LS carried out with platelet counts between 10 and 50×10^9/L did not differ in terms of blood loss, operative time or postoperative complications as compared with the outcomes of LS with platelet counts $>50 \times 10^9$/L. However, platelet counts $<10 \times 10^9$/L had an important impact on perioperative outcome, with significantly greater intraoperative blood loss, longer operative time and prolonged hospital stay [20].

32.5.6 Preoperative Risk Calculation

Currently, little information is available regarding the grade of technical difficulty in performing LS for non-traumatic diseases. In order to predict the surgical difficulty and postoperative outcome for patients undergoing LS for hematological/oncological disorders, we developed a grading system based on preoperative parameters: age, gender, type of pathology, and spleen weight [21]. The minimum possible score is 2 and the maximum is 10. In this grading system, patients older than 60 years are given 2 points (maximum for age), patients with malignant diseases are given 2 points (maximum for type of pathology), and 5 points for patients whose spleen weight is >1000 g (maximum for weight). The bottom line is that patients undergoing LS for hematologic malignancies are usually older, frail, and their malignancy is often associated with splenomegaly, thus a more difficult procedure and a troubled outcome may be expected in this setting, according to the preoperative grading system.

32.5.7 Essential Equipment for LS

LS does not require any special equipment. The use of two video monitors is recommended and improves surgeon's comfort and efficiency (Videos 32.1 and 32.2). We routinely use a set of three to four trocars. Our preference lies on an angled 30° laparoscope, which is often repositioned depending on the step of the procedure to improve visualization. Most grasping, dissecting, and cutting instruments are 5 mm in diameter. It is not uncommon, particularly for large spleens, that 10-mm instruments are required to facilitate retraction.

To seal and divide vessels, a combination of clip appliers, endovascular stapling devices, monopolar, and bipolar cautery is used. The harmonic scalpel is also a very useful device to dissect the spleen. Endovascular staplers are very useful, particularly in controlling the splenic hilum. Clips should only be placed in areas where no stapler is to be needed because as they will prevent proper closure and thus malfunctioning of the stapling device. A durable specimen retrieval bag is key equipment for LS. It has to be able to withstand the morcellation process prior to specimen extraction.

32.6 Surgical Technique

Antibiotic prophylaxis is given preoperatively. LS is always performed under general anesthesia. An oral gastric tube (OGT) is inserted to empty the stomach, which will greatly improve the visualization in the left upper quadrant. We remove the OGT upon completion of surgery. A Foley catheter should also be placed due to the length of the procedure.

32.6.1 Patient Positioning

Since LS was first described, several techniques and ways to position the patient have been reported; all aimed at best controlling the hilar vessels. The most difficult part of the procedure is the mobilization of the spleen toward the midline. Patient positioning on the operating table will depend on surgeon's preference and on the size of the spleen. The patient can be placed in a low lithotomy position and further tilted laterally to elevate the left upper abdomen. The lateral tilt may be increased to 45°, if necessary. Some surgeons prefer to start the procedure in the French position and then moving to the side, if needed. Currently the most accepted position is full lateral at 90°. We prefer the 90° full lateral approach in cases of a normal-sized spleen or moderate splenomegaly. A supine or semi-lateral position is deemed more suitable in cases of massive splenomegaly or when the median border of the spleen crosses the midline when palpated preoperatively (Fig. 32.3).

32.6.2 Anterior Approach

The patient is placed supine or in Fowler position according to surgeon's preference. A sand bag is placed underneath the left upper quadrant. After establishing the pneumoperitoneum, the

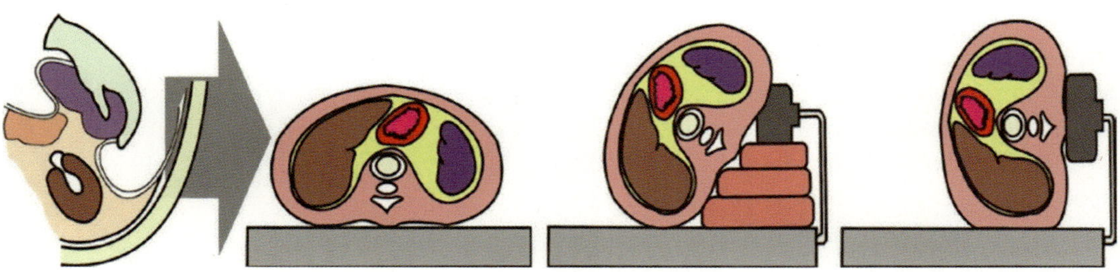

Fig. 32.3 Progressive lateral approach for LS: The spleen can be mobilized with lateral tilt taking advantage of gravity

first trocar is inserted at the umbilicus and an exploratory laparoscopy is performed. Three more trocars are inserted, one in the subxiphoid area, one in the midepigastrium, and the last one in the left iliac fossa. The scope is introduced through the midepigastric trocar. The subxiphoid trocar and umbilical port are used for grasping and dissecting instruments. The table is then tilted to the right and brought into reverse Trendelenburg position. The lesser sac is opened, and the short gastric vessels are divided with the harmonic scalpel or bipolar cautery.

Several techniques to dissect the splenic hilum are described in the literature. The splenic vessels can either be controlled at their main trunk or a segmental devascularization near the splenic parenchyma may be performed. The remaining short gastric vessels are divided with the harmonic scalpel after division of the main splenic vessels. Close attention must be paid not to injure the pancreas by carefully dissecting off the main vessels. Takedown of the splenic flexure gives access to the posterior attachments of the spleen, which may be divided using harmonic scalpel.

32.6.3 Lateral Approach

The patient is placed in right lateral decubitus position on the operating table. The table is flexed 20°–30° and brought into moderate reverse Trendelenburg position. This maximizes the window of access between the patient's left iliac crest and the costal margin. Three to four trocars are then inserted in the patient's left upper abdominal quadrant. A 12-mm port is inserted at the anterior axillary line, above the anterior superior iliac spine and is used for the endovascular stapler and final specimen removal. In pediatric and non-obese patients, we place the camera port at the level of the umbilicus. In obese patients, it is often necessary to move this site to the left upper quadrant. Subcostal and subxyphoid trocars are used for retraction and dissection. Finally, a 2- to 5-mm trocar is placed under direct vision below the 12th rib at the mid- to post-axillary line. This trocar is used to retract and elevate the lower pole of the spleen.

Dissection starts with mobilization of the splenic flexure of the colon using a combination of sharp dissection and ultrasonic energy. The lateral peritoneal attachments of the spleen are incised as a second step. A cuff of peritoneum is left alongside the spleen for further safe mobilization. This maneuver avoids grabbing the spleen directly and greatly reduces the risk of splenic tears. Dissection of the splenic hilum starts from the lower pole and progresses cephalad. An accessory splenic artery is sometimes encountered at the lower pole and should be divided between clips or with the harmonic scalpel.

After mobilization of the lower pole of the spleen and division of the polar vessels, it is possible to access the lesser sac with ease. With the spleen elevated, the short gastric vessels and main vascular pedicle are tented up. The short gastric vessels can be divided either with the harmonic scalpel, between clips, or using an endovascular stapler. The tail of the pancreas is often visible at this point of the dissection. Once the vascular pedicle is well exposed and the main artery and vein dissected off of the pancreas, they are divided by two separate firings of the endovascular stapler (white loads) (Fig. 32.4).

It is important to point out a few technical aspects concerning approach to the splenic vessels. Prior to mobilization of the spleen, we rou-

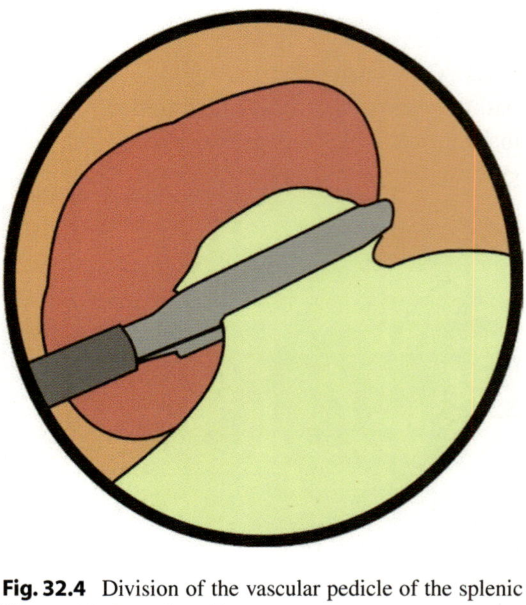

Fig. 32.4 Division of the vascular pedicle of the splenic hilum with the endostapler

tinely attempt to ligate the artery within the lesser sac in order to reduce spleen size, facilitate auto-transfusion, and decrease the risk of hemorrhage. The full lateral approach is especially useful to identify the splenic pedicle. We prefer to transect the hilar vessels with an endostapler, thus avoiding excessive intra-operative hemorrhage. In cases of non-Hodgkin lymphomas it is often possible to encounter large lymph nodes in the hilum, which makes it more difficult to identify the vascular structures. In this case, the endostapler is fired near the hilum, leaving the lymph nodes behind, avoiding unnecessary dissection and the risk of bleeding.

32.6.4 Extraction of the Specimen

After the splenic hilar and short gastric vessels are divided, the uppermost part of the splenophrenic ligament is left undivided. This serves to hold the spleen in its normal anatomic position and facilitates introduction into the retrieval bag. The specimen retrieval bag is introduced, opened, and placed under the relatively immobile spleen. The remaining splenophrenic attachments are now divided and the bag closed. The neck of the bag is withdrawn through the 12-mm trocar site and the spleen is morcellated within the bag and extracted in pieces. Careful attention is needed to insure not to rupture the bag and to avoid spillage and subsequent splenosis. Once the entire specimen and bag are withdrawn, we perform a final laparoscopic inspection of the left upper abdomen and irrigate the surgical field with normal saline. If the spleen has to be extracted intact, an accessory incision is made by enlarging the umbilical trocar site, or through a separate Pfannenstiel incision.

32.6.5 Hand-Assisted Laparoscopic Splenectomy (HALS)

LS is challenging when spleen size is significantly increased. In some cases the size of the spleen does not allow enough intra-abdominal space for manipulation and elevation of the organ, and conversion is unavoidable. HALS may be justified when an accessory incision is needed to retrieve an intact organ or when there are major difficulties in placing the spleen into the retrieval bag. Several non-randomized series have shown the potential advantages of HALS for splenectomy in cases of splenomegaly [22, 23].

The main indication for a hand-assisted laparoscopic splenectomy (HALS) procedure is a patient with massive splenomegaly [22]. Position of choice is right lateral decubitus (Fig. 32.5a). Pneumoperitoneum is created using a Veress needle inserted into the right iliac fossa, a good distance away from the spleen. A 12-mm camera port is inserted in the periumbilical area to perform an exploratory laparoscopy and to select the best site for the hand-port, which usually requires an incision of 7–7.5 cm in length. The most common site is the right epigastrium (Fig. 32.5b), but in cases of massive splenomegaly, it may be placed in the right subcostal area or in the right iliac fossa. Several devices are commercially available (Lapdisc™, Ethicon, USA; Omniport™, Advanced Surgical Concepts Ltd., Dublin, Ireland; Handport™, Smith Nephew, MA, USA). The left hand is inserted into the abdomen to examine the shape of the spleen and surrounding anatomy. A second 12-mm trocar is inserted laterally to the laparoscope port under guidance of the intra-abdominal hand. All further instruments are introduced through this trocar (Fig. 32.5b). If additional retraction is needed, a 5-mm trocar is placed at the left flank and an endoretractor (Endoflex™, Genzyme, Tucker, GA, USA) is inserted to expose the anterior aspect of the spleen.

As a first step in the procedure, we incise the gastro-splenic ligament to gain access to the retro-gastric plane. The opening of the lesser sac is widened, and the short gastric vessels are divided with the ultrasonic shears (Ultracision™, Ethicon, USA) or Ligasure™ (Valley lab, USA). The splenic artery is directly palpated at the upper border of the pancreas, and a ligature or clip is placed to interrupt the inflow to the spleen. With the hand in place, we mobilize the spleen medially to expose its

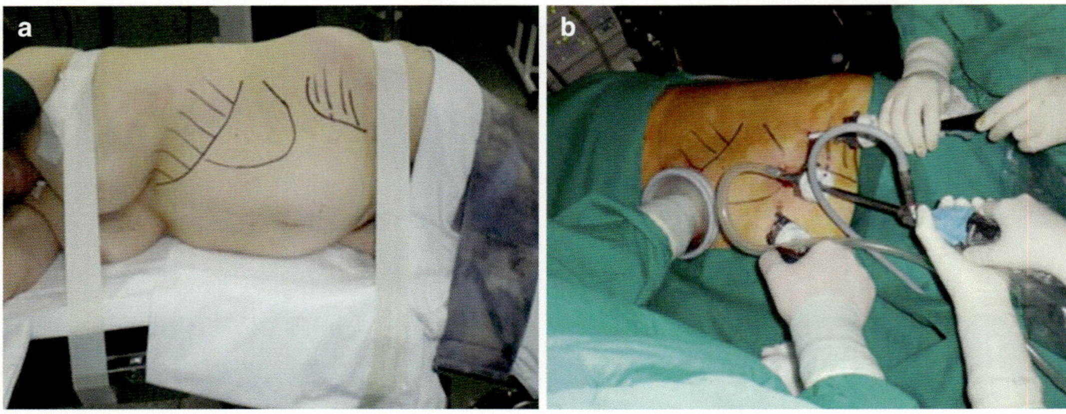

Fig. 32.5 HALS: full lateral approach, intermediate splenomegaly: (**a**) Patient positioning (**b**) trocar placement

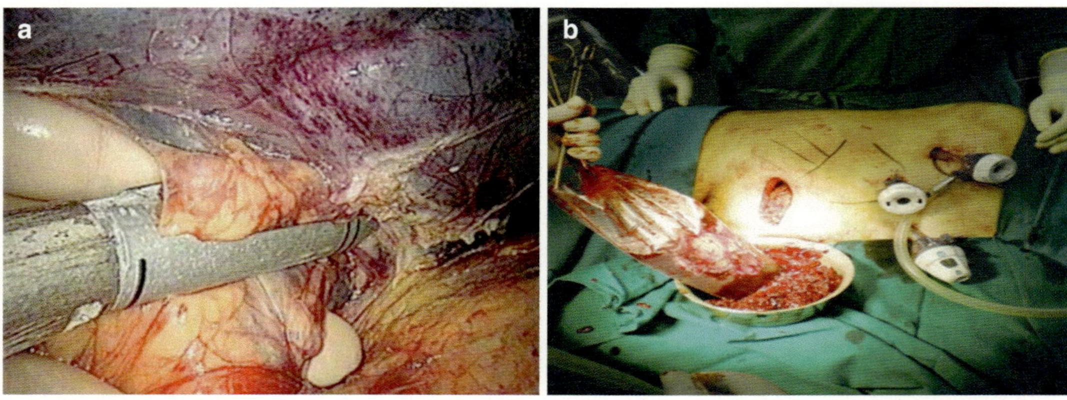

Fig. 32.6 HALS. (**a**) Dissection of the splenic hilum; the inserted hand guides the endostapling device; (**b**) Specimen extraction

posterior aspect and divide the retroperitoneal adhesions. The splenic hilum and pancreatic tail are bluntly dissected with the hand. This way, we are able to place the stapling device in the splenic hilum so that it can be fired without tension and the pancreatic tail is spared (Fig. 32.6a). Once the hilar vessels are divided, we dissect the upper pole from all posterior attachments which frees the spleen entirely. In most cases, the spleen is retrieved intact through the accessory incision. However, in cases of massive splenomegaly, a sterile plastic bag (Endocatch II™, Tyco, (Norwalk, USA)) is introduced and the spleen morcellated. The larger pieces are removed through the 7-cm incision (Fig. 32.6b).

In our experience (Table 32.2), the main advantages of HALS were shorter operative time and lower operative blood loss. One interesting observation in the HALS group is that overall morbidity was lower when compared to conventional LS. This indicates that surgical trauma during HALS is less significant and potential advantages of a laparoscopic approach are maintained despite more intense intra-abdominal manipulation. In this way, the use of HALS may be indicated in many splenic malignancies (Table 32.3).

Table 32.3 Summary of the role of LS in the management of hematological malignancies

Indication	Clinical situation	Comment
Diagnosis	Cases of moderate splenomegaly suggesting malignancy, specially if all other diagnostic studies, such as biopsy of peripheral lymph node or bone marrow biopsy are negative.	Radiological imaging does usually not allow narrowing the spectrum of differential diagnoses.
Therapeutics	• Primary splenic lymphoma.	• LS may be curative in cases of splenic lymphoma.
	• Splenomegaly-associated thrombocytopenia.	• LS can reduce transfusion needs, thus increasing quality of life.
	• Autoimmune thrombocytopenia	• LS is specially useful in the setting of CLL-associated thrombocytopenia.
Palliative	Symptomatic splenomegaly:	To relieve symptoms secondary to massive enlargement of the spleen (e.g. pain in left upper quadrant, fullness, fatigue, easy bleeding, etc.)
	• Acute myeloid leukemia	
	• Chronic myeloid leukemia	
	• Chronic myelomonocytic leukemia	
	• Myelofibrosis	
	• Non-Hodgkin's lymphoma	
Staging	Hodgkin's disease	LS is sometimes used to stage or re-stage Hodgkin's disease if noninvasive staging modalities are inconclusive

32.7 Complications Associated with LS

32.7.1 Bleeding

In cases of malignancy, there are several potential perioperative complications that the surgeon should be aware of and able to treat [24]. The most likely problem is bleeding, which is usually located at three distinct sites: (1) short gastric or polar vessels, (2) hilar vessels, or (3) splenic parenchyma.

Although not life-threatening, the first may be a considerable problem since rapidly accumulating blood may hinder adequate visualization of the operative field. In most of the cases, it can be easily stopped with clips, electrocautery, or ultrasonic dissector. Bleeding from larger vessels may require immediate conversion to laparotomy. The best way to prevent this complication is by carrying out a delicate dissection of the splenic artery and vein to avoid tearing of smaller splenic and pancreatic blood vessels. The dissected splenic artery and vein should then be clipped prior to attempting further mobilization of the spleen. Injury to these vessels can occur simply due to the rigidity of the clamping instruments. Bleeding from the parenchyma is less dangerous and can be managed either by clamping the artery, applying slight pressure with a gauze, or by using electrocautery.

32.7.2 Pancreatic Tail Injury

Another potential complication of LS is injury to the tail of the pancreas. This can be avoided by proper dissection and placement of the endostapler when dividing the hilar vessels. This may be cumbersome in cases of malignancy due to extensive surrounding lymphadenopathy. The lateral approach to LS allows placing the stapling device more safely thanks to a better exposure of the splenic hilum. Should pancreatic tail injury occur and is identified intraoperatively, it is wise to place a drain in the left upper abdominal quadrant close to the pancreatic tail in order to monitor and control any pancreatic leak.

32.7.3 Perforation of the Diaphragm

This could happen during dissection of the superior pole of the spleen. This lesion may worsen rapidly due to development of a capno-thorax. A capno-thorax is different from a pneumothorax in that the underlying cause is not an injury to the lung itself. It can be controlled in two ways: intraoperatively by sealing the opening of the diaphragm over a suction catheter, or postoperatively by temporary placement of a pleural drain. The pleural drain can then be removed in the OR after full lung expansion is confirmed on a chest X-ray.

32.7.4 Portal Vein Thrombosis

CT or ultrasonography in the immediate postoperative period suggests that the risk of portal thrombosis increases after LS, and this has been directly related to the laparoscopic approach [25, 26]. Prolonged intra-abdominal pressure is associated with markedly lower portal blood flow and may trigger this complication, especially in cases of massive splenomegaly and hypercoagulability. Although there are only a few cases reported in the literature, this complication should be taken into account in the event of unexplained postoperative abdominal pain after LS.

32.7.5 Miscellaneous Complications

Other complications reported with LS include: deep vein thrombosis, pulmonary embolus, wound infections, among others.

Conclusion

Splenectomy is a really good indication for minimally invasive approach, and the application of this technique in a more challenging subgroup of patients requiring splenectomy as are those with malignant conditions, permits to these patients more frail and usually with splenomegaly, to extraordinarily benefit of this surgical option.

References

1. Park A, Targarona EM, Trias M. Laparoscopic surgery of the spleen: state of the art. Langenbecks J Surg. 2001;386:230–9.
2. Habermalz B, Sauerland S, Decker G, et al. Laparoscopic splenectomy: the clinical practice guidelines of the European Association for Endoscopic Surgery (EAES). Surg Endosc. 2008;22:821–48.
3. Weiss 3rd CA, Kavic SM, Adrales GL, et al. Laparoscopic splenectomy: what barriers remain? Surg Innov. 2005;12:23–9.
4. Kaban GK, Czerniach DR, Cohen R, et al. Hand-assisted laparoscopic splenectomy in the setting of splenomegaly. Surg Endosc. 2004;18:1340–3.
5. Targarona EM, Balagué C, Trias M. Is the laparoscopic approach reasonable in cases of splenomegaly? Semin Laparosc Surg. 2004;11:185–90.
6. Kant JA, Hubbard SM, Longo DL, et al. The pathologic and clinical heterogeneity of lymphocyte-depleted Hodgkin lymphoma. J Clin Oncol. 1986;4:1419–20.
7. Moulin-Romsee G, Hindié E, Cuenca X, et al. (18)F FDG PET/CT bone/bone marrow findings in Hodgkin's lymphoma may circumvent the use of bone marrow thephine biopsy at diagnosis staging. Eur J Nucl Med Mol Imaging. 2010;37:1095–105.
8. Jost LM, Stahel RA, ESMO Guideline Task Force. ESMO minimal clinical recommendation for diagnosis, treatment and follow up of Hodgkin's disease. Ann Oncol. 2005;16:i54–5.
9. Multani P, White CA, Grillo A. Non-Hodgkin lymphoma: review of conventional treatments. Curr Pharm Biotechnol. 2001;2:279–91.
10. Palma M, Kokhaei P, Lundin J, et al. The biology and treatment of chronic lymphocytic leukemia. Ann Oncol. 2006;17:x144–54.
11. NCCN. Clinical practice guidelines in oncology™. Non-Hodgkin's Lymphoma. V.3.2007. www.nccn.org.
12. Hunter T. Treatment for chronic myelogenous leukemia: the long road to imatinib. J Clin Invest. 2007;117:2036–43.
13. Hehlmann R, Hochhaus A, Baccarani M. European leukemia net. Chronic myeloid leukaemia. Lancet. 2007;370:342–50.
14. Arana-Yi C, Quintás-Cardama A, Giles F, et al. Advances in the therapy of chronic idiopathic myelofibrosis. Oncologist. 2006;11:929–43.
15. Dingli D, Mesa RA, Tefferi A. Myelofibrosis with myeloid metaplasia: new developments in pathogenesis and treatment. Intern Med. 2004;43:540–7.

16. Lopez Monclova J, Targarona Soler E, Peraza Solis Y, et al. Laparoscopic approach for isolated splenic metastasis: comprehensive literature review and report of 6 cases. Surg Laparosc Endosc Percutan Tech. 2013;23:21–4.
17. Heniford T, Walsh M. Laparoscopic splenectomy for malignant diseases. In: Greene FL, Heniford B, editors. Minimally invasive cancer management. 1st ed. NY: Springer; 2001. p. 143–55.
18. Comperat E, Bardier-Dupas A, Camparo P, et al. Splenic metastases: clinicopathologic presentation, differential diagnosis, and pathogenesis. Arch Pathol Lab Med. 2007;131:965–9.
19. Iwase K, Higaki J, Yoon HE, et al. Splenic artery embolization using contour emboli before laparoscopic or laparoscopically assisted splenectomy. Surg Laparosc Endosc Percutan Tech. 2002;12:331–6.
20. Martin Arnau B, Turrado Rodriguez V, Tartaglia E, et al. Impact of preoperative platelet count on perioperative outcome after laparoscopic splenectomy for idiopathic thrombocytopenic purpura. Cir Esp. 2016;94:399–403.
21. Rodriguez-Otero Luppi C, Targarona Soler EM, Balague Ponz C, et al. Clinical, anatomical, and pathological grading score to predict technical difficulty in laparoscopic splenectomy for non-traumatic diseases. World J Surg. 2017,41:439–448, doi:10.1007/s00268-016-3683-y.
22. Targarona EM, Balagué C, Trias M. Hand-assisted laparoscopic splenectomy. Semin Laparosc Surg. 2001;8:126–34.
23. Targarona EM, Balague C, Cerdan G, et al. Hand-assisted laparoscopic splenectomy (HALS) in cases of splenomegaly: a comparison analysis with conventional laparoscopic splenectomy. Surg Endosc. 2002;16:426–30.
24. Targarona EM, Cerdan G, Trias M. Complications of laparoscopic splenectomy. Probl Gen Surg. 2002;19:72–9.
25. Ikeda M, Sekimoto M, Takiguchi S, et al. High incidence of thrombosis of the portal venous system after laparoscopic splenectomy: a prospective study with contrast-enhanced CT scan. Ann Surg. 2005;24:208–16.
26. Targarona EM. Portal vein thrombosis after laparoscopic splenectomy: the size of the risk. Surg Innov. 2008;15:266–70.

Part VII

How to Learn These Techniques?

33 Mastering Major Minimally Surgery

Miguel A. Cuesta, Nicole I. van der Wielen, Jennifer Straatman, and Donald L. van der Peet

New teaching programs in Minimally Invasive Surgery (MIS) require mentoring. We see that once a new MIS procedure has been validated by evidence, we can expect many surgical teams wanting to adopt the new procedure. The issue is how doing this according to best standards of practice is best learned. Commonly, the teaching programs in MIS may range from the institutionalized programs involved in the residency period to the quick one-or-two-days courses organized by Surgical Departments or companies targeting (young) surgeons desirous but still unable to operate by the new MIS approaches. While these opportunities offer interesting displays of new MIS, yet effective teaching programs in MIS developments are very variable and ad hoc.

Because of years of experience in teaching MIS, we argue that learning the new procedures could profit from proper assistance by an experienced team or particular a mentor. Given our experience as teacher mentor in Minimally invasive Esophageal and Gastric surgery to many apprentice surgeons, we argue that MIS of technically demanding procedures such as these Upper Abdominal procedures is best mastered by apprentice surgeons participating in the entire procedure involving the whole team at mentor's hospital, including anaesthesiologist and OR nurses, and thereby being assisted in carrying out procedures by the same mentor in one's own hospital. Hence, in this chapter a program of teaching Minimally Invasive Upper GI surgery is evaluated, where mentoring had been practiced.

33.1 Historical Background

At the VUmc, we started the MI Esophageal program in 1998 by using the laparoscopic transhiatal approach for distal and gastro-esophageal junction cancers (GEJ) [1, 2]. Then, aiming for more radicality and an adequate lymphadenectomy, in 2006 we started with the thoracoscopic approach in lateral position [3]. After a limited number of cases, and after watching the prone position approach live in a surgical congress, we then switched to the right thoracoscopy in prone position. In 2007, we performed the first interventions assisted by a thoracic surgeon who was already performing the VATS for lung cancer.

After five MIE in prone position, without any conversion and only one postoperative respiratory infection, we then felt that we could properly perform MIE through this approach. Consequentially, we continued operating all patients through this approach, with the exception of patients included in the CROSS trial [4]. The department's participation in the CROSS trial since 2005 implied that

M.A. Cuesta (✉) • N.I. van der Wielen • J. Straatman
D.L. van der Peet
Department of Surgery, VU University Medical Center (VUmc), Amsterdam, The Netherlands
e-mail: ma.cuesta@vumc.nl

M.A. Cuesta (ed.), *Minimally Invasive Surgery for Upper Abdominal Cancer*,
DOI 10.1007/978-3-319-54301-7_33

all those patients in this trial were approached by open procedure. By 2009 we considered that enough experience with this approach had been accumulated at the department, 80 operated patients, for us to engage in evaluation. Our search for evidence led to a randomized controlled trial, the TIME trial, where we compared the total open procedure by thoracotomy and laparotomy with the total MIE by right thoracoscopy in prone position and laparoscopy after neoadjuvant chemoradiotherapy according to the CROSS Scheme [5]. Since 2009, we instituted the teaching program of MIE, at first doing so in the Netherlands and later elsewhere.

33.2 Experience with Mastering

Since 2009, we have taught the MIE approach in our own department to four young fellows and in 18 centres located in Europe, Latin America and India. From the beginning our teaching strategy differentiated between teaching situations; namely (a) centres already using MIE and harbouring initial experience, and (b) centres with no experience in MIE but having enough volume of patients.

Of these, 12 centres had *no previous* MIE experience. The other six centres already had some *previous* experience with the MIE, but wanted to gain competences in the prone thoracoscopy or aimed by means of proctoring and a master class to gain the required proficiencies.

Criteria for teaching at a centre involved having a sufficient volume of patients with esophageal cancer, at least 20 cases per year, and having at least two surgeons whom were dedicated, totally or partially to upper Gastrointestinal Surgery (upper GI).

We also adopted the teaching policy to ask the whole team of those centres with *not previous* experience to visit our centre in Amsterdam for watching at least two whole procedures performed at the operating room. A whole team would include the two surgeons, the anaesthesiologist involved with the procedure and one or two scrub nurses. After some weeks, the mentor assisted the surgeons to be proctored in a variable number of procedures whereby the initial intention was doing five.

Regarding the centres with some *previous* experience with MIE a visit was arranged for operating together with the corresponding team, and involving one or more procedures as master class training.

Our protocol included that each to-be-treated patient was discussed beforehand and accepted as a good candidate for the operation. In the beginning stage I and II patients with esophageal cancer were chosen, later on no selection is made after proper response of neoadjuvant therapy. All patients had given informed consent; the mentor had been introduced to and had spoken with them before the operation. Moreover insurance items were arranged properly.

Reimbursement for the mentor was usually arranged for travel, hotel if necessary and payment for each operation, in some cases through the intervention of a commercial company.

Moreover, other items such as the way to do the cervical anastomosis, the use or not of a fast track program after MIE, and the treatment of major postoperative complications were broadly discussed.

Considering the prominent role of mentoring in our teaching strategy, we are interested in knowing whether the proctored centres had continued with the MIE programs after the provided mentoring and what significance the mentoring could be said to have had for the acquisition of requisite skills. Of the 12 centers with no previous experience only two terminated the mentory program. Moreover in the six centers with previous experience the taught MIE interventions not only involved the 3 stage procedure but also the 2 stage Ivor Lewis procedure by thoracoscopy in prone position.

33.3 Discussion

Surgical residents and (young) surgeons are the principle targets for learning advanced Minimally Invasive Surgery such as colorectal surgery. It is obvious that the majority of surgical residents with institutional programs will learn this approach during their residency period or during a fellowship period, but still there are residents and surgeons to be taught, various newly developed MIS procedures mostly by quick courses or by mentoring programs [6–10]. For other minimally invasive interventions such as gastric and esophageal, but also for pancreatic and hepatic MIS resections there are no regular programs involved with the teaching programs guided by dedicated mentors. It is obvious that MIE taught to fellows in an experienced hospital will be the favourite choice, but not always available [11]. Apart of the fellowship institutional programs, there are other didactic courses including hands-on cadaver courses, live surgery courses, and two-day courses organized by surgical academic departments frequently in cooperation with the industry where the attendees will be limited in number and previously selected. Moreover, accordingly to the 2014 report of SAGES continuing education committee two of the most desired topics have been the introduction of new procedures into clinical practice and the management of complications [12].

As explained in this article above, the mentoring programs in laparoscopic colorectal surgery had not only gained optimal results, but also disclosed that the mentor pupil relationship serves as the most optimal manner to learning this complicated approach [11, 13]. Our experience in implementing mentorship since 2009 confirms how ideal this approach is. The specific problems in our approach for MIE concern foremost, the following: (1) the requisite features of the centres involved, (2) the characteristics of the mentor(s) engaged to proctor, (3) the volume of surgeries that the teams are doing, (4) the number of surgeons involved, and (5) determining which procedure to start with. Moreover, concerns also include the financial aspects and insurances holding for the mentors. All these factors must be accounted for. Nevertheless, it is clear that the teaching program involving the type of mentoring we provided, does assure a more than sufficient introduction of new procedures with good results in patients outcomes [14]. Questions that must still be addressed are which Organization or Surgical Society will appoint centres for implementation of the program and how qualified mentors can be selected. Given our positive experience, we argue that our teaching model involving mentoring should also be applied for teaching major surgery of the upper abdomen such as gastric, pancreatic and hepatic by laparoscopy and robot assisted programs.

33.4 Recommendations

Upper Abdominal Minimally Invasive Surgery is best taught to those Surgical Units having certain properties. To start with, there must be enough volume of specific cancer patients. Moreover, the willingness to master MIS must include the conviction that its advantages are evidence-based. The units must have at least two dedicated surgeons in the correspondence surgery, comprising experience with Minimally Invasive Surgery. Furthermore, the whole team must be supportive, whilst the acquaintance of the entire Surgical Department and the Hospital's board may necessarily include collaboration. Finally, these programs should be taught by an experienced mentor.

References

1. Scheepers JJG, Mulder CJJ, van der Peet DL, et al. Minimally invasive oesophageal resection for distal oesophageal cancer: a review of the literature. Scand J Gastroenterol. 2006;243:123–34.
2. Scheepers JJG, Veenhof AAFA, van der Peet DL, et al. Laparoscopic transhiatal resection for malignancies of the distal esophagus. Surgery. 2008;143:278–85.
3. Scheepers JJG, van der Peet DL, Veenhof AAFA, Cuesta MA. Thoracoscopic resection for esophageal cancer: a review of literature. J Minim Access Surg. 2007;5:149–60.
4. van Hagen P, Hulshof MCCM, van Lanschot JJB, et al. Preoperative chemoradiotherapy for esophageal or junctional cancer. N Engl J Med. 2012;366:2074–84.
5. Biere SSAY, van Berge Henegouwen MI, Maas KW, et al. Minimally invasive versus open oesophagectomy for patients with oesophageal cancer: a multicentre, open-label, randomised controlled trial. Lancet. 2012;379:1887–92.
6. Fleshman J, Marcello P, Stamos MJ, Wexner SD. Focus group on laparoscopic colectomy education as endorsed by the American Society of Colon and Rectal surgeons (ASCRS) and the Society of American Gastrointestinal and Endoscopic Surgeons (SAGES). Dis Colon Rectum. 2006;49:945–9.
7. Verheijen PM, vd Ven AW, Davids PH, et al. Teaching colorectal surgery in the laparoscopic era. Is it safe? J Surg Educ. 2010;67:217–21.

8. Fowler DL, Hogle NJ. The fellowship council: a decade of impact on surgical training. Surg Endosc. 2013;27:3548–54.
9. Palter VN, Grantcharov TP. Development and validation of a comprehensive curriculum to teach an advanced minimally invasive procedure: a randomized controlled trial. Ann Surg. 2012;256:25–32.
10. Bosker R, Groen H, Hoff C, et al. Effect of proctoring on implementation and results of elective laparoscopic colon surgery. Int J Colorectal Dis. 2011;26:941–7.
11. Rossidis G, Kissane N, Hochwald SN, et al. Overcoming challenges in implementing a minimally invasive esophagectomy program at a Veterans Administration Medical Center. Am J Surg. 2011;202:395–9.
12. McLemore EC, Paige JT, Bergman S, et al. Ongoing evolution of practice gaps in GI and endoscopic surgery: 2014 report from the SAGES continuing education committee. Surg Endosc. 2015;29:3017–29.
13. Dominguez EP, Barrat C, Shaffer L, et al. Minimally invasive surgery adoption into an established surgical practice: impact of a fellowship-trained colleague. Surg Endosc. 2013;27:1267–72.
14. Birch DW, Asiri AH, de Gara CJ. The impact of a formal program for minimally invasive surgery on surgeon practice and patient outcomes. Am J Surg. 2007;193:589–91.

Part VIII

Final Considerations

34 Final Considerations

Miguel A. Cuesta

The objective of this book was to depict the current situation of the Minimal Upper GI surgery in Oncology. Our philosophy has been, that once a good indication exists for surgery, the combination of an optimal use of neoadjuvant therapy with Minimally Invasive Surgery will achieve the best outcome for the patient offering a high quality of life. We explained how achieving an optimal oncological resection by a perfect knowledge of the surgical anatomy leads to performing the necessary steps for an adequate resection by established planes and a reconstruction by perfect anastomoses.

We have made clear that an extensive knowledge of the surgical anatomy requires information gathered on the practice of minimally invasive surgery. This knowledge gives the surgeon the best prospect for doing perfect oncological surgery by being able to dissect through surgical planes. We take into regard that Upper GI oncological procedures—especially the esophageal and gastric resections, but also the hepatic and pancreatic—are implemented less frequently than the colorectal procedures and may be more complex. We delineated that decisions to implement these procedures can be based on the short-term advantages obtained after a perfect conducted minimally invasive procedure. The long-term advantages including survival and other oncological outcomes are not expected to be distinctive from the advantages obtained by using the counterpart open approach.

Consequently, in order to operate correctly in the particular MIS way as we have depicted, a surgeon's gaining an adequate training is paramount. Young surgeons and residents need to learn and continue to relearn MIS proficiencies. Accompanying implementation of Upper abdominal MIS, surgeons need to engender dedication to these procedures as carried out in high-volume centres and through continual training. This entails the need for initial training in the laboratory using models and cadavers and then advancing in skills through adequate programs in which the role of a mentor is crucial.

Moreover, the surgical robot has been implemented in many fields of complex MIS and provides important advantages when performing difficult dissections in difficult places and in difficult anastomoses.

All authors and contributors to this book demonstrated success with MIS, thereby prompting some considerations regarding proficiencies, permanent learning and progress, which I would like to share.

M.A. Cuesta
Emeritus professor, Department of Surgery, VU University Medical Center (VUmc), Amsterdam, The Netherlands
e-mail: ma.cuesta@vumc.nl

M.A. Cuesta (ed.), *Minimally Invasive Surgery for Upper Abdominal Cancer*,
DOI 10.1007/978-3-319-54301-7_34

34.1 Proficiencies

The model adopted in this book encompasses what we think are the most appropriate proficiencies to perform complex surgery once a good indication comes about. Foremost is the aptitude of wanting to know and being passionate about surgical anatomy of a specific area, in this case the upper abdomen. We encourage this propensity strongly for without adequate knowledge it is impossible to do a good oncological resection through adequate planes, thus preventing avoidable risks. Such good practice is based on description of surgical anatomy as portrayed in this book and which was carried out mainly in the Department of Anatomy in Utrecht Medical Center (UMC), head: Prof. R. Bleys. Moreover, surgical anatomy of different organs has been depicted by Dr. T. Weijs and Dr. H. Brenkman. The importance of neoadjuvant treatment is paramount for these dedicated oncologists, radiotherapists and surgeons. We see this demonstrated in the chapters dedicated to esophageal surgery (Prof. J. van Lanschot), gastric surgery (Prof. C. van de Velde), and pancreatic surgery (Prof. C. van Eijck). Moreover, comparison of the known evidence between the counterpart open approach and MIS is covered by respectively Prof. B. Wijnhoven, Dr. N. van der Wielen, Prof. B. Edil and Prof. R. Ciria, shows us the advantages of doing MIS. Description of specific Minimally invasive procedures has been treated by surgeons and theirs teams with a long-time dedication to these procedures, such as Prof. B. Weusten, Prof. J. Luketich, Prof. H. Osugi, Prof. D. van der Peet, Prof. C. Mariette, Prof. S. Gisbertz, Prof. M. van Berge Henegouwen, Prof. R. van Hillegersberg, Prof. A. Talvane, Prof. H. K. Yang, Prof. W. J. Hyung, Prof. C. Moreno, Prof. U. Boggi, Prof. M. Abu Hilal, Prof. M. Besselink, Prof. T. Cheung, Prof. A. Sa Cunha, Prof. A. Tsung, Prof. T. Keck, Prof. E. Targarona, and our surgical group with contributions of Prof. J.W. Dekker and Prof. J. Scheepers.

34.2 Permanent Learning

Remarkably, all authors expressed their willingness to engage in permanent learning regarding all aspects of surgery. Our shared philosophy is that continual changes in surgery require an augmented search for minimizing the operative trauma, increasing its oncological efficiency and decreasing the complication rate. All the while, a (re)learning of MIS continuously seeks high evidence. Fitting this aim, the inclusion of videos per chapter of all procedures has added important information regarding MIS. The paramount quality of the videos is magnificent and is conducive for continual learning.

34.3 Progress

Reflecting on this development, I consider this book as a good summary of the progress of surgery; yet I am aware that in the coming years the contents of this book will undergo changes. My advice for residents and young surgeons is to learn the techniques we covered in this book and to do so deeply by drawing on the motivation to improve the life expectations of our patients and to reduce their suffering.

Finally, we must recognize with distinction the essential role of the anaesthesia and intensive-care personnel on whom all of us rely day in and day out for performing the challenges of major surgery. Our communal effort, made manifest by authors and contributors to this book, continue to inspire us to persevere in gaining the best outcome for the patient offering a high quality of life.

Printed by Printforce, the Netherlands